Aesthetic Facial Plastic Surgery

A Multidisciplinary Approach

Aesthetic Facial Plastic Surgery

A Multidisciplinary Approach

Thomas Romo, III, MD, FACS

Chief, Facial Plastic and Reconstructive Surgery
Lenox Hill Hospital;
Co-Director, Facial Plastic and Reconstructive Surgery
New York Eye and Ear Infirmary;
Director, Facial Plastic and Reconstructive Surgery
Manhattan Center for Facial Plastic and Reconstructive Surgery
New York, New York

Arthur L. Millman, MD

Director of Oculoplastic Surgery
Lenox Hill Hospital;
Director of Oculoplastic and Cosmetic Surgery
Manhattan Center for Facial Plastic and Reconstructive Surgery;
Assistant Professor
New York Eye and Ear Infirmary
New York, New York

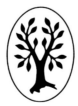

2000
Thieme
New York • Stuttgart

Thieme New York
333 Seventh Avenue
New York, NY 10001

Editorial Director: Avé McCracken
Editorial Assistant: Michelle Schmitt
Developmental Manager: Kathleen P. Lyons
Director, Production and Manufacturing: Anne Vinnicombe
Marketing Director: Phyllis Gold
Sales Manager: Ross Lumpkin
Chief Financial Officer: Seth S. Fishman
President: Brian D. Scanlan
Medical Illustrator: Anthony M.Pazos
Cover and Icon Designer: Michael Mendelsohn at MM Design 2000, Inc.
Compositor: Preparé
Printer: Canale
Cover, chapter openers, and icons: All art is from *Planet Art: The Impressionists*, from Planet Art Classic Graphics.™
Cover, facial plastic surgery icon, and openers for Chapters 1, 7, 9, 11, 14, 16, 18, 19, 22, 24, and 26 are *Irma Brunner*, Manet, 1880;
plastic surgery icon and openers for Chapters 2, 3, 4, 8, 10, 12, 20, and 25 are *Female Nude*, Renoir 1876; oculoplastic surgery icon
and openers for Chapters 13, 15, 17, 21, 22, 23, 28, and 30 are *At the Ball*, Morisot, 1875; and the dermatology icon and openers
for Chapters 5, 6, 27, and 31 are *Folies Berger*, Manet 1881; and the anesthesiology icon is *Rake*, Vincent Van Gogh, 1889.

Library of Congress Cataloging-in-Publication Data is available from the publisher.

Important note: Medical knowledge is ever-changing. As new research and clinical experience broaden our knowledge,
changes in treatment and drug therapy may be required. The authors and editors of the material herein have consulted
sources believed to be reliable in their efforts to provide information that is complete and in accord with the standards
accepted at the time of publication. However, in view of the possibility of human error by the authors, editors, or publisher of
the work herein, or changes in medical knowledge, neither the authors, editors, publisher, nor any other party who has been
involved in the preparation of this work, warrants that the information contained herein is in every respect accurate or
complete, and they are not responsible for any errors or omissions or for the results obtained from use of such information.
Readers are encouraged to confirm the information contained herein with other sources. For example, readers are advised to
check the product information sheet included in the package of each drug they plan to administer to be certain that the
information contained in this publication is accurate and that changes have not been made in the recommended dose or in the
contraindications for administration. This recommendation is of particular importance in connection with new or infrequently
used drugs.

Some of the product names, patents, and registered designs referred to in this book are in fact registered trademarks or proprietary names even though specific reference to this fact is not always made in the text. Therefore, the appearance of a name
without designation as proprietary is not to be construed as a representation by the publisher that it is in the public domain.

Printed in Italy
5 4 3 2 1

TNY ISBN 0-86577-807-8
GTV ISBN 3-13-111431-2

Dedication

To the most influential surgeon of my personal life and my professional career, Thomas Romo, Jr., MD.

Thomas Romo, III

To the true power and machinery behind the throne, the woman behind the man, my wife. If not for the constant support of my wife and family, my professional and personal life would grind to a halt. I am forever thankful.

Arthur L. Millman

Contents

Foreword

This superb textbook on aesthetic facial plastic surgery presents a unique and refreshing educational approach—namely, the comparison of surgical techniques for a specific procedure by subspecialty area. This unique approach allows the reader to benefit from the training and background of each specialty practitioner. Although much of the education and management principles have a common foundation among the specialties, the reader has the opportunity to appreciate some of the subtle differences in practice philosophy. These practice philosophies may represent, in part, the education and training of the specialists. For instance, an oculoplastic surgeon is trained first in medical and surgical diseases of the eye and surrounding structures, so that they can help us better understand how to evaluate, protect, and care for the functional implications of perio-orbital surgery. Plastic surgeons have a firm foundation in surgical techniques, wound healing, and total body surgery, owing to their general surgery background. Because of their knowledge in head and neck surgery and functional surgery of the upper aerodigestive tract, facial plastic surgeons are well-grounded in the anatomy and physiology of the face, scalp and neck. Our dermatology colleagues are quite knowledgeable about the function and physiology of the skin and its appendages, and how to protect its integrity during surgical procedures. To have the combined perspectives of these four specialties in one textbook greatly increases its educational worth.

The reader will appreciate the clear illustrations and pertinent figures in each chapter. The psychosocial aspects of the surgical procedures are attended to as important aspects of the care of the aesthetic facial surgery patient. In particular, the "Pearls" section of each chapter contains the top salient points for consideration when performing these aesthetic procedures. They represent the specific recommendations for consideration after many years of surgical experience by the authors. The surgical techniques are clearly presented and easily understood—a tribute to the authors for their treatment of difficult and complicated procedures.

I believe such a format of multidisciplinary authors is exemplary and should be emulated more frequently in the future. The reader will be pleased to benefit from these surgeons' expertise and perspective. This textbook will be a cherished reference for both resident and practicing surgeons, and especially for those who have limited their practice to aesthetic facial surgery, and wish to appreciate a variety of surgical approaches and specialty perspectives.

G. Richard Holt, MD, MSE, MPH

Foreword

In the recent decades, the popularity of facial aesthetic surgery has blossomed in the United States perhaps more than in the remainder of the world. Certainly the favorable economic climate in this country combined with a cultural resistance to the body changes inflicted by *Anno Domini* has contributed to our enthusiasm for this surgery of facial enhancement. Partially as a response to demand, and also as a natural spinoff of other surgical activities, improvements in surgical technique and technology pertaining to aesthetic surgery have been rapid, occur almost yearly, and make the field a competitive one.

Historically, facial aesthetic surgery has been performed by different surgical subspecialties, and although the notion of what constitutes the desired result in facial aesthetic surgery may be uniform, the different surgical specialties, by necessity, have variations in their approach to the aesthetic patient. The differences in heritages of the subspecialities are reflected in their perspective of priorities, and in some cases the specific tools of surgical technique.

A convergence of these various surgical disciplines can only clarify and produce the soundest approach to this ever increasing field of surgery and Drs. Millman and Romo have produced a book, devoted entirely to aesthetic facial plastic surgery, that brings together the viewpoints and the strengths of each subspeciality. The editors have included chapters written by experienced surgeons, noted and esteemed in their respective fields, who present the viewpoints of each of the specialities. Plastic surgeons, oculoplastic surgeons, facial plastic surgeons, and dermatologists, all have contributed to this comprehensive volume and bring the specifics of their surgical experience and variation in surgical techniques from their own surgical discipline to the reader. The latest techniques of endoscopic-assisted procedures, redraping procedures, laser-assisted procedures, and skin care are presented in a detailed and thorough manner. For each surgeon performing facial enhancement surgery, a "state-of-the-art" awareness of concepts and surgical techniques in this field is an obligatory need in this consumer-driven arena and this is found in the chapters of this book. *Aesthetic Facial Plastic Surgery: A Multidisciplinary Approach* is a volume that should be very helpful and practical to any surgeon performing aesthetic facial surgery.

Clinton D. (Sonny) McCord, MD

Preface

Aesthetic Facial Plastic Surgery: A Multidisciplinary Approach broaches the subject of aesthetic facial surgery in all of its manifestations in the most up-to-date and comprehensive manner possible at the turn of the twentieth century. Cosmetic facial surgery has indeed undergone a very gradual but very definite evolution, if not revolution, over the last thirty years. Over the last three decades the student and practitioner of facial surgery has no doubt realized the dramatic change in technique, technology, and surgical approaches that are now used to develop aesthetic rejuvenation of the facial area.

Some generalizations regarding this 30-year evolution became apparent to us on review of the literature and previous textbooks on the subject. Perhaps an oversimplification of this change over time can be summarized as follows. The 1970s was dominated by a concept of "beauty is only skin deep," which symbolized the general usage of cutaneous skin resectional procedures for facial reconstruction. At this time direct and coronal browlifting with large resections of scalp and frontal tissue was utilized. Reconstruction of the eyelids was characterized by a skin-only plane dissection with resection of both upper and lower eyelid skin. Midfacial and lower facial reconstruction was dominated by skin flap facelifting. The procedures were characterized by large skin resections and lateral tension.

The 1980s brought the "age of fascial awareness" with careful identification of the musculocutaneous fascial planes of the facial region and the evolution of fascial-based surgery, which took advantage of the intrinsic anatomy of the facial structures. Examples can be found in a change of blepharoplasty technique utilizing myocutaneous flaps, and the increased utilization of the underlying deep structures of the eyelid and orbit, including the lid retractors. In the upper lid, levator aponeurosis isolation and fixation and lower lid transconjunctival and lid retractor and capsulopalpebral fascial-based surgery became the standard. In the mid and lower face, facelifting procedures became SMAS-based. Thus, the age of the deep plane facelift was born, enabling surgeons to mobilize large composite areas of the facial musculoskeleton, musculocutaneous infrastructure to allow for greater mobilization of tissue, enhanced natural aesthetic effect, and a decreased reliance on skin resection procedures.

The 1990s brought the "subperiosteal revolution." The introduction of endoscopic surgical technique and the further isolation and utilization of subperiosteal planes revolutionized surgery with the creation of the endoscopic forehead, browlift, and face. The revolution continued with the increased utilization of the subperiosteal midface and cheeklift used alone and in combination with endoscopic upper and midfacial subperiosteal planes for midfacial rejuvenation. Endoscopic technique also allowed the surgeon to use minimal incisions and to avoid of skin or tissue resectional techniques, with a greater emphasis on natural resuspension and natural rejuvenation of upper, middle, and lower cervical facial structures.

Finally, as we head toward the millenium, fantastic changes in technology allow for adjunctive procedures to further enhance and to increase safety. The introduction of multiple new laser modalities, the use of pharmacologic agents such as botulinum, and the emergence of myriad of bioactive and biocompatible materials for three-dimensional tissue augmentation and facial implants have increased the efficacy of surgical reconstruction. Finally, liposuction technique and technology has improved dramatically with the introduction of very small caliber cannulae and ultrasonic techniques to allow for manipulation of the underlying lipoadipose tissue of the face and neck, further allowing the surgeon to sculpt and fine tune his or her aesthetic technique.

The last and perhaps most important evolution in facial surgery, and that which is most specifically addressed by this textbook, is the interdisciplinary synergy that has evolved in the last decade. A number of surgical specialties, including facial plastic, oculoplastic, plastic, dermatologic, and oral and maxillofacial fields, have brought tremendous expertise to bear on the subject of facial rejuvenation. Each regional specialty has introduced unique training, surgical expertise, and companion technology toward various areas of facial aesthetic surgery to create a broad and expansive array of surgical specialists whose whole is certainly greater than the sum of its parts.

Finally, the multiauthored format of this textbook has many strengths, although some weaknesses. The reader is urged to read the textbook as a whole, as the editors have taken great care to include a broad array of subjects. We have attempted to bring together authors who truly represent the pioneers and leaders in their various fields of aesthetic facial surgery. We have assigned each topic in general to two authors of two differing orientations or specialties. This allows at least two viewpoints to be published on a given subject. We have taken great care to try and minimize overlap and redundancy, although some element of repetition is both proper and unavoidable. Most importantly, every surgical specialty has much to learn from the others and we hope that this textbook allows that synergy of technique and expertise to come together under one cover.

As we enter the new millenium it is a most exciting time to be alive and to be a facial surgical specialist. The rapid changes in technique and its infrastructure of technology, bioengineering, and biomaterials have given the surgeon greater control, power, and efficacy to achieve unparalleled aesthetic results with greater levels of consistency and safety than ever before in the modern epoch. We hope you find this textbook as illuminating and worthwhile as it was to bring together.

Thomas Romo, III, MD, FACS   *Arthur L. Millman, MD*

About This Book

A few points of interest to the reader of *Aesthetic Facial Plastic Surgery: A Multidisciplinary Approach.*

This text is somewhat unusual in that it brings four specific specialties together to produce a collaboration of information on surgical and aesthetic treatment of the face. The book's authors derive from four surgical specialties that are denoted by specific icons.

Readers who are interested in specific opinions from specific authors or specific specialties can look to the Table of Contents for immediate graphic representation of the information therein. The editors would, however, urge various specialists to specifically read opinions and techniques of other specialties, as there is the most fecund source of new information that can modify established techniques in a constructive manner.

Additionally, each chapter is presented with "Pearls" which are the author's own interpretations of the very concise specifics that they feel meld to a more perfect surgical outcome. A refreshing summary of each chapter is, thereby, accomplished through the "Pearl" section.

Finally, the book is well invested with color photography and schematic illustrations by a single artist. Great care was put into creating a comprehensive and complete photographic documentation of all surgical procedures, including pre- and postoperative results, so that the reader can further gain by the visual aspects of a visual field.

We hope this text is as easy and useful to read as it was enjoyable to produce.

Indicates chapters written by facial plastic surgeons (see Chapters 1, 7, 9, 11, 14, 16, 18, 19, 21, 22, 24, and 26)

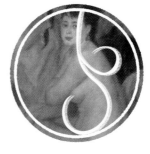

Indicates chapters written by plastic surgeons (see Chapters 2, 8, 10, 12, 20, 25, and 30)

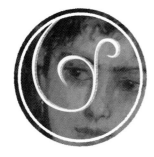

Indicates chapters written by oculoplastic surgeons (see Chapters 13, 15, 17, and 31)

Indicates chapters written by dermatologists (see Chapters 23 and 27)

Acknowledgments

The editors would like to acknowledge the incomparable support that each have received from their office staff in the preparation of these manuscripts and coordination of contributing authors. Without their constant efforts, chaos would have reigned. The constant professionalism of Avé McCracken and Kathleen Lyons who first envisioned this project and brought it to fruition is much appreciated. Lastly, our thanks is extended to all our contributing authors who put in extra-ordinary effort to bring unique material into an unusual context for this one-of-a-kind text.

Contributors

George J. Beraka, MD
Attending Plastic Surgeon
Lenox Hill Hospital
New York, New York

Leonard J. Bernstein, MD
Laser and Skin Surgery Center of New York
New York, New York

Jim L. English, MD
Assistant Clinical Professor
Department of Otolaryngology–Head and Neck Surgery
University of Arkansas Medical Sciences
Little Rock, Arkansas

Steven Fagien, MD
Private Practice
Aesthetic Eyelid Plastic Surgery
Boca Raton, Florida

Richard T. Farrior, MD
Clinical Professor
Department of Otolaryngology
University of Florida, Gainesville;
Clinical Professor
Department of Otolaryngology
University of South Florida
Tampa, Florida

Richard W. Fleming, MD
Clinical Professor
Division of Facial Plastic and Reconstructive Surgery
Department of Otolaryngology–Head and Neck Surgery
University of Southern California School of Medicine
Los Angeles, California

Craig A. Foster, MD, DDS, FACS
Surgeon
Department of Plastic Surgery
Manhattan Eye, Ear, and Throat Hospital
New York, New York

Robert M. Freund, MD, FACS
Assistant Attending Surgeon
Department of Plastic Surgery
Manhattan Eye, Ear, and Throat Hospital
New York, New York

Richard M. Galitz, MD
Clinical Assistant Professor
Department of Otolaryngology/Facial Plastic Surgery
University of Miami School of Medicine/Jackson
   Memorial Hospital
Aventura, Florida

Renée Garnes
Make-up Artist
Warren-Tricomi Salon
New York, New York

Roy G. Geronemus, MD
Director
Laser and Skin Surgery Center of New York
New York, New York

Alvin I. Glasgold, MD
Clinical Professor of Surgery
Division of Otolaryngology
Robert Wood Johnson Medical School and Hospital
New Brunswick, New Jersey

Mark J. Glasgold, MD
Clinical Assistant Professor
Division of Otolaryngology
Robert Wood Johnson Medical School and Hospital
New Brunswick, New Jersey

Robert Alan Goldberg, MD
Chief, Orbital and Ophthalmic Plastic Surgery
Associate Professor of Ophthalmology
Jules Stein Eye Institute
University of California, Los Angeles
UCLA School of Medicine
Los Angeles, California

G. Richard Holt, MD, MSE, MPH
Director
Division of Facial Plastic and Reconstructive Surgery
The Johns Hopkins Medical Institutions
Baltimore, Maryland

Robert W. Hutcherson, MD, FACS
Assistant Clinical Professor of Surgery
Department of Facial Surgery
UCLA Hospital and Clinics
Santa Barbara, California

Frank M. Kamer, MD, FACS
Clinical Professor of Surgery
Department of Surgery
Division of Head and Neck Surgery
University of California, Los Angeles
UCLA School of Medicine
Los Angeles, California

Gregory S. Keller, MD
Assistant Clinical Professor of Surgery
Department of Facial Plastic Surgery
UCLA Hospital and Clinics
Santa Barbara, California

David A. Kieff, MD
Medical Director
Premier Image Cosmetic and Laser Surgery
Atlanta, Georgia

Randall C. Latorre, MD
Otolaryngology/Facial Plastic Surgery
Tampa Facial Plastic Surgery
Tampa, Florida

Toby G. Mayer, MD
Clinical Professor
Division of Facial Plastic and Reconstructive Surgery
Department of Otolaryngology–Head and Neck Surgery
University of Southern California School of Medicine
Los Angeles, California

Clinton D. McCord, MD
Paces; Plastic Surgery and Recovery Center
Atlanta, Georgia

Arthur L. Millman, MD
Director of Oculoplastic Surgery
Lenox Hill Hospital;
Director of Oculoplastic and Cosmetic Surgery
Manhattan Center for Facial Plastic and Reconstructive
    Surgery;
Assistant Professor
New York Eye and Ear Infirmary
New York, New York

Arshad R. Muzaffar, MD
Senior Resident
Department of Plastic Surgery
University of Texas Southwestern
    Medical Center at Dallas
Dallas, Texas

Sheldon Opperman, MD
Medical Director
Ambulatory Surgery
Department of Anesthesiology
Lenox Hill Hospital
New York, New York

Andrew Paul Ordon, MD, FACS
Assistant Clinical Professor of Plastic Surgery
Dartmouth Medical School
Hanover, New Hampshire;
Assistant Clinical Professor of Plastic Surgery
University of Connecticut School of Medicine
Farmington, Connecticut;
Associate Attending Surgeon (Plastic)
Lenox Hill Hospital
New York, New York;
Associate Attending Surgeon (Head and Neck)
The New York Eye and Ear Infirmary
New York, New York;
Assistant Attending Surgeon (Plastic)
Beth Israel Medical Center
New York, New York

David S. Orentreich, MD
Associate Director
Orentreich Foundation for the Advancement
    of Science Inc.;
Assistant Clinical Professor
Department of Dermatology
The Mount Sinai Hospital
New York, New York

Norman Orentreich, MD, FACP
Clinical Professor
Department of Dermatology
New York University School of Medicine;
Associate Attending
Department of Dermatology
University Hospital
New York University Medical Center;
Associate Attending
Department of Dermatology
Bellevue Medical Hospital Center;
Consultant in Dermatology
    and Gerontology
The Animal Medical Center;
Medical Director
Orentreich Medical Group, LLP;
Director
Orentreich Foundation for the Advancement
    of Science Inc.
New York, New York

Louisa E. Pazienza, PME
Founder
Center for Aesthetic Rehabilitation;
Instructor in Medical Esthetics
Manhattan Center for Facial Plastic and Reconstructive
    Surgery
New York, New York

Stephen W. Perkins, MD, FACS
Associate Professor
Department of Otolaryngology–Head
    and Neck Surgery
Indiana University School of Medicine
Indianapolis, Indiana

Patrick G. Pieper, MD
Clinical Assistant Professor
Department of Otolaryngology–Head and Neck Surgery
University of Southern California School of Medicine
Los Angeles, California

Allen M. Putterman, MD
Professor of Ophthalmology and Director
    of Oculoplastic Surgery
University of Illinois at Chicago College of Medicine;
Clinical Professor of Maxillofacial Surgery
Northwestern University;
Chief of Ophthalmology
Michael Reese Hospital Medical Center;
Consultant in Oculoplastic Surgery
Mercy Hospital, West Side Veterans Administration
    Hospital, and Illinois Masonic Hospital
Chicago, Illinois

Oscar M. Ramirez, MD
Clinical Assistant Professor
Department of Surgery
Plastic Surgery Division
Johns Hopkins University School of Medicine
Baltimore, Maryland

Rod J. Rohrich, MD, FACS
Professor and Chairman
Holder of the Crystal Charity Ball Distinguished
    Chair in Plastic Surgery
Department of Plastic and Reconstructive Surgery
University of Texas Southwestern Medical School
    at Dallas
Dallas, Texas

Thomas Romo, III, MD, FACS
Chief, Facial Plastic and Reconstructive Surgery
Lenox Hill Hospital;
Co-Director, Facial Plastic and Reconstructive Surgery
New York Eye and Ear Infirmary;
Director, Facial Plastic and Reconstructive Surgery
Manhattan Center for Facial Plastic and Reconstructive
    Surgery
New York, New York

Paul Sabini, MD
Clinical Instructor
Division of Otolaryngology
University of Rochester Medical Center
Rochester, New York

Ali Sajjadian, MD
Medical Director
Premier Image Cosmetic and Laser Surgery
Atlanta, Georgia

William E. Silver, MD
Clinical Instructor
Emory University School of Medicine
Atlanta, Georgia;
Associate Clinical Professor
Department of Surgery (Otolaryngology)
Medical College of Georgia School of Medicine
Augusta, Georgia;
President
Premier Image Cosmetic and Laser Surgery
Atlanta, Georgia

Anthony P. Sclafani, MD
Director of Facial Plastic Surgery
Department of Otolaryngology–Head and
    Neck Surgery
New York Eye and Ear Infirmary;
Associate Professor
New York Medical College
New York, New York

Robert M. Scolnick, MD
Private Practice
Bedford, New York

Nicolas Tabbal, MD, FACS
Attending Surgeon
Department of Plastic Surgery
Manhattan Eye, Ear, and Throat Hospital
New York, New York

M. Eugene Tardy, Jr., MD, FACS
Professor of Clinical Otolaryngology
University of Illinois College of Medicine
Chicago, Illinois

Edward Tricomi
Co-owner/Creative Director
Warren-Tricomi Salon
New York, New York

Joel Warren
Co-owner/Color Director
Warren-Tricomi Salon
New York, New York

Tadeusz Wellisz, MD
Clinical Associate Professor
Plastic and Reconstructive Surgery
University of Southern California School
    of Medicine
Los Angeles, California

Preoperative Evaluation

Although this may be thought of as a mandatory chapter in all plastic surgery textbooks, it is in fact the most critical chapter and the most important step in the beginning of making a surgical plan for a patient.

The chapter, written by Dr. Anthony Sclafani, a facial plastic surgeon with extensive intellectual and scientific background. It focuses on many of the technical aspects of preoperative patient evaluation and, again, on the key to a successful surgical result. As will become apparent to the reader later in the text, by a review of the surgical "revision chapters," revisional surgery would frequently not be necessary had a more perfect preoperative evaluation occurred. It is more likely interview and preoperative evaluation, as opposed to surgical plan and its technical execution by the surgeon, that result in consistent patient satisfaction.

The wonderful companion chapter is written by Dr. Craig Foster, has been superbly written and clearly is the result of a surgeon with profound experience and profound insights into the process. Dr. Foster explains how surgery actually starts with the patient's first phone call to the office and proceeds through the evaluation process and to the actual surgery itself. A view of the subtle and not so subtle aspects of patient management that are critical to a successful surgical outcome is insightful.

Preoperative Evaluation

Aesthetic Facial Plastic Surgery, edited by Thomas Romo, III, and Arthur L. Millman, Thieme Medical Publishers, Inc., New York, New York, Copyright © 2000.

CHAPTER I

A Facial Plastic Surgeon's Perspective

ANTHONY P. SCLAFANI

Although many patients seeking facial plastic surgery will come to the preoperative consultation with specific and comprehensive desires, a great number of patients will present with unclear goals. Moreover, patients frequently focus on a specific area but neglect to consider how changes in one area interrelate with another. A complete preoperative evaluation and facial analysis are necessary to ensure the specific surgical goal blends harmoniously with the patient's facial—and general—appearance. Both the emotional and physical needs of the patient must be fully addressed to ensure a result acceptable to both patient and surgeon.

SOURCES OF INFORMATION

The surgeon must be ready to glean information about the patient from any and all reliable sources. Attentive office personnel and professional nursing staff have the opportunity to observe and interact with the patient in less formal circumstances (e.g., in telephone conversations, in encounters in reception rooms). An effective facial plastic surgery office will take advantage of all staff; indeed, a cohesive team approach allows the ancillary staff to (consciously or unconsciously) interpret the patient's demeanor, body language, and attitude as the physician does, thus acting as a true extension of the surgeon. Often the patient is on his or her "best behavior" for the physician but will act aggressively; be inappropriately demanding or dependent; or betray deep-seated fears, apprehension, or inappropriate motivating factors to the staff. These staff observations should be respected and may warrant additional discussions with the patient to avoid potential perioperative emotional conflicts.

GENERAL ASSESSMENT

Although the main focus of the consultation is the aesthetic evaluation, a conscious effort should be made to begin the interview as a physician. The general health of the patient should be ascertained, as well as complete surgical and medical histories. Equally important are current medications (including aspirin and any other anticoagulants and isotretinoin (Accutane) within the past 12 months) and any history of adverse drug or anesthetic reactions. Finally, a pertinent social history should be obtained, including past or present tobacco, alcohol, illicit drug, or topical nasal drug use. Not only does this information help avoid potentially serious operative complications, but it also allows the surgeon to assess whether the patient will be able to physically tolerate the stress of surgery. The time spent on this portion of the examination also stresses to the patient that the surgeon will assume the position of a total physician and not merely that of a technician. This portion of the consultation should be used to cement the physician-patient bond.

The physician should ask about the pattern and time course of the patient's healing, while emphasizing that facial wounds do not always behave like other wounds. However, if the patient has a prior history of unacceptable scarring, some general sense can be obtained regarding the likelihood of delayed or suboptimal healing. In addition, a patient who describes a well-healed scar from prior trauma or surgery as unsightly may later complain about a well-healed and well-camouflaged scar from aesthetic surgery, making this patient an inappropriate selection for an aesthetic procedure. The patient's demeanor should be observed because this is as important (sometimes more important) as the actual answers to the questions.

GENERAL DEMEANOR

Recent studies in psychology suggest that first opinions can be highly accurate. A general survey of the patient's appearance and demeanor is warranted. Although it is common for a patient to be nervous and self-conscious, the patient who displays these qualities may need additional attention; some of these patients may view aesthetic surgery as a solution to issues other than appearance. At a minimum, consideration should be given to a mandatory follow-up consultation because the patient's anxiety level may impede retention and comprehension of the achievable goals, benefits, and possible complications of surgery.

In addition, a patient's attention to postoperative details of personal appearance can often be inferred from the patient's preoperative behavior. Excessive attention or obsession over minute details should trigger the physician's suspicions, as should the lack of attention displayed by the disheveled patient. These patients should be scrutinized for acceptability as surgical candidates and whether their surgical goals are achievable.

PSYCHOLOGICAL EVALUATION

The emotional well-being of the patient can have a serious impact on the perioperative course and the patient's interpretation and satisfaction with the surgical results. The process of elective surgery emotionally stresses even the most stable patients. Although the patient may not express this to the surgeon (even one with whom he or she has an excellent rapport), he or she may succumb to feelings of embarrassment, foolishness, and poor self-worth. Before surgery, well-intentioned family members and friends often tell the patient that he or she "looks great" and "doesn't need surgery." In the immediate postoperative period, the patient sees little to no improvement in appearance and experiences discomfort and bruising; at this stage, the patient frequently questions the decision to undergo elective, nonfunctional surgery. A significant proportion of patients will display depressive symptoms after elective facial surgery.

Opinions vary as to the appropriate level of preoperative psychological screening that should be performed on potential aesthetic surgery patients. Some physicians require formal psychiatric evaluations. Most surgeons rely on a "gestalt" approach in attempting to categorize the patient as emotionally appropriate or inappropriate for surgery. Some authors have described "patient types" to be wary of, including "obsessive," "dependent," "demanding," and "secretive." At the opposite extreme, some surgeons believe that anything less than frank psychosis should not be a contraindication to surgery. Standardized psychiatric evaluations have been advocated, but these are usually lengthy and require professional administration and interpretation. We recently reported our results from an examination of a specific programmed psychiatric analysis (Prime-MD, Biometrics Research Department, New York State Psychiatric Institute, NY, NY). Although relatively simple to administer and easy to incorporate into a facial plastic surgery practice, no significant correlation was found with the physicians' assessments. However, the test did detect psychiatric illness in patients who had been deemed acceptable candidates by the surgeons. Although significant diagnoses were not addressed by this test, Prime-MD might be a useful supplement to the physician evaluation. The factors statistically associated with a high likelihood of a physician rating the patient's psychiatric status unfavorably were the following.

1. A patient's inability to articulate the desired surgical outcome (physician's assessment)
2. A patient's unrealistic surgical goals (physician's assessment)
3. Staff suspicion of the patient's emotional or psychological instability
4. A patient's displeasure with the results of prior surgery
5. A patient known to have psychiatric illness
6. A patient's use of psychiatric medication

Regardless of the approach, the prudent surgeon should feel that the patient's goals are related to structure and function (not emotion), that the surgeon can reasonably achieve these goals, that the patient understands the associated limitations and possible complications, and that the patient possesses the emotional and psychological fortitude to undergo the procedure. If the surgeon is unable to affirm each of these points, the surgery should be deferred until these issues are resolved.

PHYSICAL EVALUATION

Although specific guidelines for facial analysis are covered in other chapters, it is important to note certain general guidelines. Before the consultation, we provide our patients with preprinted procedure brochures. This helps the patient focus on the specific areas treated by different procedures. The typical patient will, in very general terms, express the areas of interest. When asked to point to the specific features of concern, the patient often resorts to "hand waving." To stress to the patient how precise the surgeon's eye must be, we give the patient a cotton applicator and ask him or her to point to the exact areas he or she would like addressed. This simple exercise usually cues the patient to the specificity needed in the consultation. Should this fail, we demonstrate the facial subunits (and, if necessary, the subdivisions of each unit) to the patient, and ask the patient to describe his or her features one subunit or subdivision at a time.

The physician must recognize and resist the natural tendency to immediately focus on the area of the patient's interest. A complete aesthetic assessment of the face should proceed in a crescendo-like fashion. General facial appearance and shape should be noted. Skin complexion, tone, elasticity, pigmentation, and any scars should be discussed with the patient. Areas not specifically mentioned by the patient should be examined and reviewed with the patient, as should favorable findings and areas that might benefit from surgery. This evaluation proceeds in a centripetal fashion around the area of the patient's stated interest. It is incumbent on the surgeon to instruct the patient on the interrelation of various facial structures in creating a harmonious facial synthesis. If one yields to the natural tendency to immediately examine and discuss the patient's major concern, the surgeon will find it difficult to redirect the patient's attention toward associated (and sometimes quite important) features, because the patient will interpret the associated features as secondary once the discussion has focused on the perceived defect. The surgeon should pay particular attention to any functional consequences of preoperative conditions (e.g., nasal valve collapse); not only does this help avoid any inappropriate postoperative complaints, it again emphasizes that the surgeon is interested in improving the patient's quality of life, as well as his or her appearance.

Ancillary procedures that the surgeon believes would improve the results of the primary procedure (e.g., augmentation mentoplasty in a patient with microgenia whose primary request is a reduction rhinoplasty) should be mentioned as an option that the patient should consider. However, unless failure to perform the ancillary procedure will significantly compromise the results of the primary surgery, this additional surgery should be pre-

sented only as an option. For patients who are candidates for multiple complementary procedures, we try to rank these options in order of the most to least significant effect on the condition of which the patient initially complained. A patient with brow ptosis, periorbital rhytids, and mechanical blepharoptosis who initially sought a blepharoplasty for "aging eyes" would be offered, in some instances, primarily a browlift, possibly supplemented by a blepharoplasty and laser resurfacing. Demonstrating the results of each of these procedures in isolation or together, using either a hand mirror or computer imaging system, can help educate the patient enough to make an informed decision.

COMPUTER IMAGING

At present, we use two imaging systems during patient consultations. The Mirror Image System (Virtual Eyes, Kirkland, WA) is a powerful system with excellent resolution, large storage capacity, real-time imaging, and user-friendly controls for morphing. We use the Niamtu Classic Imaging System (Niamtu Imaging Systems, Richmond, VA) at a satellite office. It is a smaller system with good image resolution, fair storage capacity, and several morphing and storage functions that, although perhaps not as easy to use as the Mirror system, is learned relatively easily. Each system has its advantages: the Mirror system can archive, retrieve, and reproduce (with appropriate developing hardware and software) a higher quality image more easily. The Niamtu system takes up less space and is significantly less expensive. If the surgeon is interested in purchasing a computer imaging system, it is necessary to determine the relative merits of each system in the surgeon's practice.

We have incorporated computer imaging into our initial consultation. All new patients are required to sign consent forms for photography and computer imaging (Fig. 1–1). After the initial physical examination, standard photographic views are obtained relative to the procedure(s) contemplated. After we have acquired all appropriate views, we review the frontal view with the

CONSENT FOR PHOTOGRAPHY

I, the undersigned, _____, am a patient of Anthony P. Sclafani, MD and consent to be photographed as relates to my treatment. This may be performed before, during or after treatment, in either the physician's office or operating room.

In the course of consultation and discussions with Dr. Sclafani and his staff, I may have been shown or provided certain brochures, pictures of actual patients or pictures of myself on an electronic imaging device. I do understand that those pictures and alterations of these pictures seen are solely for the purpose of illustration, discussion and to provide improved communications with medical professionals. I do understand that the outcome of any type of surgical procedure is directly related to my individual characteristics and health. I further understand and acknowledge that because of the obvious significant differences in how living tissues react to surgery, there may be no relationship between the electronic images created, and my actual final surgical result. Use of the computer imaging system offers an opportunity for me to discuss my desires and to allow improved communication with the medical staff.

I certify my understanding that there is NO WARRANTY, expressed or suggested, as to my own final appearance after elective surgery by the use of these electronically altered images.

The undersigned grants to Dr. Sclafani the on-going and unrestricted use of the undersigned's photographs and altered electronic images for general information, education, scientific and medical purposes at any time during or after treatment, with complete confidentiality of the my identity.

The undersigned further acknowledges that he/she relinquishes all right, title, and interest in these photographs, or any right to profit or gain directly or indirectly realized through the use of these photographs.

This consent may only be revoked in writing, signed by the undersigned and delivered to Dr. Sclafani at his office. Such revocation shall thereafter be effective as to any further use not already committed to by Dr. Sclafani. This consent is in consideration of services performed and consultations conducted or to be performed or conducted by Dr. Sclafani, and there have been no representations or inducements concerning this consent except as set forth herein.

_____	_____
Signature	Date
_____	_____
Witness	Date

Figure 1-1. Standard consent for photography and computer imaging should specify that image modifications are for demonstration purposes only and are not implied results.

patient, if only to demonstrate facial asymmetries. We briefly mention the classical aesthetic norms (rules of "thirds" and "fifths"), as well as any facial blemishes, scars, or defects.

We then perform various modifications on the images. It is essential that the original image is available for viewing; frequent "toggling" between the original and modified images helps the patient understand and appreciate even the subtlest changes. Multiple modified images can assist the patient in whom ancillary procedures are suggested. For example, if augmentation mentoplasty is recommended concurrent with a reduction rhinoplasty, three simultaneous lateral images are useful: the original, the modification with dorsal nasal reduction only, and a modified view with nasal reduction and mentoplasty. The patient can immediately see the benefit of the additional surgery; conversely, the patient can more easily decide whether the additional work is important.

Any image modification system can generate any degree of physical change, regardless of what is possible in the operating room. The surgeon must be cautious, showing on the computer only those changes that he or she believes can be achieved. Displaying changes on the computer image that are not possible surgically will only disappoint the patient and embarrass the surgeon. We describe the final image on the computer monitor as the *optimal* result. The essential function of computer imaging in our practice is to ensure that both patient and surgeon agree on what is considered an acceptable result. Occasionally, patients will point to the final modified image and request a greater degree of change. The surgeon must make only those changes on the screen that he or she believes are possible (as well as desirable) in the operating theater. However, computer imaging technology is a powerful tool to bring the expectations of surgeon and patient closer together.

PERIOPERATIVE COURSE

Once the surgery is planned, the surgeon should enumerate succinctly the operative goals. This is followed by a discussion of the operative procedures specific to each goal, as well as appropriate surgical risks. At this stage, recommendations for the operative setting (office, ambulatory surgical suite, hospital), type of anesthesia, approximate length of the procedure, and length of time the patient will stay in the facility (including preoperative and postoperative care) are discussed with the patient.

The patient should be informed of the general recovery period, specifically detailing pain, bruising, and discomfort, and the length of time with dressings or splints. The type of dressing and/or packing used postoperatively (if any) and the timing of suture removal (if any) are discussed with the patient. The importance of a proper postoperative skin care regimen (including sun avoidance and the use of appropriate sunblocks) is reviewed with patients who have had skin resurfacing. Patients are warned that each person recovers at a unique pace, but patients are informed of the typical lengths of time required before resumption of the following.

1. Showering and/or shampooing
2. Engaging in light activity at home
3. Wearing eyeglasses (postrhinoplasty) or contact lenses (postblepharoplasty)
4. Making brief excursions from home wearing a hat, sunglasses, and the like
5. Hair coloring and/or styling
6. Returning to work (wearing camouflage makeup)
7. Attending social events
8. Traveling

NURSING INTERVIEW

The nursing exit interview is essential for the team approach to facial plastic surgery to be effective. Although the surgeon will assume overall control and responsibility for patient care, an efficient office will use the skills and services of a competent nursing staff. Allowing the nurse to interact with the patient preoperatively fosters the development of a nurse-patient relationship, which enables the nurse to handle small perioperative details because the patient is less likely to insist on speaking with the surgeon about details that the nurse is capable of handling. This relationship also promotes an open dialogue between patient and nurse; we have encountered patients who have expressed major concerns only to the nursing staff because they thought they were unimportant or "did not want to bother" the surgeon.

Patient Consent Form for Operation or Special Procedure

PATIENT_____AGE_____

CHART #_____

1.   Permission.   I hereby authorize Doctor_____(and other such physician(s)
at the Hospital as he/she may designate) to perform upon _____ the
following operation(s):   myself (or name of patient)

_____

_____
(please print or type)

2.   Unforeseen Conditions.   If any unforeseen condition arises in the course of the operation or procedure for
which other procedures, in addition to or different from those above contemplated, are necessary or
appropriate in the judgment of the said physician or his designee(s), I further request and authorize the
carrying out of such operation or procedures.

3.   Anesthesia.   I consent to the administration of anesthesia under the direction of the Department of
Anesthesiology of the New York Eye and Ear Infirmary. I understand that certain risks and complications
(including damaged teeth) may result from the administration of anesthesia.

4.   Specimens.   Any organs or tissues surgically removed may be examined and retained by the Hospital
for medical, scientific or educational purposes and such tissues or parts may be disposed of in accordance
with accustomed practice and applicable State laws and regulations.

5.   Photographing, Videotaping, etc.   I consent to the photographing, videotaping, televising or other
observation of the operation or procedures to be performed; including appropriate portions of my body,
for medical, scientific or educational purposes; provided my identity is not revealed by the pictures or
descriptive texts accompanying them.

6.   Explanation of Procedure, Risks, Benefits and Alternatives.   The nature and purpose of the operation/
procedure, possible alternative methods of treatment, the expected benefits and complications, attendant
discomforts and the risks involved have been fully explained to me. I have been given an opportunity to
ask questions and all my questions have been answered fully and satisfactorily.

7.   **I further consent to the administration of blood or blood products as may be considered necessary. I
recognize that there are always risks to health, associated with the administration of blood or blood
products and such risks have been fully explained to me.**

Figure 1–2. (A) Standard institutional consent (Courtesy of The New York Eye & Ear Infirmary, NY) and **(B)** an individual consent, which lists specific pertinent complications, are signed and witnessed at the consultation visit. *(Figure continued on next page)*

The nurse confirms that the patient understands what the planned surgery is intended to achieve. He or she reviews complete and detailed surgical consents (a standard operative consent from the facility and a second completed by the surgeon (Fig. 1–2) with the patient and witnesses the patient's signature. A review of the preoperative activities and required consultations and tests (including blood work, chest x-ray, electrocardiogram,

8. <u>Cornea Transplants.</u> I consent to the release of information to the eye bank that supplied the tissue used for corneal transplant surgery. I understand that for my own health protection it may be necessary for the eye bank to contact me.

9 <u>No Guarantees.</u> I acknowledge that no guarantee or assurance has been made to me as to the results that may be obtained.

_____

I CERTIFY THAT I HAVE READ AND FULLY UNDERSTAND THE ABOVE CONSENT TO OPERATION THAT THE EXPLANATIONS THEREIN REFERRED TO WERE MADE, AND THAT ALL THE BLANK SPACES ABOVE HAVE BEEN COMPLETED PRIOR TO MY SIGNING.

Patient/Relative/Guardian*: _____
(signature)

_____
(print name)

Relationship, if other than patient signed: _____

Interpreter, if required: _____
(signature)

_____
(print name)

Witness: _____
(signature)

_____
(print name)

Date: _____

* The signature of the patient must be obtained unless the patient is an unemancipated minor under the age of 18 or is otherwise incompetent to sign.

PHYSICIAN'S CERTIFICATION

I hereby certify that I have explained to the patient the nature, purpose, benefits, risks of and alternatives to the procedure/operation, have offered to answer any questions and have fully answered such questions. I believe that the patient [relative/guardian] fully understands what I have explained and answered.

_____ Date_____
Physician's Signature

_____
Print Physician's Name

NOTE: THIS DOCUMENT MUST BE MADE PART OF THE PATIENT'S MEDICAL RECORD.

Figure 1-2A. *(continued)*

CONSENT FOR SURGERY

I, the undersigned, _____, am a patient of Anthony P. Sclafani, MD. I have been informed of the surgical and non-surgical options for treatment of my condition,_____

_____.

I understand that the treatment recommended by Dr. Sclafani for this condition is:

_____

_____

_____.

I have discussed with Dr. Sclafani these options, and the possible benefits, risks, potential complications and limitations of these options, including, but not limited to, bleeding, infection, risk of complications from anesthesia, death, unsightly scar formation, and

_____

_____

_____

_____.

Dr. Sclafani has discussed with me my treatment options and the attendant risks; I have been given the opportunity to ask questions, and these have been answered to my satisfaction. I understand the risks, benefits and limitations of the proposed procedure and desire surgery.

_____
Signature

_____   _____
Print Name   Date

_____   _____
Witness   Date

Figure 1–2B. (continued)

when applicable) is also reviewed with the patient. The patient is instructed to avoid (unless medically contraindicated) any medicine that will promote bleeding such as aspirin, vitamin E (in amounts exceeding the usual dose in a standard multivitamin supplement), garlic tablets, and the like. The nurse will also review postoperative care, which previously was reviewed by the physician. "How to Prepare for..." and "What to Expect After..." sheets specific to the contemplated procedure(s) are given to the patient. This redundancy is well worth the effort. Many patients are so preoccupied with asking questions about one aspect of the surgery that they cannot concentrate on other important details. We have found that with succinct and gentle repetition, the patient is allowed multiple opportunities to hear, understand, and question each aspect of the cosmetic surgery process. This reduces the number preoperative phone calls because patients are more comfortable with their understanding of the surgery. If, at any time, the nursing staff believes that the patient is not properly prepared, a second preoperative consultation is planned, at no charge to the patient.

FINANCIAL COUNSELING

Our surgical fee schedule is fixed, and a financial counselor is responsible for reviewing the patient's financial responsibilities. The patient is informed of the financial responsibility for not only the surgical fee but also facility and anesthesia costs. The patient is told that these charges are separate from the surgeon's fee and are collected by the facility. We have found that explicit discussion of these costs has reduced postoperative calls from patients requesting explanation of "other bills" that they receive from the facility.

We also provide a summary of the surgeon's exact charges, with a brief explanation that the facility charges are separately billed by the hospital. The patient is asked to sign and date this sheet and is given a copy. It is

explained that, should the patient defer surgery, the surgeon's fees quoted on the sheet will be honored for 12 months (Figs. 1–3 and 1–4).

Finally, we do not offer "installment payment plans." With such a system, we found that, at best, the surgeon's office becomes a "bill collector" in the patient's mind. At worst, the surgical results need to be justified with each check written. In general, the time expended administering these accounts is not worth the possible additional income. At present, we use a financing company (Unicorn Financial Services, Inc., Mesa, AZ) to provide services for interested patients. Typically, the reimbursement to the physician is slightly, but not significantly reduced compared with the additional expense of monthly billing and nonpayment of physician payment plans. The company pays the physician immediately on completion of the surgery, whereas the patient pays the financing company on a monthly basis. This arrangement has allowed us to provide services to patients who could not have otherwise afforded the service. Most importantly, the relationship between physician and patient remains medical, not financial.

The one issue that patients raise regarding the finances of cosmetic surgery that the surgeon should address personally is the issue of additional charges for revision surgery. For primary procedures, we inform the patient that if both the surgeon and patient agree to the need for revision surgery (after the appropriate postoperative waiting period), the surgical fee is waived. We believe it is imperative that the patient understands that the surgeon's goal is to achieve the preoperatively discussed result. If we truly believe that the result of a primary procedure is suboptimal, it is in the best interest of the practice to perform the necessary revision surgery. Not only is the undesirable result corrected (no longer acting as a "bad advertisement" for our practice), but the patient is better served and remains favorably disposed to our practice. We inform the patient preoperatively that although the surgical fee for this revision is waived, the facility fee is fixed and beyond our control. This residual fee usually discourages unfounded and inappropriate

Financial Counseling Form

Patient's Name: _____

Patient's Address: _____
_____

Procedure Code:	Fee:	CPT
_____	_____	_____
_____	_____	_____
_____	_____	_____
_____	_____	_____

Total Fee: _____

Down Payment: _____

Balance Due: _____

By signing below, I am affirming that I have been given an explanation of the surgical fees for the above listed procedure(s). I understand that if I schedule surgery, I must pay the balance in full at least 14 days prior to surgery. If payment is not received at least 14 days before surgery, the surgery will be postponed and will have to be rescheduled. I also understand that in addition to the surgeon's fee, I will be charged for the use of the operating suite and for the anesthesiologist's services. I understand that these are separate from the surgeon's fees. I also affirm that I have been given a copy of this form.

_____   _____
    (Date)   (Signature of Patient)

_____   _____
    (Date)   (Witness)

Figure 1–3. The patient, who is given a copy, signs "Financial Counseling" form, with quoted surgical fees; the original is filed in the office chart.

postoperative complaints. This offer, rarely used, also helps establish in the patient's mind that the surgeon is truly acting as his or her advocate.

SUMMARY

The initial consultation is a complex interaction. The patient must describe to the surgeon the specific physical changes he or she desires. The physician must decide whether surgery can achieve the patient's desired outcome and whether the patient has the physical health and psychological stability to endure the stresses of surgery. The physician must accurately describe to the patient the process involved in the surgery, as well as the risks and possible complications. The physician must demonstrate to the patient an achievable surgical goal. The properly

Financial Policy for Cosmetic Surgery

I, the undersigned, _____, have requested Dr. Sclafani perform on me the following procedure(s):

_____

_____

_____

_____

_____

I also understand that these procedures are completely cosmetic in nature. I understand that the costs of this/these procedure(s) is/are not covered by my health insurance, and that I solely am responsible for full payment to Dr. Sclafani prior to the surgery. I also understand that the costs of anesthesia, facility charges, laboratory charges, etc. are billed to me by hospital or surgi-center, that Dr. Sclafani is not involved in these charges, and that my insurance company will not pay for these charges either.

Furthermore, I understand that if non-cosmetic procedures are performed at the same time, my insurance company will be billed for these as is customary. Only medically necessary procedures will be billed to my health insurance. The usual procedure will be followed for pre-certification; if my insurance company determines these procedures to be non- covered services, I understand that I will be billed and it is my responsibility to pay in full for these services. While Dr. Sclafani's office may assist in appealing this determination by the insurance company, I understand that appeal and payment are solely my responsibility.

I wish Dr. Sclafani to perform the procedures listed above. I agree with, and agree to abide by the stipulations above.

_____   _____
(Patient)   (Date)

_____   _____
(Witness)   (Date)

Figure 1–4. "Financial Policy for Cosmetic Surgery" form is signed by the patient (who is given a copy) and filed in the office chart. This form details the responsibilities of the patient, surgeon, and any third-party payer.

prepared patient proceeds through the process of elective aesthetic surgery understanding and anticipating the reasonably anticipated phases of surgery and recovery. The patient will not interpret normal postoperative events (pain, bruising, drains, erythema, etc.), however unpleasant, as complications; he or she will be better able to adjust to these changes because she or he was prepared and anticipated them. Patients respond more favorably when they choose to accept the surgery with its attendant sequelae. We prefer when patients tell us, "It was not as bad as I thought it would be," rather than "I never knew it was going to be this bad." Finally, the physician's office staff must provide a readily available, comfortable, and nurturing environment for the patient in an emotional, medical, and financial sense. The prudent surgeon who attends to each of these needs for his or her patient sets the stage for a productive physician-patient relationship.

PEARLS

- A team approach to patient evaluation is imperative because in their interactions with patients, office personnel, and nursing staff may glean information about the patient's health, disposition, and so forth that the patient would not discuss with the surgeon.
- Beware the patient who is obsessive, dependent, demanding, or secretive.
- The patient who is knowledgeable about the postoperative surgical course is less likely to interpret the sequelae—including pain, bruising, drains, and erythema—as complications.
- Having a financial counselor on staff to review and discuss all fees with a patient before surgery is an excellent way to educate the patient of future payments while enabling the surgeon to focus on treating the patient.

ACKNOWLEDGMENTS

The author would like to acknowledge the assistance of Jennifer Hind, RN and Sandra Prescott for their contribution and nursing perspective.

SUGGESTED READINGS

Bradbury E. The psychology of aesthetic plastic surgery. *Aesth Plast Surg.* 1994; 18:301–305.

Edgerton MT, Langman MW, Pruzinsky T. Plastic surgery and psychotherapy in the treatment of 100 psychologically disturbed patients. *Plast Reconstr Surg.* 1991; 88:594–608.

MacGregor FC, Schaffner B. Screening patients for nasal plastic operations. *Psychosom Med.* 1950; 12:277–291.

Meyer E, Jacobson WE, Edgerton MT, Canter A. Motivational patterns in patients seeking elective plastic surgery. *Psychosom Med.* 1960; 22:193–203.

Facial Plastic and Reconstructive Surgery. Papel ID, Nachlas NE, eds. St. Louis: Mosby–Year Book, Inc.; 1992.

Sarwer DB, Pertschuk MJ, Wadden TA, Whitaker LA. Psychological investigations in cosmetic surgery: a look back and a look ahead. *Plast Reconstr Surg.* 1998; 101:1136–1142.

Facial Aesthetic Surgery. Tardy ME, Thomas JR, Brown RJ, eds. St. Louis: Mosby–Year Book, Inc.; 1995.

Wright MR. The male aesthetic patient. *Arch Otolaryngol Head Neck Surg.* 1987; 113:724–727.

Wright MR, Wright WK. A psychological study of patients undergoing cosmetic surgery. *Arch Otolaryngol.* 1975; 101:145–151.

Preoperative Evaluation

Aesthetic Facial Plastic Surgery, edited by Thomas Romo, III, and Arthur L. Millman, Thieme Medical Publishers, Inc., New York, New York, Copyright © 2000.

CHAPTER 2

A Plastic Surgeon's Perspective

CRAIG A. FOSTER

Patients who present for facial plastic surgery often have specific concerns that they would like addressed and specific reasons for having facial plastic surgery, some of which may not be acceptable to the surgeon. The surgeon and office staff must work together to determine whether a patient is a suitable surgical candidate both physically and psychologically. This process begins with the initial telephone interview and continues through to the consultation. A thorough consultation is key in determining a patient's suitability for surgery and satisfying the patient. The patient's medical history and appearance must be evaluated, and preoperative and postoperative issues, including anesthesia and surgical course, must be discussed in detail. The surgeon should be wary of certain kinds of patients who may be difficult to treat because of psychological problems or unrealistic expectations. In time, the physician and office staff will come to recognize and therefore avoid treating these patients.

INITIAL CONTACT

Because the patient's first contact with the plastic surgeon is invariably made over the telephone, office personnel should be familiar with the proper technique of handling telephone conversations. Telephone manner is as important as the information conveyed in the initial telephone contact. Our employees are encouraged to be friendly and responsive to prospective patients and express an interest in helping them. An experienced receptionist can often spot a difficult patient during the initial phone contact. We have found that if the office personnel suspect that the new patient will be a problem, the patient invariably is a problem. Our office personnel are given specific information to supply over the telephone, such as when appointments can be scheduled, the cost of consultation, and what general areas of plastic surgery are performed or not performed by the surgeon. They do not give medical advice or quote specific surgical fees but rather give a general range of costs. The question of quoting surgical fees over the telephone has engendered a diversity of opinions. Although quoting specific prices for individual procedures is generally not a good idea, we instruct our personnel to quote a range of fees and explain to the prospective patient that the exact fee cannot be determined until a physical examination has been done and the patient has been properly evaluated. Patients are entitled to know approximately what the fee may be because if it is totally out of their range, it will save the embarrassment of discovering in the office that they cannot afford the service.

INITIAL CONSULTATION

The initial consultation is vitally important because it establishes the relationship between surgeon and patient. No substitute exists for a thorough interview before surgery. The purposes of the initial consultation are to establish communication between surgeon and patient, diagnosis, and treatment planning.

Adequate time must be set aside for the initial consultation. Usually 20 to 30 minutes is more than adequate. Difficult or complicated cases that require more consultation time should have a second consultation.

The initial consultation allows the surgeon and the patient to evaluate one another. It is the surgeon's responsibility to accept or reject the patient's surgical request on the basis of technical feasibility, the surgeon's competence in the desired procedure, the patient's expectations, and the likelihood of achieving those expectations. The art of plastic surgery and the achievement of happy patients depends as much or more on complete preoperative consultation, evaluation, and patient education as it does on the technical skill with which the surgery is performed.

MEDICAL HISTORY

The initial consultation should begin with a thorough review of the patient's family, medical, and surgical histories; allergies, medication use, and smoking, and alcohol habits. The patient provides this information on an uptake sheet (Fig. 2–1). Obtaining patient histories is important for a number of reasons. First, it demonstrates to the patient that you are concerned with him or her as a total patient. It also identifies situations with specific impact on potential complications (i.e., aspirin use or smoking) or patient suitability for surgery (i.e., significant heart disease). Unfortunately, significant omissions by the patient of important information on the uptake sheet (e.g., previous cosmetic surgery) is not uncommon. This should alert the surgeon that the patient is not completely forthcoming and should encourage the surgeon to more closely question and evaluate the patient.

The next step is to ask the patient to describe specifically those features that the patient finds bothersome. Often the patient will say, "You are the doctor. I want you to tell me what you see." Numerous reasons exist for not falling into this trap. First, what the surgeon thinks is an obvious problem, for example protruding ears, may not bother the patient at all. This may lead the patient to question, "Why doesn't he see my problem" and may plant the seeds of dissatisfaction with heretofore acceptable features. If the patient cannot describe in reasonably precise terms the feature or features with which he or she is dissatisfied, the patient is not a good surgical candidate.

NAME_____MR / MRS / MISS / MS DATE OF BIRTH ____/____/____

ADDRESS_____ CITY _____

STATE_____ ZIP CODE_____ SS #_____

EMPLOYER_____ OCCUPATION _____

HOME PHONE ( )_____ BUSINESS PHONE ( )_____

MEDICAL HISTORY

LIST **ANY** ALLERGIES TO MEDICATIONS _____

LIST **ALL** MEDICATIONS YOU ARE TAKING _____

_____

ARE YOU TAKING ___ HEART MEDICATIONS ___ DIET PILLS ___ ACCUTANE ___ TRANQUILIZERS

___ DIURETICS ___ BLOOD PRESSURE MEDICATION ___ ANTIDEPRESSANTS ___ ALCOHOL

DO YOU SMOKE AND HOW MUCH?_____

SIGNIFICANT FAMILY HISTORY_____

_____

LIST PREVIOUS SURGERY & ILLNESSES WITH DATES_____

_____

_____

DO YOU HAVE A HISTORY OF:
___ HEART DISEASE
___ DIABETES
___ ASTHMA
___ HEPATITIS
___ LUPUS
___ ARTHRITIS
___ EPILEPSY
___ DEPRESSION
___ BLOOD DISORDERS
___ LYME DISEASE
___ HIGH BLOOD PRESSURE
___ BRONCHITIS / EMPHYSEMA
___ HEART MURMUR
___ FACIAL PARALYSIS
___ MITRAL VALVE PROLAPSE
___ ALCOHOLISM
___ DRUG ABUSE
___ TUBERCULOSIS
___ BREATHING PROBLEMS
___ NOSE BLEEDS
___ DRY EYE
___ STOMACH PROBLEMS
___ HEADACHES
___ THYROID PROBLEMS
___ SEIZURES
___ COLD SORES
___ BAD SCARRING
___ EASY BRUISING
___ PROLONGED BLEEDING
___ BLOOD CLOTS
___ CANCER _____

HAVE YOU HAD AN ADVERSE REACTION TO:
___ ASPIRIN
___ XYLOCAINE / NOVOCAINE / EPINEPHRINE
___ CODEINE
___ DEMEROL
___ PENICILLIN
___ ADHESIVE TAPE
___ MORPHINE
___ ANTIBIOTICS
___ ANESTHESIA
___ VALIUM
___ IODINE
___ CAT GUT
___ OTHER_____

REASON FOR CONSULTATION:
___ FACELIFT
___ EYELID SURGERY
___ BROWLIFT
___ NASAL SURGERY
     HAVE YOU HAD PRIOR NASAL SURGERY? ____/____/____
___ LIPOSUCTION
     WHAT AREAS?_____
___ ABDOMINOPLASTY
___ BREAST REDUCTION
___ BREAST LIFT
___ CHEMICAL PEEL
___ COLLAGEN
     DATE OF LAST COLLAGEN TREATMENT ____/____/____
___ CHIN IMPLANT
___ OTHER _____
     _____

WHO REFERRED YOU? _____

PATIENT SIGNATURE_____ DATE_____

Figure 2-1. Medical history.

APPEARANCE

The most important thing the surgeon can do during this phase of the initial consultation is listen. Careful, intuitive listening affords the surgeon an ideal opportunity to learn about the patient and his or her expectations. Short, pointed questions can direct the flow of information, but digressions should be allowed because they are often revealing. In addition to intuitive listening, the surgeon must practice intuitive observation of the patient. Is the patient's dress provocative and alluring? Does the patient shrink from physical contact? Is the patient reluctant to make eye contact? Observe the patient's grooming, hygiene, and dress. Is the patient's affect flat and voice a monotone, or is the patient overly anxious and excitable? These and other intuitive observations go a long way in forming a view or gestalt of the patient as an acceptable candidate for surgery.

PATIENT EDUCATION

The next phase of the initial consultation revolves around patient education. As the initial phase is being completed, diagnosis and treatment planning should be forming in the surgeon's mind. Addressing the patient's primary complaints and concerns, the surgeon should educate the patient about the various options available to treat those features that the patient wants corrected. These options should include whether the patient is a candidate for office surgery or whether the procedure should be done in the hospital. The type of anesthesia required should be discussed, along with a short description of the procedure (e.g., local anesthesia, IV insertion, sedation, or general anesthesia). The patient's expectations and fears should be discussed and allayed.

The length of the surgery and anesthesia time, recovery time, and expected time of discharge should be discussed. A short, not overly technical description of the surgical procedure is offered. Things important to stress are incision placement, resultant scars and their visibility, sutures and their removal, dressings, and drains. The possibility of postoperative pain or discomfort, nausea and vomiting, and the duration and treatment of all of these should be mentioned. A short list of the most frequent complications and sequelae should be discussed.

Most importantly, an honest discussion of postoperative recovery, including pain, discomfort, swelling, bruising, and time until the patient will be comfortable in a social setting, should be stressed. This phase should end with a short discussion enumerating the high points of the previous phase. A few well-chosen sentences usually completes this, something to the effect of: "Office operation, local with sedation, 1 hour surgery, in and out of the office in 3 or 4 hours, limited activity for 10 days, acceptable appearance in 10 to 14 days, back to work in 10 to 14 days, exercise in 2 to 3 weeks."

The next phase of the initial consultation addresses any questions the patient may have. These are usually few if the surgeon has done an adequate job in the preceding phase of patient education. Extensive lists of questions covering previously answered points or repeating the same questions several times should alert the surgeon to the fact that the patient is not listening or is incapable of grasping certain important concepts. Assuming the surgeon has communicated properly, this calls the patient's acceptability as a candidate for surgery into question.

PAYMENT

The last phase of the initial consultation lies with the office manager. The primary responsibilities of the office manager are full and complete disclosure of the patient's financial responsibilities, including itemized surgical fees, anesthesia fee, and facility or hospital charges. Method and timing of payments are discussed. Scheduling parameters are discussed; if the patient has a specific date in mind, all attempts are made to accommodate the patient. Demanding and inflexible patients who cannot be accommodated without significantly disrupting normal practice procedure are refused surgery. Patient education continues in the form of written materials that describe in detail preoperative preparation, including laboratory work and pictures, descriptions of the surgical procedure, and postoperative care requirements, including special duty nurses. Preoperative and postoperative pictures that demonstrate results of the same procedure(s) on other patients may be shown. A second consultation or preoperative visit is not only encouraged but required. The second consultation is extremely helpful to both surgeon and patient to ensure both are "on the same wavelength."

This consultation should occur after the pictures have been taken and are available for viewing with the patient. This visit begins with a short recap of the proposed procedure, a description of the events of the day of surgery, and what the patient can expect. With the patient photos and these preoperative forms and figures, a more detailed discussion of risks, complications, and limitations of the proposed procedure ensues. Questions are encouraged and answered. Patient signatures on a photo consult (Fig. 2–2), risks and complications (Fig. 2–3), and informed

---

Patient Name: _____ Date: _____

EYELID DEFORMITIES:

- ☐ Crows Feet
- ☐ Blepharopigmentation
- ☐ Ptosis - Left Upper Lid
- ☐   - Right Upper LId
- ☐ Herniated orbital fat
- ☐ Xantholasmas
- ☐ Malar bags
- ☐ Permanent eyeliner
- ☐ Lower lid laxity
- ☐ Dry eye syndrome
- ☐ Visual acuity
- ☐ Nerve weakness

- ☐ Edema
- ☐ Allergies
- ☐ Lesions
- ☐ Thyroid condition
- ☐ Scleral show
- ☐ Hollow orbits
- ☐ Prominent orbital rim
- ☐ Ectropion
- ☐ Previous eyelid scars
- ☐ Muscle festoon
- ☐ Contact lens wearer

BROW DEFORMITIES:

- ☐ Glabellar crease
- ☐ Horizontal rhytides
- ☐ Brow ptosis - Left
- ☐ Brow ptosis - Right

- ☐ Eyebrows shape
- ☐ Hairline position
- ☐ Vertical wrinkles across nasion
- ☐ Asymmetry

FACE & NECK DEFORMITIES:

- ☐ Jawline
- ☐ Neck
- ☐ Fat Deposits
- ☐ Asymmetry
- ☐ Platysma bands
- ☐ Perioral rhytides
- ☐ Naso labial folds
- ☐ Commissures
- ☐ Witches chin
- ☐ Microgenia

- ☐ Bells Palsy
- ☐ Hairline
- ☐ Earlobe - Left
- ☐   - Right
- ☐ Facial nerve weakness
- ☐ Larynx position
- ☐ Previous facelift scars
- ☐ Lesions
- ☐ Aging lip
- ☐ Submandibular gland position

SKIN EVALUATION:

- ☐ Type   I   II   III   IV
- ☐ Smoker
- ☐ Sun Damage
- ☐ Thickness
- ☐ Elasticity
- ☐ Wrinkles

- ☐ Scarring
- ☐ Hypopigmentation
- ☐ Hyperpigmentation
- ☐ Hypertrophic scarring
- ☐ Acne prone
- ☐ Telangiectasia

Dr. Foster has reveiwed these findings with me. I understand that the above noted pre-existing deformities may be present after surgery.

Patient Signature: _____ Date: _____

Figure 2–2. Photo consult sheet, reviewing the patient photos, stressing certain individual characteristics, asymmetries, and skin types.

Patient Name: _____   Date: _____

RISKS / COMPLICATIONS:
GENERAL:
☐ Bleeding
☐ Hematoma (blood collection that may need to be drained)
☐ Infection
☐ Wound separation (incisions that do not heal well)
☐ Sensory change (numbness/pain)
☐ Skin loss around an incision (especially smokers)

☐ Asymmetry (ALL people are asymmetrical)
☐ Loss of hair around an incision
☐ Poor scars (ALL scars are permanent)
☐ Delayed healing (how well you heal cannot be predicted)
☐ Reaction to medications (rash, nausea, vomiting)
☐ Additional surgery needed (scar revision, secondary procedure)

SPECIFIC:

FACELIFT / BROWLIFT / TEMPLE LIFT
Skin loss (especially in smokers)
Hair loss
Earlobe distortion
Residual fat, laxity
Facial paralysis (rare)
Widened or raised scars
Skin discoloration
Persistent numbness, pain
Asymmetry

RHINOPLASTY
Internal scarring
External scarring (alar bases, columella)
Asymmetries tend to persist after surgery
Persistent swelling, stiffness in tip
Persistent breathing problems (turbinate
    enlargement, deviated septum)
Sinus obstruction
Extrusion of graft or nasal implant
Septal perforation
Persistent bump or curve of nasal tip
Irregularities of bone, cartilage
Not enough change/too much change
Infected graft/implant (may have to be removed)

BREAST REDUCTION / LIFT
Poor scars (red, raised, painful, thick)
Weight gain after surgery will distort result
Pregnancy/breastfeeding may create sagging
Loss of sensation in nipple
Inability to breast feed
Loss of pigmentation in nipple areola complex
Nipple retraction
Poor contour, persistent sagging
Skin loss (nipple, around incisions)
Asymmetry
Not enough tissue removal/too much tissue removal

BLEPHAROPLASTY
Persistent dryness
Corneal abrasion or irritation
Widened or depressed scars
Ectropion (lower lid retraction)
Blepharopigmentation
Skin deficiency
Visual disturbance
Residual skin, wrinkling, fat bags

CHEMICAL PEEL
Pigmentation
Irritation
Scarring (deep peels)
Visible line of demarcation
May need to be repeated to achieve best result
Photosensitivity

FACIAL IMPLANT
Numbness
Infected implant (may have to be removed)
Malpositioned implant
Implant too large/too small
Pain
Implant may slip or move

LIPOSUCTION
Excess skin
Contour or surface irregularities
Poor scars
Not enough fat removal/too much fat removal
Areas of depression, rippling
Cellulite or dimpling will not improve
Weight gain after surgery will distort results
Pulmonary embolus (rare)
Fat embolus (rare)
Persistent numbness
Skin discoloration (rare)

Even though the risks and complications listed above occur infrequently, they are the ones that are peculiar to the operation or of greatest concern. Other risks and complications can occur, but are even more uncommon. The practice of medicine and surgery is not an exact science. Although good results are expected, there cannot be any guarantee nor warranty, expressed or implied, by anyone as to the results that may be obtained.

A copy of this sheet, a detailed Preoperative Instruction sheet, individual Postoperative Instructions sheets for each procedure I am having done, and ASPRS brochures for each procedure I am having done, have been given to me and explained fully.

_____   _____
Patient signature   Date

Given by: _____

Figure 2–3. Risks, complications, limitations sheet, delineating some, but not all, potential complications.

surgical consent are then obtained by the surgeon and witnessed by an office staff member. The patient is then seen by the office manager, and all financial scheduling and nursing matters are concluded.

Further preoperative education and preparation is carried out by staff nurses over the phone. At all points along this continuum, the staff, including the front desk staff, office manager, and nurses, are participating in the preoperative evaluation of the patient as a suitable candidate for surgery. The office staff are valuable allies and sources of information concerning the potential patient. Many times patients will be more open or less guarded with staff and will relate pertinent information they forget or deliberately withhold from the surgeon. Office staff should be encouraged to communicate this information or any concern they may have about the patient directly to the surgeon. In this way, the staff can be invaluable in protecting the surgeon from accepting an inappropriate patient.

PROBLEM PATIENTS

The following are examples of "red flags" or problem patients. Some of these are obvious, but many are not. These are the patients who require a more finely developed sixth sense, honed through intuitive listening and intuitive observation. The surgeon is well advised to develop and deepen these valuable tools. Not all surgeons are well equipped with these senses but can develop them with attention to detail. Unfortunately, most of us learn by making mistakes. By all means, learn from them and develop a good sixth sense. It is invaluable in avoiding grief both to you and your potential patients.

OVERCONCERN WITH MINOR DEFORMITY

These patients, who are relatively easy to identify, are difficult to please. Such patients have an unrealistic self-image and therefore correction of the minor defect will not satisfy the patient.

INABILITY TO DESCRIBE PROBLEM OR A DESIRED CHANGE

It is extremely important to get the patient to verbalize in a coherent fashion the feature(s) with which he or she is dissatisfied. The patient also should have a concept of what the desired change should provide. If the surgeon is unable to determine these two things, the patient should not be accepted as a surgical candidate.

UNREALISTIC EXPECTATIONS

The patient who expects the surgeon to change his or her life will not be satisfied. Expectations of a new life, new job, or new lover are unrealistic, and such a patient does not make a good surgical candidate. These patients will often confide these expectations to the staff, nurses, or office manager rather than the surgeon.

PERFECTIONIST PATIENTS

Perfectionist patients are usually recognized by highly detailed and probing questions, evidence of extensive research into procedures, and detailed descriptions of what they want done. They often bring in pictures, medical photographs, and drawings detailing their exact specifications. Usually these patients are demanding, time-consuming, and fussy. They are likely to be unsatisfied with the minor details of the operation but in the end are often pleased with the overall result. Superperfectionists cannot be pleased and should not be considered as surgical candidates. Somewhat perfectionist patients can be pleased but require more time, attention, and education. They often require several consults and careful education into the inadequacies, shortcomings, and unpredictability of the results. They will also require more frequent postoperative visits, hand-holding, and reassurance in the postoperative period.

INAPPROPRIATE PATIENT MOTIVATION

The patient who is seeking surgery at the behest of a friend or relative and who is not convincingly self-motivated is a questionable candidate. Every attempt should be made to ensure that these patients truly want the procedure for themselves. Strength of motivation is positively correlated with less postoperative pain, a shorter postoperative course, and greater satisfaction.

THE INDECISIVE PATIENT

This patient is often prone to miss scheduled appointments and does not follow-up on laboratory work, pictures, or consultations. They also often miss payment deadlines. This behavior usually denotes ambiguity or guilt about the proposed procedure. Sometimes these patients will ask whether the surgeon believes the procedure is necessary. This patient is usually seeking a way out. It is judicious to say that no one "needs" these procedures, and that it would not hurt to wait another year or so before proceeding. These patients are often grateful for the advice and usually return later more motivated to have the procedure.

THE SPECIAL PATIENT

Beware of any patient who by means of his or her wealth, standing in the community, celebrity, or relationship to the surgeon (e.g., family friend or colleague) attempts to disrupt the normal functioning and structure of the office. Such individuals often intimate or guarantee a deluge of referred patients on successful completion of their surgery. They often ask for or demand specific financial consideration. Of course, the surgeon can modify the usual fees to fit certain circumstances such as family and friends but should be advised that this behavior or modification rarely is kept confidential and often leads to a deluge of other individuals who expect the same consideration. Circumventing or ignoring standard office practices established with good reason, over years of experience, will often lead to disaster.

THE SECRETIVE PATIENT

The obvious example is that of a wife who does not tell or want her spouse to know of the surgery. Such an arrangement is essentially impossible to guarantee. It indicates a high degree of guilt about the procedure and often leads to conflict with the party kept in the dark.

THE DISAPPROVING FAMILY

Although it is true that patients should be self-motivated to have these procedures done, strong family disapproval is a harbinger of trouble ahead. These patients will lack critical support in the early postoperative phase when a casual or deliberately hurtful remark can destroy the patient's confidence, accentuate guilt, and deepen depression.

THE PATIENT THE SURGEON DOES NOT LIKE

The experienced surgeon can usually determine within a few minutes of intuitive listening and observation whether he or she and the patient will get along. All experienced surgeons can recall experiences of "bad vibes" with such a patient. If such an event occurs, the wise surgeon will listen to that sixth sense and not accept the patient.

THE "SURGIHOLIC"

Beware of the patient who has had multiple repeated cosmetic surgeries. These patients usually have internally distorted body images to go along with their usually distorted external images. Nothing that even the most experienced surgeon can do will improve either.

THE HYPERCRITICAL AND LITIGIOUS PATIENT

Early on in the consultation these patients will criticize the work of other surgeons, find fault with everything done for them, and often refuse to divulge the names of any previous operating surgeons. It is imperative to determine who the previous surgeons were and communicate with them directly. They will often be among your more respected colleagues, and therefore failure to elicit their names from the patient should be grounds to proceed no further. The patient may have been involved in litigation against others, which often is withheld from you. Attempts may be made to massage your ego as the only one who can rectify the situation. Do not believe this because it is much more likely that you will become the latest surgeon to be criticized or sued. These patients usually cannot be satisfied and should be avoided.

The following are often-cited examples of patients to be avoided but who can be successfully treated if approached and evaluated with the care and concern that should be afforded to all.

MALE PATIENTS, ESPECIALLY RHINOPLASTY PATIENTS

Male cosmetic surgery patients probably comprise no more than 10% of such patients in most practices but have been blamed for a higher percentage of problems. Experience had taught that this does not have to be the case and that rewarding relationships and results can be accomplished. Most conflicts arise when a female aesthetic is imposed on the planning and performance of male aesthetic surgery. The key to satisfied male patients is application of a different aesthetic thought process. This resolves around less aggressive, more conservative approaches, for example leaving skin fold on the upper lid or leaving some nasal hump behind. If the surgery is carefully planned, male facelift patients are usually easier to please than female facelift patients.

PATIENTS WHO HAVE HAD OR ARE IN PSYCHOTHERAPY

This group includes patients taking antidepressants such as fluoxetine (Prozac™) or sertraline (Zoloft™). In most major metropolitan areas a significant number of patients are taking such medications and are not necessarily poor candidates for surgery. Support and approval from the therapist is of great value. However, patients who want to keep such things from their therapists or who refuse to let the surgeon contact their therapists should be treated cautiously or refused surgery.

PATIENTS WHO HAVE HAD POOR EXPERIENCE WITH OTHER SURGEONS

Not all patients who criticize other plastic surgeons or who have had bad experiences are poor candidates. They may be justified in their criticisms. They usually respond well when treated like all other patients. You may perform a great service for the other plastic surgeons and plastic surgery in general by converting a disgruntled patient to a happy one. However, beware the hypercritical, chronically dissatisfied patient who goes from surgeon to surgeon as was mentioned earlier. These patients can usually be distinguished from those who have had poor results or bad relationships elsewhere but can still be satisfied happy patients.

SUMMARY

The key to successful preoperative evaluation of patients is to develop and to establish a system that is adhered to without exception and that allows maximal evaluation and information gathering to ensure, as much as possible, a relationship and outcome that satisfy both the surgeon and patient. This evaluation begins with the initial phone contact with the patient and includes all staff members in the patient evaluation. The initial consultation has five phases: (1) review of the patient's medical and surgical history; (2) the patient's explanation as to what bothers him or her; (3) diagnosis, treatment planning, and patient education of the proposed procedure and its implications; (4) patient questions; and (5) office manager's review of financial responsibility, scheduling, and continued patient education.

A second consultation or preoperative visit is required, which should briefly recap the initial consultation. Within this framework, the single most important thing for the surgeon to do is to intuitively listen and observe. Successful preoperative evaluation and patient selection depends on the development of an all-important sixth sense. The surgeon who develops and nurtures this intuitive sense will be more successful in selecting patients who are appropriate for his or her personality, skill level, and technical expertise.

PEARLS

- If the office staff suspect that a patient will be a problem, the patient invariably is a problem.
- The surgeon is responsible for accepting or rejecting a patient's request for surgery on the basis of technical feasibility, the surgeon's competence, the patient's expectations, and the likelihood of achieving those expectations.
- Significant omissions from a patient's medical history are not uncommon. This circumstance should prompt the surgeon to question the patient more closely because this may be the first sign of a problem patient.
- The surgeon should listen intuitively to a patient and always observe the patient's appearance and mannerisms. What the patient is *not* saying and how he or she acts will help the surgeon decide whether a patient is an appropriate surgical candidate.
- Although men present for cosmetic surgery far less often than women, they are frequently difficult to satisfy. The key to successful male cosmetic surgery is the application of an aesthetic thought process that differs from that used for women.

SUGGESTED READINGS

Baker TJ, Gordon HL. *Surgical Rejuvenation of the Face.* St. Louis: C.V. Mosby Co.; 1986.

Edgerton MT, et al. Surgical results and psychosocial changes following rhytidectomy. *Plast Reconstr Surg.* 1964; 33:503.

Fisher S, Cleveland SE. *Body Image and Personality* (2nd rev. ed.), New York: Dover; 1968.

Goin JM, Goin MK. *Changing the Body: Psychological Effects of Plastic Surgery.* Baltimore: Williams & Williams; 1981.

Goin JM, Goin MK. *Psychological Aspects of Aesthetic Plastic Surgery in the Art of Aesthetic Plastic Surgery.* Boston: Little Brown & Co.; 1989.

Goin MK, Burgoyne RW, Goin JM. Facelift operation: The patient's secret motivations and reaction to "informed consent." *Plast Reconstr Surg.* 1976; 58:273.

Goldwyn RM. *The Patient and the Plastic Surgeon.* Boston: Little Brown & Co.; 1981.

Goldwyn RM. *The Unfavorable Result in Plastic Surgery, Avoidance and Treatment.* Boston: Little Brown & Co.; 1984.

Gorney M. *Patient Selection: An Ounce of Prevention.* In: Corirro EH, ed. *Male Aesthetic Surgery.* St. Louis: C.V. Mosby Co.; 1982.

Gorney M. *Guidelines for Preoperative Screening of Patients.* In: Lewis JR, ed. *The Art of Aesthetic Plastic Surgery.* Boston: Little Brown & Co.; 1989.

Jacobson WE, et al. Psychiatric evaluation of male patients seeking cosmetic surgery. *Plast Reconstr Surg.* 1960; 26:356.

Leeb D, Bowers DG, Jr, Lynch JB. Observations on the myth of informed consent. *Plast Reconstr Surg.* 1976; 58:280.

Lewis JR. *The Art of Aesthetic Plastic Surgery.* Boston: Little Brown & Co.; 1989.

MacGregor FC, Schaffner B. Screening patients for nasal plastic operations. *Psychosom Med.* 1950; 12:227.

MacGregor TC. Social and psychological considerations in aesthetic plastic surgery: Old trends and new. In: Rees TD, ed. *Aesthetic Plastic Surgery.* Philadelphia: W.B. Saunders; 1980.

Rees TD. *Aesthetic Plastic Surgery.* Philadelphia: W.B. Saunders; 1980.

Wright MR, Wright WK. A psychological study of patients undergoing cosmetic surgery. *Arch Otolaryngol.* 1975; 101:141.

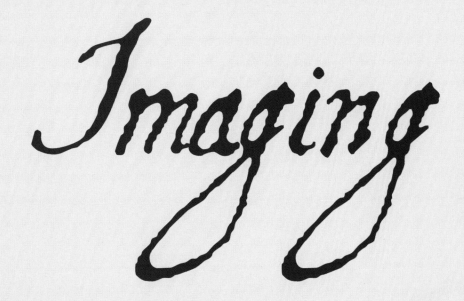

Imaging

The chapters by Dr. Galitz and the editors represent the gamut of preoperative and postoperative imaging of the aesthetic facial surgery patient. Dr. Galitz has written an extraordinarily precise and informative chapter that the reader is well advised to simulate, if not duplicate, in his or her office. Dr. Galitz has taken great trouble to give both room specifications and photographic specifications to all aspects of preoperative and postoperative photography from intricate details of lighting and camera positioning to the most appropriate view ports for given surgical procedures.

We provide a chapter on computer imaging because we have found that computer imaging in the practice of facial surgery is an excellent method for "communication" in preoperative evaluation of the patient. It should be emphasized that imaging should not be used as a sales tool or to create unrealistic expectations. Consequently, the ability to accurately discuss and use an image to convey concepts and expectations, both on the surgeon's part and on the patient's part, helps determine whether goals are realistic and what the exact intent is for the given facial surgery.

It is clear that one of the most important steps, both for documentation and the process of evaluation and postoperative finalization of a procedure, is the photographic documentation of the patient and the patient's final results. These are critical in the surgeon's own archives for his ability to objectively review his results and to modify his procedures in the process of a lifetime of technique improvement.

Imagine

Aesthetic Facial Plastic Surgery, edited by Thomas Romo, III, and Arthur L. Millman, Thieme Medical Publishers, Inc., New York, New York, Copyright © 2000.

CHAPTER 3

Traditional Photo Documentation

RICHARD M. GALITZ

Standardized and highly accurate photography of patients undergoing facial plastic surgery is of paramount importance to both surgeons and patients. This part of the surgical process should never be overlooked or approached half-heartedly. Single preoperative Polaroid photographs in frontal and side views taken by an office worker is a great disservice to a patient and can be a potential catastrophe for a surgeon. The most important aspect of surgical photography is documentation, and this documentation must be beyond reproach by a court of law, a patient, colleagues, and other involved professionals. To achieve this goal, surgical photography must be held to the highest standards of integrity and quality, no different than that applied to the surgical procedure itself. Proper equipment and setup, along with strict adherence to basic standardized principals of surgical photography, will ensure honest, reproducible, preoperative and postoperative photographs. These same photographs will be able to serve many uses, such as documentation, education, and even marketing.

Video imaging, which will be discussed later in the chapter, has become an important and widely used tool in the past 5 years. The process that has been a boon to many surgical practices has brought with it a totally new and different dynamic regarding the documentation and integrity of visual imagery in facial plastic surgery. This will be discussed later, but the same principles of standardization and honesty must still be applied here. Unfortunately, the ability of a surgeon to alter the dynamic of the photographic process in video imaging is far greater than it is in standard photography, and if abused, the potential to mislead and to subsequently alter documented work can occur.

Even today some in the surgical community believe that the temptation to be less than honest in representing the expected surgical results with the imaging process is a drawback to its use. In my own office, video imaging has been excellent for both the patient and for my practice. I apply the same honest approach to video imaging as I do to all other aspects of the surgical process.

SETUP

Proper equipment and setup is the best way to achieve standardized and accurate patient photography. All photographic systems begin with a studio (i.e., space). It must be large enough to accommodate all necessary photographic equipment, it must be removed from unnecessary light sources, it must not alter the arrival of proper lighting in the area being photographed, and it must be comfortable for the patient. To this end a single-purpose room without windows, devoid of reflective objects, and at least 9 ft × 12 ft (preferably larger) will be sufficient. Shuffling cameras and light sources around examination room chairs, pulling a backdrop down in front of a window, and making obvious double duty of an office space intended for other uses looks unprofessional and detracts from a patient's confidence level. A single-purpose photographic space with high-quality equipment helps to ensure its use and adds to the overall professionalism of any office.

It is probably an unnecessary and added expense to set up a separate studio space for video imaging. In my office standard photography and video imaging are done in the same room. I have a computer-type work desk along one wall and a wall-mounted swing arm for the video camera that swings into proper position and then moves away when not in use. I use the same lighting system for both standard and imaging photographic processes. Depending on one's own equipment, necessary alterations to this setup can still usually be done in a single space.

LIGHTING

The approach to the light source in medical photography varies, depending on the available space, cost, and type of photography to be taken. Through the years many surgeons have grown accustomed to a particular type of light source and, as with many things in surgery, find it difficult to change in midstream.

However, it is important to remember that personal habits and idiosyncrasies lead away from standardization. Unlike the art world, the very best surgical photography shows no personal stamp whatsoever.

The simplest light sources are ring lights and strobe lights attached to the camera. More complex but by far the best and most desirable is full studio lighting. The ring light is relatively inexpensive and generally ensures that light reaching the subject comes in at the proper angle. The main drawback to ring lighting is flat lighting. The camera mounted strobe light, which is the kind of lighting most people are familiar with, does not produce flat lighting. However, a single camera-mounted strobe light has a tendency to artificially highlight and shadow a subject if the angle of the strobe is not correct or consistent. Again, for standardized and accurate patient photography the single-mounted strobe lighting system is less than ideal.

The studio lighting system ensures the most standardized, accurate, and professional photographic results. The purpose of studio lighting is to remove any artificial shadowing and highlights while allowing for the accurate depiction of natural contours. Studio lighting involves right and left main lights in front of the subject and some form of backlighting. Backlighting can involve right and left lights or can be accomplished as a setup with a single slave-type flash properly positioned toward the backdrop. I have found that backlighting serves mostly to remove any shadowing behind the patients and that its use in separating the subject from the background is of minor importance (Fig. 3–1).

My office setup uses right and left umbrella flashes with incorporated modeling lights. The modeling lights

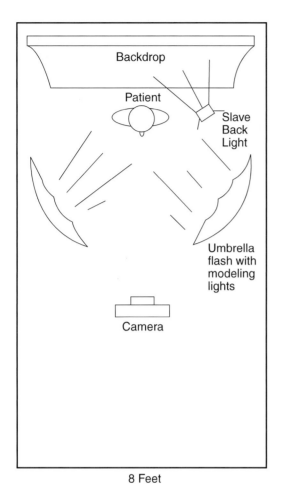

Figure 3–1. Medical photographic studio showing backdrop, right and left umbrella flashes with built-in modeling lights, and slave backlight flash.

keep an even and continuous flow of light on the subject and remove the need for backlighting all together.

Any shadowing created by the right and left umbrella strobe flash is diffused by the modeling lights. The modeling lights also help to tone down undesirable highlighting created by oily or shiny skin.

As a backdrop, I use heavy-grade paper with a black matte finish. I have had the same paper hanging for 10 years and it has held its shape. I prefer a black background because it tends to show much less shadowing than many of the lighter blue backgrounds. It also gives more contrast and definition to the subject. It will not clash with a patient's clothing or hair color. A black background will show up in standard photographs as a medium dark gray with proper lighting and a normal F stop.

EQUIPMENT

Anyone interested in a detailed description of the many camera types and lenses available for photographic work should refer to the suggested readings at the end of this chapter. For the purpose of standard patient photography the discussion will be limited the 35-mm single-lens reflex camera. Polaroid photographs may be convenient but are not appropriate for the purposes discussed here. Larger film format cameras used in professional portrait photography have certain advantages regarding aspects of definition and eventual print size but again are unnecessary in a plastic surgery setting. A 35-mm single-lens reflex camera affords a large enough film format for high-resolution printing of prints up to 11 inches × 14 inches and the ability to change and use many different lenses. A high-quality, reliable, full-sized 35-mm camera body without motorization or other unnecessary options will cost most surgeons between $250 and $600. Because the camera is to be used in a simple repeatable fashion, any options or frills to the basic system are unnecessary.

A telephoto lens (90 to 110 mm) will work well within the studio space described and will afford a normal rendition of facial features. This same setup with a macro lens will allow close-up focus work.

This is very important to surgeons removing skin lesions or doing scar work, which may need close skin photography to accurately describe the pathological condition present. As a point of reference, in my practice I use a Pentex K-1000 body with a Pentex-A macro lens 1 : 2.8 100 mm. With this setup I am able to reproduce high-quality 5-inch × 7-inch prints or slides as desired and excellent close-up photography to within a few inches of a patient's face.

It is important to maintain one setup if it is to be used in preoperative and postoperative photography. Different lens sizes and configurations can result in misleading and potentially dishonest information. (I once had a patient who refused to believe that she had significant improvement on her postoperative rhytidectomy photos. When I showed her the original preoperative photography, she accused me of having switched lenses from one that artificially adds wrinkles to one that artificially removes them. She was actually claiming that her surgical results were nothing more than a clever manipulation of camera lenses.)

PRINTS

I believe all photography should be color photography and prints should be at least 5 inches × 7 inches. Smaller print sizes are less expensive but do not show facial features as well. Larger print sizes are unnecessary unless requested by the patient or to be used for analytic design purposes by the surgeon. Early in my career I made slides of every patient, but this became very expensive and most patient photographs were never used in a teaching or lecture situation requiring slide presentations. I now catalog the negatives of my 5-inch × 7-inch prints and have slides made from these if necessary.

THE PATIENT

Taking photographs for documentation and recording accurate visual data require removal of all possible visual distractions. Makeup, jewelry, distracting apparel, and hair should be removed or rearranged. Special attention should be paid to the patient's hair. Hair can be both visually distracting and misleading to the patient's overall visual image.

However, it is also important to maintain an honest representation of the patient's true hairline. Foreheads, brows, ears, and even the mandible and neck line are visually intregrated with the patient's hair line. Patients must also feel at ease during photography, so that any unnatural representation of their appearance or excessive removal of clothing should be avoided.

VIEWS

A full-on front view of the face should include the entire circumference of the head to just above the sternal notch. The patient should be looking directly into the camera lens, which is at eye level. (Fig. 3–2).

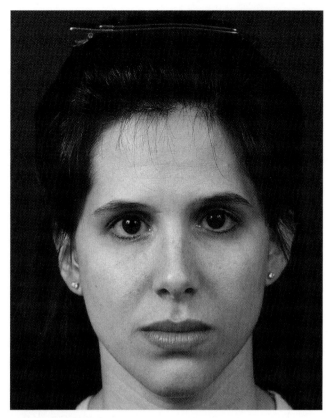

Figure 3–2. Full-face front view. Note that the entire head is depicted. The hair has been elevated off the forehead and the eyes are at camera-lens level. The head is erect and the ears and jawline are symmetrical.

Good posture should be maintained with the head in proper position above the shoulders. Some patients find it unnatural to look directly into the camera and try to offset themselves slightly right or left. Meticulous care should be taken to avoid this. Eye levels and the ears serve as a good guide to prevent this problem.

The facial profile in Figure 3–3 includes the top of the head to just above the sternal notch. The neck outline should be visualized by pulling the hair back. If the occiput is significant, the nasal tip can be brought closer to the edge of the photograph; however, a visually acceptable space must be left between the nasal tip and the edge of the photograph.

The oblique view also includes the entire head down to the sternal notch. This view is best standardized by aligning the nasal tip with the outline of the cheek (Fig. 3–4).

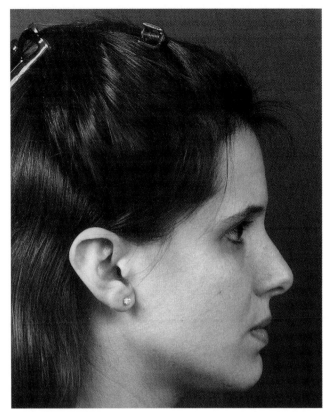

Figure 3–3. Profile. Adequate space is left between the nasal tip and the photograph margin. Note that visually obstructing hair has been pulled back, but the natural hairline has been maintained.

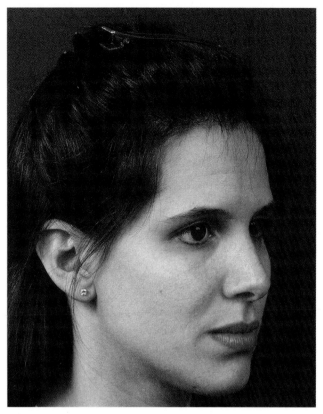

Figure 3–4. Oblique view. Standardization of the oblique view is best accomplished by aligning the nasal tip with the outline on the cheek.

Close-up views of the nose, both frontal (Fig. 3–5A) and profile (Fig. 3–5B), should include the eyebrows and the lips. In these views the level of the lens is at the center of the subject to avoid any artificially introduced angular irregularities. Close-up views of the nose are particularly helpful in depicting subtle irregularities of the nasal anatomy and aspects of skin texture.

Close-up oblique views of the nose follow the same rules as the frontal and lateral views. (Fig. 3–5C)

The chin-up view (Fig. 3–6A), depicting the nasal vertible, is an excellent view to document preoperative asymmetry of the nostrils, caudal septal dislocations, and nasal tip width. This view is absolutely necessary when any procedures to reposition the nasal ala are being considered.

The ear should be shown in the standard face views—frontal, oblique, profile—and should also include a rear view (Fig. 3–6B), oblique rear view (Fig. 3–6C) and

close-up view (Fig. 3–6D). The full rear view and oblique rear view are excellent views to show the relative position of the pinna to the scalp. These views are important both for documentation and analysis in any patient undergoing reconstruction of the external ear or otoplasty. It is important to maintain a visible hairline in all these views.

Proper visualization of the eyes should include a close-up view with the eyes both open (Fig. 3–7A) and shut (Fig. 3–7B). These views should include at least part of the forehead, the eyebrows, and most of the nose. They should extend outward to the lateral outline of the temporal region. The lens should be at the level of the eyes to prevent the patient from looking either up or down.

Views of the lower face (Fig. 3–8) must include the nasal tip, the earlobes, and some space between the outline of the chin and the edge of the photograph. The preceding applies to both the frontal and lateral views.

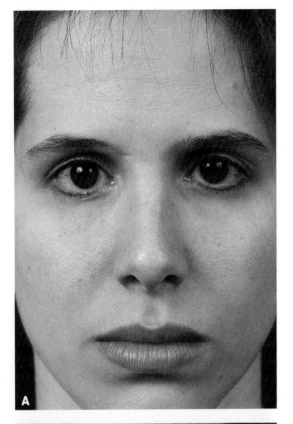

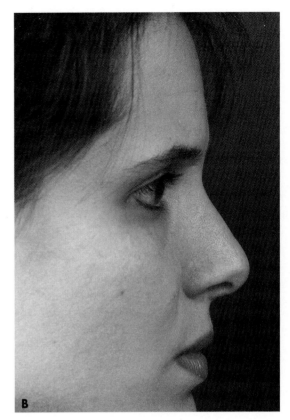

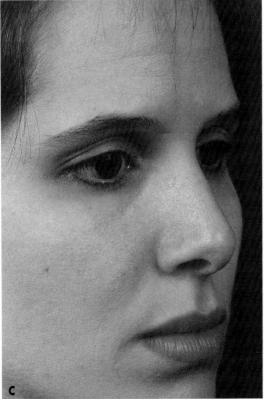

Figure 3–5. Close-up of nose. **(A)** Frontal view. The camera lens is at the center of the subject (not eye level) to prevent angular distortion. The nasal cartilages and skin texture are clearly demonstrated. **(B)** Profile. Note the inclusion of the eyebrows, eyes, and lips. **(C)** Oblique view. Excellent visualization of the lower lateral cartilages. Standardization is accomplished through allignment of nasal tip and cheek outline.

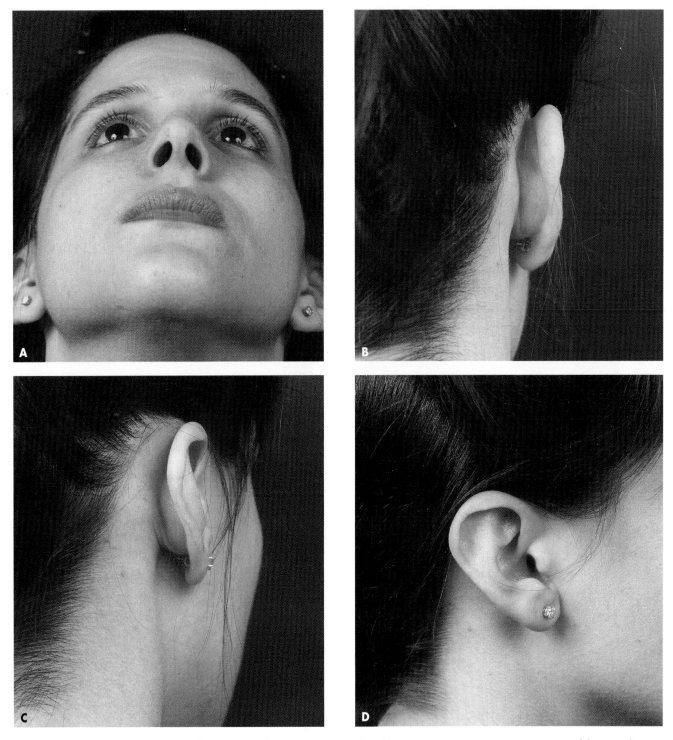

Figure 3–6. Close-up of ear. **(A)** Chin-up view. This view is essential to document any preoperative asymmetry of the nostrils, caudal septal dislocations, and nasal tip width. **(B)** Rear view. This view demonstrates the position of the pinna in relation to the scalp. **(C)** Oblique rear view. Excellent depiction of the ear relative to the hairline is visualized by adjusting the hair back without distorting it. **(D)** Profile view. Close-up demonstration of the ear and its anatomic landmark.

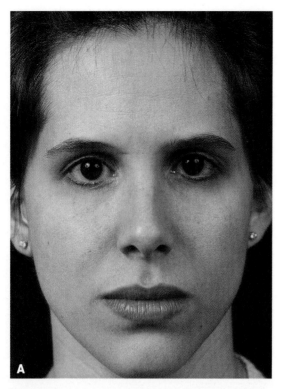 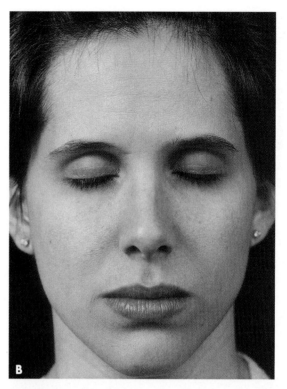

Figure 3–7. Close-up of eyes. **(A)** Open. The lens should be at the level of the eyes. The view should extend outward to the lateral outline of the temporal region. **(B)** Closed. The eyes should be closed in a relaxed fashion.

If the lips are the main focus of the views, a close-up photograph may be taken with acceptable sacrifice of the lateral mandible and earlobe areas.

The views described here are for standard aesthetic and reconstructive procedures of the face and neck. Many other views exist both for documentation and analyses; some highly specialized views are necessary for many other procedures. These other views are best described in the context of those specific procedures. However, the basic principle of standardization, integrity, and accuracy will still apply.

COMPUTER IMAGING

Computer-assisted imaging systems are now a major part of the surgical consultation process. Our office receives calls every day for consultations, and the first question asked is whether we have computer imaging available. Regardless of the merit the public is now aware of its availability, and many people believe their consultation is incomplete without it.

Early on I had reservations about computer-assisted imaging, believing it was far more a marketing tool than one of analysis or education. Having used a high-quality system for the past 5 years, I now believe it has a valuable place in the consultation process and physician-patient relationship. The ability to mislead a patient and display unrealistic potential surgical results exists. However, this is a problem with the surgeon not the machinery or process.

What I have found more than anything else in the past few years is that a picture is worth a thousand words. Many patients, no matter how well counseled, never visualize the aesthetic changes being discussed. This can lead to the classic words we are all familiar with. "I would like to do my nose, but I'm just afraid of what I might look like." With computer-assisted imagery we can now give anyone an accurate visual representation of what they might look like after surgery.

It is also easier to get feedback from patients regarding our suggested aesthetic alterations. A secondary procedure such as augmentation mentoplasty or liposuction

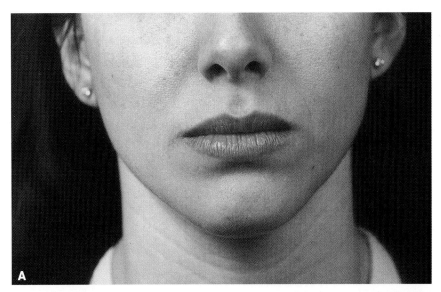

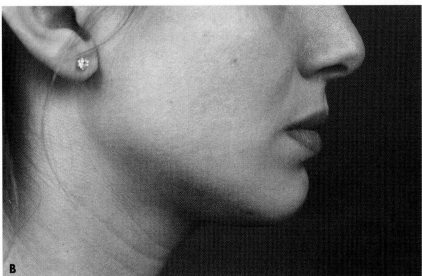

Figure 3–8. Lower face. **(A)** Frontal. Lower face view should include the nasal tip, earlobes, and some space between the outline of the chin and the edge of the photograph. **(B)** Profile. This view clearly visualizes the line of the mandible and must include the earlobe, neck, and nasal tip.

of the neck is easy to depict with the imaging process. Before this, patients requesting a primary procedure were often skeptical about the suggestion of a second or third cosmetic procedure that they had not fully visualized in their minds eye.

When using a computer imaging system, it is not enough to simply say that any adjusted image is a hoped-for result and not guaranteed. Any unrealistic postoperative change should never be depicted because this image will stay with the patient regardless of any warning or disclaimer and can lead to eventual unhappiness and confrontation. Most systems have disclaimers in the software package that display on the screen that a projected image may vary in actual result.

The decision to invest in a computer-assisted imaging system is more complex than that for standard photography. First, any high-quality system will cost between $25,000 and $45,000. Second, as with the computer industry in general, hardware is continually evolving, making it more difficult to buy one system for the long run. Third, software is very complex, has a potential for break down, and needs to be periodically upgraded. All this means that from who and where your equipment is purchased is very important.

HARDWARE

The basic hardware should include (1) Central processing unit (CPU) of 166 Mhz or more (dual CPU's are better); (2) 32 MB RAM (64 MB RAM is better); (3) 2 GB hard disk or larger; (4) dual floppy drives; (5) super VGA card; (6) Windows NT drive system; (7) 17-inch monitor with 0.27 mm dot pitch or less, and a high refresh rate to eliminate visual flicker; (8) Hi 8 camcorder; (9) tripod, wallmount, or other camera stabilizing system; (10) drawing tablet with cordless pen; (11) modem; (12) CD ROM drive; (13) imaging software; (14) constructive and training; and (15) professional video board with a minimum of 16 MB RAM.

The CPU determines the basic speed at which your software will run. CPUs are rapidly evolving in power and speed. Most software systems will run well on a single 166 MHz CPU. Dual processors and those higher than 166 MHz will usually run the software faster and more reliably.

All monitors should be at least 17 inches in size, with a low dot pitch of less than 0.27 mm. This will result in a large and very sharp image. A high refresh rate reduces screen flicker and eases viewing.

A high-quality video camera mounted securely to a swing arm or tripod is absolutely necessary. As with all photography systems, the visual image quality is determined by the weakest link in the system. If the camera cannot produce a high-quality image under available lighting conditions, the quality of the rest of the equipment cannot be brought into play. I recommend using a professional grade Hi 8 video camera in spite of the added expense. High-quality digital still cameras and video cameras may be interfaced with the computer and software removing the need for a camcorder.

Systems that run professional graphics or video imaging software need high-end video boards with at least 16 MB of VRAM or DRAM. The board should also support S-Video.

SOFTWARE

The imaging software is the heart of the package; it is what separates one company from another and what determines the imaging ability. Software should be reliable, user-friendly, and have the ability to perform all the imaging chores the practice requires. It is highly recommended that the software from a number of different suppliers be sampled before choosing any particular unit. It is also important that a company offer software upgrades on a reliable basis and at a reasonable price. If upgrades to both the software and hardware are not made available, the equipment can become rapidly obsolete.

MISCELLANEOUS

Instruction and training should be available from any reputable company so that prior computer expertise need not be necessary to get a system up and running in the office.

I recommend that computer-assisted imagery never be done by anyone other than the surgeon who will be performing the actual procedure. It is unconscionable that anyone not fully qualified to perform the actual surgery or who will not be performing the actual surgery should assist in designing it.

Some systems have video print machines that can produce a photograph of the preoperative and projected postoperative results for the patient. I do not use one in my office. Despite frank discussions about not guaranteeing results, patients will come back and complain if the actual results do not look like the computer-projected postoperative picture.

As in the discussion of standard office photography, principles of integrity, accuracy, and standardization must be applied to computer-assisted visual imagery.

CONCLUSIONS

A facial plastic surgeon who desires to use photography in either the office setting or in a clinical and scientific forum must apply the strictest principles of integrity, accuracy, and standardization. Any variations in the parameters of lighting, patient position, or lenses, or the addition of artificially enhancing elements such as makeup, will produce preoperative and postoperative photographs that are unacceptable to both patients and colleagues. Reviewers and audiences at scientific conferences will consider such photographic misrepresentation as a lack of professional integrity or incompetence. The inability of a trained facial plastic surgeon to obtain these standards is not acceptable. The inability to produce accurate documentation for the medical record is not only unacceptable but leaves a physician much more vulnerable in a malpractice claim.

High-quality, standardized and accurate patient photography will provide a great service to both the surgeon and the patient. It will also be a superb addition to the overall professionalism of an office and present the opportunity to show work in a highly scientific fashion to both colleagues and other professionals.

PEARLS

- It is essential that the surgeon removing skin lesions have a high-quality lens that allows close-up photography to accurately document the pathologic lesions.
- Maintaining an honest representation of the patient's hairline is important for documentation, especially in patients undergoing otoplasty. Therefore all views taken for such patients should include the hairline.
- Because many patients find it unnatural to look directly into the camera, it is imperative that the surgeon take care to properly position the patient for frontal views.

SUGGESTED READINGS

Buck G. *Contributions to Reparative Surgery: Showing Its Applications to the Treatment of Deformities Produced by Destructive Disease or Injury; Congenital Defects from Arrest or Excess of Development; and Cicatricial Contractions from Burns.* New York: D. Appleton; 1876.

Chapple JC, Stephenson KL. Photographic misrepresentation. *Plast Reconstr Surg.* 1970; 45:135.

Clinical Photography in Plastic Surgery. Arlington Heights, Ill.: American Society of Plastic and Reconstructive Surgeons, Inc.; 1995.

DiBernardo BE. Standardized photographs in aesthetic surgery [letter]. *Plast Reconstr Surg.* 1991; 88:373.

DiBernardo BE, Gianpapa VC. Standardized Hair Photography. In: Unger WP, ed., *Hair Transplantation,* 3rd ed. Toronto, Ontario, Canada: Marcel Dekker; 1995:70.

Dickason WL, Hanna DC. Pitfalls of comparative photography in plastic and reconstructive surgery. *Plast Reconstr Surg.* 1976; 58:166.

Duguid K, Ollerenshaw R. Standardization in records of the foot. *Med Biol Illustr.* 1962; 12:241.

Ellenbogen R, Jankauskas S, Collini FJ. Achieving standardized photographs in aesthetic surgery. *Plast Reconstr Surg.* 1990; 86:955.

Flowers RS, Flowers SS. Diagnosing photographic distortion: Decoding true postoperative contour after eyelid surgery. *Clin Plast Surg.* 1993; 20:387.

Gilson C, Parbhoo S. Standardized serial photography in the assessment of treatment of advanced breast cancer. *J Audiovis Media Med.* 1981; 4:5.

Gunter JP. A graphic record of intraoperative maneuvers in rhinoplasty: The missing link for evaluating rhinoplasty results. *Plast Reconstr Surg.* 1989; 84:204.

Hallock GG. Multipurpose background for standardization in medical photography. *Ann Plast Surg.* 1985; 15:177.

Jemec BIF, Jemec GBF. Suggestions for standardized clinical photography in plastic surgery. *J Audiovis Media Med.* 1981; 4:99.

Jemec BIF, Jemec GBF. Photographic surgery: Standards in clinical photography. *Aesthetic Plast Surg.* 1986; 10:177.

Karlan MS. Contour analysis in plastic and reconstructive surgery. *Arch Otolaryngol.* 1979; 105:670.

Kirwan L. Photographing patients for liposuction [letter]. *Plast Reconstr Surg.* 1995; 95:942.

Lockwood T. Lower body lift with superficial fascial system suspension. *Plast Reconstr Surg.* 1993; 92:1112.

Loughry CW, Sheffer DB, Price TE, Jr. et al. Breast volume measurement of 248 women using biostereometric analysis. *Plast Reconstr Surg.* 1987; 80:553.

Marshall RJ, Marshall BM. Routine medical photography with 35 mm black and white film. *Med Biol Illustr.* 1975; 25:115.

Matarasso A. The anatomic data sheet in plastic surgery: Graphic and accurate documentation for standardized evaluation of results. *Plast Reconstr Surg.* 1993; 91:734.

McCausland T. A method of standardization of photographic viewpoints for clinical photography. *J Audiovis Media Med.* 1980; 3:109.

McDowell F. On the necessity of precision photographic documentation in plastic surgery. *Plast Reconstr Surg.* 1976; 58:214.

Mladick RA. Sequential compression devices for postoperative lipoplasty of the calves and ankles [letter]. *Plast Reconstr Surg.* 1991; 87:585.

Mladick RA. Circumferential "intermediate" lipoplasty of the legs. *Aesthetic Plast Surg.* 1994; 18:165.

Morello DC, Converse JM, Allen D. Making uniform photographic records in plastic surgery. *Plast Reconstr Surg.* 1977; 59:366.

Photographic Standards in Plastic Surgery. Arlington Heights, Ill.: Plastic Surgery Educational Foundation, Clinical Photography Committee; 1991.

Pitman GH, Grazer FM, Lockwood T, et al. Liposuction: Problems and techniques. *Perspectives Plast Surg.* 1993; 7:73.

Rathjen AH. The Equipment: Film. In: *Clinical Photography in Plastic Surgery.* Arlington Heights, Ill.: American Society of Plastic and Reconstructive Surgeons, Inc.; 1995.

Rogers GW. Standard view in oral photographic practice. *Med Biol Illustr.* 1971; 21:134.

Rogers BO. The first pre- and post-operative photographs of plastic and reconstructive surgery: Contribution of Gurdon Buck (1807–1877). *Aesthetic Plast Surg.* 1991; 15:19.

Rogers BO, Rhode MG. The first Civil War photographs of soldiers with facial wounds. *Aesthetic Plast Surg.* 1995; 19:269.

Schwartz MS, Tardy ME. Standardized photodocumentation in facial plastic surgery. *Facial Plast Surg.* 1990; 7:1.

Stenstrom W. Guidelines for external eye photography. *J Biol Photogr Assoc.* 1978; 46:155.

Vetter J. Standardization for the biomedical photographic department. *J Biol Photogr.* 1979; 47:3.

Vetter JP. *Biomedical Photography.* Stoneham, Mass.: Butterworth-Heinemann; 1992.

Wallace AF. The early history of clinical photography for burns, plastic and reconstructive surgery. *Br J Plast Surg.* 1985; 38:451.

Zarem HA. Standards of photography. *Plast Reconstr Surg.* 1984; 74:137.

Zarem HA. Standards of medical photography. In: *Clinical Photography in Plastic Surgery.* Arlington Heights, Ill.: American Society of Plastic and Reconstructive Surgeons, Inc.; 1995.

Imagine

Aesthetic Facial Plastic Surgery, edited by Thomas Romo, III, and Arthur L. Millman, Thieme Medical Publishers, Inc., New York, New York, Copyright © 2000.

CHAPTER 4

Computer Imaging Documentation

THOMAS ROMO, III AND ARTHUR L. MILLMAN

Computer imaging is a recent advent of the personal computer revolution. Desktop computers and "morphing" software have allowed the cosmetic surgeon to use a digital video capture camera to input digital images into a desktop computer and then manipulate those images to demonstrate cosmetic surgical techniques to any area of the body, specifically, the face. As with any technique, be it surgical or photographic, accuracy and consistency of technique and meticulousness are the key to successful use.

The first goal in computer imaging is to use it as a tool for proper pre-surgical consultation with a patient. Computer imaging enables the surgeon to use a two-dimensional image rather than verbal description to discuss three-dimensional concepts. As the old proverb goes "a picture is worth a thousand words." This goal, therefore, is aimed at creating a realistic postoperative image, not an unrealistic or self-unfulfilling prophecy. It should absolutely not be used as a "sales tool." This can only lead to both patient and surgeon dissatisfaction. For that reason, the surgeon should personally review all imaging done in the office and make sure that it accurately represents what is intended to be done and what is possible in the surgical process. A careful explanation to the patient that the image is a forecast and by no means a definition of future reality is imperative.

Asian eye. I find it particularly useful in Asian patients because the concept of Westernization versus maintenance of an Asian crease is critical to patient satisfaction, and this can best be demonstrated by allowing the patient to draw in their own crease on the computer screen. We have found that this is the most reliable method for accomplishing the surgical goal. In addition, it allows discussion of certain difficult-to-treat areas such as malar festoons, brow ptosis, eyelid ptosis, and other critical points of blepharoplasty (Figs. 4–1 and 4–2).

In upper facial evaluation, as already eluded to in the previous paragraph, the need to identify patients who require blepharoplasty versus brow lifting or both can sometimes best be explained to the patient (the pros and cons of each procedure and their combination) by showing intended results with and without blepharoplasty and brow lifting (see Figs. 4–1 and 4–2).

BLEPHAROPLASTY

In blepharoplasty the goal is to discuss specific points of interest, including where herniated orbital fat will be removed, amount of excess skin or dermatochalasia to be removed from the upper lid and, most importantly, identification of the upper eyelid crease and where the eyelid crease should be postoperatively. This is imperative in both Western or Caucasian eyes and in the Eastern or

RHINOPLASTY

Computer imaging allows rhinoplasty patients to see themselves with subtle to dramatic changes of the nasal contour in the frontal and side views. This is an important step in the preoperative rhinoplasty assessment because it allows the surgeon and the patient to come to some agreement on the amount of nasal profile thinning, dorsal hump reduction, and nasal tip rotation that can be achieved.

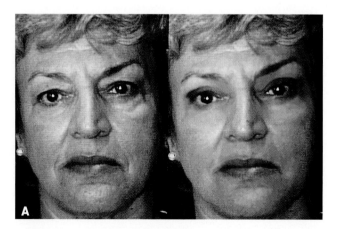
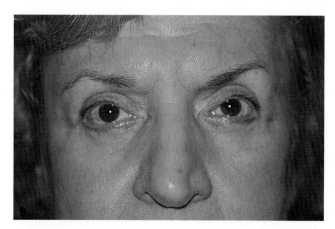

Figure 4–1. (A) Preoperative (*left screen*) and projected postoperative (*right screen*) computer captures. Pertinent findings include brow ptosis, malar festoon, and placement of upper lid creases. **(B)** Actual postoperative result after upper lid blepharoplasty and laser resurfacing to lower lid and festoon.

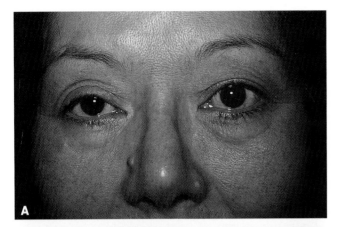

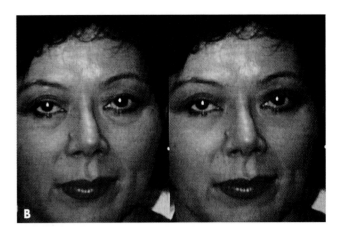

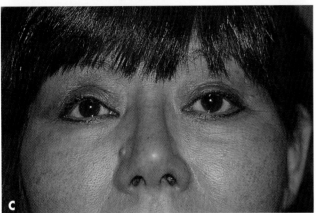

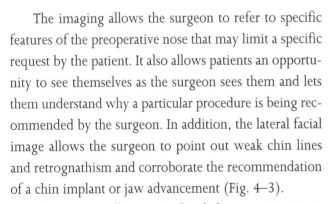

Figure 4–2. (A) Preoperative view of Asian patient who had upper lid blepharoplasty that resulted in asymmetric crease and lid level. **(B)** Computer capture of preoperative (*left screen*) and projected postoperative results (*right screen*) of upper lid blepharoplasty revision and lower lid ptosis and crease repair. **(C)** Actual postoperative result shows successful upper lid blepharoplasty with lower lid ptosis and upper lid crease fixation with levator supratarsal fixation.

The imaging allows the surgeon to refer to specific features of the preoperative nose that may limit a specific request by the patient. It also allows patients an opportunity to see themselves as the surgeon sees them and lets them understand why a particular procedure is being recommended by the surgeon. In addition, the lateral facial image allows the surgeon to point out weak chin lines and retrognathism and corroborate the recommendation of a chin implant or jaw advancement (Fig. 4–3).

Once an overall image is decided on, most patients experience a reduction in anxiety concerning their postoperative rhinoplasty result.

OTHER PROCEDURES

For surgical procedures for the aging face, computer imaging allows the surgeon to show the amount of improvement that may occur in the ptotic neck and lower face and limitations on improving effacement of the upper nasolabial folds. Midface ptosis can also be presented to the preoperative patient (Fig. 4–4).

The newer computer imaging software packages also can demonstrate subtle changes from facial rejuvenation techniques such as fillers into the nasolabial folds and marionette lines, lip augmentation, and rhytid elimination with laser resurfacing.

CONCLUSIONS

The bottom line in using computer imaging in preoperative assessment is to improve communication about what the patient desires as a possible postoperative facial aesthetic surgery result.

SUGGESTED READING

Papel ID, Schoenrock LD. *Computer Imaging: Principles of Facial Plastic and Reconstructive Surgery.* St. Lousis: Mosby–Year Book; 1992.

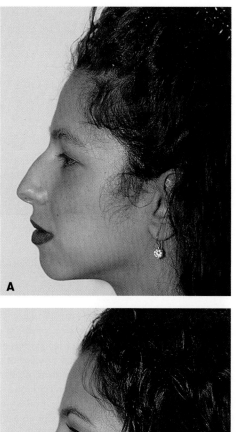

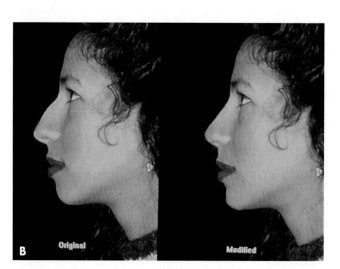

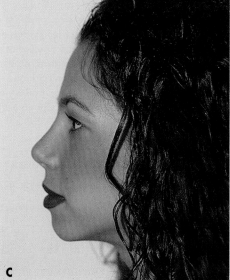

Figure 4–3. (A) Preoperative view of patient presenting for rhinoplasty. **(B)** Preoperative (*left screen*) and projected postoperative (*right screen*) computer capture. **(C)** Actual postoperative result.

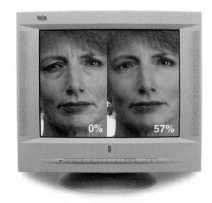

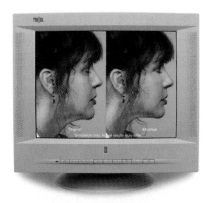

Figure 4–4. (A) Preoperative (*left screen*) and projected postoperative (*right screen*) computer captures of a patient presenting for facelift. **(B)** Preoperative (*left screen*) and projected postoperative (*right screen*) computer captures of a patient presenting for facelift and blepharoplasty.

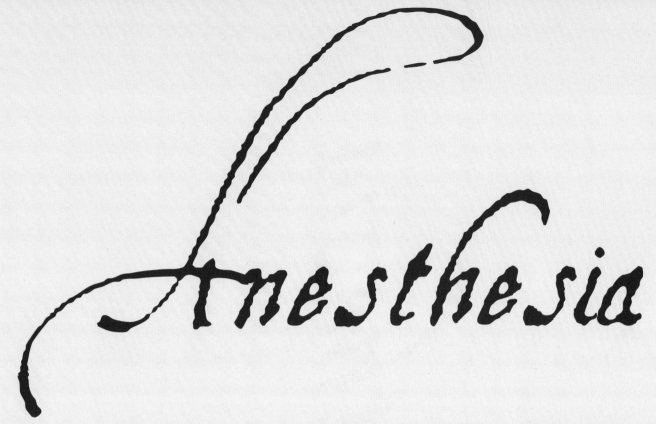

Anesthesia

This interesting section is written by two prominent anesthesiologists, Dr. Opperman and Dr. Scolnick. Both surgeons work closely with the editors, however, in two distinct environments. Dr. Opperman is a hospital-based physician, who specializes in elective anesthetic surgical services, and Dr. Scolnick is an office-based anesthesiologist, who also specializes in elective anesthetic surgical services.

A review of their chapters brings forth peculiarities in technical details needed to adapt to the different surgical environments: the modern, institutional-based operating room expertise and the private office. Dr. Opperman's chapter provides many technical considerations for preoperative medical clearance, evaluation of medical status, and avoidance of medical contraindications to the administration of anesthesia for cosmetic patients. It is interesting that these are, of course, very much the focus in hospital settings, rather than what might be considered the softer side of anesthesia. This softer, interpersonal component of patient anxiety reduction, hand holding, and verbal communication with operating room staff and anesthesiologist at all times, in addition to technical considerations, are stressed by Dr. Scolnick. Although excellent care can be delivered in either modality, sometimes a surgeon's ability to control the environment of his private operating room and office allows for more individualized care of the emotional and psychological needs, as well as the technical and medical needs of the aesthetic patient.

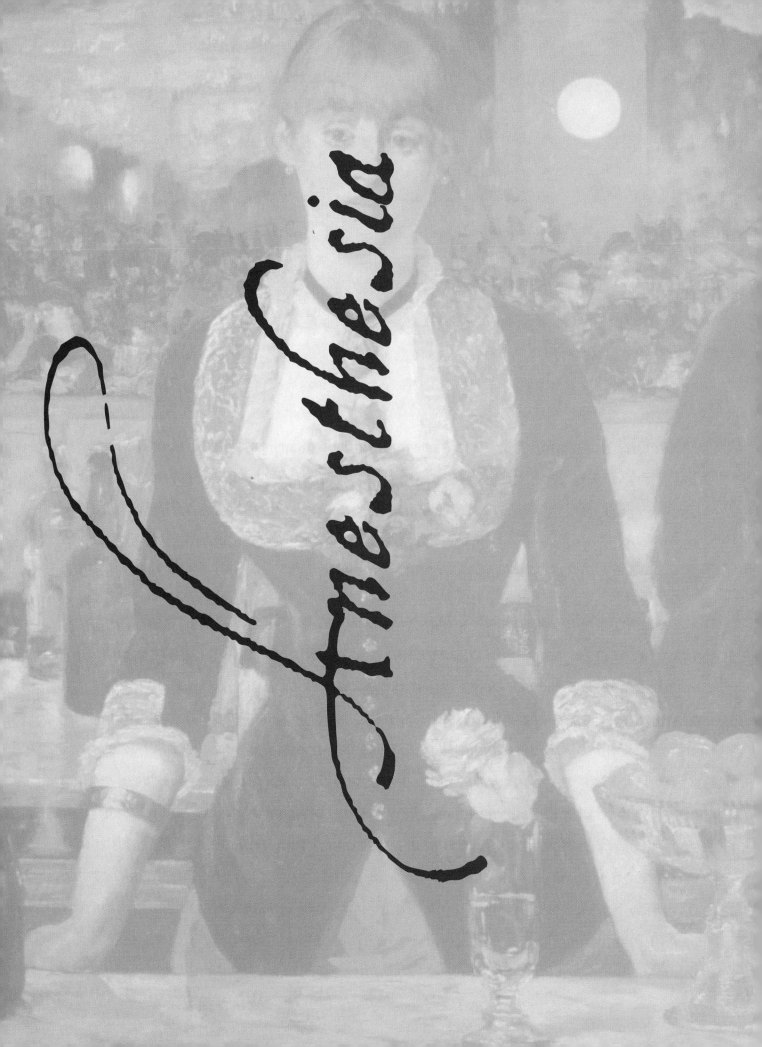

Anesthesia

Aesthetic Facial Plastic Surgery, edited by Thomas Romo, III, and Arthur L. Millman, Thieme Medical Publishers, Inc., New York, New York, Copyright © 2000.

CHAPTER 5

Hospital-based Approach

SHELDON OPPERMAN

Over the past 20 years, a dramatic shift in patient care has taken place from the inpatient setting for surgical procedures to the ambulatory or outpatient facility. This is the result of the importance of providing cost-effective care. Approximately 60% of surgical cases in 1996 were outpatient procedures. This has allowed a reduction in the cost of surgical care and a decrease in long waiting lists for surgical procedures in many fields, including the field of facial plastic surgery. This shift to ambulatory procedures, whereby the patient is discharged home or to a recovery facility on the same day as the surgery, has been achieved by the development of minimally invasive surgical techniques and newer and safer anesthetic drugs with minimal side effects. Although the focus of this chapter is geared to the ambulatory patient, most of the guidelines presented here can be extended to all patients presenting for facial plastic surgery.

PATIENT SELECTION

Successful outpatient surgery depends on patient selection. Therefore it is of the utmost importance that a reliable and accurate method is in place for the preoperative assessment of outpatients. The traditional preoperative visit by the anesthesiologist on the night before surgery is usually not done for this type of surgery. Therefore reducing patient anxiety and conducting a proper medical evaluation of the surgical patient has become more of a challenge.

It is not in the interest of the surgeon, anesthesiologist, or patient to cancel surgery at the last minute. Many ways of properly evaluating the patient preoperatively exist, including a call by the anesthesiologist the night before surgery. In this way the anesthesiologist can adequately assess the patient's medical condition and discuss the appropriate anesthetic expectations for the surgery. This would include explanations of preoperative, intraoperative, and postoperative procedures.

In general, the patient should have no medical condition that has not been evaluated or addressed. The American Society of Anesthesiologists (ASA) has defined a classification of physical status (Table 5–1). Outpatients should be ASA status I or II. Considerations can be given to physical status III or IV if the disease process is under control.

Table 5–1 ASA Physical Status Classification

ASA Class	Description
I	No organic disease
II	Mild or moderate systemic disease without functional impairment
III	Organic disease with definite functional impairment
IV	Severe disease that is life-threatening
V	Moribund patient, not expected to survive

SPECIFIC CONSIDERATIONS FOR THE PREOPERATIVE ASSESSMENT

A preanesthetic assessment of all patients is a requirement of the ASA (Table 5–2). This standard ensures that an anesthesiologist is responsible for the review of all pertinent information regarding the patient and for the determination that the candidate is ready to undergo the proposed anesthesia and surgery. In some of the following instances, it is best that a procedure is performed on an inpatient basis.

Table 5–2 Basic Standards for Preanesthesia Care
(American Society of Anesthesiologists)

These standards apply to all patients who receive anesthesia or monitored anesthesia care. Under unusual circumstances (e.g, extreme emergencies), these standards may be modified. When this is the case, the circumstances shall be documented in the patient's record.

Standard I: An anesthesiologist shall be responsible for determining the medical status of the patient, developing a plan of anesthesia care, and acquainting the patient or the responsible adult with the proposed plan.

The development of an appropriate plan of anesthesia care is based upon

1. Reviewing the medical record
2. Interviewing and examining the patient to
   a. Discuss the medical history, previous anesthetic experiences, and drug therapy
   b. Assess those aspects of the physical condition that might affect decisions regarding perioperative risk and management
3. Obtaining and/or reviewing tests and consultations necessary to the conduct of anesthesia
4. Determining the appropriate prescription of preoperative medications as necessary to the conduct of anesthesia

The responsible anesthesiologist shall verify that the above has been properly performed and documented in the patient's record.

From American Society of Anesthesiologists. Approved by House of Delegates on October 14, 1987, with permission.

1. In general, age should not be a consideration; there should be no upper age limit as long as the patient's medical condition is optimal for surgery. However, specific pediatric problems may best be dealt with if the child is an inpatient.

2. If the proposed surgery may cause significant blood loss, consideration must be given to inpatient rather than outpatient surgery.

3. If severe postoperative pain is anticipated, inpatient surgery would best suit the needs of the patient.

4. The duration of surgery should not be considered a contraindication to outpatient surgery. However, proper and adequate staffing considerations must be considered.

5. If the patient requires special monitoring intraoperatively because of pre-existing disease, the hospital setting would be more appropriate.

LABORATORY TESTING

Although in the past preanesthetic testing involved routine blood and urine testing, electrocardiogram (ECG) and chest radiograph, this is no longer the case. The ASA recommends that no routine screening tests be done for the preanesthetic evaluation. Instead, specific indicators relevant to each patient should guide laboratory test: A test should be ordered if the result of the test might alter the anesthetic management of the patient.

However, practice groups might adopt some guidelines. Some consideration for hemoglobin testing might be indicated for instance in all menstruating women, as would pregnancy testing if this could not be ruled out by history. Routine ECG testing might be considered for all men older than 45 and for women older than 55. It is important that laboratory testing is patient guided and is performed on the basis of a test's potential usefulness to the anesthesiologist.

PRE-EXISTING DISEASE

A large study of more than 13,000 outpatients showed that the incidence of complications in patients with pre-existing disease was the same as a healthy population undergoing the same procedures. What is most important

is that all pre-existing disease processes be optimally controlled before surgery.

Circulatory System

Hypertension

Hypertension is defined as a blood pressure greater than 160 mm Hg systolic and/or 95 mm Hg diastolic. The major organ systems that are at risk in the hypertensive patient are the heart, brain, and kidneys. Most authorities would agree that for elective procedures the blood pressure should be controlled preoperatively to achieve pressures less than 195 mm Hg systolic and/or 110 mm Hg diastolic.

Coronary artery disease

Although still controversial, most would agree that patients with preoperative untreated myocardial ischemia are at increased risk for postoperative cardiac complications. It also has been shown that patients who had recent (less than 6 months before the current surgical procedure) myocardial infarcts are at increased risk for reinfarction postoperatively. After 6 months, the reinfarction rate drops significantly. Therefore it is prudent to wait at least 6 months after a myocardial infarction before planning elective surgery.

Respiratory System

Brochospastic disease

The patient with well-controlled brochospastic disease should present little problem for elective surgery. Continuation of all medications and administration of steroids perioperatively for the steroid-dependent patient is important.

Upper respiratory infections

Upper respiratory infections (URIs) are common and much controversy exists as to whether surgery should be postponed in patients who have an URI. Even after resolution of symptoms, the airway remains reactive for several weeks. Most authorities would agree that procedures that do not require tracheal intubation might be tolerated in a patient whose respiratory symptoms are resolving.

Endocrine Disease

Diabetes mellitus

Diabetic patients whose disease is well controlled should have little problem tolerating anesthesia and surgery. The anesthesiologist must monitor perioperative glucose levels. Preoperative considerations of insulin use must be addressed and adjusted accordingly.

Thyroid disorders

Most patients with thyroid disorders are well controlled with medication. As long as the euthyroid state has been achieved these patient should be at no greater risk.

PATIENT PREPARATION

Optimal patient preparation should allay patient anxiety with both medication and nonpharmacologic means. Some of the more common concerns of patients scheduled for surgery deal more with the anesthesia than the actual surgical procedure. Postoperative pain, awareness under anesthesia, side effects including nausea and vomiting, and oversedation are some of the most common patient fears.

It is the responsibility of the anesthesiologist to deal with these concerns. Talking to the patient preoperatively to explain the entire perioperative experience is one of the most important means in helping patients deal with the stress of surgery. Short-acting benzodiazepines, including 1 to 2 mg of midazolam IV in the preinduction period can alleviate anxiety, can cause sedation and amnesia, may be given without delaying patient discharge from the recovery room.

NPO ORDERS

The once strict NPO after midnight order for all surgical procedures in children and adults has been modified because of many studies that have shown this to be unnecessary. It has been shown that the patient may take clear liquids up to 2 hours before surgery without increasing the gastric volume. It has been shown in other studies that allowing intake of clear fluids may even stimulate gastric secretions and empty the stomach more quickly. Allowing the patient to have clear fluids up to 2 hours preoperatively helps reduce anxiety and reduces thirst and hunger.

It is also important to communicate to the patient that medications usually taken can be taken with a sip of water up to 1 hour before surgery.

SUMMARY

Outpatient anesthesia has gained popularity in all fields of medicine. However, not all patients are candidates for outpatient procedures. Successful outpatient anesthesia depends on proper patient selection. The ASA's guidelines suggest that blood loss, severe postoperative pain, and the need for special monitoring may require that a procedure be performed in the hospital setting. Although age is not generally a consideration, pediatric patients may fare better in an inpatient setting. In addition, laboratory testing should be patient guided and take into consideration any pre-existing medical conditions. If a patient scheduled for outpatient surgery has a pre-existing disease, the surgical team must be certain that it is controlled. Finally, patients about to undergo surgery experience a great deal of stress. The anesthesiologist should talk with the patient about the procedure to allay any fears and, if necessary, provide a pharmacologic means of alleviating anxiety.

PEARLS

- A phone call on the evening before a planned procedure will serve to reduce patient anxiety and enable the anesthesiologist to assess the patient's medical condition.
- Pre-existing disease need not be a contraindication to outpatient surgery, but to decrease the chance for complications, it is imperative that the condition be controlled.
- A patient's fears of impeding surgery often center around the anesthesia. It is important that these fears are addressed before surgery to alleviate the patient's stress.

SUGGESTED READINGS

Longnecker, Tinker, Morgan. *Principles and Practice of Anesthesiology*. St. Louis: Mosby; 1998.

White PF. *Preoperative Evaluation of Ambulatory Patients*. ASA Refresher Courses in Anesthesiology; 1991.

White PF, Smith I. *Patient Selection and Anesthetic Techniques for Ambulatory Surgery*. ASA Refresher Courses in Anesthesiology; 1995.

White PF. *Ambulatory Anesthesia and Surgery*. Philadelphia: WB Saunders; 1997.

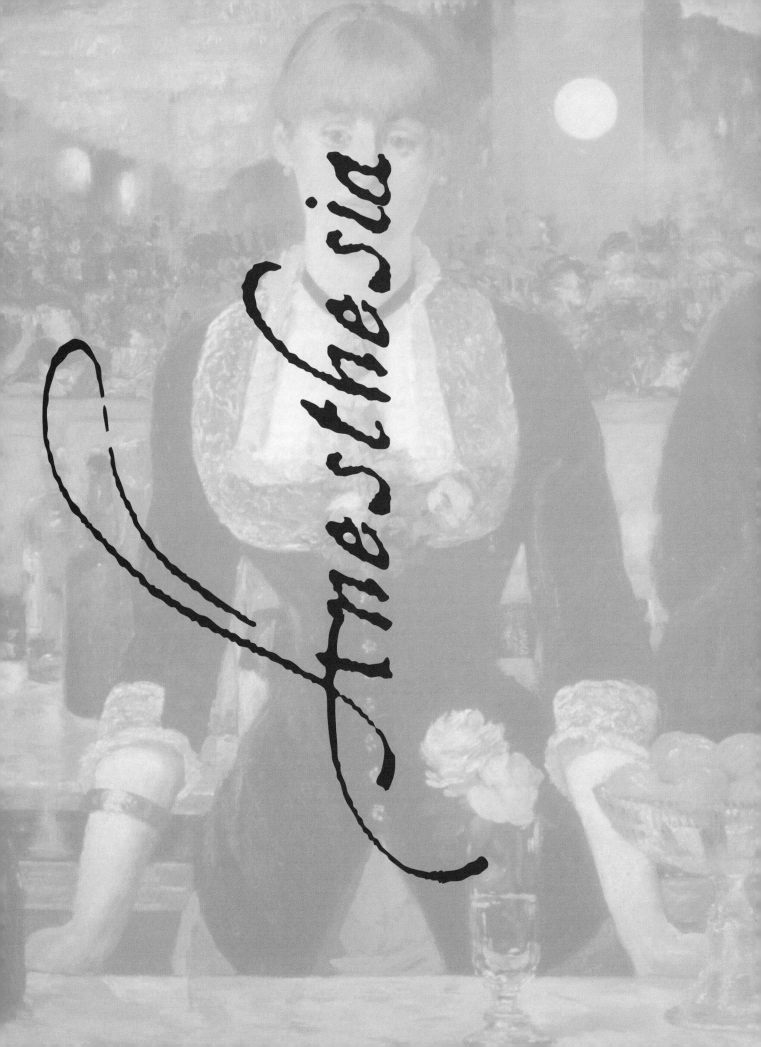

Aesthetic Facial Plastic Surgery, edited by Thomas Romo, III, and Arthur L. Millman, Thieme Medical Publishers, Inc., New York, New York, Copyright © 2000.

CHAPTER 6

Office-based Approach

ROBERT M. SCOLNICK

In the past few years we have witnessed enormous improvements in anesthetic agents and in patient monitoring, which have resulted in a more rapid recovery with fewer side effects delivered with a greater margin of safety. Whether a general anesthetic or local anesthetic with sedation is administered, a plan of action must be previously determined by the surgeon, anesthesiologist, and patient. The anesthetic technique chosen should have the following criteria: rapid induction, anesthetic maintenance with minimal physiologic change, and rapid emergence with quick recovery and discharge.

MONITORING

Patient safety and comfort are the primary concerns of the anesthesiologist during all phases of the intraoperative and postoperative periods. It is imperative that the patient be monitored according to American Society of Anesthesia standards, which include noninvasive blood pressure, ECG, pulse oximetry, and, when applicable, temperature and end tidal CO_2.

Constant clinical assessment is vital to endure a safe outcome and be alerted to signs of airway obstruction, hyperventilation, or regurgitation. Unfortunately, changes in vital signs occur late in the chain of events. Often, hypoxia can be avoided with the use of supplemental oxygen. The use of an oral or nasal airway may keep the airway patient avoiding either a partial or total airway obstruction. If airway obstruction is present change of head position is required. If this does not suffice a jaw thrust to lift the tongue off the palate should be attempted. Manual ventilation will be necessary if previous methods fail. Finally, if the airway is comprimised the insertion of an LMA or endotracheal intubation must be performed.

A precordial stethoscope is a simple device that should be used to assess heart and lung sounds. The ECG is used for the detection of dysrhythmias and left ventricular ischemia, which will be manifested by ST-T segment changes.

Temperature monitoring is important for the detection of malignant hypothermia (MH). MH is a rare complication of general anesthesia and is usually triggered by succinylcholine and volatile anesthetic gasses, which result in muscle rigidity, tachycardia, increased end tidal CO_2, increased blood pressure, and increased body temperature, which is reflective of a hypermetabolic state. If general anesthesia is being administered, an MH protocol should be on hand and dantrolene available to initiate therapy.

Heat loss during surgery is quite common and is caused by cooled operating rooms and poorly insulated patients. During anesthesia the patient produces less heat, resulting in decreased body core temperature. Simple methods such as heating IV solutions and placing a heating blanket or heating device over the patient can prove beneficial. Hypothermia is manifested by shivering, which not only can cause discomfort to the patient but can elevate blood pressure and increase oxygen consumption. Finally, emergency medication must be available, as should resuscitative equipment including an AMBU-bag and oxygen.

ANESTHESIA
GENERAL ANESTHESIA

General anesthesia with endotracheal intubation or laryngeal mask airway (LMA) can be used to maintain an airway, have a quiet surgical field, and reduce the risk of aspiration. Maintenance of anesthesia can be achieved with any potent inhalational agent (desflurane, sevflurane, isoflurane, enflurane) or with propofol and a narcotic. General anesthesia can cause a sore throat associated with intubation but has a superb track record of safety and efficacy.

Anesthetic techniques that use sedation have gained enormous popularity in recent years. Many patients will not endure the discomfort and awareness associated with local anesthesia and for this reason monitored anesthesia care is used. It furnishes patients with analgesia, anxiolysis, and amnesia, which are critical to a positive anesthetic experience.

The art of sedation is a balancing act between administering the proper amount of medication required for safety and comfort, and avoiding cardiorespiratory depression or prolonged emergence from anesthesia.

It is imperative that we realize that sedation represents a continuum and that vigilance must be paramount when we administer these potent medications. Conscious sedation is a term that implies a slightly altered state in which a patient can respond to verbal commands and maintain protective reflexes. Deep sedation can be produced when the patient is unresponsive or unarousable and may lose the protective reflexes and the patency of the airway. If the patient is determined suitable for sedation, medications should be titrated to achieve a satisfactory end point.

Tranquilizers

Diazepam is a benzodiazapine that produces sedation, anxiolysis, and amnesia shortly after injection. It usually is administered in 2.5-mg increments. Pain can be caused by venous irritation, so injections should be slow and hand veins avoided. Midazolam is much more potent than diazepam, has a much shorter duration of action, and produces no pain on injection. One to 2-mg increments are usually administered over 2 to 3 minutes. When either drug is used in concert with an opoid, barbituarate, or propofol, care must be taken because these medications act synergistically and can cause respiratory depression and hypoxia.

Propofol is a sedative hypnotic drug that has become popular because of its rapid clearance from the body, resulting in quick anesthetic emergence and discharge.

Serious mishaps during anesthesia can be averted by exercising diligence and careful monitoring when sedating patients. Administration of small titrated doses is preferable to large intermittent boluses. Cardiovascular and respiratory depression can occur during sedation, which may result in obtunded laryngeal and esophageal reflexes and hypoxia and hypercarbia.

LOCAL ANESTHESIA

Local anesthesia containing epinephrine is routinely used and has an extraordinary record of safety. Unfortunately, the physician can be lulled into complacency regarding these agents because they do possess systemic toxicities. Toxicity occurs when the rate of absorption is greater than the rate of degradation. This can be due either to excessive volume or concentration or both. It is important to know the particular toxic levels of the agents being used and the signs and symptoms of systemic toxicity. The observable signs of toxicity include drowsiness followed by light-headedness, numbness around the mouth, ringing in the ears, and blurred vision. If the symptoms intensify, the patient will appear confused and have slurred speech, nystagmus, and muscle tremors or twitches. Down this cascade, unconsciousness and seizures will become manifest. Ventilatory and circulatory collapse will ensue with resulting hypoxia, hypercarbia, hypertension, or hypotension.

Should the patient have a mild reaction oxygen given by face mask should be initiated. If frank convulsions occur, oxygen given by AMBU- bag and administration of diazepam, 5 to 15 mg IV, or thiopental, 50 to 100 mg IV may be required. Should cardiorespiratory collapse occur, IV access should be established and the patient supported with fluids and vasopressors. Local anesthetic solutions may contain adrenaline and can result in tachycardia and hypertension along with cardiac dysrhythmias so the physician should be prepared for complications in these cases.

RECOVERY ROOM

After the surgical procedure is completed, the patient is brought to the recovery room to allow the affects of the anesthesia to dissipate and allow the patient to return to normal function. Some of the postoperative problems faced in the recovery period include elevated blood pressure, hypotension, postsurgical pain, and nausea and vomiting.

Nausea and vomiting postoperatively are more prevalent in patients who are obese, are female, have a history of motion sickness or previous history of nausea and vomiting from anesthesia, or use narcotics, and have increased gastric volume. The type of surgery and amount of pain also may affect postoperative nausea and vomiting. A number of useful antiemetics are available (Table 6–1).

Table 6–1 Antiemetics

Generic Name	Trade Name	Dose	Route of Administration
Droperidol	Inapsine	0.6–1.2 mg	IV or IM
Perchlorperazine	Compazine	5–10 mg	IV or IM
Trimethobenzamide	Tigan	100–200 mg	IV, IM, or PR
Promethazine	Phenergan	25–50 mg	PO or PR
Hydroxyzine	Vistaril	25–50 mg	IV or IM
Diphenhydramine	Benadryl	10–50 mg	PO, IV
Odansetron	Zofran	2–4 mg	IV
		8–16mg	PO

ZOFRAN

Postsurgical pain must be treated promptly and a host of medications are presently available. These include opioids and nonsteroidal anti-inflammatory drugs (NSAIDs). Fentanyl and meperidine are the parenteral narcotics of choice. Minor oral analgesics such as codeine, propoxephene (Darvon), or NSAIDs can provide good postoperative pain relief.

DISCHARGE

The recovery room allows the day surgery patient to return to consciousness, regain protective reflexes, take in fluid, void, and regain psychomotor skills. Postanesthesia scoring systems allow us to evaluate patients so they can be discharged to their homes. The patient must have stable vital signs for 1 hour with no evidence of respiratory depression. They must be oriented to person, place, and time; coordinated enough to dress themselves, and be able to walk out. The patient should also have minimal physical discomfort, relatively clean surgical sites, and a minimal amount of nausea.

Patients are expected to be escorted home by a responsible adult, and a postoperative call should be made by the office to ascertain their condition. Patients find this reassuring, and if any problems exist, they can be addressed immediately. Patients are advised to recuperate at home, not to drive or drink alcohol, and not make any important decisions.

Day surgery has enjoyed enormous popularity from the public because it delivers high-quality care in a cost-effective fashion.

SUMMARY

Whether anesthesia is general or local, its induction must be rapid, it must be maintained with as little physiologic change as possible, and emergence to recovery and discharge must be quick. Whether the surgery is performed in a hospital, free-standing surgical facility, or private office, the monitoring standard includes blood pressure, ECG, pulse oximetry, and, when applicable, capnography and temperature.

General anesthesia with endotracheal intubation or LMA is a proven method of anesthesia administration.

The use of monitored anesthesia care further reduces any discomfort. Although local anesthesia has proven to be effective, especially for outpatient procedures, these anesthetic agents can produce systemic toxicities. As with general anesthesia procedures, emergency medications and resuscitative equipment must remain on hand in the event that systemic toxicity occurs. Nausea and vomiting is the most common postoperative concern in the recovery room and usually can be controlled with antiemetics. Patients undergoing day-surgery procedures are released only when they meet specific discharge criteria.

PEARLS

- The art of sedation is a balancing act between administering the proper amount of medication required for safety and comfort and avoiding cardiorespiratory depression or prolonged emergence from medication.
- Constant vigilance is imperative to ensure that vital signs remain stable throughout the anesthetic course.
- It is preferable to administer small, titrated doses than to administer large intermittent boluses. Administering large boluses can lead to cardiovascular and respiratory depression.
- Although local anesthesia with epinephrine has been proven safe, the anesthesiologist must watch for signs of toxicity. The operating room should be equipped with all necessary emergency medications and resuscitative equipment in the event of such an untoward reaction

SUGGESTED READINGS

Barash P, Cullen B, Stoelting R. *Clinical Anesthesia.* Philadelphia: Lippincott-Raven; 1990.

Wetchler B. *Anesthesia for Ambulatory Surgery.* 2nd ed., Philadelphia: Lippincott.

White P. *Outpatient Anesthesia.* N.Y., Edinburgh, London: Churchill Livingstone; 1990.

Whitham E. *Day Care Anesthesia.* London, Edinburgh: Blackwell Scientific; 1994.

Rhinoplasty

This section on aesthetic rhinoplasty features two internationally known leaders in the field with extensive experience and profound academic publications on this topic. Dr. Eugene Tardy, a facial plastic surgeon, initially emphasizes preoperative evaluation of the nasal form. He presents an elegant and thorough review of this topic, including inspection and palpation of the preoperative nasal anatomy to gain increased knowledge of the nasal architecture. This he states leads to proper diagnosis and a better postoperative result. The chapter has a thorough review of anesthetic techniques. Dr. Tardy emphasizes conservation of nasal tip surgery and the maintenance of tip supports. He thoroughly reviews the indications for different surgical techniques in approaching the nasal tip. The concept of finesse rhinoplasty is further illustrated by demonstrating minimally traumatic osteotomy techniques. Dr. Tardy is well known for his endonasal approach to nasal rhinoplasty and emphasizes the need to evaluate patients with long-term follow-up of between 5 and 10 years to gain a more accurate understanding of the postoperative result.

Dr. Rohrich, who is a plastic surgeon, thoroughly reviews his procedure for preoperative rhinoplasty analysis and surgical planning. He emphasizes that the external rhinoplasty approach allows for precise intraoperative analysis of traumatic and iatrogenic deformities and the subsequent accurate correction of these anomalies. This approach ensures a more consistent and superior result in rhinoplasty. The advantages and disadvantages of the open rhinoplasty approach are thoroughly reviewed.

Rhinoplasty

Aesthetic Facial Plastic Surgery, edited by Thomas Romo, III, and Arthur L. Millman, Thieme Medical Publishers, Inc., New York, New York, Copyright © 2000.

CHAPTER 7

A Facial Plastic Surgeon's Perspective

M. EUGENE TARDY, Jr.

Universal agreement exists that aesthetic rhinoplasty poses the most challenging and difficult of all facial plastic surgery procedures. The standard of excellence required and demanded is high and continues to rise with each decade.

The most capable surgeons find this procedure highly fulfilling but constantly vexing because tolerances of less than 1 mm can render the ultimate surgical outcome ideal or disappointing. The nasal plastic surgeon must learn not only how to control the operative event but also how to manipulate and control the dynamics of the postoperative healing process. Such skills do not come easily, but are accumulated over years of study and experience as the surgeon witnesses, analyzes, and modifies his or her surgical outcomes. Fortunately, teaching and learning rhinoplasty allow the surgeon to continue refining the technique.

The final result of any rhinoplasty is the consequence of the limitations of the individual patient's anatomy as much as the surgeon's skill. No two noses are ever quite alike; it follows then that no single, standard procedure suffices to reconstruct every nose perfectly. The ability to accurately diagnose the possibilities and limitations inherent in each patient is an absolute prerequisite to achieving consistently outstanding results while avoiding complications.

Patients with relatively minor deformities are almost always the best candidates for ideal surgical outcomes because less surgery (and therefore less trauma) is necessary for desired improvements.

This group of patients, however, expects and demands perfection because of the minimal nature of the problem. In patients whose deformity demonstrates a significant departure from the aesthetic ideal (a large hump, an elongated drooping nose, a twisted nose), more dramatic surgical results are possible. This latter group of patients may tolerate possible minor imperfections because the overall improvement is indeed a significant one. It is the fundamental responsibility of the surgeon to balance the wishes and desires of the patient with what is realistically possible given the anatomic limitations (or possibilities) inherent in each nose.

Misguided attempts to create more than the condition of the nasal tissues will allow (overoperating) inevitably leads to the all-too-frequent complications seen after overaggressive rhinoplasty.

Time-honored and contemporary principles and techniques that are recognized as effective and safe for rhinoplasty surgery are presented.

PATIENT SELECTION AND PREOPERATIVE EVALUATION

From the outset of the evaluation process, patient motivations and expectations and all surgical possibilities and limitations must be analyzed by developing an open and easy communication with the patient. If the surgical possibilities are limited by anatomic restrictions or the surgeon's understanding of the problem, rhinoplasty is probably best not undertaken.

The patient should be capable of pointing out, in a three-way mirror or on a medical photograph, *exactly* what is disliked or in need of surgical alteration. The surgeon must balance these wishes with what is surgically possible given the individual anatomic component characteristics of each nose.

Surgeons should develop an orderly and compulsive analytic evaluation of the nose and the surrounding facial feature proportions. An appreciation for facial "ideal normal" will provide the surgeon with a visual baseline from which to interpret the findings. Careful interpretation of the infinite variations in anatomy characterizes the experienced surgeon, progressively mentally planning during the physical and visual examination what can and cannot be reasonably accomplished. *Inspection and palpation* are the hallmarks of the nasal examination.

It is helpful to conceive of the nose as being composed of a series of interrelated *nasal anatomic components*, which include the covering epithelium, the bony pyramid (maxillary ascending process, nasal bones, and bony septum), the cartilaginous pyramid (the quadrangular cartilage and attached upper lateral cartilages), and the mobile nasal tip (paired alar cartilages and surrounding soft tissues) (Figs. 7–1 and 7–2). Topographic subunits within the nasal tip or base include the infratip lobule, the alar sidewalls, and the columella.

An essential indicator of the eventual surgical outcome is the quality and thickness of the skin-subcutaneous complex; it plays a significant role in preoperative planning. Extremely thick skin, rich in sebaceous glands and subcutaneous tissue, is the least ideal skin for achieving desirable refinement and definition. Although ideal for achieving critical definition, thin skin with sparse subcutaneous tissue provides almost no cushion to hide even the most minute of skeletal irregularities or contour imperfections and therefore demands near-perfect surgery to achieve the desired natural result. The ideal skin type falls somewhere between these two extremes, being neither too thick and oily nor too thin and delicate. Evaluation of skin type is made by inspection and palpation—rolling the skin over the nasal skeleton and gently pinching it between the examining fingers to determine the skin-subcutaneous tissue complex thickness.

In each patient it is essential to evaluate the critical factors relating to the inherent *strength and support* of the nasal tip, referred to as the *tip recoil*. Finger depression of the tip toward the upper lip provides a quick and reliable

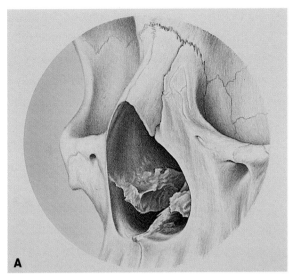
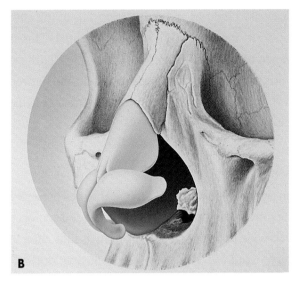

Figure 7–1. (A) The bony vault of the nose, including the paired nasal bones and ascending processes of the maxilla. **(B)** The cartilaginous vault of the nose is securely affixed to the undersurface of the nasal bone and is comprised of the paired upper lateral cartilages and cartilaginous septum. The free-floating alar cartilages are mobile and, in the young, generally overlap the caudal margins of the upper lateral cartilages.

test of the ability of the mobile tip structures to spring back into position. The size, shape, attitude, symmetry, and resilience of the alar cartilages may be estimated also by palpation or "ballottement" of the lateral crus between two fingers surrounding its cephalic and caudal margins. During this assessment the surgeon makes the all-important

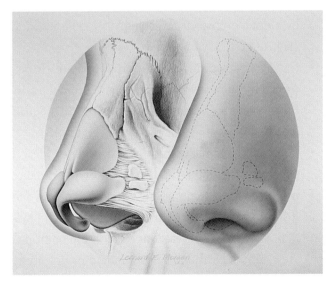

Figure 7–2. The subcutaneous structure of the nose is covered by the superficial musculoaponeurotic system (*SMAS*) of the nose in association with the overlying epithelium. The thickness of this overlying canopy essentially dictates the course of long-term healing, as the overlying skin envelope "shrink-wraps" around the altered nasal skeleton.

preoperative decision about the need to surgically *enhance, reduce, or carefully preserve* the tip projection.

The length of the nasal bones may be palpably determined with relative ease, along with the ratio of bony to cartilaginous hump. The external topography of the subcutaneous bony-nasal skeleton can be reliably mapped within tolerances of 1 to 2 mm for future surgical orientation.

Palpating the internal vestibules of the nose with the thumb and forefinger surrounding the columella detects twists and angulations of the nasal septum, and the width and length of the columella, and provides important information about the potential of the tip to undergo (or resist) desirable cephalic rotation.

This information is supplemented by careful examination of the nasal cavities before and after shrinkage of the mucosa and turbinates to determine subtle deflections of the nasal septum, mucosal abnormalities, the size and shape of the turbinates, and the condition of the internal nasal valves on quiet and forced inspiration.

Finally, the position and inclination of the nasofrontal and nasolabial angles, the shape and size of the alae, the overall width of the middle and upper thirds of the nose, and the relationship of the nose to the remainder of the facial features and landmarks are evaluated.

Facial asymmetries and the relationship of the chin projection to the nose should be documented. This is the time to make the patient aware of any and all limitations that the existent anatomy imposes on the desired surgical outcome; a three-way mirror enhances this understanding.

SURGICAL ANATOMY

Interpretation of the individual surgical anatomy possessed by each patient is essential to determine the ideal approach and technique to be used. Nasal anatomy is illustrated in Figures 7–1 and 7–2. Reduction, augmentation, or reorientation of the individual anatomic components of the nose will determine the outcome of each surgical procedure. *Conservative changes* devoted to balancing the size and proportional relationships of these components during nasal surgery invariably lead to superior results.

AESTHETIC CANONS OF PROPORTIONALITY

Balance and proportion combine to create the aesthetically pleasing face. Although no set of mechanical measurements may be used to define beauty, the rhinoplasty surgeon must possess the inner vision of the "ideal normal" when planning facial and nasal improvement (Fig. 7–3A):

- Vertically the frontal face approaches balance and harmony if equal fifths, sited at the junctions of known facial landmarks, exist.
- Horizontally the face may be conveniently divided into aesthetic thirds, bounded by the frontal hairline, glabella, subnasale, and menton.
- On lateral view the ideal nasal length is slightly less (43%) than the distance from the subnasale to menton (57%). The vertical length of the upper lip comprises only $\frac{1}{3}$ of the subnasale-menton distance.
- Symmetry of the four quadrants of the face characterizes the "ideal normal" but seldom perfectly exists in even the most attractive faces.

- On frontal view, ideal nasal contours are favorable if an imaginary unbroken line courses gracefully from the infrabrow region across the nasal root concavity into the lateral nasal dorsum, ultimately gently flaring to the end in the tip-defining points of the alar cartilages (Fig. 7–3B).
- The nasal tip appearance is ideally represented by four key landmarks characterized by three prominences (the bilateral tip defining points and the columellar-lobule junction), and upper midline site of the supratip break. The former three prominences may reflect light and therefore demonstrate symmetry (or lack thereof), whereas the latter reflects no light.
- An oblique view the same landmarks may be appreciated. The line flowing from the brow region along the nasal dorsum should ideally terminate in the right tip-defining point, imparting elegant projection to the nasal tip.
- An ideal nasal profile demonstrates a definite beginning at the nasofrontal angle, courses along a straight or slightly convex nasal dorsum, lifts forward or anterior 1 to 2 mm at the supratip break to encounter the well-projected nasal tip-defining point, then curves gently into the columella, characterized best by a double-break at the columella-lobule junction (Fig. 7–4).
- Nasal tips possessing elegant projection are characterized by ratios in which the distance from the alar-facial junction to the tip-defining point (CD) equals 0.55 and 0.60 of the nasal dorsum length (AB).
- Columellar-alar relationships are considered ideal if equal vertical lengths are occupied by the distance from the tip-defining points to the alar margin and from the alar margin to the columellar-lateral junction. Figure 7–4B reveals this relationship on frontal view, in which the infratip lobule dips gracefully only slightly below the alar margins ("gull in flight" appearance). Exaggerated convexity or "hanging" of the body of the gull imparts an unpleasant dependent infratip lobule to the nose.

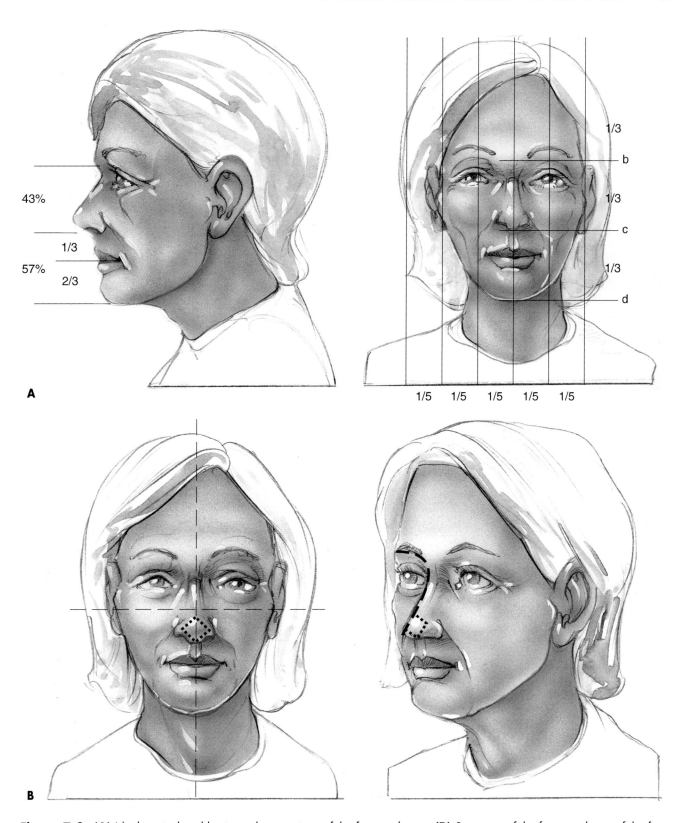

Figure 7–3. (A) Ideal vertical and horizontal proportions of the face and nose. **(B)** Symmetry of the four quadrants of the face characterizes the "ideal normal" but seldom perfectly exists in even the most attractive faces. On frontal and oblique views, an unbroken line (the brow-tip aesthetic line) courses from the eyebrow medially along the radix and along the nasal dorsum to end at the tip-defining points.

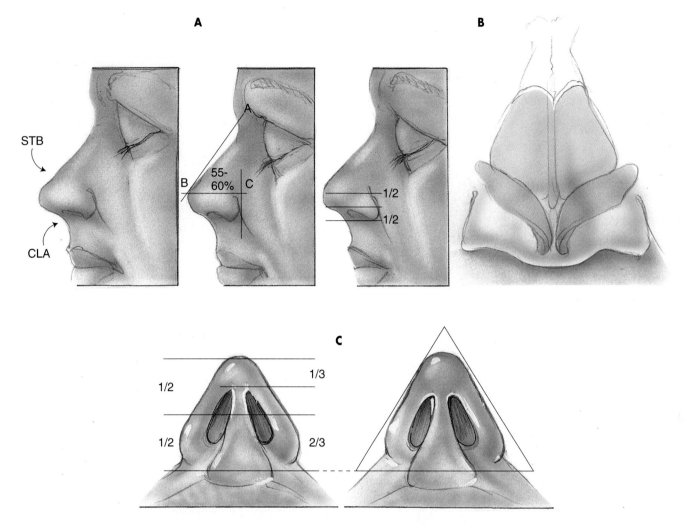

Figure 7–4. (A) Ideally, a supratip break (*STB*) characterizes the relationship of the nasal tip to the immediate supratip dorsum. The columellar-labial angle (*CLA*) should describe a gentle curve at the junction of the base of the columella and upper lip. Ideal nasal tip projection exists when the line B–C is 55% to 60% of line A–B (the length of the nasal dorsum). **(B)** Alar-columellar relationships are considered within normal limits if equal vertical lengths are occupied by the distance from the tip-defining points to the alar margin and from the alar margin to the columellar-labial junction. On frontal view, this appearance should approximate a gentle "gull-in-flight" appearance. **(C)** On base view the ideal nose reveals a lobule-columellar ratio of $\frac{1}{3}$ to $\frac{2}{3}$, and nasal base is essentially triangular.

• On basal view the ideal nose reveals a lobule-columella ratio of $\frac{1}{3}$ to $\frac{2}{3}$, and the nasal base is essentially triangular (Fig. 7–4C).

PHOTODOCUMENTATION

Standard and uniform color photographs (35-mm color transparency slides) of the rhinoplasty patient, recorded before and serially after the surgical event, constitute critical guides to operative planning and execution, definitive records for evaluation by the surgeon and patient, invaluable teaching tools, and vital medicolegal records. A dispassionate critical evaluation of long-term uniform postoperative photographs allows successes to be noted and useful techniques reinforced; errors in judgment and/or technique can be identified and discarded from the surgical repertoire.

Standard views in rhinoplasty photography include full frontal, basal, right and left lateral, and right and left oblique views. Optional close-up and smiling views may be vital in certain patients.

By use of a fast 105-mm portrait lens with dual flash strobe units and an overhead slave "key" flash, standardized shadow-free accurate representations of facial features may be easily recorded from sitting to sitting. A background that complements skin tones (light blue, green, or gray) serves best; pure white, black, or cluttered backgrounds should be avoided. Accurate positioning of the patient's head in all views with the Frankfort horizontal plane as a guide is vital to achieving consistency and standardization. This plane is parallel to the floor and courses from the top of external auditory canal along the orbital rim.

PSYCHOLOGICAL CONSIDERATIONS

Critical to the successful outcome of any aesthetic operation is the development of easy and thorough communication between surgeon and patient. The surgeon must be assured that the patient's outcome expectations are in fact realistic, that the motivations expressed are appropriate, and that the patient's anatomy is amenable to the desired changes. The patient, understandably anxious, must be reassured that a safe and relatively pain-free procedure may be carried out, resulting in a natural and improved condition. Verbal and written educational materials not only serve to inform and reassure patients but also allow them to form a knowledge base from which may spring important questions in later discussions. Initially, the surgeon must be a good *listener*, drawing out the patient's concerns with open-ended and then more specific questions. It is *vital* to learn *why* each individual seeks aesthetic surgical changes and *critical* to understand *what is expected*.

The types of patients in whom caution should be exercised before undertaking surgery are: (1) the patient with unrealistic expectations; (2) the obsessive-compulsive, perfectionistic patient; (3) the "sudden whim" patient; (4) the indecisive patient; (5) the rude patient; (6) the overflattering patient; (7) the overly familiar patient; (8) the unkempt patient; (9) the patient with minimal or imagined deformity; (10) the careless or poor historian; (11) the "VIP" patient; (12) the uncooperative patient; (13) the overly talkative patient; (14) the surgeon shopper; (15) the depressed patient; (16) the "plastic surgiholic"; (17) the price haggler; (18) the patient involved in litigation; (19) the patient whom you or your staff dislikes. Second and even third interviews are useful in such patients; if any doubts exist regarding the appropriateness of such individuals in seeking surgical changes, the operation is best postponed or avoided.

INDICATIONS

Nasal surgery is carried out to improve or correct the *appearance* and *function* of the nose; commonly these two features are closely interrelated and are best achieved in a single operation. Precise indications for nasal corrective surgery include congenital, developmental, traumatic, and iatrogenic (revisional surgery) deformities.

GOALS OF THE OPERATION

Simply stated, the ideal outcome of nasal corrective surgery results in a normally functioning nose possessing a natural, nonoperated appearance. The surgeon must determine, by exacting evaluation, what can and what cannot be achieved given the anatomic limitations encountered. Every effort should be expended to orchestrate a tidy, minimally traumatic operation, *preserving* the normal and ideal nasal anatomy while *correcting* aberrant and displeasing features. The avoidance of complications is critical because revisional rhinoplasty invariably becomes more difficult, given the scarring and altered anatomy resulting from primary procedures.

PREOPERATIVE PREPARATION

Before surgery the following may be considered the minimum evaluation and preparation necessary.

- Thorough preoperative informed consent discussions
- Documentation of all medications taken routinely
- Complete examination of the internal and external nose
- Standardized photodocumentation
- Operation rehearsal with patient photograph evaluation
- Hematologic profile, including coagulation studies
- Pertinent history and physical examination
- Sinus radiographs or CT scans (optional) where indicated
- Facial cleansing with antibacterial soap the evening before and the morning of surgery

The patient arrives at the hospital the morning of surgery, where the present physical condition is again reviewed. An intravenous line is established and the patient is positioned comfortably on a cushioned operating table, maintaining the head in a slightly elevated horizontal position.

ANESTHESIA AND ANALGESIA

Just as multiple rhinoplasty techniques exist, varied approaches also exist to nasal anesthesia and patient analgesia. Both endotracheal and monitored intravenous analgesia with local topical and infiltration anesthesia are suitable for this operation, representing a fundamental, safe, and reliable method for achieving the goals of nasal anesthesia: (1) a comfortable, relaxed, and responsive patient; (2) a bloodless operative field; and (3) minimal distortion of the nasal tissues.

Topical Anesthesia

Before infiltration of local anesthesia, the nasal mucous membranes are anesthetized with 4% color-coded cocaine solution, which is deposited in each nasal fossa on a single neurosurgical cottonoid. The cottonoids further act as excellent tampons, retarding the flow of blood and nasal secretions into the pharynx.

Intravenous Analgesia

For ultimate safety, it is important that the patient not receive a great many different families of drugs during surgery. The intravenous titrated administration of reversible drugs is ideal, allowing greater control over the depth of sedation. Any potential drug reaction from the use of multiple families of pharmacologic agents is confusing to treat and may be impossible to counteract intelligently. Close cooperation between the surgeon and anesthesiologist is important at this time, as well as throughout the operation. Each is responsible for the patient's safety and well-being, and each catalyzes the operative process by a healthy respect for the other's responsibilities.

Before drug administration, automated vital sign monitors providing constant readouts of patient pulse, electrocardiogram, blood pressure, and oxygen saturation are secured.

Innovar (a combination of a potent narcotic and phenothiazine—fentanyl and droperidol) has been found to be safe and reliable for inducing a state of relaxed sedation. Infused intravenously in *small titrated increments*, patient comfort is safely established. The powerful antiemetic effect of droperidol has largely eliminated the problem of postoperative nausea.

In addition, small increments of an ultra-short-acting barbiturate (methohexital [Brevital, Surital]) may be given just before local anesthetic infiltration and osteotomy maneuvers to render the patient more soporific and amnestic. Some anesthesiologists prefer Diprivan (Propofol) as the intravenous anesthetic of choice. Midazolam (Versed) used in combination with these agents lends relaxation and amnesia for the procedure. General inhalation anesthesia is preferred by many surgeons.

Infiltration Anesthetic

The goal of infiltration anesthesia is to render the nose completely anesthetic and intensely vasoconstricted with the least possible distortion of normal anatomy; 1% lidocaine with a 1 : 100,000 to 1 : 50,000 dilution of epinephrine, *freshly mixed*, is preferred for infiltration anesthesia (the weaker solution is used in older patients or in those with possible cardiovascular abnormalities). Except in unusual cases, a total of 3.5 to 5.0 mL of the solution, injected sparingly into the *proper surgical planes*, is sufficient to produce profound vasoconstriction and complete nasal anesthesia. No effort is made to block specific nerves. If septal reconstruction is to be carried out, an additional 2 mL of the anesthetic is injected into the septal submucoperichondrial and subperichondrial planes to aid, by hydraulic dissection, the elevation of the septal flaps.

The infiltration of the local anesthetic is initiated by retracting the ala cephalically with thumb and forefinger, exposing the caudal edge of the upper lateral cartilage. A long 27-gauge needle is placed parallel to the long axis of the exposed upper lateral cartilage and, with a quick stabbing motion, the needle penetrates the epithelium, usually with minimal sensation to the patient. Any sensation of the needle stick may be masqueraded by bluntly pinching the skin elsewhere in the face simultaneously, a technique referred to as "lateral inhibition." The needle is advanced along the lateral wall of the dorsum, hugging the perichondrium of the upper lateral cartilages and the periosteum of the nasal bones, *thus remaining in the proper plane*. Approximately 0.5 mL is deposited into this plane as the needle is withdrawn to, but not beyond, the point of initial penetration. The procedure is repeated over the dorsum and on the opposite side. Infiltration of the nasal base, columella, and tip follows. Anesthetic may now be deposited along the course of the lateral osteotomies or, if desired, delayed until later in the operation. The needle is inserted at the pyriform aperture near the insertion of the inferior turbinate and advanced *lateral and medial to the ascending process*, depositing 0.5 mL on either side. A vasoconstricted pathway for the lateral osteotomy is thus established. Infiltration of the nasal septum follows.

After infiltration anesthesia, it is critical that the surgeon wait 10 to 15 minutes before proceeding with the operation, allowing vasoconstriction to reach its maximal effectiveness.

The ingredients considered essential for a comfortable and successful procedure are illustrated in Figure 7–5.

This method of infiltration anesthesia ensures patient comfort, provides for constant patient monitoring, limits the number of needle penetrations, minimizes the

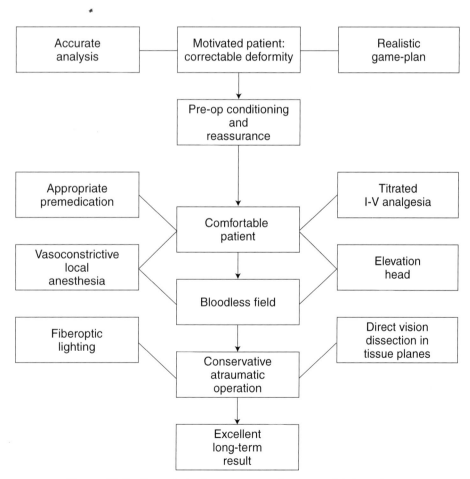

Figure 7–5. The principal components of a successful rhinoplasty.

amount of anesthetic, and avoids tissue distortion. In most operations, little if any bleeding occurs during the procedure, and postoperative ecchymosis is minimal or nonexistent. All these factors help to permit the precise, bloodless dissection of nasal structures that is essential for the carefully controlled rhinoplasty operation.

INTRAOPERATIVE TECHNIQUE
TOPOGRAPHIC LANDMARK IDENTIFICATION

Sketching the topography of the nasal skeleton on the nasal surface, indicating key landmarks, is especially helpful for the neophyte surgeon. It reinforces a thoughtful preview, through palpation and inspection, of the location and size of the individual nasal anatomic components to be modified. Critical decisions about planned tissue excisions, augmentations, and reorientation of nasal structures can thereby be supported by visual illustration on the nose itself.

SCULPTURE OF THE NASAL TIP

Experienced surgeons regard surgery of the nasal tip as the most challenging and exacting aspect of nasal plastic surgery. The surgeon is confronted by nasal anatomic components that are essentially *bilateral* (demanding symmetric surgical technique and healing), animate, and mobile, which may require reduction, enhancement, or simply preservation of existing projection.

Surgeons have gradually come to understand that radical excision division and extensive sacrifice of alar cartilages and other tip support mechanisms all too frequently result in eventual unnatural or "surgical" tips.

A philosophy of a *graduated incremental anatomic approach* to tip surgery is highly useful to achieve consistently natural results (Fig. 7–6). Conservative reduction of the volume of the cephalic margin of the lateral crus, thus preserving a substantial complete, undisturbed strip of residual alar cartilage, is a preferred operation in individuals in whom nasal tip

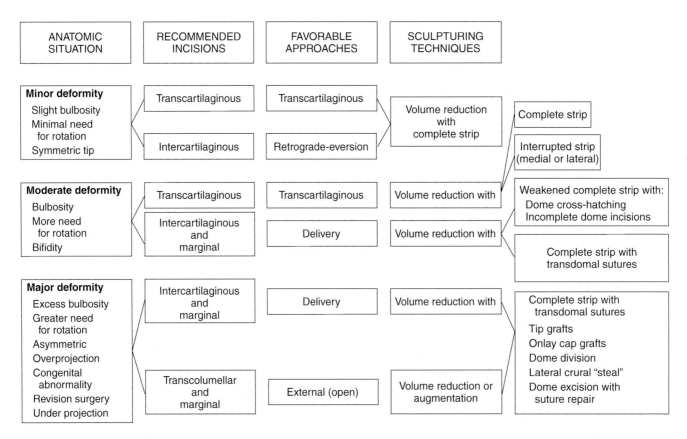

Figure 7–6. Algorithmic representation of the graduated anatomic systematic approach to the nasal tip. As the anatomy encountered becomes more abnormal, the magnitude of the surgical approach and techniques selected increases accordingly. The procedure selected is then dictated by the presenting anatomy *only*. Minimal deformities are corrected with less invasive, less risky procedures, whereas major deformities are approached more aggressively.

changes need not be profound. As the tip deformity encountered becomes more abnormal, more aggressive techniques are required from *weakened complete strip* techniques to significant *interruption of the residual complete strip* with a profound alteration in the alar cartilage size, shape, and attitude.

Tip sculpture cannot be successfully undertaken, let alone mastered, until the *major and minor tip support mechanisms* are appreciated, respected, and preserved (or reconstructed). Loss of tip support in the postoperative healing period is one of the most common surgical errors in rhinoplasty.

In most patients the *major tip support mechanisms* consist of size, shape, and thickness of the alar cartilages; attachment of the medial crural footplates to the caudal septum; and attachment of the upper lateral cartilages to the alar cartilages. Compensatory re-establishment of stable tip support should be considered if during the operation any or all of these major tip support mechanisms are significantly compromised.

Minor tip support mechanisms, which in certain anatomic and ethnic configurations may assume *major* support importance, include (1) the dorsal cartilaginous septum, (2) the interdomal ligament, (3) the membranous septum, (4) the nasal spine, (5) the investing skin and soft tissues, and (6) the alar sidewalls.

Given this knowledge, the appropriate tip incisions and approaches should be planned to *preserve as many tip supports as possible*. No routine tip procedure is ever used; instead the appropriate incisions, approaches, and tip sculpturing techniques are selected *entirely on the basis of an analysis of the varying tip anatomy encountered*. Several factors are important to assess before selecting the appropriate tip procedure. The surgeon must determine whether the tip requires a change in the *attitude* and *orientation* of the alar cartilages, a change in *tip projection*, a *cephalic rotation* of the tip, or a narrowing of over-wide domal angles.

SURGICAL APPROACHES TO THE TIP

Approaches to the nasal tip are simply a method to *gain access* to the tip structures and should not be confused with *techniques*. Ideally, normal and aesthetically pleasant tip structures should remain undisturbed if at all possible during surgical approaches.

NONDELIVERY APPROACHES

In nasal tips where only minimal conservative volume reduction is indicated, nondelivery approaches allow minimal disturbance of normal structures and thus provide the surgeon with greater control over healing.

Transcartilaginous Approach

Because of its atraumatic simplicity and ease of use, the *transcartilaginous approach* is preferred when conservative tip refinement is indicated (Fig. 7–7). This approach is useful in patients whose tip anatomy is fundamentally satisfactory, requiring only volume reduction to accomplish a thinning sculpture of the cephalic-medial margin of the lateral crus, preserving a generous residual complete strip. The initial incision penetrates only the vestibular skin underlying the lateral crus; the skin flap is easily dissected and preserved *before* continuing the incision through the alar cartilage.

Retrograde Approach

This conservative, atraumatic approach is similar to the transcartilaginous approach except that an intercartilaginous incision is used, dissecting beneath the vestibular skin flap in retrograde fashion to expose and reduce the size of the alar cartilage (Fig. 7–8).

DELIVERY APPROACHES

Delivering the alar cartilages as individual bipedicle chondrocutaneous flaps or through an open (external) approach allows full exposure of the anatomy and is used when the tip cartilages are asymmetric or in need of more profound alterations. Significant narrowing refinements are facilitated through these approaches; however, more tissue trauma results. Delivering the alar cartilages is useful when nasal tip bulbosity or bifidity exists, when the paired domal angles are excessively broad, and when alar cartilage asymmetry exists.

Alar Cartilage Delivery Approach

Carried out through intercartilaginous and marginal incisions, delivery of the alar cartilages provides a binocular

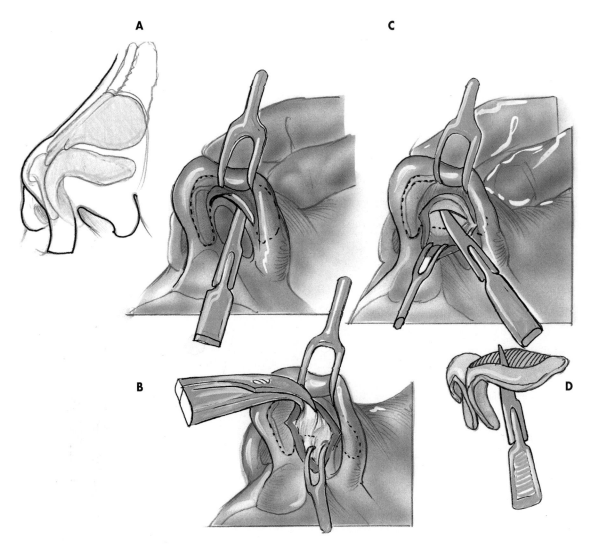

Figure 7–7. The transcartilaginous (cartilage splitting) approach to the nasal tip, with calculated volume reduction of the cephalic margin of the lateral crura.

view of the tip anatomy and affords the added ease of bimanual surgical modification (Fig. 7–9). If on frontal and basal view the alar cartilages flare or diverge unpleasantly, if tip triangularity is unsatisfactory, or if the tip appears too amorphous and bulbous, a delivery approach should be considered. Transdomal suture narrowing of broad domes and interrupted strip techniques are best effected through delivery approaches.

EXTERNAL (OPEN) APPROACH

The external or open approach to the nasal tip is in reality a more aggressive form of the delivery approach,

requiring an external incision irregularized across the waist of the columella, and is chosen with discretion in very specific nasal tip deformities. The anatomic view is unparalleled through this approach, affording the surgeon diagnostic information unavailable through traditional closed approaches. These technical virtues must be balanced with the potential disadvantages of an enlarged scar bed, slightly delayed healing with some prolongation of tip edema, and an increased operating time. Clearly when subtle and conservative tip surgery is indicated by the patient's existent anatomy, the open approach is unnecessary.

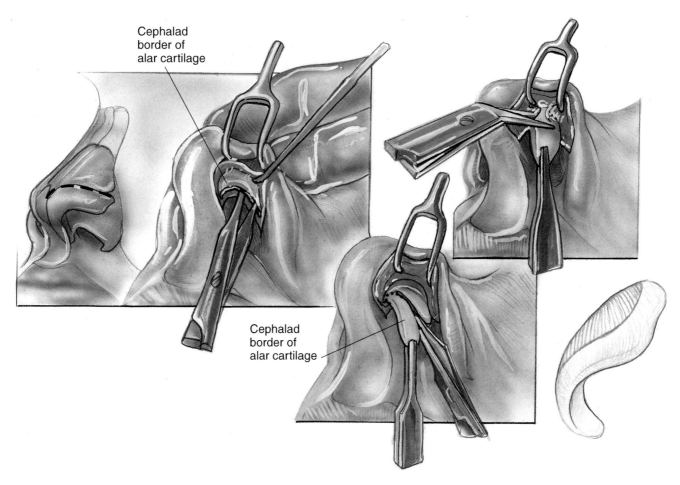

Figure 7–8. The retrograde approach to the cephalic margin of the alar cartilages accessed through an intercartilaginous incision.

The open approach is facilitated if bilateral marginal incisions are created at the outset with a 15c blade, carrying the incision down the columella along the caudal aspects of the intermediate and medial crura to the site of the eventual external columellar incision. The alar cartilages are then dissected free from their investing soft tissue attachments *before* the irregularized columellar incision is executed. This sequence of dissection adds a degree of safety to the procedure, helping to avoid trauma or tears to the dissected skin flap (Fig. 7–10). The open approach facilitates the suturing of cartilage grafts to the tip and dorsum, allows unparalleled assessment and correction of tip asymmetries, and can be helpful in difficult revision surgery.

TIP SCULPTURE TECHNIQUES

The choice of the technique used to modify the alar cartilages and the relationship of the nasal tip to the remaining nasal structures should be based entirely on *the anatomy encountered* and the predicted result desired as defined from the known dynamics of long-term healing. The astonishing diversity of tip anatomy encountered demands a broad diversification of surgical planning and execution.

Four broad categories of nasal tip sculpturing procedures may be identified. Although additional subtle technical variations exist, these include (1) volume reduction with residual complete strip, (2) volume reduction with weakened or suture-narrowed residual complete strip, and

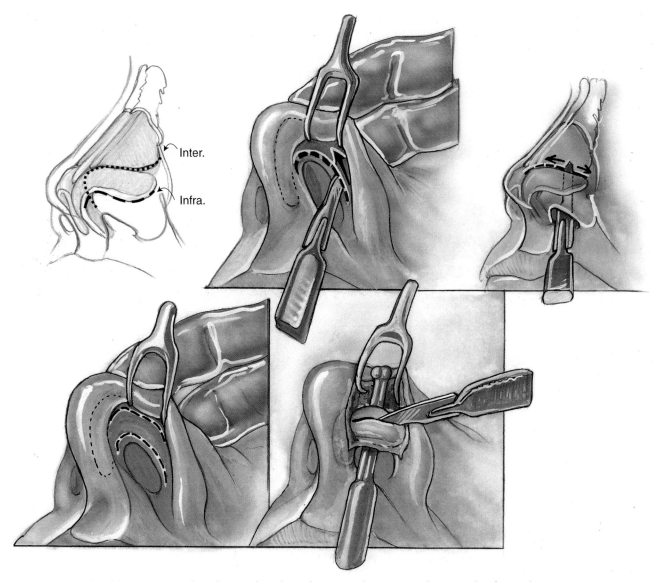

Figure 7–9. The delivery approach to the nasal tip through intercartilaginous and marginal (infracartilaginous) incisions.

(3) volume reduction with interrupted strip, and cartilage tip grafting.

Complete Strip Technique

Preserving the major portion of the residual complete strip of the alar cartilage is always preferred when the anatomy of the alar cartilages and their surrounding soft tissue investments will allow. This preservative approach retains the supportive advantage of the intact cartilage strip (thus "mimicking" nature), discourages cephalic rotation when it is undesirable, eliminates many of the potential hazards of more radical techniques, and tends to produce a more natural final result.

Accomplished either by means of a nondelivery or delivery approach, a portion of the cephalic margin of the lateral crus and dome is excised, preserving the underlying vestibular skin. To preserve existing tip projection, a portion of the medialmost aspect of the lateral

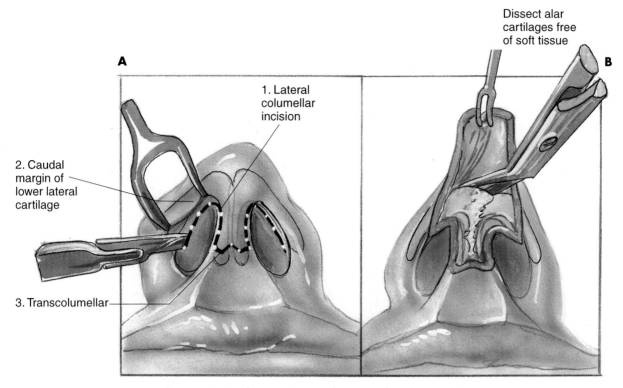

Figure 7–10. The open (external) approach to the nasal tip.

crus responsible for tip projection is preserved. The normal contour and shape of the cartilage is retained while reducing its overall size (Fig. 7–11). The medial crura or domes may be sutured together to further refine and strengthen the tip projection and favorably narrow domal angles that are too broad.

Weakened Complete Strip

Techniques involving a weakened (or reoriented) residual complete strip possess all the positive virtues noted previously, while in addition allow the surgeon to effect reorientation of the attitude of the dome, projection modification, and narrowing refinement so desirable in the ideal postoperative appearance. After preservation of a generous complete strip, the lateral crus is slightly weakened and attenuated by noncoalescent alternating partial-thickness incisions along its extent (Fig. 7–12A–D). This maneuver allows improved narrowing refinement to occur as healing progresses. Optional

sutures uniting the medial crura or domes assist in stabilizing the repair.

The lateral crus may be further weakened, if indicated, by serial partial-thickness cuts across its entire width. Greater risk of asymmetric healing exists whenever the integrity of the modified complete strip is compromised.

Complete Strip with Transdomal Sutures

In nasal tips characterized by broad domal angles and bifidity of the intermediate crura with marked lateral divergence, imparting a bulky, trapezoidal configuration to the tip shape, horizontal mattress sutures spanning the dome and encircling both the medial and lateral crura (transdomal sutures) provide favorable narrowing refinement and improved long-term tip support (Fig. 7–13). Properly positioned, they can also increase tip projection by 2 to 3 mm.

After any delivery approach and alar cartilage modification, it is vital that the sculpted cartilages be replaced

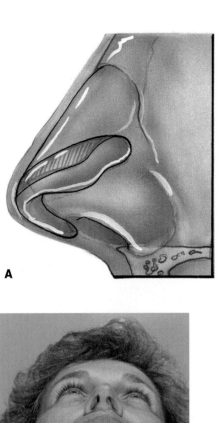

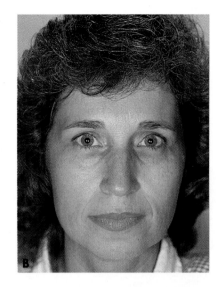

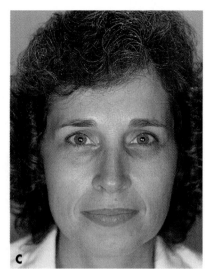

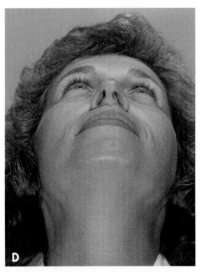

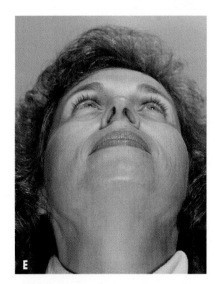

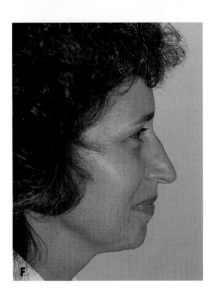

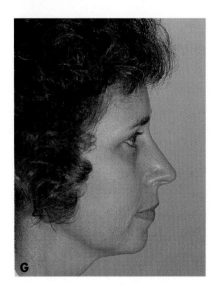

Figure 7–11. (A) Volume reduction of the cephalic margin of the lateral crus, preserving a complete intact strip of alar cartilage of at least 50% of the cartilage. Preoperative **(B)** and postoperative **(C)** views of a patient operated on through a transcartilaginous approach by use of a volume reduction, complete strip operation. Preoperative **(D)** and postoperative **(E)** base view. Preoperative **(F)** and postoperative **(G)** lateral view.

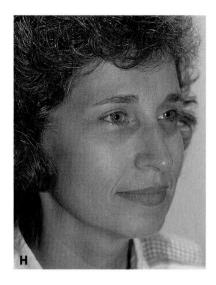 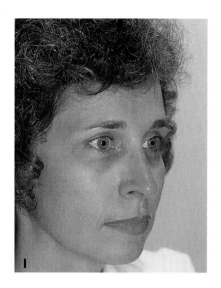

Figure 7–11. *(continued)* Preoperative **(H)** and postoperative **(I)** oblique view.

precisely in their previous soft tissue beds and incisions repaired with 5-0 chromic catgut sutures.

Interrupted Strip Techniques

The integrity of the residual complete strip cannot always be maintained because of more profound abnormalities and asymmetries encountered in certain unusual tip configurations, including marked overprojection, severe underprojection, or asymmetry. In these instances the alar cartilage must be interrupted in a vertical fashion somewhere along its extent to achieve maximal refinement, enhance cephalic rotation, and improve or reduce tip projection.

The risks of *asymmetric healing* are greater when interrupted strips are created; however, and initial *loss of tip support* occurs immediately. The latter deficiency must be recognized and countermeasures taken during surgery to ensure that sufficient tip support is reconstituted with columellar struts, infratip lobule cartilage tip grafts, or transcrural sutures.

Through a delivery approach, the alar cartilages are presented and volume reduction is accomplished. Interruption of the complete strip is carried out medial to or lateral to the tip-defining point, depending on the anatomy encountered (Fig. 7–14A). Vestibular skin is

religiously preserved. To improve projection of the tip, cartilage may be "borrowed" from the lateral crura to lengthen the medial crura. Stabilizing suture(s) effects final tip reconfiguration (Fig. 7–14B). This form of interrupted strip technique is reserved for patients with thick skin and subcutaneous tissues whose projection is poor. Tip grafts may also be considered.

TIP ROTATION TECHNIQUES

Cephalic rotation of the nasal tip complex (alar cartilages, columella, and nasal base) assumes a major role in many patients undergoing rhinoplasty, whereas in others the *prevention of upward rotation* is vital. The planned degree of tip rotation depends on a variety of factors, which often include the nasal length, the length of the face, the height of the patient, the length of the upper lip, facial balance and proportion, the patient's aesthetic desires, and the surgeon's aesthetic judgment.

An important distinction must be drawn between *tip rotation* and *tip projection*. Although certain tip rotation techniques may result in desirable increases in tip projection, the converse is not true. Tip rotation and projection are in fact complementary to each other, and their proper achievement in individual patients is constantly interrelated.

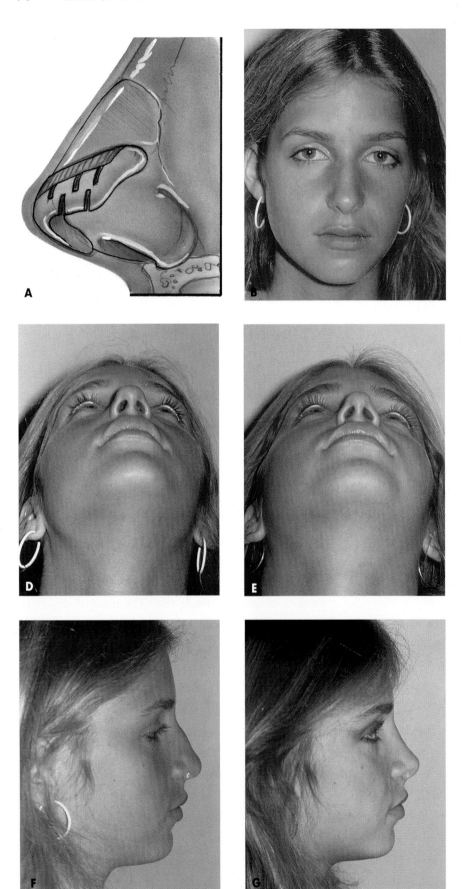

Figure 7-12. (A) Weakening of the residual complete strip of strong alar cartilages by means of non-coalescent partial incisions. Preoperative **(B)** and postoperative **(C)** views of patient operated on with a volume reduction, weakened complete strip procedure. Preoperative **(D)** and postoperative **(E)** base views. Preoperative **(F)** and postoperative **(G)** lateral views.

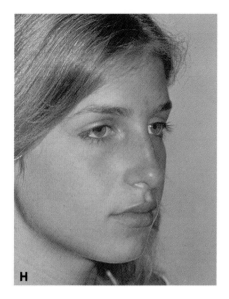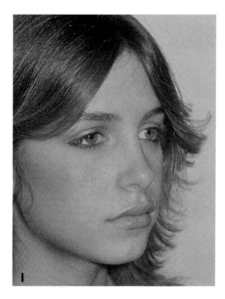

Figure 7–12. *(continued)*
Preoperative **(H)** and postoperative
(I) oblique views.

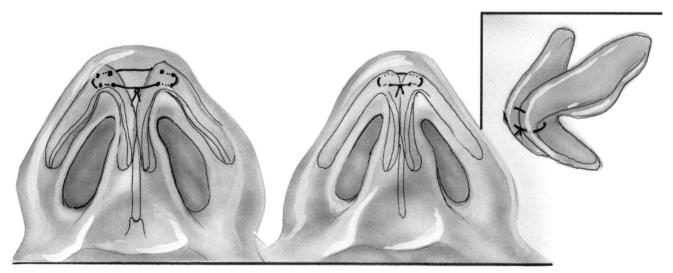

Figure 7–13. Transdomal suturing of the domes of the alar cartilages, correcting bifidity, boxy deformity of the nasal tip, and excess domal angulation.

Most tip rotation techniques may be incorporated in an organizational scheme that includes three procedures preserving a complete, intact strip of alar cartilage (Fig. 7–15A) and three additional procedures involving interrupted strip techniques (Fig. 7–15B).

Volume reduction of the alar cartilage results in a tissue deficit of minimal, moderate, or maximal proportions, depending on the degree of cartilage removal indicated or desirable. Essentially no cephalic tip rotation results from minimal volume reduction alone (the com-

plete strip tends to *resist* cephalic rotation, whereas the greater tissue void resulting from maximal volume reduction tends to produce slightly more cephalic rotation [Fig. 7–15A]). Therefore, when complete strip techniques are selected, substantial planned tip rotation depends on the addition of *adjunctive rotation techniques* to achieve desired tip rotation. These include (Fig. 7–16A) caudal septal shortening, reduction of excess caudal upper lateral cartilage, high septal transfixion with septal wedge excision, reduction of overly convex medial crura, cartilage struts, and

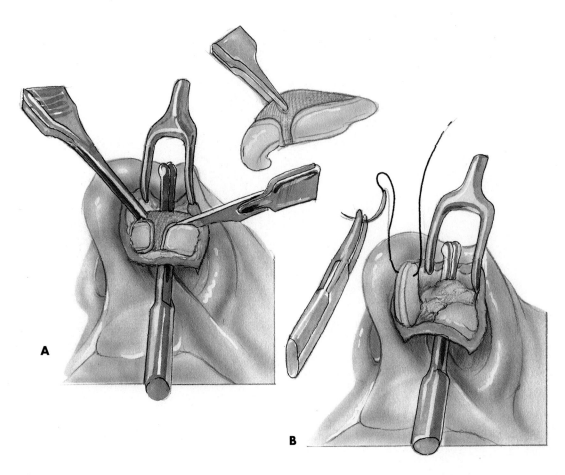

Figure 7-14. **(A)** Interruption of the residual complete strip just lateral to the dome. **(B)** The intermediate crura are reflected medial and sutured together to increase projection of the nasal tip. Such operations, which divide the complete strip, are reserved only for certain revision procedures and in patients with thick skin who require additional projection.

cartilage plumping grafts (to provide *illusion* of rotation).

Interrupted strip techniques combined with volume reduction of excessive alar cartilage tend to result in a more substantial degree of cephalic rotation of the tip complex, fostered by virtue of upward scar contracture forces acting inexorably on divided alar cartilage segments, which are now more flail and less well supported.

Medial interruption techniques will predictably lead to some degree of tip rotation but are reserved almost exclusively for patients with thicker skin and supporting structures to minimize potential undesirable asymmetric healing and an unnatural tip appearance.

Lateral interruption techniques are preferred in patients in whom cephalic rotation is desirable and the anatomy of

the bridge between the lateral and medial crus ("dome") is aesthetically pleasing. The lateral interruption allows the reduced alar cartilage to be pulled moderately upward by scar tissue contracture during healing, but because the dividing cut is sited more laterally and therefore more deeply in the soft tissues of the tip, notching, pinching, and asymmetries are essentially prevented.

Maximal predictable rotation is predictably realized by combining *lateral strip interruption* with a calibrated *triangular excision of cartilage laterally* and stabilization of the cut cartilage edges with *fine suture fixation* (Fig. 7-16B). The degree of rotation realized here is controllable by the surgeon, essentially eliminates most of the undesirable sequelae of interrupted strip techniques, and changes in a predictable

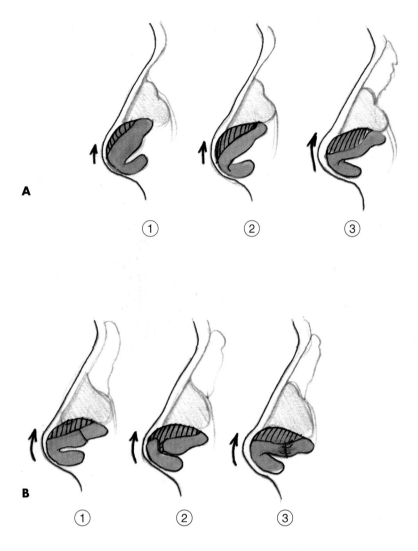

Figure 7–15. (A) As the amount of volume reduction of the cephalic margin of the alar cartilage increases, a tendency exists for additional rotation to occur in the postoperative period. **(B)** Interruption of the residual compete strip at any of several regions along its extent tends to create a more flail residual lower lateral cartilage, which may promote cephalic rotation during healing.

and permanent way the attitude of the alar cartilages. The suture fixation helps to diminish loss of tip support inherent in interrupted strip techniques. In individuals with thin skin with more delicate cartilages, this method is highly predictable and desirable (Fig. 7–16C).

Correction of Inadequate Tip Projection

In addition to the creation of narrowing refinement and symmetry of the operated nasal tip, which are most evident in the frontal view, appropriate *tip projection* must be preserved or created anew to set the tip subtly but distinctly apart from the nasal supratip region. Ptotic or poorly projected tips produce a snubbed and indistinct appearance typical of nonskillful rhinoplasty.

Reorientation of the alar cartilages with transdomal suture fixation or by rotating a portion of the lateral crus into the medial crus to gain projection have been previously discussed (Figs. 7–13 and 7–14).

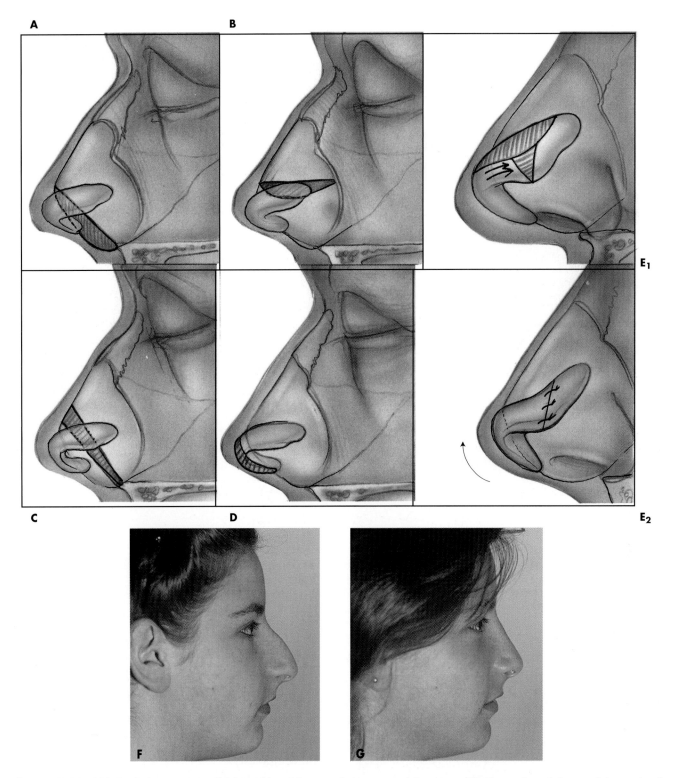

Figure 7–16. (A) Cephalic rotation is facilitated by reduction of excess caudal septum. **(B)** Shortening of the caudal margin of the upper lateral cartilages may assist in facilitating cephalic rotation. **(C)** Cephalic rotation of the entire tip may be accomplished by a resection of a segment of the septum through a high transfixion incision. **(D)** A dependent nose as a result of excessive convexity of the medial and intermediate crura may be elevated by direct shaving of the caudal margins of the intermediate and medial crura. **(E)** A reliable method of cephalic tip rotation is by removal of a triangle (based upward) in the lateralmost extent of the lateral crus, resuturing the cartilaginous segments together with fine suture. This maneuver reliably results in a cephalic repositioning of the nasal tip in selected patients. Preoperative **(F)** and postoperative **(G)** views of a patient in whom modest cephalic rotation and retropositioning of the nasal tip is accomplished by the maneuvers described in Figure 7–16E.

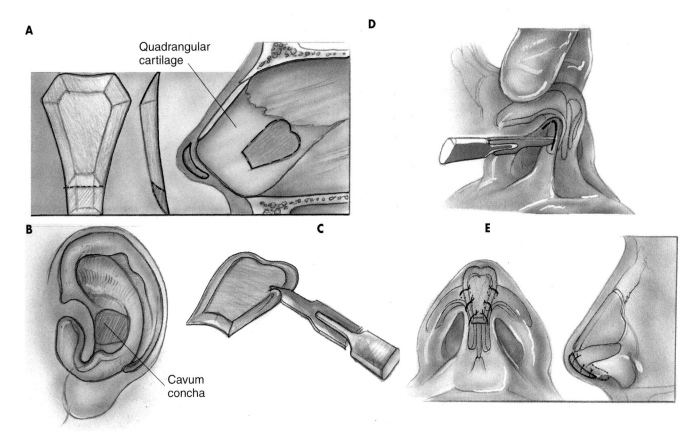

Figure 7–17. (A) Sculptured tip grafts are best harvested from the intact quadrangular cartilage. **(B)** Tip grafts may be created from the auricular cartilage located just posterior to the ear canal. **(C)** Beveling and shave excision of the margins of tip grafts is carried out with the No. 15 blade. **(D)** Tip grafts may be inserted through bilateral marginal incisions. **(E)** Sutured-in-place tip grafts provide the most reliable stability and projection to the nose, particularly when associated with cartilaginous strut support to the nasal tip.

Tip cartilage grafts serve admirably to redefine and contour the skeletal anatomy of the deficient tip, providing quantifiable degrees of stable tip projection. Harvested from the nasal septum (Fig. 7–17A) or auricular cartilage just posterior to the ear canal (Fig. 7–17B), their edges must be scalpel-beveled to avoid detection beneath the tip soft tissues (Fig. 7–17C, D).

Carved in shieldlike or triangular shapes, the grafts may be successfully inserted into precise pockets created in the infratip lobule through *bilateral* marginal incisions beneath each dome; suture fixation is unnecessary if pockets are precisely dissected. When the external rhinoplasty approach is chosen, tip grafts (single or laminated) may be accurately sculpted and sutured to the alar cartilages in the infratip lobule region to impart stable projection to the reconstructed tip (Fig. 7–17E).

If additional projection or tip support is required, it may be achieved with autogenous cartilage columellar struts (Fig. 7–18A), plumping cartilage grafts at the nasolabial angle (Fig. 7–18B), or suture-apposition of divergent medial crura. (Fig. 7–18C). Tip grafts should be avoided (or used cautiously) in patients with extremely thin skin.

Correction of the Overprojecting Tip

The nose that projects too far forward of the anterior facial plane results in significant facial disharmony. Any one or a combination of nasal anatomic components may be responsible for overprojection, and therefore no single surgical technique is uniformly useful in correcting all the problems responsible for the various overprojection

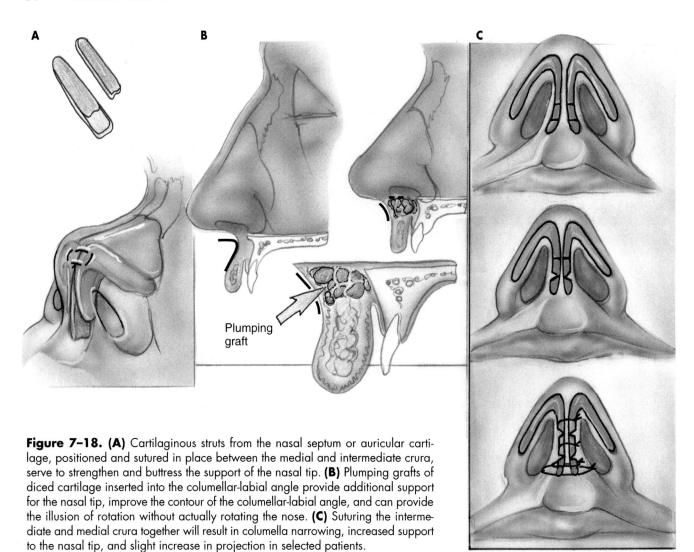

A **B** **C**

Plumping
graft

Figure 7–18. (A) Cartilaginous struts from the nasal septum or auricular cartilage, positioned and sutured in place between the medial and intermediate crura,
serve to strengthen and buttress the support of the nasal tip. **(B)** Plumping grafts of
diced cartilage inserted into the columellar-labial angle provide additional support
for the nasal tip, improve the contour of the columellar-labial angle, and can provide
the illusion of rotation without actually rotating the nose. **(C)** Suturing the intermediate and medial crura together will result in columella narrowing, increased support
to the nasal tip, and slight increase in projection in selected patients.

abnormalities. Accurate diagnosis will lead to the development of a logical *individualized strategy for correction. In
almost every instance, weakening or reducing normal tip support
mechanisms is required to initiate retroprojection by use of
a complete transfixion incision to divide the medial crural footplates from
the caudal septum.*

Overdevelopment of the alar cartilages, commonly associated
with thin skin and large nostrils, is a common cause of tip
overprojection. The hypertrophied cartilages must be
delivered, their abnormalities clearly diagnosed, and
overall volume and shape reduction of the lateral and
medial crus accomplished (Fig. 7–19).

Overdevelopment of the caudal and dorsal quadrangular cartilage
frequently results in an overprojected nose. The tip

anatomy may be otherwise normal, but the overlarge
quadrangular cartilage produces webbing of the
nasolabial angle because of septal elongation, and the
high anterior septal angle lifts the nasal tip into an abnormally forward position, tenting the nose and lip under
some degree of tension. Reduction of the supratip cartilaginous dorsuin along with significant nasal shortening
by excision of the overlong caudal quadrangular cartilage allows the tip to be positioned in a more normal
attitude (Fig. 7–20).

An overlarge nasal spine may be responsible for tip overprojection; it is almost always associated with overdevelopment of the caudal septum. The nasolabial angle is
blunted, appearing full, webbed, and excessively obtuse,

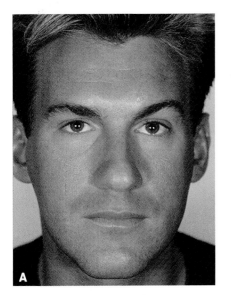

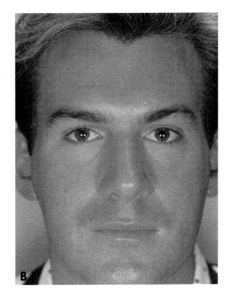

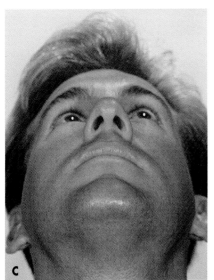

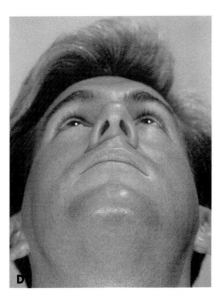

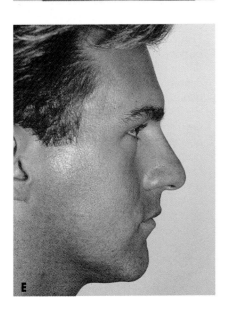

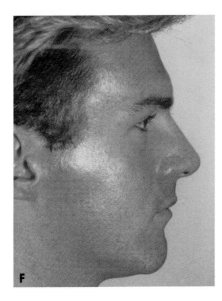

Figure 7–19. Preoperative and postoperative views of a patient presenting with overdeveloped alar cartilages with consequent nasal tip overprotection, a boxy appearance to the nasal tip, and bifidity. A transdomal suture repair through a delivery approach provides improvement. Preoperative **(A)** and postoperative **(B)** frontal views. Preoperative **(C)** and postoperative **(D)** basal views, demonstrating improved triangularity and correction of bifidity. Preoperative **(E)** and postoperative **(F)** lateral views.

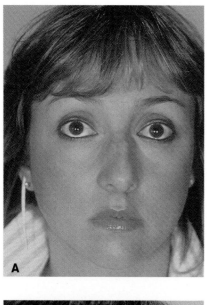
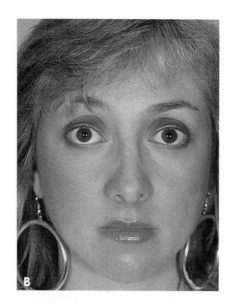
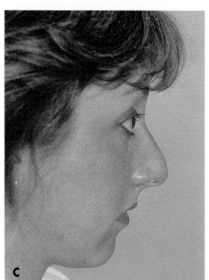
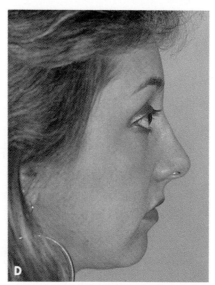
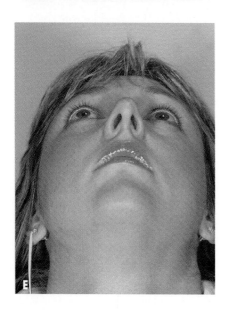
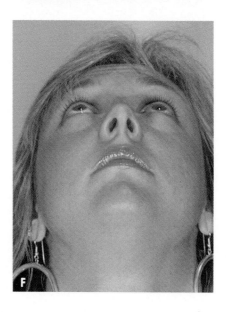

Figure 7–20. Preoperative and postoperative views of the patient, demonstrating overprojection as a consequence of an overdeveloped quadrangular cartilage, both dorsally and caudally. The nose is deviated with significant nasal obstruction. Correction is accomplished through retropositioning of the nasal tip, sculpturing of the overlarge nasal tip cartilages, and straightening of the nose and septum. Preoperative **(A)** and postoperative **(B)** frontal views. Preoperative **(C)** and postoperative **(D)** lateral views. Preoperative **(E)** and postoperative **(F)** basal views.

with no obvious demarcation between the lip and columella. The upper lip may appear short, tethered, and tense, often exposing excessive gingiva in facial repose and in animation. Rongeur or osteotome reduction of the spine and caudal septum is a surgical prerequisite to tip retroprojection.

Overprojection may occur as the result of an *overly long columella* associated with *excessively long medial crura*. In this deformity the infratip lobule is commonly insufficient, creating the effect of extremely large and disproportionate nostrils. The use of the open approach is suggested here to shorten the columellar soft tissue length and that of the medial crura.

If an overdeep nasofrontal angle exists in tandem with the overprojected nose (a common finding), cartilage graft augmentation of this region serves to improve overall nasal proportions.

Retropositioning of the overprojected nose ordinarily leads to alar base flaring, suggesting the need for *alar base reduction* procedures to normalize the tip appearance. Alar wedge excisions of various geometric designs and dimensions are illustrated in Figure 7–21. The exact and extremely varied anatomy of the alar base, alar sidewalls, and nostril sill will determine the proper type of alar base reduction.

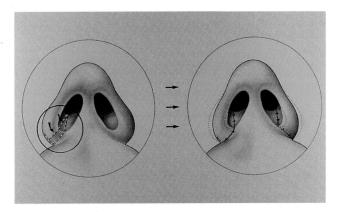

Figure 7–21. A typical form of alar base reduction-excision to narrow and refine the alar base and nasal sidewalls. The exact anatomy of the excision will depend on the anatomy of the lateral alar sidewall, the internal alar sidewall, the nostril sill, and the nostril floor.

ELEVATION OF NASAL SOFT TISSUES

Surgical access to the nasal dorsum is gained through the transcartilaginous, intercartilaginous incision, or open approach incisions, depending on which approach was used during tip refinement. Commonly the chosen incision is slightly extended around the anterior septal angle and into the membranous septum for a distance of 5 to 8 mm to provide full visualization of the nasal dorsum. Routine complete transfixion incisions are unnecessary.

The tissue plane used for elevation of the nasal soft tissues is vital for several important reasons. A *relatively avascular potential plane* exists just intimate to the perichondrium of the cartilaginous vault and just beneath the periosteum of the bony vault. Elevating the tissue flap in this important plane preserves the thickest possible epithelial soft tissue covering to ultimately cushion the newly formed bony and cartilaginous profile. Only sufficient skin is elevated to gain access to the profile, avoiding more traditional wide lateral undermining techniques.

The soft tissues over the cartilaginous dorsum are elevated by scalpel dissection with a No. 15c blade (Fig. 7–22A and B), whereas the periosteum over the bony pyramid is lifted from its bony attachment with the sharp Joseph elevator (Fig. 7–22C). Because the periosteum inserts into the internasal suture line in the midline, the periosteum is first lifted on either side of this suture and the elevated spaces then brought into continuity with the sharp scissors. Little or no bleeding should ensue during dissection in this plane, allowing direct vision assessment of the anatomy encountered.

PROFILE ALIGNMENT

Three anatomic nasal components are responsible for the preoperative profile appearance: *the nasal bones, the cartilaginous cartilages, and the alar cartilages.* Generally all three must undergo modification to create a natural profile alignment.

The ultimate intended profile is visualized in the surgeon's mind's eye, extending from the nasofrontal angle

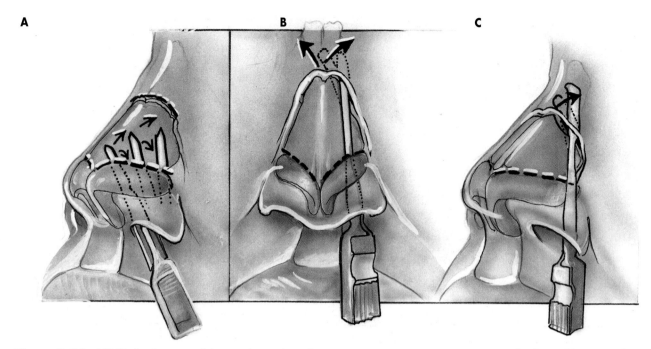

Figure 7–22. (A) Knife elevation of the overlying skin-subcutaneous tissue canopy, remaining in the favorable tissue plane intimate to the cartilaginous dorsum. **(B, C)** Elevation of the periosteum overlying the nasal bones, just sufficient to gain access to any existing nasal hump.

to the tip-defining point. The extent of reduction of bone, cartilage, and soft tissue will always depend and be guided by *stable tip projection*; thus positioning the projection of the tip at the outset of the operative procedure is beneficial. Because the thickness of the investing soft tissues and skin varies at different areas of the profile and from patient to patient, dissimilar portions of cartilage and bone constituting the nasal hump must be removed to result ultimately in a straight or slightly concave profile line. Aesthetics are generally best served when profile reduction results in a high, strong, straight-line profile in the male patient, with the leading edge of the tip just slightly higher in the female.

Either of two methods of profile alignment are preferred: *incremental* or *en-bloc*. In the former method the cartilaginous dorsum is reduced by incremental shaving maneuvers of the cartilaginous profile until an ideal tip-supratip relationship is established (Fig. 7–23A), followed by sharp osteotome removal of the residual bony hump. If en-bloc hump removal is contemplated, the knife is positioned at the osseocartilaginous junction and plunged through this area, then advanced caudally to and

around the anterior septal angle of the caudal septum as indicated by the degree of reduction desired.

In large cartilaginous profile reduction a portion of the upper lateral cartilage attachment to the quadrangular cartilage will out of necessity be removed with the dorsal septum, leaving these two cartilaginous components attached by the intact underlying mucoperichondrial bridge. A sharp Rubin osteotome (honed to razor sharpness at the operating table), seated in the opening made by the knife at the osseocartilaginous junction, is driven gently cephalically to remove the desired degree of bony hump in *continuity with the cartilaginous hump* (Fig. 7–23B). The hump is then removed en-bloc as a single segment.

Any irregularities remaining are corrected under direct vision with a knife or sharp tungsten rasp (Fig. 7–24A). Palpating the skin of the dorsum with the examining finger *moistened with peroxide* will often provide clues to unseen irregularities (Fig. 7–24B), as will intranasal palpation of the newly created profile with the noncutting edge of the No. 15 blade.

Except in very large or severely twisted noses, it is unnecessary and potentially harmful to separate the upper

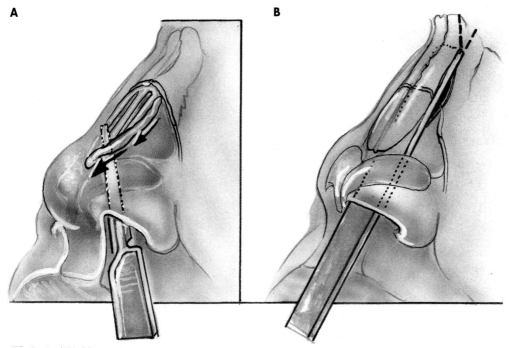

Figure 7–23. (A) Knife reduction of the cartilaginous dorsum, ordinarily created in small increments. **(B)** En-bloc resection of the nasal hump, created by incising the cartilaginous dorsum at the osteocartilaginous junction and inserting a Rueben osteotome into the mortis joint thus created.

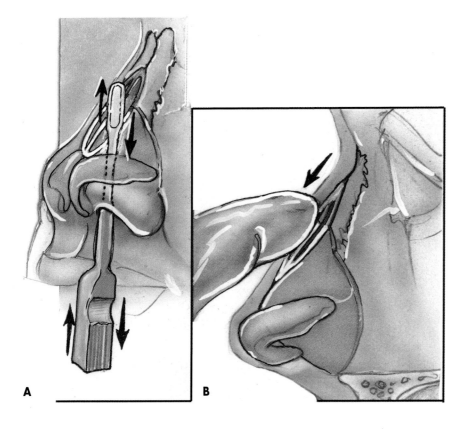

Figure 7–24. (A) Smoothing of the rusal bone surfaces with a sharp tungsten carbide rasp, carried out either manually or with a power-driven rasp. **(B)** Palpation of the nasal profile after alignment with a moistened finger provides a most accurate assessment of regularity.

lateral cartilages from the septum by cutting through the mucoperichondrial bridge of tissue connecting them at the nasal valve.

On occasion in the long "hourglass"-shaped nose characterized by a narrow middle vault and short nasal bones, cartilage spreader grafts sutured between the septum and upper lateral cartilages should be contemplated for both functional and aesthetic improvement.

NASOFRONTAL ANGLE ALIGNMENT

In patients in whom the nasofrontal angle is poorly defined or in need of repositioning, weakening of the bone in the desired area is accomplished before bony hump removal. At the exact site in the midline where the new nasofrontal angle is desired, *a 2-mm osteotome is driven transcutaneously* into the midline of the nasal bone (Fig. 7–25A). By angulating this small osteotome later-ally on either side, the exact cephalic extent of bony hump removal may be controlled by scoring the bone in a horizontal line. Thus during the bony hump removal phase of profile alignment, the nasal bones fracture cephalically where this weakening maneuver has established a bony dehiscence, allowing the surgeon some additional control over the ultimate site of the nasofrontal angle.

In patients in whom the nasofrontal angle is over deep, augmentation with residual septal cartilage grafts or remnants of the excised alar cartilages provides a beneficial aesthetic refinement, raising the nasal bony profile to achieve a more elegant, strong profile (Fig. 7–25B, C). Further profile enhancements may be favorably developed with contouring cartilage grafts positioned along the dorsum, supratip area, infratip lobule, columella, and nasolabial angle (Fig. 7–25D).

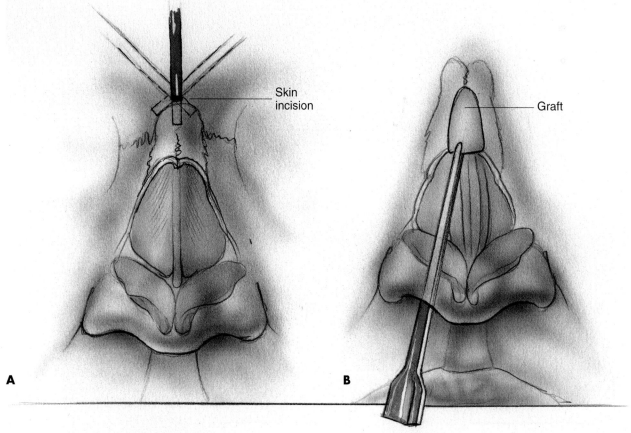

A

Skin
incision

B

Graft

Figure 7–25. (A) To precisely determine the cephalic extent of hump removal, a 2-mm osteotome is tapped transcutaneously through the skin and into the nasal bones at the nasion. Scoring of the bone is then carried out by angulating the 2-mm osteotome to create weakening of the bone at the level desired. **(B)** Augmentation of the overdeep, nasal frontal angle with a cartilage graft is indicated in patients in whom the root of the nose is overdeep.

BONY PYRAMYID NARROWING AND ALIGNMENT

Osteotomies, the most traumatic of all surgical maneuvers during nasal surgery, are best delayed until the final step in the planned surgical sequence, when vasoconstriction exerts its maximal influence and the nasal splint may be promptly positioned. Swelling and ecchymosis are thus diminished or avoided entirely.

During the typical reduction rhinoplasty, hump removal inevitably results in an excessive plateaulike width to the nasal dorsum, requiring narrowing of the bony and cartilaginous pyramids to restore a natural, more narrow frontal appearance to the operated nose.

The lateral bony sidewalls (consisting of the nasal bones and maxillary ascending processes) must be *completely mobilized* by nongreenstick fractures and moved medialward (exceptions may exist in older patients with more fragile bones in whom greenstick fractures may be acceptable or even preferable to prevent excessive instability of more brittle bones). The upper lateral cartilages are also moved medially because of their stable attachment cephalically to the undersurface of the nasal bones.

MEDIAL-OBLIQUE OSTEOTOMIES

To facilitate atraumatic low lateral osteotomy execution, *medial-oblique osteotomies* angled laterally 15 to 20 degrees from the vertical midline are preferred unless the bones are very short or thin (Fig. 7–26A). By creating an osteotomy dehiscence at the intended cephalic apex of the lateral osteotomy, the surgeon exerts added control of the *exact site of back-fracture* in the lateral bony sidewall during low lateral osteotomy.

A 2 to 3 mm unguarded sharp micro-osteotome is positioned intranasally at the cephalic extent of the removal

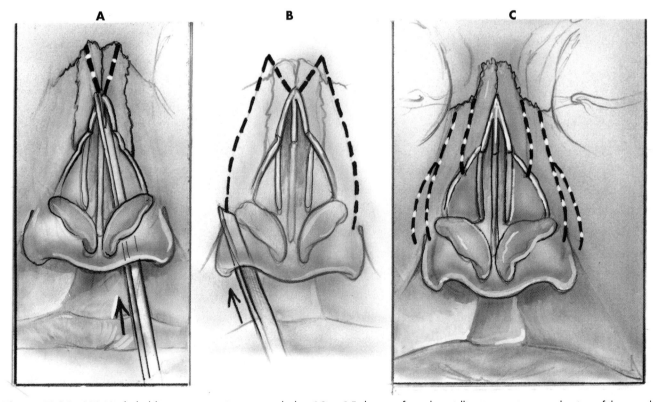

Figure 7–26. (A) Medial oblique osteotomies are angled at 12 to 15 degrees from the midline to create a weakening of the nasal bones to control the site of exact back-fracture. **(B)** Curved low lateral osteotomies are created with a 2- or 3-mm osteotome along the ascending process of the maxilla to meet the weakened segment of bone created by the medial oblique osteotomies. Lateral infracture of the sidewalls is thus controlled by the surgeon, and aberrant fractures are uncommon. **(C)** Multiple osteotomies at different levels may be required to adequately infracture and straighten nasal bones, particularly when the nasal bony sidewalls are asymmetric.

of the bony hump; if no hump removal has been necessary, the site of osteotome positioning is at the caudal extent of the nasal bones in the midline. The osteotome is driven cephalomedially to the intended osteotomy apex at an angle of 15 to 20 degrees, depending on the shape of the nasal bony sidewall. Little trauma results from medial-oblique osteotomies, which prevent the ever present possibility of eccentric or asymmetric surgical fractures developing when lateral osteotomies alone are performed.

LOW LATERAL CURVED MICRO-OSTEOTOMIES

Use of small micro-osteotomes to accomplish the desired infracture of the lateral bony sidewalls results in a *significant reduction of surgical trauma*. Furthermore, no need exists for traditional elevation of the periosteum along the pathway of the lateral fractures because the small osteotomes require little space for their cephalic progression. Appropriately, the intact periosteum stabilizes and internally splints the complete fractures, facilitating controlled and precise healing.

The low curved lateral osteotomy is initiated by pressing the sharp osteotome through the vestibular skin to encounter the bony margin of the pyriform aperture at or just above the inferior turbinate attachment. Beginning the osteotomy at this site preserves the bony sidewall width along the floor of the nose (where narrowing would achieve no favorable aesthetic improvement but might compromise the lower nasal airway without purpose). The osteotome is then driven in a slightly curved direction, first toward the base of the maxilla, curving next up along the nasomaxillary junction to encounter the previously created medial-oblique osteotomy. A complete, controlled, and *atraumatic* fracture of the bony sidewall is thus created, allowing infracture without excessively traumatic infracture pressure maneuvers (Fig. 7–26B). *Immediate finger pressure* is applied bilaterally over the lateral osteotomy sites to forestall further any extravasation of blood into the soft tissues. In reality, no bleeding ordinarily occurs during lateral osteotomy performance because the soft tissues embrac-

ing the bony sidewalls remain essentially undamaged by the diminutive osteotomes.

In most rhinoplasty procedures, controlled nasal fractures as the result of osteotomies should create definite mobility of the bony sidewalls stabilized by the internal and external periosteum, which bridges the nasal fragments on either side of the osteotomy pathway. Large guarded osteotomes destroy this vital periosteal sling, potentially rendering the bony fragments unstable and susceptible to eccentric or asymmetric healing.

MULTIPLE OSTEOTOMIES

In deviated noses characterized by essentially convex or concave bony asymmetries, excessively wide or extremely thick bones (including certain revision rhinoplasties), *double lateral osteotomies* may be necessary for improved mobilization and regularization of the nasal bony sidewalls. In such cases the higher (more anterior) osteotomy cut should be accomplished before the low curved lateral osteotomy (Fig. 7–26C).

ALAR REDUCTION TECHNIQUES

Usually the final step in the sequence of surgical steps in rhinoplasty, *alar base reduction and sculpturing*, must be considered when the alae are overlarge, flare excessively, or are asymmetric. Alar wedge excisions of various geometric designs and dimensions are necessary to improve nasal balance and harmony (Fig. 7–21). These excision dimensions are determined by the present and intended shape of the nostril aperture, the degree and attitude of the lateral alar flare, the width and shape of the nostril sill, and the thickness of the alae.

Whenever possible, conservative internal nostril floor excisions are preferred to avoid cutting across the nostril sill and leaving a visible scar. If more substantial alar excisions are required, the incision should be sited 1 to 2 mm *above the alar-facial crease*, rather than placing the incision exactly within the crease. This allows improved suture repair with 5-0 *mild chromic catgut sutures*, reinforced by tissue glue, and significantly diminishes the appearance of any suture marks after healing. Closure may be alternately carried out with tissue glue for exact epithelial apposition after buried deep suture(s) of 5-0 polydioxanone (PDS) have closed the alar wound.

NASAL TOILETTE, DRESSINGS, AND SPLINT

Final subtle nasal refinements are now completed, which may include caudal septal reduction, resection of excessive vestibular skin and mucous membrane, trimming of the caudal margins of the upper lateral cartilages (only if overlong or projecting into the vestibule), columellar narrowing, and final inspection and refinement of the nasal profile. These final maneuvers are effected with the assistant maintaining constant finger pressure over the lateral osteotomy sites to prevent even minimal oozing and intraoperative swelling.

All incisions are now closed completely with 4-0 or 5-0 chromic catgut sutures. No permanent sutures are used. Transcolumellar incisions used in the open approach require *meticulous closure with 7-0 nylon.*

Nasal dressings are immediately applied. *No intranasal dressing or packing is necessary in routine rhinoplasty.* If septoplasty has been an integral part of the operation, a folded strip of Telfa is placed into each nostril along the floor of the nose to absorb any drainage (transseptal quilting mattress sutures act as the sole internal nasal splint for the septum, completely obliterating the submucoperichondrial dead spaces and fixing the septal elements in place during healing).

The external splint consists of a layer of compressed Gelfoam placed along the dorsum and stabilized in place with flesh-colored Micropore tape, extending over and laterally beyond the lateral osteotomy sites. A small aluminum and Velcro (Denver) splint applied firmly over the nose and maintained for 5 to 7 days completes the splinting process.

MODIFICATIONS

Because individual nasal anatomy is marvelously varied, modifications and departures from the approaches and techniques described will be necessary on occasion. *Surgeons should base thin surgical decisions and manipulations entirely on the anatomy encountered,* enacting surgical changes on the basis of the known principles of rhinoplasty just discussed.

Commonly used modifications in rhinoplasty include the following.

- Augmentation and contouring with *septal or auricular cartilage autografts.* Supportive cartilage autografts are useful as nasal struts, tip grafts, and alar battens for correction of inspiratory alar collapse (Fig. 7–27A–C). Contouring cartilage grafts improve the over-deep nasofrontal angle, elevate the saddled nasal bony or cartilaginous dorsum (Fig. 7–28), efface depressions in the tip or supratip region, improve the angulation of the columella, and plump the nasolabial angle. Grafts commonly require beveling their cut edges to avoid creating visible or palpable step deformities beneath the overlying epithelium. Additional smoothing and burnishing is ideally accomplished by sanding with a Bovie scratch pad.
- Nasal obstruction caused by overlarge inferior turbinates is managed by a *submucous reduction of the inferior concha,* suturing the turbinate back against the lateral nasal wall to enlarge the cross-sectional airway, sacrificing only a minimum of turbinate tissue. The upper lateral cartilages are routinely left attached to the quadrangular cartilage unless they are responsible for participating in a significant twist deformity of the nose.
- *Flaring medial crural footplates and associated excess columellar soft tissue,* responsible for an overwide colummella, may be delivered through small incisions over their summits and sutured together in the midline or shave-excised to narrow the columellar base.

SURGICAL LANDMARKS AND DANGER POINTS

Landmarks of vital importance have been described under the section on surgical anatomy. The surgeon should take extra care to attend to the following.

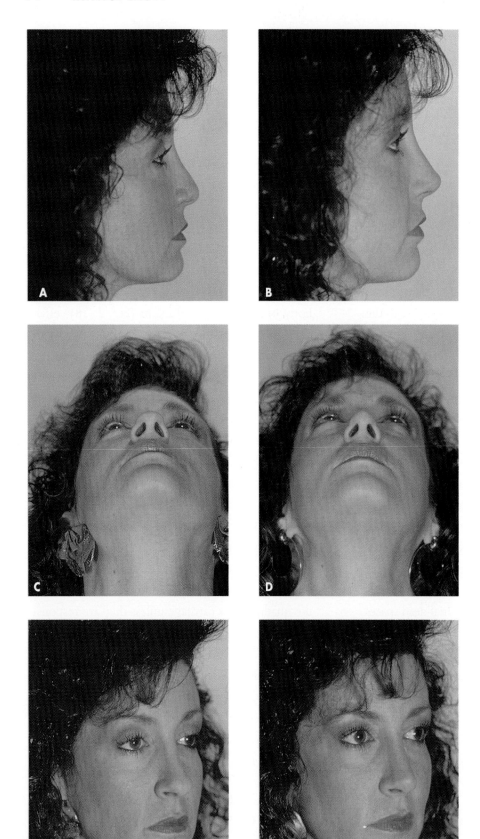

Figure 7-27. Preoperative and postoperative photographs of a patient who required a nasal tip graft, bilateral alar battens, and a cartilaginous strut to support and project the nasal tip and alar sidewalls. Preoperative **(A)** and postoperative **(B)** lateral views. Preoperative **(C)** and postoperative **(D)** basal views. Preoperative **(E)** and postoperative **(F)** oblique views.

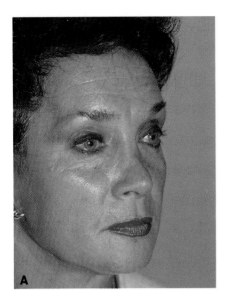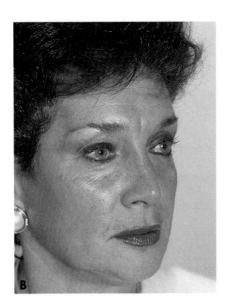

Figure 7–28. Preoperative **(A)** and postoperative **(B)** views of patient whose saddle nose deformity is corrected with a dual-layer onlay cartilage graft from the nasal septum.

- Every effort must be made to sculpture the paired alar cartilages symmetrically to control symmetric healing.
- Overaggressive sacrifice of the lateral crus and injudicious division of the residual complete strip runs the risk of eventual alar collapse with consequent airway blockade.
- Overreduction of the anterior septal angle can lead to a loss of tip support sufficient to result in tip ptosis in the early postoperative period.
- The underlapping relationship of the cephalic margins of the upper lateral cartilages to the caudal aspects of the nasal bones should be religiously preserved, avoiding avulsion deformities leading to collapse of the middle vault of the nose.
- Lateral osteotomies are best initiated high on the ascending process of the maxilla, curved lower toward the face as the bony cut proceeds cephalically, and then inclined medially and upward to meet the medial-oblique osteotomy. This maneuver thus preserves a triangle of bone along the lateral floor of the nasal vault, avoiding unnecessary airway narrowing in a region in which excessive narrowing results in little or no aesthetic improvement. The lacrimal sac is potentially at risk if osteotomy cuts are maldirected laterally; however, the thick bone of the lacrimal crest serves as a strong buttress against penetration.
- Dissecting within the established favorable tissue planes within the nose leads to minimal intraoperative bleeding, little postoperative swelling, diminished scar tissue fibrosis, and more rapid controlled healing.

POSTOPERATIVE COURSE

Strong emphasis must be placed on patient cooperation and self-discipline in the postoperative period. Because essentially no pain results from carefully performed atraumatic rhinoplasty, patients may, unless warned to the contrary, disregard important postoperative care principles. Written instructions, provided for the family and the patient, are highly useful (Fig. 7–29).

Bedrest with the head elevated 30 to 45 degrees is recommended for 24 hours. Early ambulation is beneficial, as long as no strenuous physical activities are carried out.

The intranasal dressing of rolled Telfa is removed at 12 to 24 hours after surgery; no further intranasal dressing or packing is necessary or useful. Routine antibiotics are not used unless significant autografting has been carried out; in the latter circumstance a cephalosporin (Ceclor) is given daily in divided oral doses for 5 days. Diet is not restricted; however, extensive chewing and talking should be avoided in patients in whom more extensive surgery of the tip-lip complex has been necessary. Any nose-blowing

PATIENT INSTRUCTIONS FOLLOWING NASAL PLASTIC SURGERY

A. INTRODUCTION

Please read and familiarize yourself with these instructions both <u>BEFORE</u> and <u>AFTER</u> surgery. By following them carefully you will assist in obtaining the best possible result from your surgery. If questions arise, do not hesitate to communicate with me and discuss your questions at any time. Take this list to the hospital with you and <u>begin observing these directions on the day of surgery</u>.

B. INSTRUCTIONS

1. Do not blow nose until instructed. Wipe or dab nose gently with Kleenex, if necessary.

2. Change dressing under nose (if present) until drainage stops.

3. The nasal cast will remain in place for approximately one week and will be removed in the office. <u>Do not</u> disturb it; <u>keep it dry</u>.

4. Avoid foods that require prolonged chewing. Otherwise, your diet has no restrictions.

5. Avoid extreme physical activity. Obtain more rest than you usually get and avoid exertion, including athletic activities and intercourse.

6. Brush teeth gently with a soft toothbrush only. Avoid manipulation of upper lip to keep nose at rest.

7. Avoid excess or prolonged telephone conversations and social activities for at least 10-14 days.

8. You may wash your face - carefully avoid the dressing. Take <u>tub baths</u> until the dressings are removed.

9. Avoid smiling, grinning and excess facial movements for one week.

10. Do not wash hair for one week unless you have someone do it for you. **DO NOT GET NASAL DRESSINGS WET**.

11. Wear clothing that fastens in front or back for one week. Avoid slipover sweaters, T-shirts and turtlenecks.

12. Absolutely avoid sun or sun lamps for 6 weeks after surgery; heat may cause the nose to swell. Thereafter use sunscreens.

13. Don't swim for one month, since injuries are common during swimming.

14. Don't be concerned if, following removal of dressing, the nose, eyes and upper lip show some swelling and discoloration - this usually clears in 2-3 weeks. In certain patients it may require 12 - 18 months for all swelling to completely subside.

15. Take only medications prescribed by your doctor(s).

16. Do not wear regular glasses or sunglasses which rest on the bridge of the nose for at least 4 weeks. We will instruct you in the method of taping the glasses to your forehead to avoid pressure on the nose.

17. Contact lenses may be worn within 2-3 days after surgery.

18. After the doctor removes your nasal cast, the skin of the nose may be cleansed gently with a mild soap or Vaseline Intensive Care Lotion. <u>BE GENTLE</u>. Makeup may be used as soon as bandages are removed. To cover discoloration, you may use "ERASE" by Max Factor, "COVER AWAY" by Adrien Arpel, or "ON YOUR MARK" by Kenneth.

19. <u>DON'T TAKE CHANCES!</u> - If you are concerned about anything you consider significant, call me at 773-472-7559.

20. When we remove your splint, your nose will be swollen and will remain so for several weeks. In fact, <u>it takes at least one year for all swelling to subside</u>.

Figure 7-29. Patient instructions after nasal plastic surgery.

in the first 10 days must be unilateral and gentle. Intranasal blood crusting may be softened by the use of hydrogen peroxide applied with a cotton applicator around the nostril margins only; saline nosedrops also soften intranasal collection of crusted blood.

The nasal splint is removed at 5 to 7 days by gently teasing it away from the nasal skin with a dull elevator or nonpointed scissors. Because the dorsum is covered by a layer of Gelfoam, the splint easily lifts away from the healing skin *without disturbing the epithelium or underlying layers of newly forming subcutaneous fibrosis.* Additional splinting or taping of the nose is generally without value unless abundant scar tissue has been excised in a revision rhinoplasty; compression taping of the tip and supratip regions may then be useful for several additional days.

Sun avoidance and reduction of activities that produce overheating are recommended for several weeks, along with a number of additional precautions.

Trauma must be religiously avoided; all contact sports activities are prohibited for a minimum of 6 weeks.

Patients are examined postoperatively at 1 week, 3, 6 and 12 months and at yearly intervals thereafter for as long as possible. Long-term follow-up provides an invaluable self-teaching asset to the surgeon as he or she witnesses the unfolding of longitudinal dynamics of healing over a prolonged period. Only in this manner can rhinoplasty techniques be adequately evaluated, modified, and reinforced. *The surgeon who elects not to evaluate patients over long periods is deprived of invaluable experience that is essential to a complete understanding of rhinoplasty surgery.*

COMPLICATIONS AND SEQUELAE

Because septorhinoplasty is an exacting operation, any slightly imperfect outcome may be regarded by some as a complication. In experienced hands rhinoplasty results are uniformly highly satisfactory and fulfilling; significant complications are rare. The ideal end result after rhinoplasty must produce a happy patient and proud surgeon; anything short of this outcome might be considered a complication.

Minor revision procedures after primary rhinoplasty procedures are common in anywhere from 5 to 10% of patients. Such revisions (most commonly performed under local anesthetic as a minor outpatient procedure) should be anticipated in the hands of even the most expert surgeons to place the "finishing touches" on their work. The exacting control of healing remains the most challenging problem in nasal surgery, hence minor touch-up procedures become necessary, particularly as patients become more sophisticated and demanding in the quest for perfection.

Significant postsurgical complications include bleeding, infection, prolonged swelling, airway obstruction, redeviation of a twisted nose, tip ptosis, and dorsum irregularities.

Bleeding may occur immediately after surgery or in the first several days thereafter. Most bleeding episodes become manifest when an intranasal soft clot persists, leading to annoying persist oozing. Evacuation of the clot by suction or gentle nose-blowing followed by finger compression of the nose for a full 15 minutes will control most such episodes. Brisk hemorrhage demands control by accepted principles of the treatment of epistaxis. Packing used should, if possible and practical, avoid disturbing the newly structured nasal components. Careful and complete suture closure of all nasal incisions, coupled with gentle and atraumatic surgical technique, essentially eliminates any significant postoperative hemorrhage development.

Prolonged and extensive intranasal packing sets the stage for edema, swelling, lymphatic and venous obstruction, and secretion stasis and therefore contributes to the potential for infection, which is a rare postoperative occurrence. Suture fixation of the reconstructed septum eliminates the need for traditional packing, thus effectively eliminating the causal conditions potentiating the infection process.

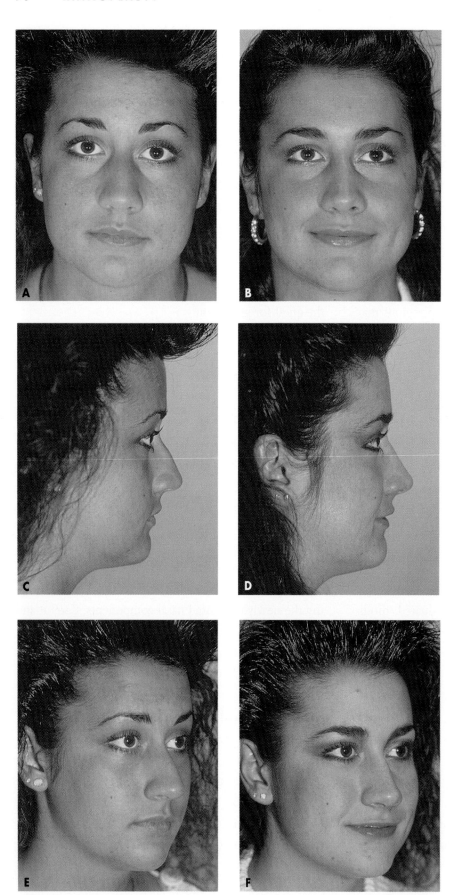

Figure 7–30. Two-year outcome in patient operated on by means of a cartilage-splitting approach, preserving a residual complete strip of 70% of the alar cartilage. Preoperative **(A)** and postoperative **(B)** frontal views. Preoperative **(C)** and postoperative **(D)** lateral views. Preoperative **(E)** and postoperative **(F)** oblique views. Preoperative **(G)** and postoperative **(H)** base views.

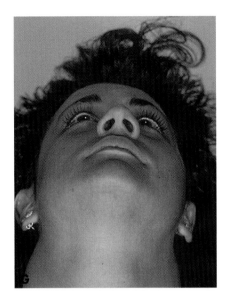
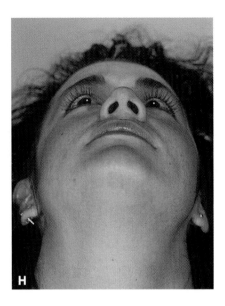

Figure 7-30 (continued)

Prolonged swelling is most common (and to be anticipated) in patients with thick, sebaceous skin. Excessively traumatic surgical technique with intraoperative swelling sets the stage for this avoidable complication.

Airway obstruction results from failure to recognize and correct bony or cartilaginous deviations, redeviation of inadequately repaired septal deformities, or overlarge nasal turbinates or occasionally alar collapse (the consequence of overaggressive excision of alar cartilages in patients with poorly supported alar sidewalls).

Re-deviation of the twisted nose is a common occurrence in patients with marked deformities and scarring of the cartilaginous and bony vaults, particularly when the inherent interlocked stresses twisted cartilage have not been properly released. Inadequate osteotomies of the greenstick variety predispose to redeviation.

Tip ptosis is the consequence of needless sacrifice of major tip support mechanisms with early or late settling of the tip and nasal base. The aesthetic relationship between the projected nasal tip and the supratip region is thus lost. In certain patients failure to recognize tip sup-

port loss and reconstitute it (cartilage struts or tip grafts) produces this all-too-common complication.

Dorsum irregularities, which are particularly common in thin-skinned patients, occur either early or late in the healing period. Small tissue fragments left behind may spoil an otherwise ideal profile, although most commonly profile problems result from inadequate smoothing of the bony and cartilaginous dorsum.

Because an infinite variety of nasal anatomic types are encountered in a diverse rhinoplasty, limitless minor complications are possible from reconstructive surgery. A nose made over-large or over-small for the patient's body and facial proportions represents a failure regardless of the beauty of the nasal outcome. Failure to proportionately reconstitute the individual anatomic component units of the nose into a harmonious blend leads to dissatisfaction. In the final analysis, judgments about the aesthetic and respiratory outcomes of septorhinoplasty emanate from the operated patient, whose happiness and nasal health stamp the outcome with approval or failure (Fig. 7-30 and 7-31).

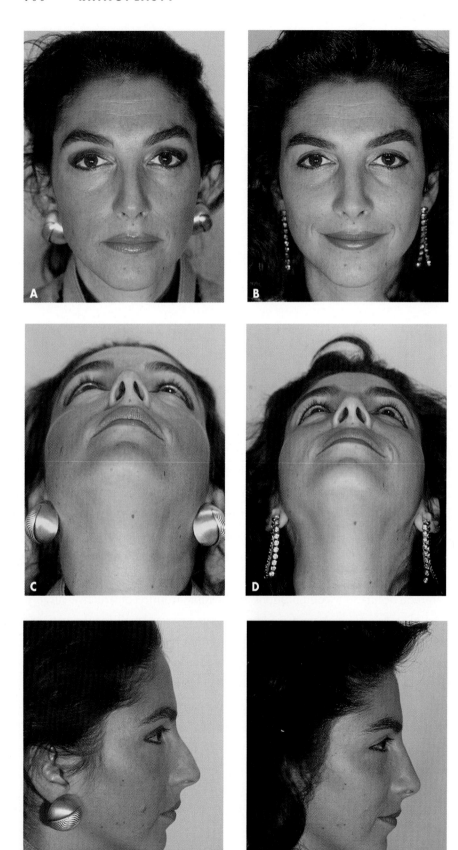

Figure 7–31. Two-year outcome of patient operated on by retrograde approach preserving most of the alar cartilages and a strong, high profile. Preoperative **(A)** and postoperative **(B)** frontal views. Preoperative **(C)** and postoperative **(D)** base views. Preoperative **(E)** and postoperative **(F)** lateral views. Preoperative **(G)** and postoperative **(H)** oblique views.

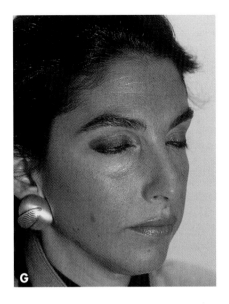
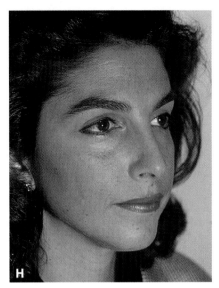

Figure 7–31. *(continued)*

PEARLS

- Exacting analysis of patient photographs (or color slides) preoperatively coupled with orchestrated step-by-step rehearsal of the procedure facilitates the surgical procedure.
- Sharp knife dissection results in less intraoperative bleeding and reduced postoperative scarring. When intraoperative bleeding does occur, it is best controlled by finger pressure for several minutes until hemostasis is complete.
- Reconstruction of the septum is usually best carried out at the outset of septorhinoplasty, particularly in twisted noses.
- Fiberoptic-lighted specula and retractors aid greatly in intranasal visualization and decision making.
- Large noses, well-proportioned after surgery, are preferable to ill-proportioned, over-reduced smaller noses.
- The alar cartilages are best preserved, conservatively reduced, or reoriented to maintain a more natural tip appearance.
- Permanent septocolumellar "orthopedic" sutures positioned to elevate the nasal tip provide little or no long-term tip support or projection; their use is discouraged.

- Revision rhinoplasty should ordinarily await tissue healing of 1 year or more. Exceptions may exist to this rule for completing a greenstick osteotomy, adding cartilaginous tip support grafts, carrying out alar reduction procedures, or correcting a deviated septum.
- Too superficial undermining of the soft tissues over the dorsum may lead to telangiectasia formation.

SUGGESTED READINGS

Brennan HG, Parkes ML. Septal surgery: The high septal transfixion. *Int Surg.* 1973; 58:732.

Fry HJJ. Nasal skeletal trauma and the interlocked stresses of the nasal septal cartilage. *Br J Plast Surg.* 1967; 20:146.

Gilbert JG, Felt LJ. The nasal aponeurosis and its role in rhinoplasty. *Arch Otolaryngol.* 1955; 61:433.

Goin MK, Goin JM. *Changing the Body.* Baltimore: Williams & Wilkins; 1981.

Goodman WS, Charles DA. Technique of external rhinoplasty. *Can J Otolaryngol.* 1978; 7:13.

Gunter JP. Anatomical observations of the lower lateral cartilages. *Arch Otolaryngol.* 1969; 89:61.

Janeke JB, Wright WK. Studies of the support of the nasal tip. *Arch Otolaryngol.* 1971; 93:458.

Natvig P, et al. Anatomical details of the osseous-cartilaginous framework of the nose. *Plast Reconstr Surg.* 1971; 48:528.

Ortiz-Monisterio F, Olmedo A, Oscoy LO. The use of cartilage grafts in primary aesthetic rhinoplasty. *Plast Reconstr Surg.* 1981; 67:597.

Padovan IF. External approach in rhinoplasty. Sur ORL Lug. 1966; 3–40:354.

Parkes ML, Brennan HG. High septal transfixion to shorten the nose. Plast Reconstr Surg. 1970; 45:487.

Smith TW. As clay in the potter's hand: A review of 221 rhinoplasties. Ohio Med J. 1967; 63:1055.

Sheen JH. Achieving more nasal tip projection by use of small autogenous vomer or septal cartilage grafts. Plast Reconstr Surg. 1975; 56:35. Discussion by Horton CE. Plast Reconstr Surg. 1975; 56:211.

Sheen JH. Secondary rhinoplasty. Plast Reconstr Surg. 1975; 56:137.

Sheen JH. Aesthetic Rhinoplasty. St. Louis: Mosby–Year Book; 1985.

Skoog T. Plastic Surgery. Philadelphia: W.B. Saunders Co.; 1975.

Straatsma BR, Straatsma CR. The anatomical relationship of the lateral nasal cartilage to the nasal bone and the cartilaginous nasal septum. Plast Reconstr Surg. 1951; 8:443.

Tardy ME. Rhinoplasty tip ptosis: Etiology and prevention. Laryngoscope. 1973; 83:923–929.

Tardy ME. Septal perforations. Otolaryngol Clin North Am. 1973; 6:711–714.

Tardy ME. Nasal reconstruction and rhinoplasty. In: Ballenger's Textbook of Otolaryngology. ed 12, Philadelphia: Lea & Febiger; 1977.

Tardy ME. Surgical correction of facial deformities. In: Ballenger's Textbook of Otolaryngology, ed. 12. Philadelphia: Lea & Febiger; 1977.

Tardy ME. Rhinoplasty in midlife. Symposium on the ageing face. Otolaryngol Clin North Am. 1980; 13:289–303.

Tardy ME. Rhinoplasty, Color Monograph. Richard's Manufacturing Co.; 1980.

Tardy ME. Rhinoplasty. Baltimore: Williams & Wilkins; 1984.

Tardy ME. Rhinoplasty. In: Cummings CW, ed. Otolaryngology–Head and Neck Surgery, vol I. St. Louis: Mosby–Year Book; 1986.

Tardy ME. Transdomal suture refinement of the nasal tip. Fac Plast Surg. 1987; 4:4.

Tardy ME. Rhinoplasty: The Art and the Science. Vols I & II. Philadelphia: W.B. Saunders Co.; 1987.

Tardy ME, Broadway D. Graphic record-keeping in rhinoplasty: A valuable self-learning device. Fac Plast Surg. 1989; 6:2.

Tardy ME, Denneny JC. Micro-osteotomies in rhinoplasty: A technical refinement. Fac Plast Surg. 1984; 1:2, 137–145.

Tardy ME, Denneny JC, Fritch MH. The versatile cartilage autograft in reconstruction of the nose and face. Laryngoscope. 1985; 95(5):523–533.

Tardy ME, Hewell TS. Nasal tip refinement: Reliable approaches and sculpture techniques. Fac Plast Surg. 1984; 1:2, 87–124.

Tardy ME, Tom L. Anesthesia in rhinoplasty. Fac Plast Surg. 1984; 1:2, 146–156.

Tardy ME, Toriumi D. Alar retraction: Composite graft correction. Fac Plast Surg. 1989; 6:2.

Tardy ME, Schwartz MS, Parras G. Saddle nose deformity: Autogenous graft repair. Fac Plast Surg. 1989; 6:2.

Tardy ME, et al. The over-projecting tip: Anatomic variation and targeted solutions. Fac Plast Surg. 1987; 4:4.

Tardy ME, et al. The cartilaginous pollybeak: Etiology, prevention and treatment. Fac Plast Surg. 1989; 6:2.

Webster RC. Advances in surgery of the tip: Intact rim cartilage techniques and the tip-columella-lip aesthetic complex. Otolaryngol Clin North Am. 1975; 8:615.

Webster RC, Smith RC. Rhinoplasty. In: Goldwyn RM, ed. Long Term Results in Plastic and Reconstructive Surgery. Boston: Little Brown & Co., Inc.; 1980.

Rhinoplasty

Aesthetic Facial Plastic Surgery, edited by Thomas Romo, III, and Arthur L. Millman, Thieme Medical Publishers, Inc., New York, New York, Copyright © 2000.

CHAPTER 8

A Plastic Surgeon's Perspective

ROD J. ROHRICH AND ARSHAD MUZAFFAR

In rhinoplasty, the difference between a good and poor result can be 1 to 2 mm. To obtain consistent results, the surgeon must perform a complete nasal history and anatomic examination to determine the patient's problems and goals and then arrive at an individualized preoperative plan. Success in rhinoplasty is best obtained at the primary procedure, and this requires accurate nasal analysis, meticulous planning and operative execution, and painstaking postoperative care.

A systematic approach by use of the open rhinoplasty technique is described to aid the rhinoplastic surgeon in obtaining optimal aesthetic and functional results in patients with primary nasal deformities. The open approach allows for a more precise intraoperative anatomic diagnosis and subsequent complete correction of the nasal deformity. Attaining consistent and reproducible functional and aesthetic results in the primary rhinoplasty patient remains a challenge. Indeed, 5 to 12% of rhinoplasty patients require secondary rhinoplasty[1]. By following a systematic approach with the full and undistorted exposure of the nasal framework afforded by the open rhinoplasty technique, the surgeon can most reliably and consistently modify the framework to achieve optimal functional and aesthetic results.

ADVANTAGES AND DISADVANTAGES

The major advantage of the open rhinoplasty approach (Fig. 8–1, Table 8–1) is that it provides unparalleled anatomic exposure and a direct binocular view of the nasal framework without distortion. If the surgeon is familiar with the effect of the underlying framework on the shape of the nose, it becomes a simple task to create the desired framework and nasal shape.

With complete exposure, the nasal framework structures can be stabilized in their correct anatomic positions. Should cartilage grafting be required, the graft can be accurately modeled and positioned. Furthermore, for teaching purposes, the entire operation is done under direct vision so that rhinoplasty techniques become much more accessible to the novice.[2,3] After reconstruction of the nasal framework, the resulting position and shape can be assessed and any residual deformities corrected. The skin is redraped to assess the effect of the new framework on the external appearance. Further adjustments can be made before to closure of the transcolumellar incision if the shape is not satisfactory.

The principal objection to the open rhinoplasty approach is the transcolumellar scar. The potential disadvantages of wound separation, prolonged operative time, prolonged tip edema, and delayed secondary healing have not occurred in our experience with the open rhinoplasty approach.

The distinct advantages provided by the 6-mm skin incision traversing the columella far outweigh its potential disadvantages in the management of patients with primary nasal deformities that require significant tip and dorsum reshaping.

PATIENT SELECTION

The initial interview allows the surgeon to determine whether the patient is a candidate for rhinoplasty. During the interview, as the history and nasal examination are performed, the patient's expectations are voiced, and the surgeon assesses the realistic possibilities for preoperative planning. The patient should specifically describe any complaints about his or her nasal appearance and function and then rate them in order of importance. The sur-

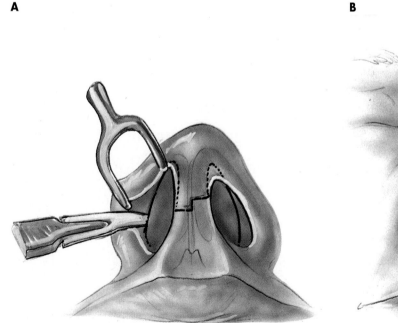

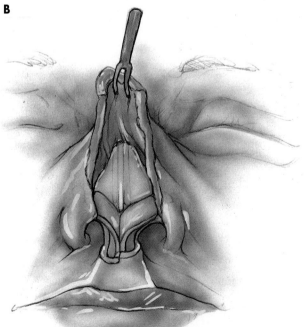

Figure 8–1. (A) The transcolumellar stairstep incision. **(B)** Exposure of the nasal framework with the open rhinoplasty approach.

Table 8–1 Open Rhinoplasty Approach Rationale

Distinct Advantages	Potential Disadvantages
Binocular visualization	External nasal incision (transcolumellar scar)
Evaluation of complete deformity without distortion	Prolonged operative time
Precise diagnosis and correction of deformities	Protracted nasal tip edema
Allows use of both hands	Columellar incision separation
More options with original tissues and cartilage grafts	Delayed wound healing
Direct control of bleeding with electrocautery	
Suture stabilization of grafts (invisible and visible)	

geon should ask the patient, "If you had only one problem that could be corrected, what would it be?" This "one thing" is then documented verbatim in the patient's notes. A patient who focuses on a minor or uncorrectable problem is most likely to be disappointed regardless of the postoperative aesthetic improvement. It may be wise to avoid operating on such patients.

Specific nasal problems such as asymmetry, tip deformities, supratip deformity, dorsum irregularities, and septal perforations must be delineated and visually shown to the patient. The patient must understand the proposed surgical plan and the potential sequelae. Complications must be completely outlined and disclosure made to obtain an informed consent for rhinoplasty and any other indicated procedure (i.e., graft harvesting).

Photographs are used to illustrate pre-existing problems that will persist postoperatively or inevitable consequences of the reconstruction, such as notches, grooves, and irregularities. Facial disproportions should be clearly pointed out to the patient with an explanation that the asymmetry will not be corrected by the surgery. Some patients may require adjunctive orthognathic or craniofacial procedures.

CHOICE OF PROCEDURE
NASAL HISTORY

A key part of any rhinoplasty planning is the nasal history. This allows the surgeon to determine whether the patient is emotionally, medically, and/or physically prepared for a rhinoplasty.

The emotional stability of the patient is a factor that greatly influences the relationship between the surgeon and the patient. One must learn to differentiate healthy and unhealthy reasons for seeking rhinoplasties. Poor results often stem from emotional dissatisfaction rather than technical failure. Obviously, not every patient seeking rhinoplasty should undergo psychiatric evaluation, but it is critical to review certain issues, such as family conflicts, inadequate feelings, major losses, divorce, immaturity, and unrealistic expectations, to ascertain whether the patient is a rhinoplasty candidate.[4,5] Most patients have realistic expectations and also understand the limitations of surgery. Patients should articulate which aspects of the nose they think should be changed and indicate their priorities in order of importance. Patients should be shown photographs of themselves in different views. These will allow them to focus on those features that most concern them.

A history of allergic disorders, hay fever, or vasomotor rhinitis should alert the surgeon to the possibility of postoperative exacerbations.[6,8] Such difficulties may last for several weeks or months, and the patient should be made aware of this. In cases with a long history of allergic rhinitis, a nasal obstruction is often found.[7,8] This nasal obstruction is primarily a result of hypertrophied inferior turbinates. When the inferior turbinates become engorged, the symptoms are exacerbated, especially at night. These patients typically use antihistamines, local decongestants, and/or different short courses of corticosteroids once or twice a year. Inadequacy of their obstructed inferior turbinate, which normally warms the inspired air, may cause headaches.

The surgeon should question the patient specifically about other illnesses, such as sinusitis, asthma, bronchitis, previous nasal trauma, or operations such as rhinoplasty, septal reconstruction, and sinus surgery. Smoking, alcohol consumption, and various drugs can complicate the operative procedure; for instance, medications containing acetylsalicylic acid may cause increased bleeding.

ANATOMIC EXAMINATION

The external anatomic examination is critical because the surface anatomy of the nose directly reflects the underlying framework. Nasal skin thickness and texture affect rhinoplasty outcomes. Patients with thick sebaceous skin will have more postoperative edema and scar formation. These changes occur late, predominately in the nasal tip area. Conversely, patients with thin nasal skin develop less postoperative edema and scarring and heal more rapidly. Normally, nasal skin is thinner and more mobile in the cephalic zone, and thicker and glandular in the nasal tip zone. The thinnest skin is found over the osteocartilaginous junction, whereas the thickest skin lies over the nasion and supratip dorsum.

To define the deformity, a systematic nasal examination must be done as follows. Starting superiorly, the nasofrontal angle position and depth are noted. The bony pyramid, upper lateral cartilages, and supratip are assessed for their height, width, and symmetry. The nasal tip is analyzed in terms of its projection, rotation, symmetry, and position of the tip-defining points. Increased width, collapse, or retraction of the alae are noted. The columella is inspected for increased or decreased show. The columellar-lobular and columellar-labial angles are measured and compared with the desired angulation.

> Nasofrontal angle position
> Bony pyramid
> Upper lateral cartilages
> Supratip area
> Nasal tip
>   Projection
>   Rotation
>   Symmetry
>   Position of tip-defining points
> Alae
>   Width
>   Collapse
>   Retraction
> Alar-columellar relationship
> Columellar-labial angle
> Intranasal examination
>   Internal nasal valves
>   Septum
>   Turbinates

Internal nasal examination defines the functional deformity. The nasal mucosa is first constricted with oxymetazoline (Afrin) nasal spray. The internal valves are examined by tilting the patient's head back and using a light source to observe narrowing or collapse of the valves with inspiration. The condition of the turbinates and the structure and amount of septum available are documented. Because the septum is the primary source of autogenous graft material, it is essential to ascertain whether the quantity and quality of the septal cartilage will be sufficient for use in reconstruction.

Finally, the overall condition of the soft tissue envelope is evaluated. The surgeon should assess the thickness of the nasal tip skin. Defatting, to re-establish tip projection or definition, must be avoided because this will compromise nasal tip vascularity. The findings of the nasal history and anatomic examination must be meticulously documented.

PHOTOGRAPHIC COMPUTER ANALYSIS

Photographic analysis is essential to rhinoplasty planning, as well as for recording "before" and "after" documentation for medicolegal purposes. Generally, surgeons need a 35-mm SLR camera, macrolens (60 to 100 mm), and dual lighting with blue or black background or digital photography to obtain a 1 : 1 reproduction ratio photograph. To develop a rhinoplasty operative plan, standardized photographic views are analyzed (Fig. 8–2).

The photographs or digital images are analyzed to determine any nonideal nasal/facial anatomic line and landmarks. Computer images can be made, comparing these lines and landmarks to the ideal obtained from our nasal analysis. Computer imaging allows the rhinoplastic surgeon to perform interactively a simulation of nasal changes seen with rhinoplasty. An accurate operative plan is detailed on the rhinoplasty worksheet and taken to the operating room with the patient's photographs and computer images. Computer analysis is used to help visually educate the patient on changes that are potentially feasible with their rhinoplasty.

AESTHETIC ANALYSIS

Aesthetic facial/nasal analysis in the rhinoplasty patient essentially involves proportions.[4,9] The typical proportions

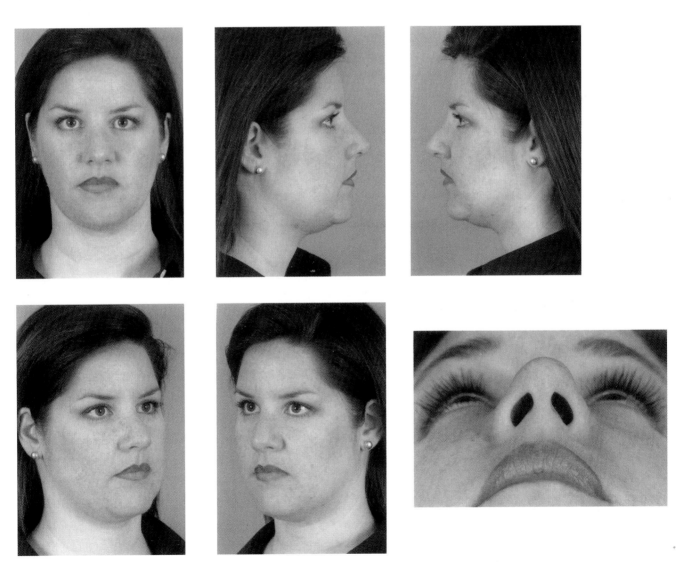

Figure 8–2. Standard photographic views for preoperative analysis.

of a Caucasian woman are used because she is the patient who most commonly seeks rhinoplasty. Variations for men are noted as appropriate.

1. Transverse lines adjacent to the mentum, subnasale, and brow at the level of the suborbital notch and the hairline divide the face into thirds. The upper third is least important for purposes of nasofacial diagnosis. The lower third of the face is split into an upper third and lower two thirds by a transverse line between the oral commissures. A transverse line through the labial mental groove divides the distance from the stomion to the menton in a 1:2 ratio. Byrd and Hobar[10] compare the facial proportions to nasal length and calculates nasal length (r-t) as equal to the distance from the stomion to the menton (s-m). Ideally, nasal tip projection (ap) equals 0.67 × ideal nasal length.

2. By drawing a line perpendicular to a plumb line superimposed over the head and the eyes in straightforward gaze, a natural horizontal facial plan is determined. This may not correspond to Frankfort's line.

3. Attention is now turned to the nose. Any sign of nasal deviation is noted. A line drawn from the midglabellar area to the menton should bisect the nasal ridge, upper lip, and Cupid's bow. In patients with a normal occlusion the midline is the vertical line that passes between the two central incisors.

4. Two slightly curved divergent aesthetic lines extend from the medial superciliary ridges to the tip-defining points to outline the nasal dorsum.

5. The width of the bony base should be 70 to 80% of the normal alar base. If the bony base is wide, however, mobilization of the bones may be necessary to narrow the dorsum.

6. The width of the alar base should approximate the intercanthal distance. If the interalar width is wider than the intercanthal width, one must determine whether this is the result of increased interalar width or alar flaring. Normal flaring in the Cau-

casian woman is 2 mm outside the alar base. If it is >2 mm, an alar base resection should be considered. This should be distinguished from excessive interalar width. If the interalar width is excessive, a nostril sill resection may be indicated. The alar rims are assessed for symmetry and should flare slightly outward in the inferior lateral direction.

7. The outline of the rims and the columella should resemble a "seagull" in gentle flight. The columella lies just inferior to the alar rims on frontal view, giving the outline of the rims and lowest portion of the columella a gentle gullwing appearance.

8. The basal view of the outline of the nasal base should describe an equilateral triangle. The lobular portion of the nose should be in a 1:2 ratio with the columella. The nostril should have a slight teardrop shape with the long axis from the base to the apex in a slight medial direction.

9. On lateral view, the position and depth of the nasofrontal angle should be noted. The deepest portion of the nasofrontal angle should fall between the upper eyelash line and supratarsal fold with the eyes in natural horizontal gaze. The aesthetic nasal dorsum should lie approximately 2 mm behind and parallel to a line from the nasofrontal angle to the tip-defining points in women, but *in men* it should be slightly higher.

10. To assess tip projection in patients with normal upper lip projection, a line is drawn from the alar-cheek junction to the tip of the nose. If 50 to 60% of the tip lies anterior to the vertical line adjacent to the most projecting part of the upper lip, tip projection is normal. If it is >60%, the tip may be overprojecting and require reduction. Ideal nasal length is assessed as a ratio of nasal length (rt) to tip projection (at), 0.67 × rt, according to Byrd's analysis.

11. The degree of supratip break is assessed when the nasal tip projection and dorsum are evaluated. A slight supratip break is preferred in women but not in men. This gives the nose more definition and distinguishes the dorsum from the tip.

12. The degree of tip rotation is assessed by measuring the nasolabial angle. This angle is formed by a straight line through the most anterior and posterior edges of the nostril that transects the plumb line. In women this angle is between 95 and 105 degrees and in men it is between 90 and 95 degrees. This is in contrast to the columellar-labial angle, which is formed at the junction of the columella with the upper lip. Increased fullness in this area usually is caused by a prominent caudal septum and gives the illusion of increased rotation even though the nasolabial angle is normal.

13. The columellar-lobular angle should normally be 45 degrees.

14. The aesthetic relationship of the lip and chin is assessed. The upper lip should project approximately 2 mm anterior to the lower lip. In women, the chin is slightly posterior to the lower lip, approximately 2 to 3 mm. In men, it should be slightly stronger.

OPERATIVE TECHNIQUE

The following technique should serve as a guide to the sequence of steps and the rationale behind them in pri-

mary rhinoplasty. The sequence is altered according to the preoperative nasal analysis and operative goals. An organized approach to the open rhinoplasty is essential in obtaining consistent results.

PREOPERATIVE PREPARATION

After induction of general anesthesia with endotracheal intubation, epinephrine-containing local anesthetic is infiltrated. We use 10 mL of 1% lidocaine with 1 : 100,000 epinephrine to infiltrate the soft tissue envelope and the intranasal mucosa. Injection begins posteriorly on the nasal septum mucosa in a submucoperichondrial plane, proceeding posteriorly to anteriorly, and includes the mucosa along the entire vertical height of the septum. Next, the soft tissue envelope is infiltrated. The infiltration should be evenly distributed. Particular attention is paid to highly vascular anatomic subunits: the midcolumella, lateral nasal walls and dorsum, nasal tip, alar base, and intranasally along the caudal margin of the lower lateral cartilages (Fig. 8–3). The anterior head of the inferior turbinate is also injected when an inferior turbinoplasty is planned.

After completion of local anesthetic infiltration, oxymetazoline-soaked cottonoid pledgets are placed

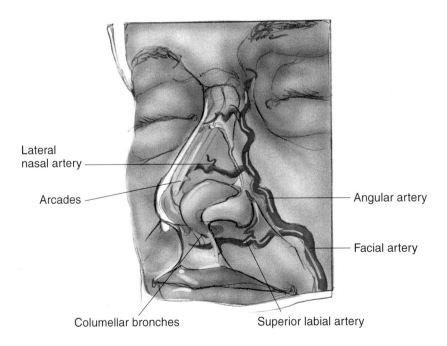

Lateral nasal artery

Arcades

Angular artery

Facial artery

Columellar bronches

Superior labial artery

Figure 8–3. Nasal tip blood supply. FA, facial artery; AA, angular artery; SLA, superior labial artery; LN, lateral nasal artery; CA, columellar artery.

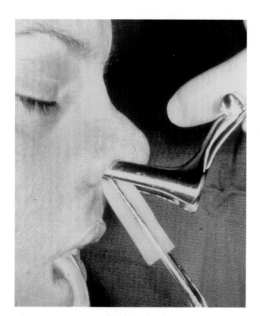

Figure 8–4. Oxymetazoline-soaked cottonoid pledgets are placed into the nose.

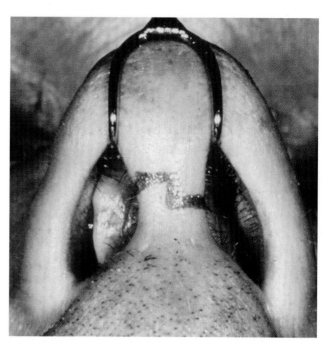

Figure 8–5. The transcolumellar stairstep incision is marked.

into the nose (Fig. 8–4). Three pledgets are placed per side along the middle turbinate, inferomedial septum, and superior nasal vault. Vasoconstriction of these areas will allow maximal intranasal visual exposure. Because the inferomedial septum houses the sphenopalatine vessels, vasoconstriction is especially important here. We prefer oxymetazoline over cocaine as a vasoconstrictive agent. Equivalent mucosal shrinkage is achieved without introducing issues revolving around the use of a controlled substance. If the patient has engorgement of the nasal mucosa or a significant septal spur that obstructs visualization of the intranasal vault, the pledgets should be placed before infiltration of the local anesthetic.

A throat pack is placed to minimize bleeding into the oropharynx. This also minimizes intragastric blood, which contributes to postoperative nausea and vomiting. In addition, blood is prevented from collecting at the endolarynx, which can cause laryngeal irritation with coughing or laryngospasm. The stomach should be suctioned with an orogastric tube before extubation.

STAIRSTEP TRANSCOLUMELLAR INCISION/APPROACH

An incision is made at the narrowest part of the columella, generally located near its midportion (Fig. 8–5). This is done superficially to prevent injury to the underlying medial crura. A stairstep incision is used to camouflage the scar, to provide landmarks for accurate closure, and to prevent linear scar contracture. The incision is extended intranasally by means of an infracartilaginous incision, which follows the caudal border of the medial crura (Fig. 8–6). This incision is continued toward the apex of the middle crus. Laterally, a separate incision is begun in the vestibule along the caudal margin of the lateral crus of the lower lateral cartilage. This is demonstrated by everting the ala with digital pressure externally against a double skin hook placed within the alar rim (Fig. 8–7). The inferior border is visibly evident with this maneuver or can be palpated with a scalpel handle. The incision is extended laterally to medially, staying along the caudal cartilage margin. The two incisions are connected at the middle crus region.

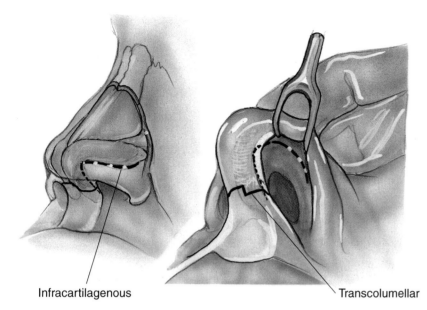

Infracartilagenous

Transcolumellar

Figure 8–6. The transcolumellar and infracartilaginous incisions are joined.

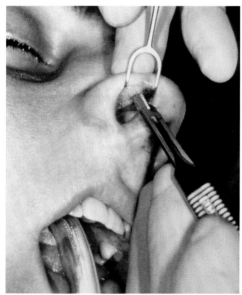

Figure 8–7. Demonstration of the caudal margin of the lateral crus of the lower lateral cartilage.

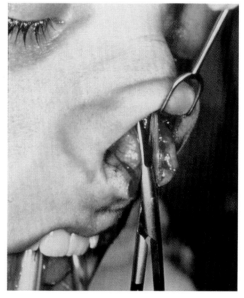

Figure 8–8. Elevation of the soft tissue envelope.

SKIN ENVELOPE DISSECTION

The soft tissue envelope is elevated sharply in a sub-musculoaponeurotic plane up to the bony pyramid (Fig. 8–8). The periosteum is sharply incised and elevated with a Joseph periosteal elevator to the radix area (Fig. 8–9). Laterally, subperiosteal dissection is limited to the extent necessary to allow for bony hump reduction, if indicated.

COMPONENT NASAL DORSUM SURGERY

Skeletonization is described earlier. It is important to maintain as much periosteal attachment of the bony sidewall as possible because it provides significant external support for the nasal pyramid after osteotomy. Likewise, an effort is made to perform an extramucosal hump excision to minimize late scarring with subsequent internal

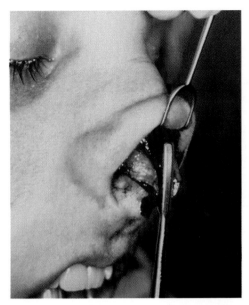

Figure 8–9. Periosteal elevator is used to establish a subperiosteal plane to the radix.

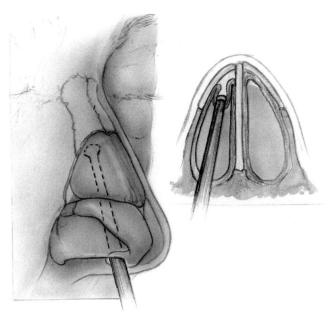

Figure 8–10. Submucosal tunnels are created below the osseocartilaginous roof.

nasal valve dysfunction and to provide a closed space for the safe placement of spreader or dorsal grafts. An extramucosal approach is ensured by initially creating submucosal tunnels beneath the osseocartilaginous roof, before modification of the dorsum (Fig. 8–10).

Dorsal humps are managed according to their size. In general, reduction of small-to-medium dorsal humps (~5 mm) is accomplished by simple rasping (Fig. 8–11). Rasping should be done in short strokes between the nondominant index finger and thumb for maximal control. An oblique angle is maintained when rasping to prevent mechanical avulsion of the upper lateral cartilage. I prefer to use a sharp down-biting Forman diamond rasp. After rasping, the superior edge of the upper lateral cartilage, which projects under the nasal bone, may require trimming to avoid lateral fullness.

Large dorsal humps (>5 mm) are expediently managed by sharp resection with a guarded osteotome. The cartilaginous dorsum is initially reduced as a separate component by lowering the septum and upper lateral cartilages in an extramucosal manner. The sharp guarded osteotome is positioned at the desired level along the cau-

dal margin of the bony pyramid and carefully driven to a predetermined point superiorly. Large hump reductions with a significant open roof deformity will require either a dorsal onlay, if the nasal base is normal, or, more commonly, a lateral percutaneous osteotomy to close the open dorsum (Fig. 8–12). The skin envelope is redraped and a three-point test is performed. The newly contoured nasal dorsum is moistened to allow a finger to glide smoothly across the skin. Three separate digital strokes palpate along the midsagittal dorsum and on either lateral side to ensure a smooth and straight nasal dorsum without irregularity or contour deformity (Fig. 8–13).[10]

After the dorsal septum is reduced to its desired height, spreader grafts are indicated if the lateral dorsal aesthetic lines are too narrow or the middle vault has an inverted V deformity. The mucoperichondrium is elevated 4 to 6 mm from the dorsal septal edge bilaterally. The mucoperiosteum is also elevated medially from the undersurface of the nasal bones and from the perpendicular plate of the ethmoid. Preferably, septal cartilage grafts are designed measuring 25 to 30 mm in length and 3 mm in width for spreader grafts to be placed either

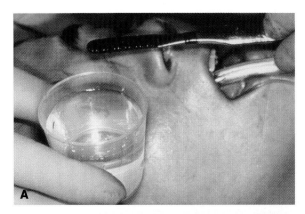

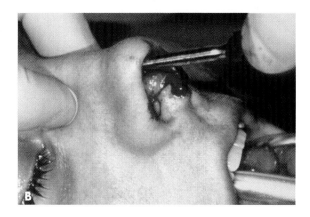

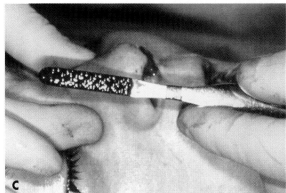

Figure 8-11. (A to C) Simple rasping of the dorsum is used to reduce small-to-medium humps.

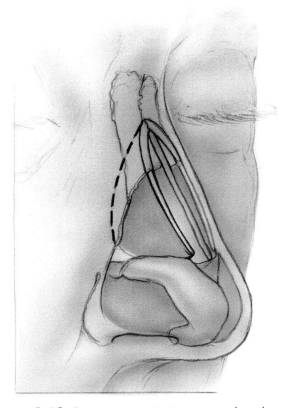

Figure 8-12. Percutaneous osteotomy is used to close the open roof.

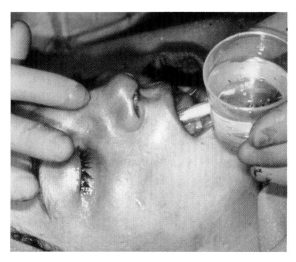

Figure 8-13. The three-point test to assess the new dorsal contour.

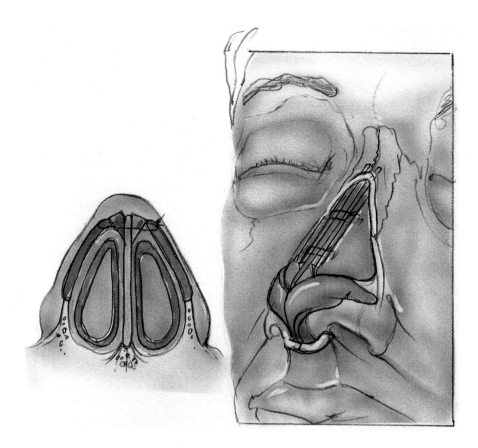

Figure 8–14. Placement of dorsal spreader grafts.

unilaterally or bilaterally, depending on the patient's nasal dorsum (Fig. 8–14).[11,12]

The dorsal cephalic edges of the grafts are obliquely resected to allow them to be placed under the bony dorsum. The grafts are positioned and sutured to the dorsal septum with two to three through-and-through horizontal mattress sutures of 5-0 polydioxanone (PDS). Should *lengthening* of the nose be desired, the caudal ends of the grafts are left long to extend past the septal angle. However, *if lengthening is not desired*, the grafts should stop at the septal angle. Furthermore, the spreader grafts can be placed higher (*visible*) or lower (*invisible*) along the dorsal septum, depending on the clinical situation. Final dorsal trimming occurs after the osteotomies are performed to infracture the nasal bones.

SEPTAL RECONSTRUCTION/CARTILAGE GRAFT HARVEST

If septal cartilage harvest or septal reconstruction is indicated, the intradomal suspensory ligament is incised to expose the anterior septal angle. Starting at the anterior septal angle, a sharp No. 15 scalpel is used to incise the perichondrium and a Cottle elevator is used to elevate the perichondrium toward the floor of the nose to the junction of the septum with the maxillary crest. The elevation is extended posteriorly along the crest. The mucoperichondrium is then elevated off the rest of the nasal septum and the perpendicular plate. This is done bilaterally (Fig. 8–15).

With a No. 15 scalpel starting at the perpendicular plate, the septal cartilage is incised 10 mm below and parallel to the dorsal septal edge down to within 10 mm of the caudal septum. At the caudal edge of the incision, the incision parallels the caudal septum, leaving a 10 mm caudal strut down to the maxillary crest area. With a sharp Cottle elevator, the mucoperichondrium is elevated off the right side of the septum and maxillary crest, but not off the caudal or dorsal septum. The septal cartilage is separated at its junction with the maxillary crest.

A

B

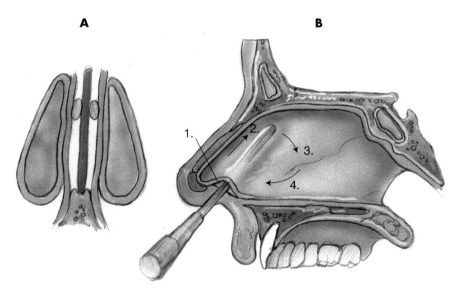

Figure 8–15. (A) The completed septal exposure. **(B)** Subperichondrial dissection of the septum proceeds in the sequence shown.

Angled septal scissors are used to extend the dorsal incision through the perpendicular plate. The septum now has three free sides. With an angled Cottle elevator, the thin perpendicular plate of the ethmoid is fractured from the posterior end of the dorsal incision down to the end of the separation of the septal cartilage from the maxillary crest. The block of septal cartilage and perpendicular plate are removed, leaving at least a 10-mm L-shaped strut attached to the mucoperichondrium (Fig. 8–16) for support of the lower nasal vault.

The excised cartilage is placed in a saline-moistened gauze sponge. Ideally, no mucosal rents are created, avoiding the need for repair and potential septal perforation. The opposing mucoperichondrial flaps can be reapproximated either by using an absorbable quilting suture or by placement of intranasal splints at the time of nasal closure.

INFERIOR TURBINOPLASTY

For patients with symptomatic obstructive hypertrophic inferior turbinates resistant to medical management, a turbinoplasty is performed.[7] The previously placed cottonoids are removed. A pinpoint electrocautery is used to incise the inferior margin of the turbinate down to conchal bone. A medial mucoperiosteal flap is elevated

Retain 10 mm of dorsal and caudal septal strut

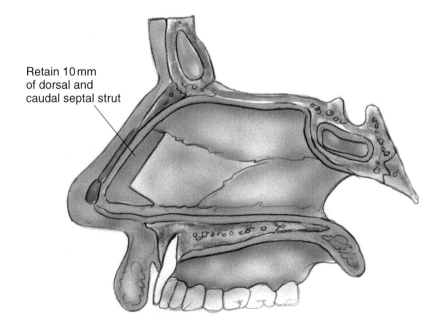

Figure 8–16. A 10-mm strut of dorsal and caudal septum must be retained.

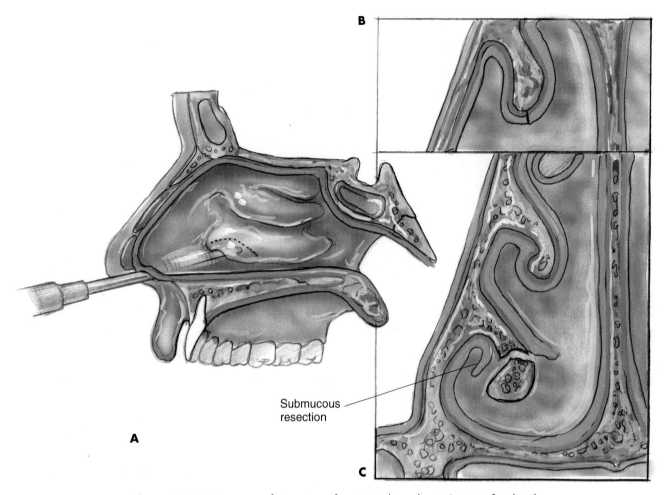

Submucous
resection

A

C

Figure 8-17. Sequence of steps in performing turbinoplasty. See text for details.

to expose the desired amount of turbinate to be resected
(Fig. 8–17). After sharp resection of the conchal bone,
the mucoperiosteal flap is replaced, taking care to cover
the cut edge of the turbinate. Any excess flap is resected.
Postoperative crusting and/or epistaxis may occur if the
cut edge of conchal bone is not covered. Sutures are not
necessary for closure because the mucoperiosteal flap will
self-adhere to the remaining underlying bone.

CEPHALIC TRIM

Cephalic trim is indicated only when the domes are bulbous or boxy, causing paradomal fullness. The cephalic
portion of the middle and lateral crura of the lower lateral
cartilage is resected, leaving at least a 5-mm rim strip.
Calipers accurately demarcate the planned incision.
Excised cartilage can then be used for tip or alar grafting
when indicated (Fig. 8–18).

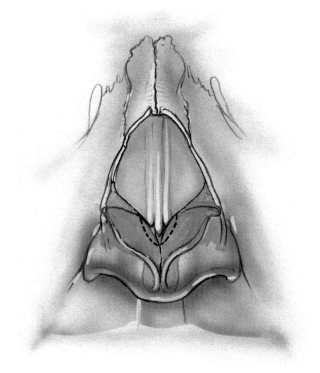

Figure 8-18. Cephalic trim of the lower lateral cartilages.

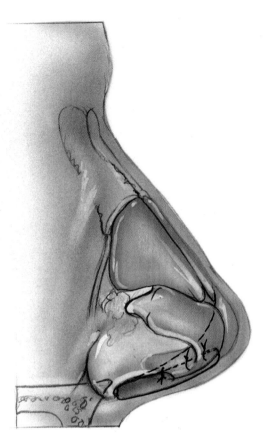

Figure 8–19. Floating columellar strut.

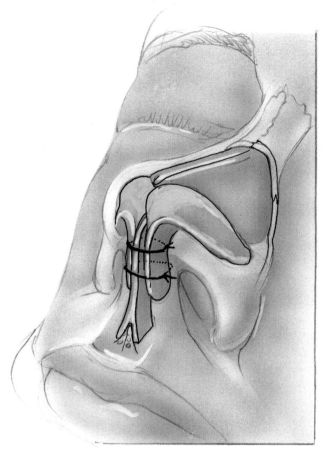

Figure 8–20. Fixed columellar strut.

NASAL TIP SUTURE TECHNIQUES/GRAFTING

A graduated approach to nasal tip surgery involves the use of *columellar struts, suture techniques, and tip grafts.*[13]

An intercrural *columellar strut* is used either to maintain or to increase tip projection. Two types of columellar struts can be used. A *floating strut* is placed between the medial crura 2 to 3 mm in front of the nasal spine (Fig. 8–19). A *fixed strut* rests on the spine itself (Fig. 8–20). The struts are secured at the junction of the medial crura with the middle crura with a 5-0 clear PDS suture.

Four primary suture techniques are commonly used. *Medial crural suture* techniques stabilize the columellar strut between or in front of the medial crura (Fig. 8–21). A columellar strut fashioned from a septal cartilage graft should measure approximately 3×25 mm. With upward traction

Medial crura

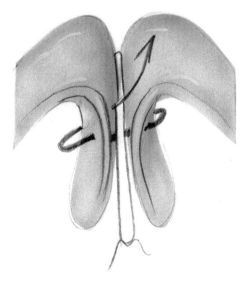

Figure 8–21. Medial crural suture.

Interdomal

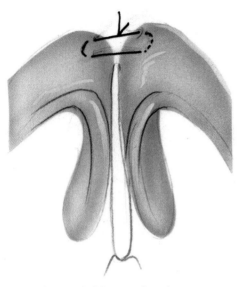

Figure 8–22. Interdomal suture.

Transdomal

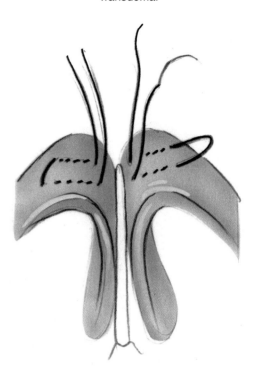

Figure 8–23. Transdomal suture.

of a hook in each vestibular apex, a tunnel or pocket is dissected in the soft tissue between the medial crura toward the nasal spine, leaving a soft tissue pad between the base of the pocket and the nasal spine. The columellar strut is positioned in the pocket, and with the tip-defining points held at the same level under slight tension, a 25-gauge needle is placed through the feet of the medial crura and the columellar strut to stabilize the strut for suturing. A 5-0 PDS suture stabilizes the medial crura to the columellar strut. Two additional superior sutures are inserted to stabilize and unify the tip complex. The sutures are inserted so that the medial portions of the domes are sutured to the columellar strut. The strut is then trimmed to its desired shape to alter or refine the infratip lobular area. *Interdomal sutures* can be used to increase infratip columellar projection and definition or to further increase tip projection (Fig. 8–22). A 5-0 PDS simple suture is placed through the medial walls of the domes and tied to narrow the interdomal distance. *Transdomal sutures* address dome asymmetry (Fig. 8–23). A 5-0 PDS horizontal mattress suture is passed from the medial surface of the dome

through the lateral surface, staying beneath the vestibular skin. It is passed back from lateral to medial. A double surgeon's knot is placed in the suture and tightened until the desired dome angulation is achieved. One end of the suture is cut short and the other left approximately 1 inch long. The same procedure is then performed on the opposite side, leaving one end of the suture long. The two long ends are tied to each other if the distance between the tip-defining parts is excessive (>5 to 6 mm) (Fig. 8–24). The knot is tightened until the desired distance exists between the tip-defining points and is then tied. This is a spanning suture to prevent alar notching and primarily should be used in thicker-skinned patients. Finally, tip rotation may be altered using intercrural *septal sutures*

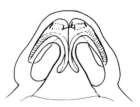

Figure 8–24. Joined transdomal sutures.

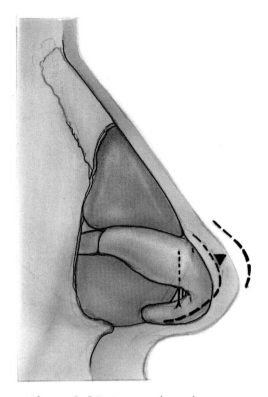

Figure 8-25. Intercrural-septal sutures.

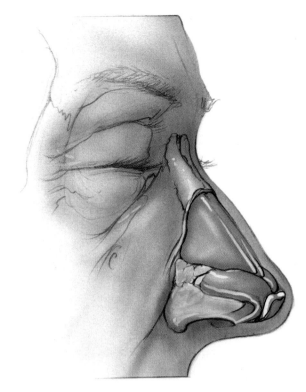

Figure 8-26. Infralobular tip graft.

(Fig. 8–25). This is the only instance in which a 5-0 clear nylon spanning suture is required for permanency.

Only if adequate tip projection, definition, or symmetry cannot be obtained with the techniques just described are visible tip grafts used. They are used infrequently in primary rhinoplasty because visible grafts over the long term can reabsorb and become asymmetric and sharply angulated, requiring revision in up to 30% of cases. The *infralobular graft* primarily increases infratip lobular definition and tip projection (Fig. 8–26). These grafts are individually shaped, depending on the nasal tip anatomy and anatomic requirements but must have smooth, tapered edges. A shield-shaped graft is cut from the septal cartilage so that the upper graft is approximately 8 mm in width. The width of the base of the graft should equal the distance between the caudal margins of the medial crura. The length of the graft is 10 to 12 mm. The graft is placed so that it extends 2 to 3 mm beyond the tip-defining points. The graft is secured with 5-0 PDS sutures at the caudal margins of the dome and medial crura. Usually four sutures are required. *Onlay grafts*

increase tip projection and tip definition. These can be stacked as needed but must be firmly suture stabilized with 5-0 PDS (Fig. 8–27). A 6 × 8-mm onlay tip graft is fashioned from the septal cartilage graft and suture

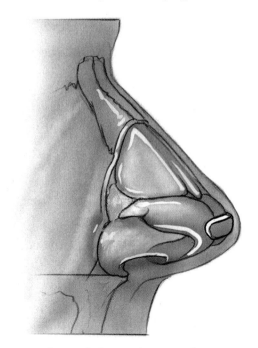

Figure 8-27. Onlay tip graft.

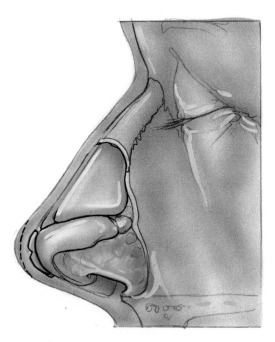

Figure 8–28. Combination tip graft.

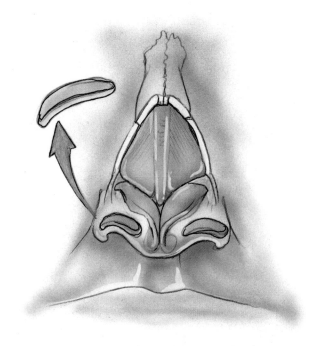

Figure 8–29. Alar contour grafts.

stabilized with two 5-0 PDS sutures to the tip-defining points of the dome. The sutures are placed in a horizontal mattress fashion with the knots tied on the underside of the dome areas. In addition, the columellar, infratip lobular, and onlay tip cartilage grafts can be fashioned into a *combination graft* (Fig. 8–28). This visible graft is reserved for the difficult primary rhinoplasty nasal tip with inadequate tip projection and/or the thick-skinned patient.

Alar contour grafts may be necessary to correct either primary alar notching or pinching resulting from correction of the tip deformity (Fig. 8–29). A subcutaneous tunnel is made with a sharp Stevens scissors below the infracartilaginous incision. The pocket should span the alar notched area, overlaying it by 2 to 3 mm on either side. A 3 × 10 mm straight graft is contoured from septal cartilage and placed into the pocket to correct the alar notch. The graft is secured medially with a 5-0 chromic suture.

PERCUTANEOUS OSTEOTOMIES

Percutaneous osteotomies are used to narrow a wide bony vault, to close an open roof defect, or to straighten deviated nasal bones. We prefer a transcutaneous discontinuous osteotomy through a lateral 2-mm incision.[14] The

incision is made in the nasofacial groove at the level of the orbital rim paralleling the face of the maxilla. This is slightly above the caudal margin of the bony pyramid (Fig. 8–30). The sharp 2-mm straight osteotome is

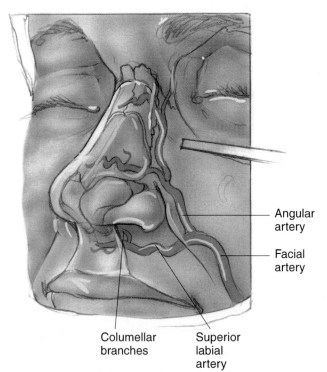

Angular artery

Facial artery

Columellar branches

Superior labial artery

Figure 8–30. Placement of osteotome for percutaneous discontinuous lateral osteotomy.

inserted through the incision down to periosteum and swept laterally to the bony nasofacial groove to avoid injury to the angular vessels. The discontinuous osteotomy is performed from inferiorly, preserving the nasal aperture, to superiorly at the level of the medial canthus. A superior oblique osteotomy is then done. To prevent a palpable or visible shadow deformity the osteotomy is generally done in a low-to-low fashion, especially in a thin-skinned patient.

Infrequently, medial osteotomies are done to narrow the bony nasal septum or if an open roof is not present after dorsal hump reduction. An Aufricht retractor is used to retract the dorsal skin. A medial osteotomy is performed on the right side, placing a 7-mm osteotome on the edge of the nasal bone at its junction with the dorsal septum, angling it laterally 15 degrees. The osteotomy is performed by lightly tapping the osteotome with a mallet, stopping at the level of the medial canthus. Once completed bilaterally, the fracture is gently completed with slight digital pressure only.

CLOSURE

All debris is carefully removed with irrigation before closure. The osseocartilaginous contour should be inspected for a smooth, harmonious appearance. A final three-point dorsum contour test is done and any irregularities or depressions corrected with morselized onlay cartilage grafts. The soft tissue envelope is redraped, and the supratip break is assessed. A 6-0 nylon suture on a PC-3 needle is used to close the transcolumellar incision centrally with two sutures at the stairstep incision followed by the lateral vestibular margin suture. This must be done meticulously to prevent notching or a noticeable scar, particularly at the vestibular margin. The infracartilaginous incision is closed with a 5-0 chromic on a PC-3 needle by use of interrupted sutures. Particular care must be taken to reapproximate the mucosa at the middle crus region. Poor healing or inadequate closure in this area can create distortion of the soft triangle and infratip area, as well as a web deformity. Internal nasal splints coated with an antibacterial ointment are

placed and secured anteriorly with a transseptal 3-0 nylon suture. The dorsal soft tissue envelope is taped, followed by placement of a dorsal nasal splint. A 2 × 2 cm gauze drip pad is placed under the alar base and fixed to the cheek with $\frac{1}{2}$-inch flesh-colored paper tape. One-inch flesh-colored paper tape over the malar areas prevents skin maceration from frequent nasal dressing changes, especially for the first 2 to 3 days postoperatively. The throat pack is carefully removed, and suction is applied to the orogastric tube as it is slowly removed to evacuate any pooled blood and secretions. This helps minimize or prevent postoperative nausea and sore throat.

DEPRESSOR SEPTI MUSCLE TRANSLOCATION

In patients with a tension tip, which on animation causes a foreshortened upper lip and decrease in tip projection, the depressor septi muscle is released through a gingivolabial sulcus approach. An 8- to 10-mm horizontal incision centered over the upper labial frenulum is made with a pinpoint Colorado tip cautery with the setting at 8. The orbicularis–depressor septi dissection is easily visualized superiorly, and the depressor septi is released from its orbicularis or periosteal insertion. The muscle is identified along its course and is released and separated with electrocautery. Once each depressor septi muscle is released and transposed end-to-end, the mucosal incision is closed vertically to further elongate and add fullness to the central upper lip.

ALAR BASE SURGERY

Abnormalities that require alar base modification include nostril flaring, elongated nasal sidewalls, widened nasal base, large alae, and alar asymmetry. Alar abnormalities are carefully analyzed preoperatively to select the appropriate alar-contouring procedure. Alar flaring is the most common indication for alar base modification. The measured alar plane and the nostril circumference dictate the surgical approach.[15]

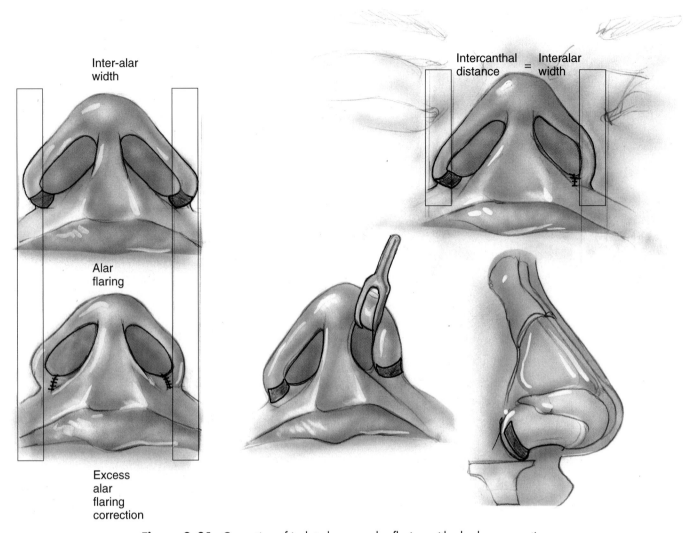

Figure 8–31. Correction of isolated excess alar flaring with alar base resection.

Alar Flaring Correction Only

To correct isolated alar flaring, alar base excision is limited to the alar flare leaving at least 1 to 2 mm of the alar base. This prevents alar base notching. The incision is not carried into the vestibule. The wound is closed with 6-0 nylon on a PC-3 needle by use of the "halving principle" because the alar groove incision is longer than the one on the alar surface (Fig. 8–31).

Alar Flaring and Nostril Shape Correction

Conversely, resecting a complete wedge extending into the vestibule reduces the nostril circumference as well when done for nostril asymmetry or excessively large nostrils

(Fig. 8–32). Straight-line closure is avoided to prevent notching or a distorted nostril. The inferior resection should extend into the nasal vestibule 2 mm above the alar groove. To make the medial incision at the sill, a No. 11 scalpel is used and angled 30 degrees laterally. This will create a small flap medially. Resection of the full-thickness lateral rim superiorly is also done. The wound edges are everted during closure by use of the "halving principle" with 6-0 nylon to avoid a depressed scar across the nostril sill.

HARVESTING AUTOLOGOUS CARTILAGE GRAFTS IN RHINOPLASTY

With increasing finesse in nasal analysis and iatrogenically induced nasal deformities, the need for augmenta-

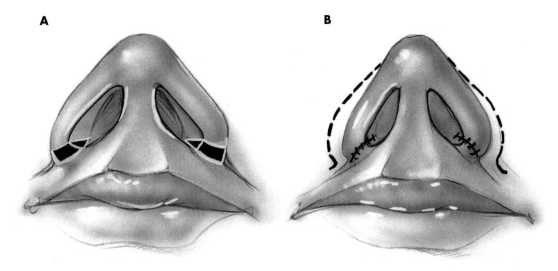

Figure 8–32. Correction of excess alar flaring and excessive nostril circumference with alar base resection extending into the vestibule.

Table 8–2 Preferred Use of Cartilage/Bone Grafts in Rhinoplasty

Septum Cartilage	Ear Cartilage	Rib Cartilage
Tip graft	Alar cartilage	Dorsal onlay
Dorsal onlay	Dorsal onlay	Columellar strut
Columellar strut	Tip graft	Tip graft
Spreader graft		Spreader graft
		Alar cartilage

tion rhinoplasty has increased. Thus, a growing requirement exists for suitable donor sites that provide consistent and effective autogenous supportive tissue. We prefer to use autogenous tissue in the nose and do not believe that alloplasts are indicated (Table 8–2).

CASE ANALYSES

CASE I. DEVIATED NOSE WITH NASAL AIRWAY OBSTRUCTION AND TIP ASYMMETRY

Patient Presentation

This 35-year-old white male presented for primary rhinoplasty with the following complaints, in order of

their importance to him: (1) nasal airway obstruction, (2) a pinched and asymmetric nasal tip, and (3) deviation of the nose to the left.

On frontal view (Fig. 8–33A), analysis reveals adequate facial proportions. The nose is deviated to the patient's left. In addition, the nasal tip is asymmetric with a concave, pinched appearance bilaterally. On lateral (Fig. 8–33B) and oblique views (Figs. 8–33C and 33D), the patient has a slight dorsal hump and a low radix. There is adequate tip projection. Tip concavity is confirmed on these views. The basal view (Fig. 8–33E) confirms the nasal deviation and also reveals a wide alar base. The lobular-columellar ratio is acceptable. The intranasal examination revealed pink mucosa with a septal deflection to the left, without perforation.

Operative Goals

1. Correct nasal airway obstruction
2. Correct tip asymmetry and increase projection
3. Correct nasal deviation
4. Correct the low radix

Surgical Plan (Figs. 8–33K and 33L)

1. External approach with transcolumellar incision and infracartilaginous extensions

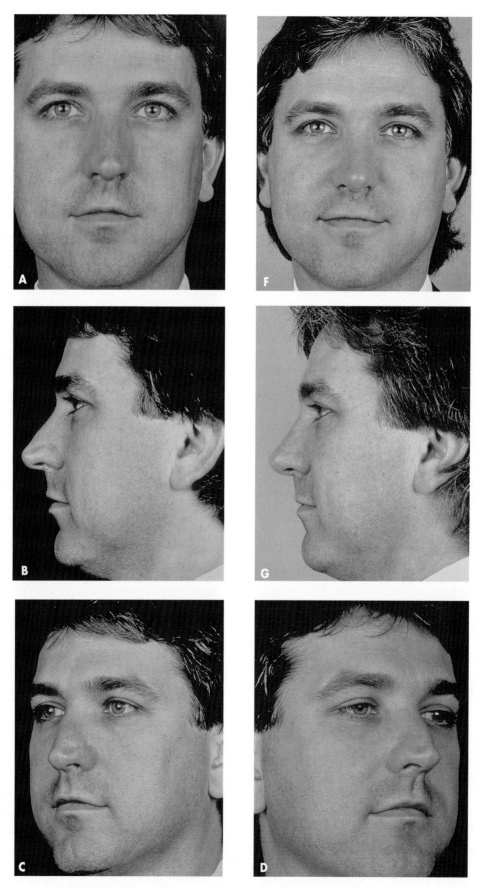

Figure 8–33.   A-D, **F**, and **G**. *(Continued on pages 127 and 128.)*

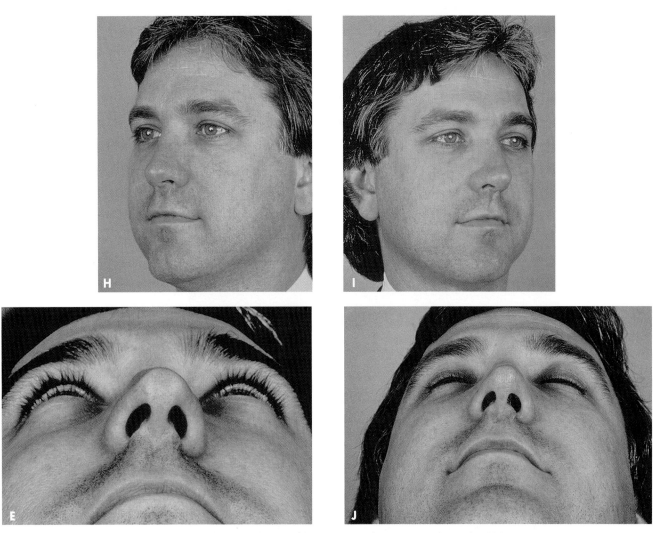

Figure 8–33.   H, I, E, and **J**. *(Continued on pages 126 and 128.)*

2. Exposure of nasal framework

3. Exposure of nasal septum and harvest of septal cartilage

4. Application of morselized cartilage onlay radix graft to correct low radix and appearance of slight nasal hump

5. Low-to-low osteotomies to reposition bony nasal base

6. Turnover flaps of cephalic portion of lower lateral cartilages to correct pinched/asymmetric appearance of tip

7. Intercrural and interdomal sutures in graduated approach to tip projection

8. Scoring of the septum and creation of a swing-door septal flap with figure-of-8 suture to contralateral periosteum of anterior nasal spine with 5–0 PDS suture to correct septal deviation

Results

The result at 5 years is shown. Analysis of the pre- (Fig. 8–33A) and postoperative (Fig. 8–33F) frontal views reveals straight dorsal aesthetic lines and a balanced tip and dorsum. The nasal tip is more symmetric. Lateral pre- (Fig. 8–33B) and postoperative (Fig. 8–33G) comparison views confirm the balance between tip and dorsum. Moreover, the low radix has been corrected, resulting in a smooth, straight dorsum. Tip projection is good, with a nasolabial angle of approximately 90

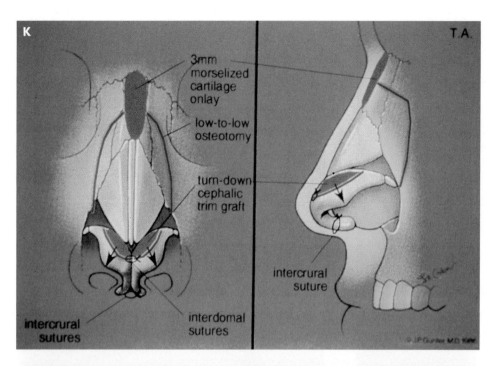

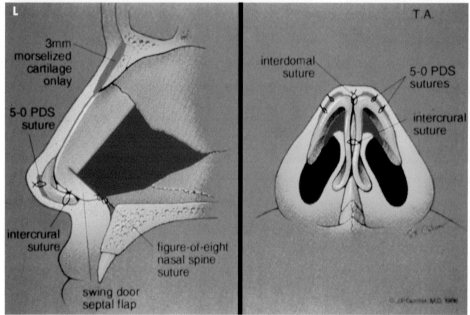

Figure 8–33. K, L. *(Continued from pages 126 and 127.)*

degrees. The alar-columellar relationship is normal. The improved nasal balance is confirmed on the oblique pre- (Figs. 8–33C and 33D) and postoperative (Figs. 8–33H and 33I) comparison views, especially in the area of the midvault. Comparison of the basal pre- (Fig. 8–33E) and postoperative (Fig. 8–33J) views demonstrate a balanced tip with a 2:1 columellar-lobular ratio. The transcolumellar scar is nearly imperceptible.

CASE 2. SHORT, WIDE NOSE WITH A BULBOUS TIP AND NASAL AIRWAY OBSTRUCTION

Patient Presentation

This 20-year-old white female primary rhinoplasty patient presented with the following complaints, in order of their importance to her: (1) nasal airway obstruction,

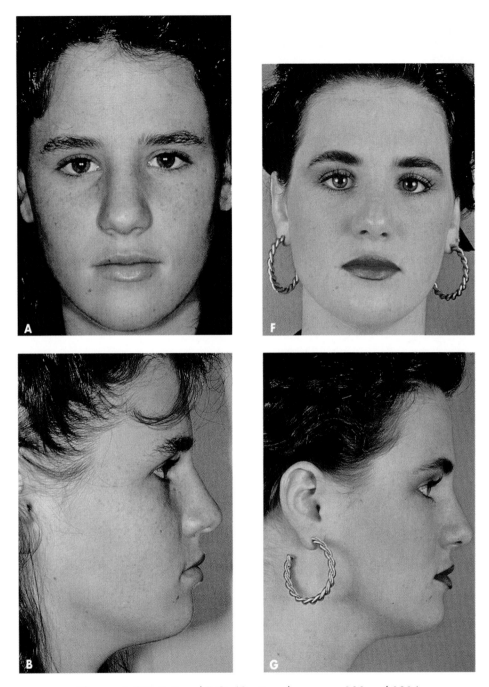

Figure 8–34. A-B and **F-G**. *(Continued on pages 130 and 131.)*

(2) short nasal length, (3) wide dorsum, and (4) an ill-defined nasal tip.

On frontal view (Fig. 8–34A), analysis reveals moderately thick skin and a normal occlusion. The patient has wide dorsal aesthetic lines and a wide bony nasal base. The nasal tip is ill-defined and bulbous. The lateral view (Fig. 8–34B) demonstrates a high radix and inadequate tip projection. These findings are confirmed on examination of the oblique views (Figs. 8–34C and 34D). On the basal view (Fig. 8–34E), the bulbous nature of the tip is apparent. The lobular-columellar ratio approaches 1:1. There is also a suggestion of a septal deviation, which is

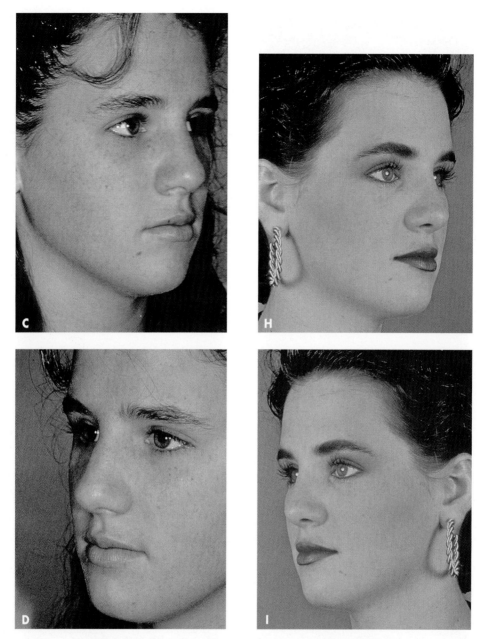

Figure 8–34. C-I. *(Continued on pages 129 and 131.)*

confirmed on intranasal examination, which reveals a left posteroinferior septal deflection.

Operative Goals

1. Correct nasal airway obstruction
2. Increase nasal length by derotating the nose
3. Narrow the bony dorsum

4. Improve tip projection and definition
5. Lower the radix

Surgical Plan (Figs. 8–34K and 34L)

1. External approach with transcolumellar incision and infracartilaginous extensions
2. Exposure of nasal framework

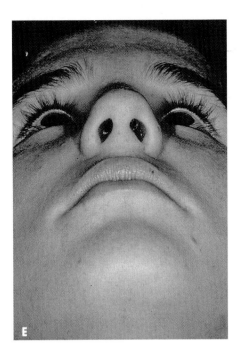

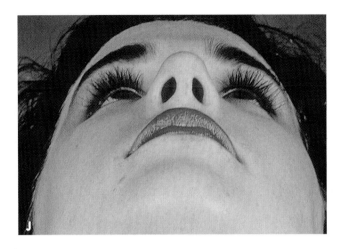

Figure 8–34. **E,J**. *(Continued on pages 129 and 130.)*

3. Exposure of the septum with separation of the upper lateral cartilages from the septum

4. Harvest septal cartilage

5. Place extended spreader grafts to define dorsal aesthetic lines, straighten the dorsum, and derotate the tip; spreader grafts placed approximately 8 mm below tip defining points to push middle crura laterally

6. Medial osteotomies and low-to-high lateral osteotomies to narrow bony nasal base

7. Lower the radix by elevating periosteum and using an oscillating dental burr with dorsal protection, resulting in a 2:1 bone-to-soft tissue alteration (4 mm bony reduction resulting in 2 mm soft tissue reduction)

8. Full-thickness cuts in the inferior 50% of the remaining septum from the deviated portion distally to correct a severe occult septal deviation

9. Mobilize the lower lateral cartilages to derotate the tip

10. Cephalic trim of lower lateral cartilages

11. Placement of columellar strut and intercrural, transdomal, and interdomal sutures in graduated approach to increase tip projection

Results

The result at 6 years is shown. Comparison of the pre- (Fig. 8–34A) and postoperative (Fig. 8–34F) frontal views demonstrate improved nasal balance with more narrow, straight dorsal aesthetic lines. Significant tip refinement is evident. Pre- (Fig. 8–34B) and postoperative (Fig. 8–34G) lateral views show that the nose is slightly longer, with improved tip projection. The radix is in good position, and there is a gentle supratip break. The nasolabial angle is appropriate, approximately 95 degrees. These findings are confirmed by comparing the pre- (Fig. 8–34C and 34D) and postoperative (Fig. 8–34H and 34I) oblique views. The pre- (Fig. 8–34E) and postoperative (Fig. 8–34J) basal views demonstrate a harmonious equilateral triangle with a lobular-columellar ratio of 1:2. The appearance of the transcolumellar scar is quite acceptable.

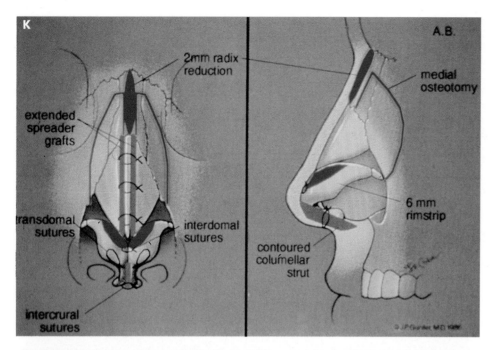

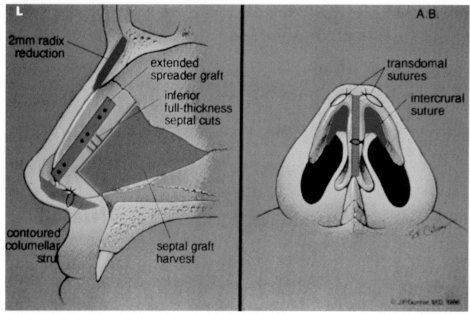

Figure 8–34. *(Continued)* K, L.

POSTOPERATIVE COURSE

All patients are given a general overview of postoperative care at the time of the initial consultation, as well as the specific preoperative and postoperative instructions. We call our rhinoplasty patients the evening after the rhinoplasty and see them 5 to 7 days postoperatively and again at the third and eighth postoperative weeks, at 3, 6, and 12 months, and annually thereafter. All patients are given the following preoperative prescriptions.

1. Cephalexin, 500 mg po q8h × 3 days postoperatively (1 g IV cephalexin is given 1 hour preoperatively)
2. Medrol Dosepak postoperatively (to minimize postoperative edema) (8 mg Decadron is given IV 1 hour preoperatively)

3. Codeine or propoxyphene for postoperative pain
4. Normal nasal saline for postoperative nasal congestion

Any prescribed pain medications may be taken every 3 to 4 hours if needed. The patient should be encouraged to take the medication after eating (e.g., crackers, jello). If the patient does not feel pain, he or she should not take the medication.

Immediately after surgery, the patient is instructed to elevate the head on at least two pillows to keep swelling to a minimum. Applying ice bags to the eyes during the day for the first 48 hours will decrease the amount of postoperative swelling. Pressure must not be put on the nasal splint. The patient must be warned that swelling may continue after the first 24 hours, reaching its peak at 48 to 72 hours.

Because patients usually have a bloody nasal discharge for 2 to 4 days after surgery, we advise them to change the drip pad under the nose as often as needed. Rubbing or blotting the nose is discouraged because this irritates it. When drainage has stopped, the patient is allowed to discard the drip pad and remove the tape on the cheeks. To avoid postoperative bleeding, the patient is instructed not to sniff or blow the nose for the first 3 weeks after surgery. If the patient must sneeze, it should be done through the mouth.

A liquid diet is preferred for the day of surgery. The patient can start a soft regular diet the next day. For 2 weeks any foods that require excess lip movement (e.g., apples, corn on the cob) should be avoided.

The nasal splints and sutures are removed 5 to 7 days after surgery in the office. At this visit, the nose (especially the tip) may appear swollen and turned up. The tip also may feel numb. Both will resolve with time. The numbness may take from 3 to 6 months to return to normal.

After the splint is removed, the nose is washed gently with soap, and makeup can be applied. Moisturizing creams can be used if the nose is dry. If a patient has oily skin, the pores may become blocked while wearing the splint. A buff puff can be used to gently clean the skin.

The inside of the nose is often swollen and results in difficulty breathing, which improves with time. A normal saltwater nasal spray (e.g., Aryr or Ocean Spray) and over-the-counter Afrin-like nasal sprays may be used to minimize nasal congestion for the first 2 weeks. Patients are encouraged to breathe through the mouth if able to get air through the splints. If the patient is very congested, we may have them come in for suctioning.

After the splint is removed, the patient cannot let anything, including eyeglasses, rest on the nose for at least 4 weeks. Glasses should be taped to the forehead. Contacts can be worn as soon as the swelling has decreased enough for them to be inserted (usually less than 5 to 7 days).

The patient is instructed to keep the inside of the nostrils and any stitches clean by applying hydrogen peroxide with a cotton swab. A thin coating of polysporin ointment also should be applied. The cotton swab can be advanced into the nose as far as the cotton on the swab, but no further.

The nasal splint must remain dry. Hair washing should be done as in a beauty salon, with the patient leaning the head backward over the sink.

Patients are instructed to restrict strenuous activity that increases heart rate greater than 100 bpm (e.g., aerobics, heavy lifting, bending over) for 3 weeks after surgery. After 2 weeks, patients may slowly increase activity so that they have returned to normal daily activities by the end of the third week.

Because the skin of the nose may be sensitive to sunlight after surgery, patients are advised to protect their nose from the sun for 3 months and to wear a wide-brimmed hat or sunscreen (SPF-15 or greater) if in the sun for prolonged periods.

Of course, the patient should take care to avoid hitting the nose for at least 4 weeks after surgery.

Swelling and discoloration are fairly normal early in the postoperative course. During postoperative visits, the surgeon must spend the time to reassure the patient that the swelling and discoloration will disappear. The surgeon also must urge the patient to be patient for the final result. Although some noses look excellent within 6 to 8 weeks, others need more time for complete healing. The nose may appear swollen for up to 1 year after surgery, but after 2 to 3 weeks it will not be obvious to anyone but the patient.

COMPLICATIONS AND SEQUELAE

AESTHETIC

Given its largely subjective character, aesthetic surgery does not lend itself easily to statistical analysis. Approximately 5.3 to 18% of patients require a revision of secondary rhinoplasty for either aesthetic or functional complications: 5 to 10% is considered an acceptable number. Most unfavorable results occur in the lower third of the nose, followed by the middle and then upper thirds. These results include knuckling of the lower lateral cartilages and hanging columella in the tip region, the polybeak and pinched supratip in the middle third, and excessive dorsal reduction and dorsal irregularities in the upper third.[1]

The incidence of significant complications after rhinoplasty ranges from 1.7 to 18%.[4] McKinney has reported more recent figures of 4 and 5%.[16] Such complications may be categorized as hemorrhagic, infectious, traumatic, or miscellaneous. Significant postoperative bleeding, which is the most common of these complications, occurs in 0.7 to 3.6% of cases reported by Goldwyn and other authors.[17] Infectious complications occur in 1.7 to 2.8% of cases reported by Klabunde[18] and Miller.[19] Traumatic complications result from damage to the nasal framework or adjacent structures; they occur in 0.4 to 1.9% of cases. Finally, miscellaneous complications represent anecdotal reports of various unusual occurrences, such as anesthetic and psychiatric complications.[1]

FUNCTIONAL

Nasal airway obstruction is the primary functional complication in rhinoplasty. In the immediate postoperative period, nasal airway obstruction results from persistent edema or crusting and is usually self-limited. Allergy or disturbance of the neuromuscular control of the nasal mucosal circulation may cause prolonged obstruction. In addition, obstructive symptoms may be due to undiagnosed or untreated turbinate hypertrophy.[1]

External valve pathology may result in long-term nasal airway obstruction. Problems with the external valve may occur after over-resection of the lower lateral cartilages and septum, resulting in loss of tip support, or after making poorly placed intranasal incisions, which cause vestibular stenosis.

Nasal airflow also may be limited by thickening of the columella, which occurs as a result of flaring of the medial crura or simply surgical trauma. Problems with the internal nasal valve can result in long-term functional abnormalities. Surgical trauma and blunting of the nasal mucosa at the angle created by the junction of the upper lateral cartilages with the septum may obstruct the internal valve. In addition, internal valve obstruction may occur after overresection of the dorsum and after collapse of the lateral nasal walls after osteotomies.

CONCLUSION

The rationale for the use of the open approach to rhinoplasty is derived from four key factors. The open approach allows the following.

1. *Maximal visual exposure* of the osseocartilaginous framework without distortion
2. Assurance of *accurate diagnosis* of nasal deformity
3. Ease of osseocartilaginous framework modification by use of native tissue
4. Increased options for framework alteration.

The open approach allows modification of the cartilaginous framework while maintaining the integrity of the framework. This is done primarily with sutures and repositioning rather than transection and resection, which are an integral part of the endonasal approach. In addition to facilitating the reshaping and repositioning of the cartilaginous framework with sutures, the open approach permits precise stabilization of the framework and grafts. The results of modifications on the osseocartilaginous framework can be continually and accurately assessed by the surgeon.

The goal in primary rhinoplasty is to consistently produce long-lasting, natural-appearing results, a goal that is optimally achieved with the open approach to rhinoplasty.

PEARLS

- Establish specific patient concerns about nasal deformity in order of importance (i.e., nasal hump, bulbous tip).

- Systematic nasal analysis is essential for accurate and detailed preoperative rhinoplasty planning.

- Use standardized preoperative photographs or computer imaging for preoperative planning patient education, and intraoperative review.

- Meticulous execution of the open approach on the basis of an organized operative plan derived from the systematic nasal analysis.

- Reproducible key operative techniques such as creating a smooth and straight dorsum, refining the tip using suture techniques primarily and invisible cartilage grafts, and maintaining nasal function.

REFERENCES

1. Teichgraeber JF. Nasal surgery complications. Dallas Rhinoplasty Symposium (14th). 1997.
2. Gunter JP, Rohrich RJ. External approach for secondary rhinoplasty. *Plast Reconstr Surg.* 1987; 80:161.
3. Goodman WS. External Approach to Rhinoplasty. *Can J Otolaryngol.* 2:3, 1973.
4. Rohrich RJ. Rhinoplasty planning. p. 47. DRS (14th), 1997.
5. Rohrich RJ, Hollier LH. Rhinoplasty with advancing age: Characteristics and management. *Clin Plast Surg* 1996; 23(2):281–296.
6. Rohrich RJ. Management of the rhinoplasty patient. p. 27. DRS (14th), 1997.
7. Pollock RA, Rohrich RJ. Inferior turbinate surgery: An adjunct to the successful treatment of nasal obstruction in 408 patients. *Plast Reconstr Surg.* 1984; 74(2):227.
8. Pownell P, Rohrich RJ. Endoscopic-assisted inferior turbinectomy. *Perspect Plast Surg.* 1994; 8(1):91.
9. Byrd HS. The dimensional approach to rhinoplasty. DRS (10th), p. 29, 1993.
10. Rohrich RJ. Dorsal Reduction and Osteotomies. DRS (12):209, 1995.
11. Gordon HL, Baker TH Jr. Primary cosmetic rhinoplasty. *Clin Plast Surg.* 1977; 4(1):9–14.
12. Daniel RK, Lessard ML. Rhinoplasty: A graded aesthetic-anatomical approach. *Ann Plast Surg.* 1984; 13(5): 436–451.
13. Rohrich RJ. Graduated approach to tip projection in rhinoplasty. DRS (14th), p. 129, 1997.
14. Rohrich RJ, Minoli JJ, Adams WP, Hollier LH. The lateral nasal osteotomy in rhinoplasty: An anatomic endoscopic comparison of the external versus the internal approach. *Plast Reconstr Surg.* 1997; 99(5):1309–1312.
15. Oneal RM. Alar base surgery. DRS (14th), p. 179, 1997.
16. McKinney P, Cook JQ. A critical evaluation of 200 rhinoplasties. *Ann Plast Surg.* 1981; 7(5):357–361.
16. McKinney P, Cook JQ. A critical evaluation of 200 rhinoplasties. *Ann Plast Surg.* 1981; 7(5):357–361.
17. Goldwyn RM. Unexpected bleeding after elective nasal surgery. *Ann Plast Surg.* 1979; 2:201.
18. Klabunde EH, Falces E. Incidence of complications in cosmetic rhinoplasties. *Plast Reconstr Surg.* 1964; 34:192.
19. Miller T. Immediate postoperative complications of septoplasties and septorhinoplasties. *Trans Pac Coast Oto-opthalmol Soc.* 1976; 57:201.

Revision Rhinoplasty

In these chapters the authors' review one of the most technically challenging surgical procedures, revision rhinoplasty. Both authors emphasize the preoperative evaluation with extensive patient assessment and maintenance of proper timing for revision nasal surgery. Dr. Tabbal, a plastic surgeon, stresses the use of autogenous material for architectural reconstruction but introduces the concept of Gortex dorsal implants used in the rare revision case.

Dr. Romo, a facial plastic surgeon, also stresses the need for the use of autogenous material in reconstructive rhinoplasty. He emphasizes the use of porous high[tr]density polyethylene for structural implants and rewiews his extensive experience. Both authors favor the external rhinoplasty approach in deference to closed surgical techniques in addition, both authors' review their surgical treatment plans on the basis of the anatomic segments of the nasal profile. Careful review of the numerous illustrations and postoperative photographs in these chapters will increase the reader's understanding.

Revision Rhinoplasty

Aesthetic Facial Plastic Surgery, edited by Thomas Romo, III, and Arthur L. Millman, Thieme Medical Publishers, Inc., New York, New York, Copyright © 2000.

CHAPTER 9

A Facial Plastic Surgeon's Perspective

THOMAS ROMO, III

Revision rhinoplasty is one of the most complicated procedures that can be performed by the aesthetic facial plastic surgeon. Not only is a secondary surgical procedure being performed on a scarred facial structure, which limits overall success, but also the patient undergoing revision rhinoplasty often has unrealistic expectations of the final results, which sets the stage for failure even when an acceptable result is achieved.

Therefore it is imperative that the revision rhinoplasty surgeon adhere to a set of rules to increase the overall success rate in this type of surgery.

PHILOSOPHY

The surgeon who wishes to perform revision rhinoplasty must develop a consistent philosophy in managing these difficult surgical cases. This philosophy will change and mature as more experience is gained in managing these cases, but several standards should routinely be observed.

First, the surgeon must be honest with himself or herself. Does he or she possess sufficient clinical and technical knowledge and the surgical skills to perform the varied techniques and procedures necessary to produce a successful result in revision rhinoplasty? Failure in this area will produce inappropriate and misdiagnosed preoperative evaluations, thereby leading to incorrect surgical procedures and ultimately a dissatisfied patient.

Second, does the surgeon understand the concerns the patient has with the present failed rhinoplasty? Are these concerns real? For example, were nasal asymmetries caused by a previous procedure or are they a natural product of the bony cartilaginous and skin structures (e.g., thick skin and therefore poor tip definition)? Failure to elicit and understand actual patient concerns will lead to procedures being performed that may never satisfy the patient or the surgeon.

Third, proper timing of planned revision nasal surgery can lead to long-term success. On the other hand, incorrect timing will lead to a misleading preoperative evaluation and ultimately a failed revision surgery. Routinely, revision nasal surgery should first be contemplated at 1 year after the prior surgical procedure. This allows for resolution of edema and shrink wrapping of the skin envelope down to the underlying bony cartilaginous structures. If surgical revision is attempted before this time, incorrect information is gleaned from the preoperative assessment, which will ultimately lead to failed revision rhinoplasty. This standard is very difficult to maintain because the patient will coerce and plead for earlier surgical intervention, but maintaining this philosophy will improve the final surgical result.

PATIENT EVALUATION

During the initial evaluation, the overall structure and contour of the nose should be delineated.[1] From the frontal view the nose should be straight or vertical, beginning at the infraglabella region or level of the superior eyelid crease (Fig. 9–1). The midnasal width should be symmetric without indentations, curves, or internal nasal valve collapse. The nasal tip should be in the midline without twists or asymmetries. In the Caucasian nose the width of the nostrils should be equal to the intercanthal distance. Nostril show should be minimal. The submental view should reveal a vertical straight midline columella progressing to a symmetric smooth rounded nasal tip (Fig. 9–2). Columella asymmetries and tip distortions are

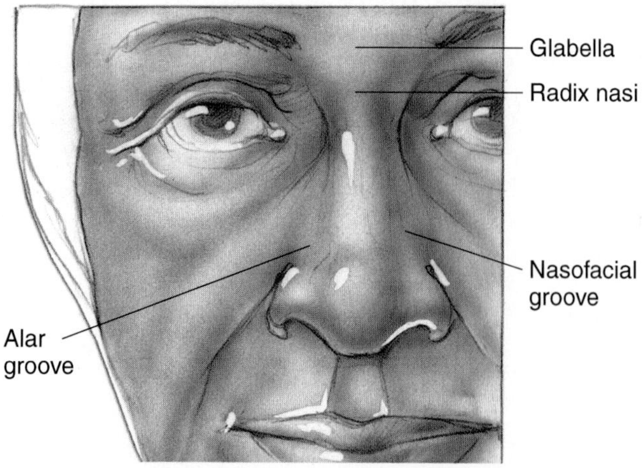

Figure 9–1. Superficial nasal anatomy, frontal view.

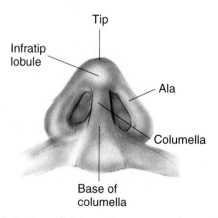

Figure 9–2. Superficial nasal anatomy, submental view.

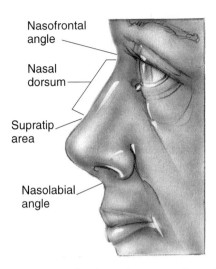

Figure 9–3. Superficial nasal anatomy, lateral view.

Nasofrontal angle

Nasal dorsum

Supratip area

Nasolabial angle

noted. Nostril shape should be slightly curved from inferior to superior and symmetric. Caudal septal deflections and widened or distorted medial crura are noted. Alar contour should progress from the nasal tip with a gentle outward curve. No pinching or collapse of the nostril should be present. A small nasal speculum can be inserted into the anterior nares to document the normal vestibular patency. Vestibular mucosal stenosis and external valve collapse are noted. From the side or lateral view the nose should again begin at the infraglabellar region, with a slight concavity just superior to this area (Fig. 9–3). The nasal dorsum should progress inferiorly at approximately a 30-degree angle and gently intersect with the nasal tip. The nasal tip should be 2 mm to 3 mm higher than the nasal dorsum, with a smooth rounded contour to intersect with the infratip lobule. In the male nose the supratip break is less defined. The infratip lobule is angulated back posteriorly to connect with a slightly inferiorly curved columella. The nasal labial angle measures 90 degrees in the male patient and 95 to 105 degrees in the female patient. The distance of the nasolabial angle to the tip of the nose should approximate the distance from the angle to the tip of the superior lip. Excessive concavity or convexity of the nasal dorsum is noted. Asymmetries of the supratip, nasal tip, and infratip lobule and columella are documented. Acute or obtuse nasolabial angles and discrepancies in tip projection are noted. Actual digital palpation of the nasal segments is then performed. This examination is critical because it provides the surgeon with more specific information about the degree of nasal soft tissue scarring and subtle structural deficiencies. All these primary impressions are documented in the patients chart. An initial treatment plan is formulated and documented in the patient chart and reviewed thoroughly with the patient. It is helpful to present anatomic templates and graphics of the planned procedure to the patient. This will help illustrate the detailed concepts of the planned surgical procedure and further facilitate patient understanding about what kind of surgical intervention is being recommended. The initial consultation is now completed.

The patient is subsequently scheduled for a second consultation before surgery is performed. During the second evaluation all pertinent previously gleaned data and treatment plans are thoroughly reviewed with the patient. Any changes in the planned procedure and patient requests are reviewed, finalized, and documented. It is imperative at this point that the surgeon is able to conclude that the patient fully understands the planned procedure and likely outcome and risks, complications, benefits, and alternatives to the planned surgery.

A detailed, attorney-generated informed consent is then reviewed and signed by the patient and the surgeon. Finally, after all the previous steps have been concluded, preoperative photographs of the frontal, three-quarter, lateral, submental, and overhead views are obtained.

GRAFTING MATERIAL

Once a complete evaluation of the nose has been performed, a plan is developed to reconstitute the nose back to a functional and aesthetic structure. Routinely overresection of the bony cartilaginous framework results in excessive shrink wrapping of the mucosa and epithelial envelope down to the underlying architecture. This process results in a smaller and usually asymmetric nasal profile. In revision rhinoplasty it is advisable to replace missing or scarred structures with like or similar tissue. If mucous membrane, cartilage, or epithelium is deficient, these structures should be replaced with like tissue. Therefore it is recommended that autogenous tissue be used whenever available. The long-term stability and resistance to infection of these structures as grafting material have stood the test of time. Autogenous septal cartilage is the ideal grafting material[2] for columella struts, tip grafts, internal and external nasal battens, and nasal dorsal grafts. On the other hand, the cartilaginous nasal septum may be a limited donor site because of prior nasal septal surgery and scarring. Therefore the next preferred donor site for cartilaginous grafts is the auricular conchal bowel. This graft may be harvested through an anteriorly or posteriorly[3] placed incision, but either approach heals relatively well. This graft is well suited for external valve battens, tip grafts, and isolated nasal dorsal deformities. The downside in the use of this donor site is that some contour changes and deformity of the residual auricular profile exist. It is not unusual for a patient to refuse the ear as a donor site when they already possess another distorted facial structure. Autogenous peripheral donor sites include the calvarium, rib, and iliac crest. These bony sites can provide large amounts of bulk augmentation grafts but may be associated with significant morbidity of the donor site. Autogenous rib grafts can supply a large amount of structural cartilage and bone. This is usually used as nasal dorsal onlay grafts but can be carved into a tongue-and-grove articulated columella and dorsal framework.

The sixth and, if necessary, seventh medial ribs are the usual donor sites. If only one long straight graft is needed, the medial aspect of the ninth floater rib can be used. Resistance to long-term resorption has been noted with autogenous rib grafts, but the occasional tendency for this graft to warp is well documented.[4] Morbidity includes a local chest wound contour deformity and the possibility of pneumothorax, necessitating chest tube insertion. These potential complications must be weighed against the need for using this graft material.

Outer table calvarial bone grafts have recently gained favor as a nasal graft material.[5] This is because only one operative site needs to be prepared. The head and face can be draped off in one surgical field. Also it has been shown that membranous bone when secured in place with wire or screw fixation has a lower resorption rate than endochondral long bone grafts. These grafts can be used as dorsal onlay, columella struts, and external batten grafts. The morbidity for using this material includes intracranial penetration, subdermal hematoma, and brain injury.

Iliac crest bone grafts can provide substantial bulk grafting material for nasal reconstruction. This graft is mainly used for nasal dorsal onlay grafts. Because the donor site morbidity includes significant pain and decreased patient mobility for up to 6 weeks, this type of grafting material has fallen out of favor.

Allografts include irradiated human rib grafts. This material handles much like autogenous rib grafts and is used for similar purposes (e.g., dorsal onlay, columella struts, and nasal valve battens). The long-term stability of these grafts is questionable, with significant absorption and warping noted in many cases.[6]

Contemporary alloplastic material for use in revision rhinoplasty consists of solid silicone rubber (Silastic), expanded polytetrafluoroethylene (e-PTFE, GorTex) and porous high-density polyethylene (Medpor) implants. Solid silicone implants have been used for nasal reconstruction for 30 years. This implant is used for dorsal onlay and columella struts. Because of the solid nature of these implants, no tissue infiltration occurs, and therefore these implants always remain mobile and have high extrusion rates. Therefore these implants have fallen out of favor as useful nasal implants.

Expanded polytetrafluoroethylene implants have gained popularity as a nasal dorsal onlay implant.[7] This material is soft and handles and carves easily. The long-term stability of implants has been documented in their use as vascular implants for more than 20 years. The pore size of this porous implant averages 25 μm, which does not allow for active infiltration of soft tissue. Therefore expanded Teflon implants are easily removed if the situation arises. Because of the soft flexible nature of this implant, its use in revision nasal surgery is limited to dorsal onlay implants. Use as columella struts and external valve battens is obviated by the lack of firm architectural structure of these implants.

Porous high-density polyethylene implants have recently gained favor as useful implants in revision rhinoplasty when autogenous material is limited or not available.[8] Because of the firm but flexible characteristics of this implant, it can be used as dorsal onlay implants and columella struts and external valve battens. The pore size of the implant averages 150 μm, which allows for aggressive soft tissue infiltration and long-term stabilization. Resistance to extrusion and infection has been noted in several studies.[9] I have used this material extensively over the past 5 years in more than 200 nasal surgeries and have found it to be an ideal implant material when autogenous grafting material is not available.

SURGICAL TECHNIQUE

The preferred approach for revision rhinoplasty is the external or decortication rhinoplasty technique. In most revision nasal surgery cases multiple grafts or implants are being exactingly placed to reconstitute proper archi-tectural support. This proper graft or implant placement is facilitated by direct exposure of the underlying overresected bony cartilaginous framework. Rarely in cases that require minimal augmentation is a closed technique used in revision nasal surgery.

By use of information gleaned from the prior consultation examinations and formulated surgical plan, definitive surgery is now begun.

Surgical alteration performed on the prior operated nose is facilitated by approaching the nose in its three basic anatomic regions.

UPPER THIRD OF NOSE

The upper third of the nose essentially consists of the paired nasal bones or nasal pyramid. From the frontal view, common postoperative rhinoplasty anomalies include overresection of one or both nasal bones. If one nasal bone is overresected, correction consists of placement of an overlying cartilaginous graft from the septum or ear. If both nasal bones are overresected, a similar augmentation of this region with a larger graft is performed (Fig. 9–4). This later defect will also be noted on the lateral view as a depression of the upper third of the nose.

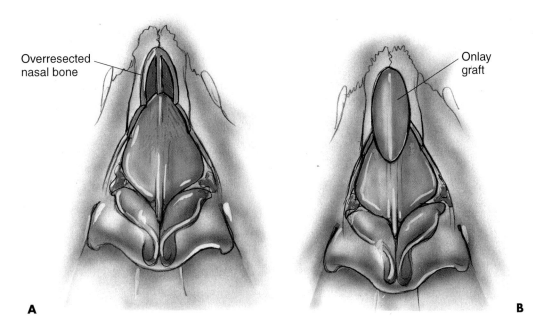

Figure 9–4. (A) Overresected nasal bone. **(B)** Defect correction with cartilage graft.

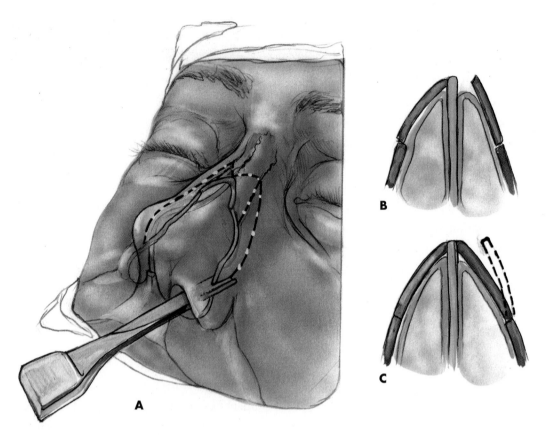

Figure 9–5. (A) Position of medial, intermedial, and lateral osteotomy. **(B)** Open-roof deformity, lateralized nasal bone. **(C)** Defect correction, medialized nasal bone.

Aggressive osteotomies may result in actual collapse of the nasal bones off the bony maxillary pyramid into the nasal vault. This condition may present unilaterally or bilaterally. Management consists of refracture of the depressed nasal bone and elevation of the nasal bone back onto the bony maxillas. The nasal bones are stabilized in position by intranasal packing and a nasal dorsal splint for 1 week.

Persistently depressed nasal bones may be additionally stabilized by elevation and fixation of the inferior attached upper lateral cartilage to the cartilaginous dorsal septum. Ultimately open reduction of collapsed nasal bones may result in subtle asymmetries of the upper third of the nose. These depressed areas are grafted with thin onlay septal cartilage grafts at the 1-year postoperative period.

Another common postoperative rhinoplasty problem seen in the upper one third of the nose is unilateral or bilateral open roof deformity. This problem results when inadequate infracturing of one or both nasal bones is produced.

Management of this problem is solved by completing the medial and then lateral osteotomy on the laterally positioned nasal bone (Fig. 9–5). Occasionally, exceedingly wide or thick nasal bones may require an intermediate osteotomy. This is always performed after the medial osteotomy and before the lateral osteotomy. This should result in adequate removal and appropriate thinning of the upper third of the nose (Fig. 9–6).

An additional postsurgical problem may present with the upper third of the nose, which may appear excessively high on lateral view, especially in relation

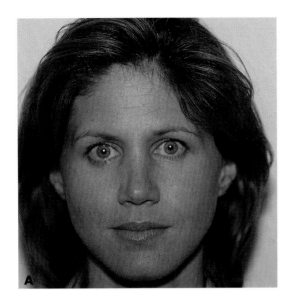
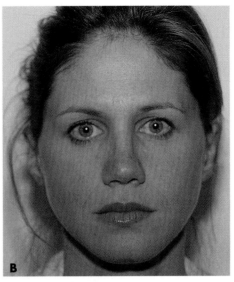

Figure 9–6.
(A) Preoperative open-roof deformity, lateralized right nasal bone.
(B) Postoperative open-roof closure, medialized right nasal bone.

to the middle third of the nose. If, in fact, the problem is excessive nasal bone height, a reduction dorsal osteotomy and possible rasping is performed to lower the bony configuration. If necessary, medial and lateral osteotomies are then completed to close the open roof deformity.

MIDDLE THIRD OF THE NOSE

Anatomically, the middle third of the nose consists of the dorsal septal cartilage and its intrinsic lateral extensions, the upper lateral cartilages. These upper cartilages form a T-shaped extension from the septum at the upper middle nasal third and progress to an inverted V in the lower middle third of the nose (Fig. 9–7). The upper cartilages extend down close to the edge of the pyriform aperture.

Common postsurgical deformities include detachment of the upper lateral cartilages from the dorsal septum and then overresection of one or both upper lateral cartilages. This can produce asymmetric or symmetric collapse and thinning of the middle third of the nose and gives the appearance of an inverted V just inferior to the nasal bones. This defect is corrected by first elevating the mucoperichondrium off the overlying dorsal septum and upper lateral cartilage intersection through an endonasal approach.

Next, by use of the open rhinoplasty approach, the collapsed upper lateral cartilage is incised from the nasal septum and lateralized. This leaves the underlying mucoperichondrium intact. Long, thin septal cartilage grafts are then suture fixated between the nasal septum and the lateralized upper lateral cartilages with 5-0

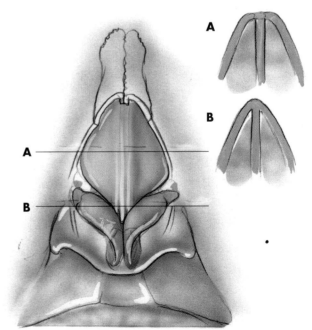

Figure 9–7. Midnasal anatomy **(A)** T-shaped upper cartilage extension. **(B)** Inverted V upper cartilage extension.

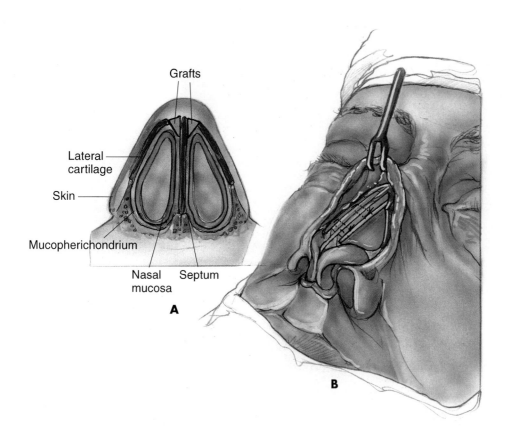

Grafts

Lateral cartilage

Skin

Mucopherichondrium

Nasal mucosa   Septum

A

B

Figure 9–8. (A) Cross-section view, spreader grafts lateralize upper lateral cartilages. **(B)** Suture secured spreader grafts open the internal nasal valve.

chromic sutures. These stents or spreader grafts widen the middle third of the nasal dorsal configuration and reopen the critically needed internal nasal valve.[10] The grafts extend from the nasal bones down to near the septal angle (Figs. 9–8 and 9–9).

Overresection of the middle nasal dorsal septal cartilage may also occur in conjunction with overresection of the upper lateral cartilages. On lateral view this configuration will appear as a depression of the middle bridge of the nose or a saddle nose deformity. Correction of this defect includes lateralizing the upper lateral cartilages as previously described with spreader grafts then augmentation of the middle nasal dorsum

with autogenous septal or auricular cartilage grafts. Not infrequently this overresection of the middle nasal dorsum is associated with concomitant overresection of the nasal bones. In this case a long onlay graft or implant is inset onto the total nasal dorsum.

If available, augmentation is accomplished with septal cartilage grafts. Split calvarium and autogenous rib grafts are acceptable alternatives but may be rejected by the informed patient. If alloplasts are used, our preference is a porous high-density polyethylene long thin nasal dorsal implant covered with an appropriately contoured 2 cm × 4 cm decellularized human dermal matrix graft.[11] This composite alloimplant provides excel-

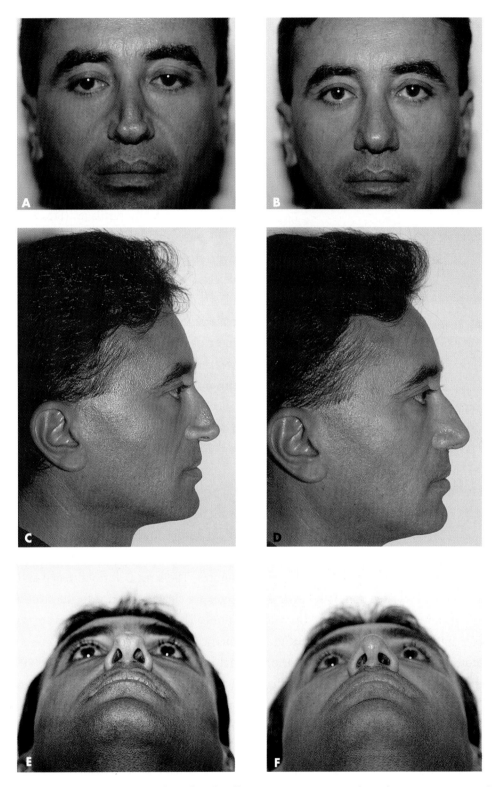

Figure 9–9. **(A)** Preoperative frontal view: midnasal vault collapse. **(B)** Postoperative frontal view: correction with spreader grafts. **(C)** Preoperative lateral view. **(D)** Postoperative lateral view. **(E)** Preoperative submental view. **(F)** Postoperative submental view.

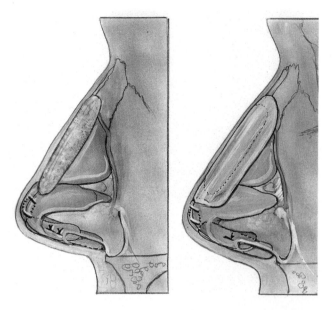

Figure 9-10. (A) Porous polyethylene dorsal implant. **(B)** Dorsal implant covered with dermal matrix graft.

lent architectural support with the addition of soft tissue dermal coverage of the implant (Figs. 9–10 and 9–11).

An additional postsurgical defect to the middle third of the nose includes insufficient reduction of the septum and upper lateral cartilages on lateral view. This problem presents as a persistent hump on the nose after rhinoplasty.

Before surgical reduction of this area is attempted, it is imperative that the position and strength of the lower third or tip of the nose be evaluated and, if necessary, corrected. A weakened and underprojected nasal tip will give the illusion of a higher middle nasal dorsum. If the nasal tip is not reprojected or augmented in this scenario, overresection of the nasal dorsal and upper lateral cartilages will result.

Therefore surgical correction of this defect requires lowering of the cartilaginous dorsal septum and upper lateral cartilages with preservation of the underlying mucoperichondrium. Rasping of these structures is usually not effective because of their cartilaginous nature.

Reduction is accomplished with a long, thin sharp-angled scissors, cutting small slivers of cartilage. This can

also be performed with a No. 11 blade and knife handle (Fig. 9–12).

LOWER THIRD OF NOSE

The lower third of the nose consists of the paired lower lateral cartilages that resemble a tripod with the central leg positioned inferiorly.[12]

Postoperative complications in this area are usually the result of inaccurate and asymmetric overresection of the lower lateral tip cartilages (Fig. 9–13).

Consequently, long-term scar contraction of the overresected tip cartilages produces several resultant defects. First, collapse of the lateral limb of the lower cartilage into the nasal vestibule results in external nasal valve collapse. Second, nasal tip bifidity and pinching become more obvious as the nasal domes lateralize in response to weakened lateral support. This process can also result in progressive loss of nasal tip support and projection. Third, circumferential scar contraction in the lateral alla as a result of the paucity of lateral limb cartilage results in superior alar retraction and excessive columella show.

Surgical management of this postoperative defect is managed in a sequential manner. First, columella support must be reestablished. This is accomplished by placement of an autogenous septal cartilage or alloplastic implant between the medial crura and fixated with 5-0 monocryl sutures. The strut is foreshortened and the dome cartilages are fixated anterior to the strut with 4-0 prolene suture. The residual tip cartilages are carved into as symmetric a shape as possible. Next, a resection of the residual lateral limb cartilage from the vestibular lining is accomplished. This is done with great care, and any rents in the mucosa are repaired with 5-0 chromic suture. These portions of cartilage are saved for possible use as additional onlay grafts.

A pocket is created as the alar cartilages are removed, and this is carried over to the pyriform aperture. Hemostasis is usually required in this portion of the dissection. Next a batten graft is placed into the lateral alar pocket. This graft sits just anterior to the pyriform aperture, superior to the alar margin, and lateral to the nasal tip carti-

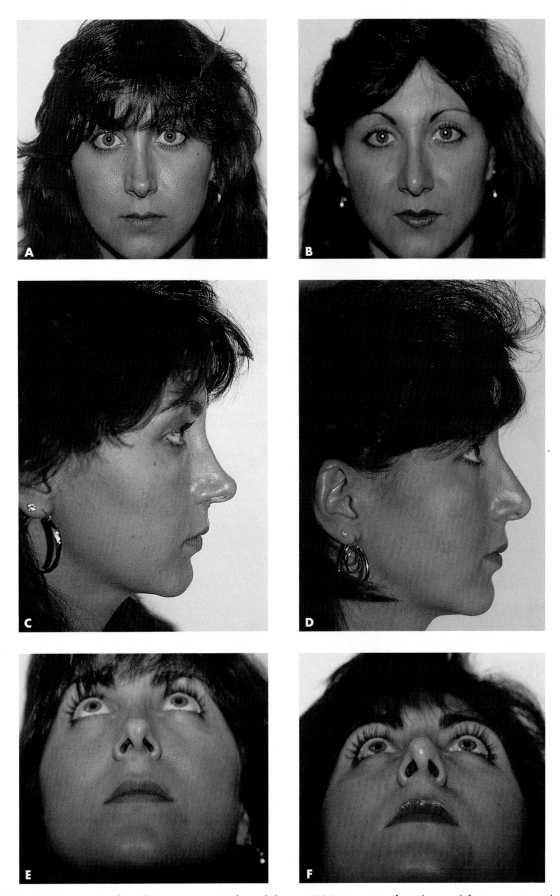

Figure 9–11. **(A)** Preoperative frontal view: overresected nasal dorsum. **(B)** Postoperative frontal view: defect correction with composite alloimplant. **(C)** Preoperative lateral view. **(D)** Postoperative lateral view. **(E)** Preoperative submental view. **(F)** Postoperative submental view.

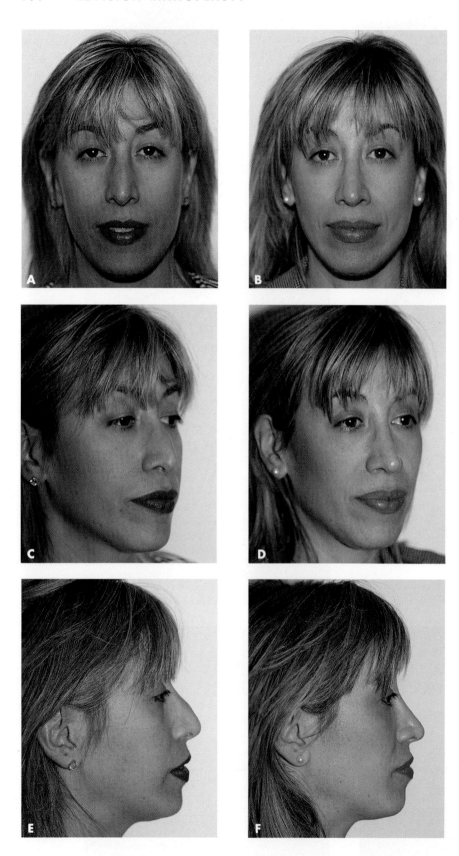

Figure 9-12. (A) Preoperative frontal view: Insufficient nasal dorsal reduction. **(B)** Postoperative frontal view: sharp scissors nasal dorsal cartilage reduction. **(C)** Preoperative three-quarter view. **(D)** Postoperative three-quarter view. **(E)** Preoperative lateral view. **(F)** Postoperative lateral view.

Normal

Collapsed lateral
nasal cartilage

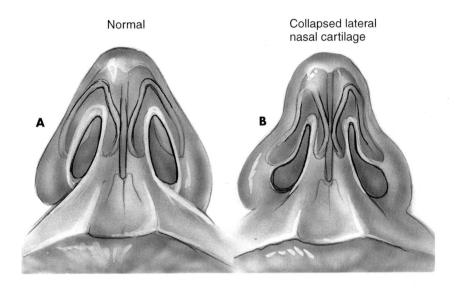

Figure 9–13. (A) Submental view: natural contour of native lower lateral cartilage. **(B)** Submental view: overresected lateral limb of lower cartilage and external valve collapse.

lages. This batten is usually harvested from the cymba and cavum conchal cartilage but may be fashioned from septal cartilage or alloplastic implants (Figs. 9–14 and 9–15).

Augmentation of the tip cartilages is now accomplished with autogenous septal cartilage. This can be fashioned as a tiered umbrella graft to increase tip projection or a tiered shield graft, which can also add length to the nasal profile (Fig. 9–16).

If excessive columella show remains, shortening of the caudal nasal septum 2 mm to 3 mm will improve this defect. Rarely, the cephalic edge of the medial crura may need to be resected to improve excessive columella show.

When severe alar retraction results because of loss of vestibular lining and excessive cartilage resection, a composite chondrocutaneous graft is harvested from the auricular concha. This graft creates a defect that requires

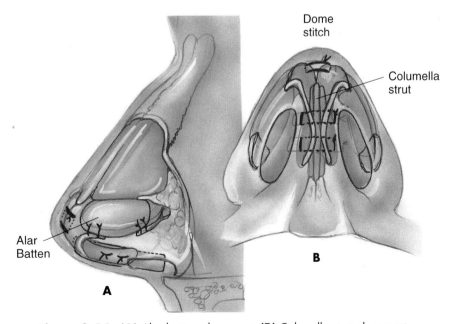

Figure 9–14. (A) Alar batten placement. **(B)** Columella strut placement.

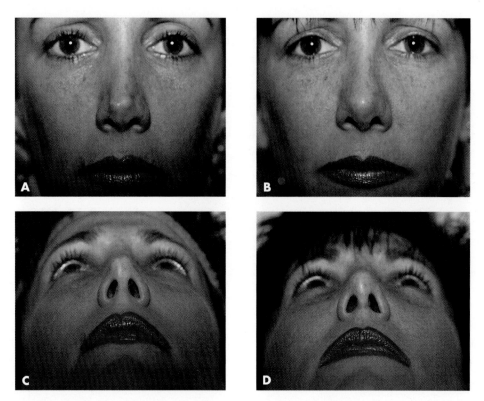

Figure 9–15. (A) Preoperative frontal view: overresected lower lateral cartilage. **(B)** Postoperative frontal view: correction of external valve collapse with alar batten. **(C)** Preoperative submental view. **(D)** Postoperative submental view.

a subsequent skin graft from the postauricular region. The composite graft is inset and suture fixated into the alar vestibular defect created by incising the vestibular mucosa and inferior retraction of the alar margin (Figs. 9–17 and 9–18).

Columella retraction and loss of columella show can be handled by placement of tiered septal cartilage strut superficial to the medial and intermediate crural cartilages. This technique can add 2 mm to 3 mm of columella show (Fig. 9–19). If excessive columella

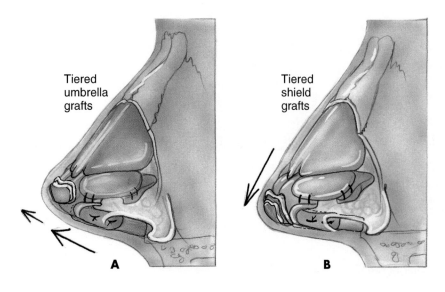

Tiered umbrella grafts

Tiered shield grafts

Figure 9–16. (A) Tiered umbrella graft adds projection. **(B)** Tiered shield graft adds projection and nasal length.

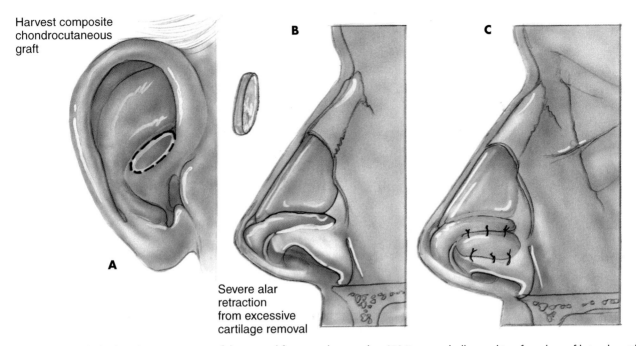

Harvest composite chondrocutaneous graft

Severe alar retraction from excessive cartilage removal

Figure 9–17. **(A)** Chondrocutaneous graft harvested from cymba concha. **(B)** Retracted alla resulting from loss of lateral cartilage and vestibular mucosa. **(C)** Chondrocutaneous graft inset into nasal vestibule recipient site.

retraction is present, a composite auricular cartilage graft is harvested and inset into the membranous septum between the caudal septum and cephalic edge of the medial crura (Fig. 9–20).

Occasionally a loss of tip projection occurs as a result of lysing of the natural tip supports and resultant scar contracture. Reprojection of the nasal tip is accomplished by placement of a columella strut between the medial crura. Medial fixation of the tip cartilages and shield tip graft fixation re-establish an adequate tip contour (Fig. 9–21).

COMPLICATIONS

By definition revision rhinoplasty is a high-risk endeavor. The probability of obtaining excellent results after one nasal reconstruction procedure is limited. Therefore in preoperative consultation the patient needs to be informed that 25% of the time a secondary procedure may need to be performed 1 year after the initial reconstruction. Even after the secondary procedure, a 10% chance exists that the postoperative result may not satisfy the patient.

CONCLUSION

The high-risk nature of revision rhinoplasty can lead to acceptable success rates if strict tenets have been applied. These include proper patient selection, with realistic goals being established. Limiting the extent of the reconstructive surgery may result in less dramatic postoperative nasal definition but usually produces a satisfactory result that the surgeon and the patient can live with. The old adage that less is more definitely applies in this situation.

PEARLS

- The surgeon must be sure that the patient fully understands the limitations of the final result before beginning revision nasal surgery.
- Allow for total healing of the nasal tissues before revision nasal surgery is attempted.
- Use autogenous donor grafting material preferentially.
- Alloplastic materials are acceptable implants when autogenous tissues are not available.
- Set conservative achievable goals; less is more.

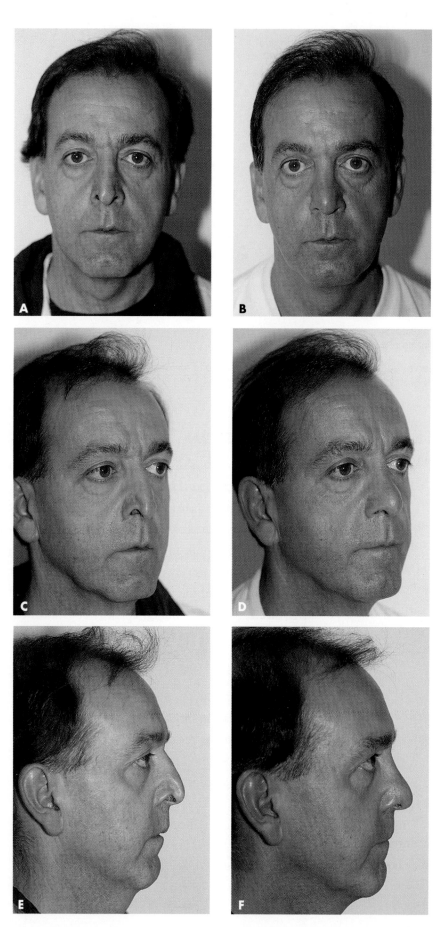

Figure 9–18. (A) Preoperative frontal views: nasal alar retraction.
(B) Postoperative frontal view: correction of alar defect with chondrocutaneous ear graft. **(C)** Preoperative three-quarter view. **(D)** Postoperative three-quarter view. **(E)** Preoperative lateral view.
(F) Postoperative lateral view.
(G) Preoperative submental view.
(H) Postoperative submental view.

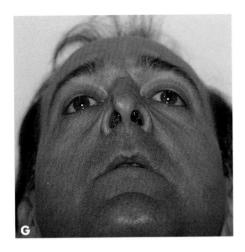

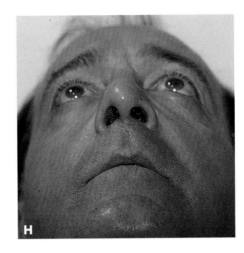

Figure 9–18. *(continued)*

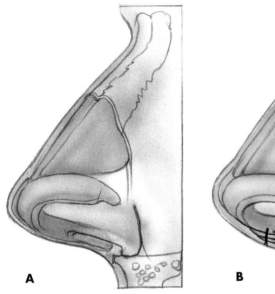

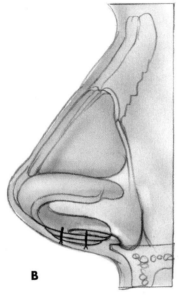

Figure 9–19. (A) Mild columella retraction.
(B) Defect correction with tiered cartilage graft
superficial to medial crura.

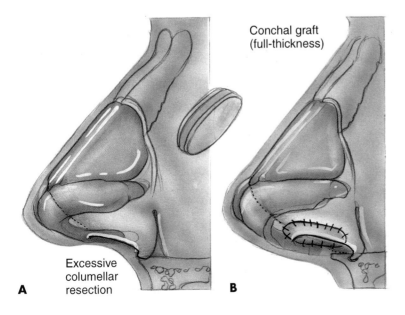

Figure 9–20. (A) Severe columella
retraction. **(B)** Full-thickness conchal graft inset
between caudal septum and medial crura.

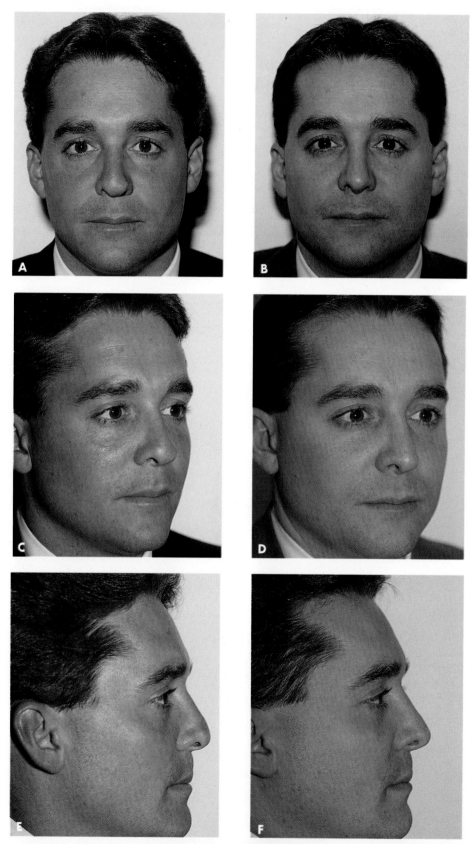

Figure 9–21. (A) Preoperative frontal view: nasal tip blunting resulting from loss of tip supports. **(B)** Postoperative frontal view: tip projection re-established with columella strut and tip grafting. **(C)** Preoperative thee-quarter view. **(D)** Postoperative three-quarter view. **(E)** Preoperative lateral view. **(F)** Postoperative lateral view. **(G)** Preoperative submental view. **(H)** Postoperative submental view.

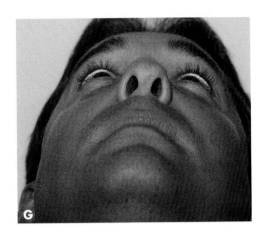

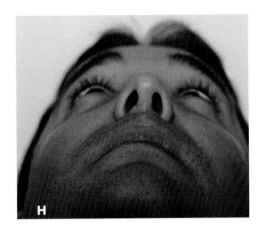

Figure 9–21. *(continued)*

REFERENCES

1. Tardy ME, Brown RJ. *Surgical Anatomy of the Nose.* New York: Raven Press; 1990; 1–23.
2. Gunter JP, Rohrich RJ. Augmentation rhinoplasty: Dorsal onlay grafting material using shaped autogenous septal cartilage. *Plast Reconstr Surg.* 1990; 86:39–45.
3. Johnson C, Toriumi DM. Open structure rhinoplasty, Philadelphia: W.B. Saunders; 1989: 99.
4. Daniel RK. *Aesthetic Plastic Surgery Rhinoplasty.* Boston: Little Brown & Co; 1993; 466.
5. Romo T, Jablonski RD. Nasal reconstruction using split calvarial grafts. *Otolaryngol Head Neck Surg.* 1992; 107:622–630.
6. Maves MD. Comment on Murakamics, Cook TA, Guida RA. Nasal reconstruction with articulated irradiated rib cartilage. *Arch Otolaryngol Head Neck Surg* 1991; 117:331.
7. Owsley TG, Taylor CO. The use of Gore-Tex for nasal augmentation: A retrospective analysis of 106 patients. *Plast Reconstr Surg.* 1994; 94:241.
8. Romo T, Sclafani AP, Sabini P. Use of porous high-density polyethylene in revision rhinoplasty and in the platyrrhine nose. *Aesthet Plast Surg.* 1998; 22:211–221.
9. Sclafani AP, Romo T, Silver L. Clinical and histological behavior of exposed porous high-density polyethylene implants, *Plast Reconstr Surg.* 1997; 99:41–50.
10. Sheen JH. Spreader graft: A method of reconstructing the root of the middle nasal vault following rhinoplasty. *Plast Reconstr Surg.* 1984; 73:230.
11. Romo T, Sclafani AP, Sabini P. Reconstruction of the major saddle nose deformity using composite allo-implants. *Facial Plast Surg.* 1998; 14:151–157.
12. Anderson JR, Ries WR. Rhinoplasty emphasizing the external approach. New York: Thieme Inc; 1986: 71.

Revision Rhinoplasty

Aesthetic Facial Plastic Surgery, edited by Thomas Romo, III, and Arthur L. Millman, Thieme Medical Publishers, Inc., New York, New York, Copyright © 2000.

CHAPTER 10

A Plastic Surgeon's Perspective

NICOLAS TABBAL AND ROBERT M. FREUND

Upon this point a page of history is worth a volume of logic.

Oliver Wendell Holmes, Jr., 1921

The art of rhinoplasty has been studied and practiced since the time of Sushruta (500 BC). Modern rhinoplasty was advanced in the 19th century when von Graefe (1787–1840) and Dieffenbach (1794–1847) published refined methods of the Indian and Tagliacotian methods of reconstructive rhinoplasty. The closed approach to cosmetic rhinoplasty was introduced by John O. Roe, an American-born otorhinolaryngologist in his classic paper in 1891, which described the removal of the bony and cartilaginous hump through an intranasal approach. Between 1928 and 1931, Jacques Joseph pioneered cosmetic rhinoplasty with his two-volume textbook on the subject.

The trend in rhinoplasty surgery has been toward a more conservative approach with more awareness of the negative structural and functional implications of reduction procedures. As a result, the aesthetic ideal nose is both natural appearing and functional. Recently, interest in the open approach originally described by Jacques Joseph in the 1930s has increased. This approach allows the surgeon more freedom to preserve anatomic structures because of increased visibility and control.

Because of the difficulty in predicting the idiosyncrasies of wound healing, even in the best of hands, the incidence of postsurgical nasal deformities requiring secondary corrections lies anywhere from 5 to 15%. Localized rasping and other minor revisions make up most of these procedures. Major revisions, such as corrections of saddle deformities and tip contractures, are decreasing in incidence because of the overall trend toward conservatism. The major deformities requiring secondary rhinoplasty can be avoided at the primary procedure with careful preoperative analysis. Furthermore, a basic understanding of the cause of secondary deformities and careful technical execution are essential components to their prevention.

PREOPERATIVE EVALUATION

HISTORY

The challenge of secondary rhinoplasty begins with a complete history. Most secondary rhinoplasty patients have specific dislikes and concerns about their nasal imperfections. In general, these patients are more skeptical of the medical profession and feel victimized by their prior experience. With this in mind, it is important to understand the nature of their complaints and treat them with an added degree of compassion.

It is important to determine whether the patient's complaint is purely an aesthetic issue or is compounded by a functional problem. The exact points of discontent, whether real or imagined, and the way in which they are expressed may provide critical information about the patient's psychologic makeup and may help determine whether their expectations are realistic.

Next, information should be obtained regarding the previous surgeries. The number of procedures and the time lapse between them is important to determine the state of wound maturation. Surgeons should resist the temptation to reoperate prematurely on patients when soft tissues have not reached their optimal state.

Finally, it is worth noting that despite detailed descriptions of septal surgery in a previous operative report, it is not uncommon to find a virgin septum during the subsequent physical examination. Such discrepancy can only be explained by the desire of the previous surgeon to get insurance coverage for a cosmetic rhinoplasty. Operative reports should be read with some skepticism because often a discrepancy exists between the narrative elegance of the described procedure and the unfavorable nature of the clinical outcome.

EXTERNAL NASAL EXAMINATION

In a systematic fashion the entire nose is visually examined. Starting at the radix, determine its depth and height relative to the supratarsal fold. Examine the bony vault for symmetry, dorsal irregularities, and stair-step deformities. Note the height and length of the dorsal profile and its relation to the lobule. Is the width of the bony vault adequate? If osteotomies were performed, are they symmetric, and if not, does the asymmetry create a visual deformity?

Next, focus attention to the middle vault, the part of the nose created by the upper lateral cartilage and the septum. A collapse of these cartilages can accentuate the caudal borders of the nasal bones, causing an "inverted v sign." Determine the symmetry of the middle vault. Dorsal septal deviations will cause a unilateral collapse of the upper lateral cartilage with visibility of the caudal border of the nasal bones, which is interpreted by the patient as a prominence.

Moving inferiorly, carefully evaluate the tip-lobule complex. Identify the tip-defining points. Are they symmetric? Is the tip boxy or bifid? Is tip projection adequate or does the patient have overprojection of the nasal tip? Examine the tip-lobule complex for alar integrity. Alar collapse will present in thin-skinned individuals as an overly pinched tip.

Next, evaluate the length of the nose. In an ideal situation, projection of the tip should make up two thirds of the dorsal length, as measured by the distance from the radix to the tip-defining points. Thus a lower radix or an overprojecting tip can accentuate the apparent shortness of the nose.

Analyze the relationship of the columella with the alar rims. A malpositioning of either structure will create a variety of abnormal relationships as described by Gunter. Note the impact of smiling on the lobule. Nasalis muscle will affect the tip during smiling by decreasing tip projection, particularly when the tip is underprojected.

In addition to the visual examination, manual palpation of the nose is critical. Determining the thickness of the skin will forecast the potential for success of any subsequent procedure. In patients with very thick nasal skin, supratip fullness correction, or enhancement of tip definition are difficult to accomplish. Thus patients' goals should be realistic. Finally, palpation should also be used to determine the presence and location of any graft material because a variety of malformations of the nasal anatomy can be caused by improper graft use or placement.

INTERNAL NASAL EXAMINATION

Examination of the septum should determine the presence of deviations and associated obstructions. In addition, because most secondary procedures require some degree of augmentation, assessing the availability of the septum as a donor site is of prime importance. Particular attention should be paid to both high septal deformity and septal spurs in the region of the hard palate. These septal spurs, if missed, result in airway compromise. High septal deviation often affects the shape of the dorsum after hump reduction and can also influence the surgeon's ability to infracture the nasal bones symmetrically. Septal perforations should be noted, and patients should

be made aware of their presence before surgery.

Internal nasal examination should also include examination of the turbinates and nasal mucosa. The mucosa and vestibular skin should be examined for previous scarring and webbing. A deficiency in lining can cause deformities such as alar retraction, short nose deformity, or columellar retraction. Look for narrowing of the internal nasal valve, the angle made by the junction of the upper lateral cartilage and the septum. This is best done when the patient is inhaling rapidly. This angle should ideally measure 10 to 15 degrees. If lateral displacement of the cheek improves the airway on that side, the presence of a valve problem is confirmed. Finally, the external nasal valve should be observed during active inspiration to assess the functional stability of the ala.

PRINCIPLES OF TREATMENT

The timing of a secondary rhinoplasty should be based on the status of the nasal soft tissues. The interval between procedures, particularly the ones involving the lobule, should be no less than 1 year. It is permissible to perform minimal rasping of the bridge, if soft tissues permit, several months after the procedure as long as the tip is not violated. Palpation of the soft tissues, especially in the lobule, for induration, thickness, and pliability will determine to a great extent the readiness of the nose for surgery.

In our opinion, secondary nasal surgery, with the exception of small revisions, should preferably be performed through an open approach. We believe that under the proper circumstances, the benefits of this technique far outweigh the liability of the columella scar.

Our material of choice for nasal augmentation is septal cartilage because of its flatness and availability. Conchal cartilage is our next choice if septal cartilage is not available. Although not ideal for dorsal augmentation, its natural curvature can be used in tip and alar rim reconstruction.

If septal or conchal cartilage is not available, rib cartilage is a third choice for nasal reconstruction. Unfortunately, this cartilage has a tendency to warp. Gunter has reduced this risk by inserting a K-wire through the long axis of the cartilage. Other autogenous tissues used for augmentation include iliac and calvarial bone. Both of these materials are best suited for dorsal reconstruction and share the problem of unpredictable resorption.

The use of synthetic material in secondary surgery should be avoided, if possible. We have, on rare occasions successfully used GoreTex grafts for dorsal augmentation in patients who already had the septum and both ears used as previous donor sites. Although these grafts generally do well on the dorsum, their use in the tip should be condemned because of tension on the overlying skin.

OPEN VERSUS CLOSED APPROACH

The closed technique is still the most commonly used approach in nasal reconstruction (Table 10–1). Its benefits include concealed scars, reduced surgical time, and decreased swelling compared with the open approach. Furthermore, this procedure allows for a good evaluation of surface aesthetics at the time of surgery. These benefits make closed rhinoplasty the procedure of choice for simple nasal problems, such as the wide nasal base, excess anterior nasal spine, minor tip revisions, dorsal irregularities, and the overprojecting tip.

Table 10–1 Open versus closed rhinoplasty

Open	Closed
Total exposure	Limited exposure
Complete analysis	Limited analysis
Anatomic manipulation	Surface aesthetics
Better use of native cartilage	Concealed scars
Columellar incision	
Increased tip edema	

The closed technique is still handicapped by the limited exposure and the inability to accurately examine the nasal architecture. Furthermore, productive manipulation of the alar remnant in secondary tip surgery is severely limited.

In contradistinction, the open technique benefits from improved exposure, thus allowing total evaluation of the anatomic deformities. Because of the better visualization, manipulation of the anatomy is more precise and meticulous. It allows preservation and better use of the native cartilage, thus minimizing the need for grafting. If used, grafts are secured with sutures under visual control, thus minimizing malposition and displacement.

The drawbacks of the open technique include the potentially visible columellar scar and possibly prolonged tip edema. In our opinion, the benefits of this procedure outweigh the potential problems because of the added improvements that are generally associated with the open approach.

SPECIFIC DEFORMITIES IN SECONDARY SURGERY
Nasal Bone Deviation

Nasal bone deviation is commonly the result of incomplete osteotomy or on rare occasions an unrecognized high septal deviation that would have prevented medial displacement of the nasal bones after osteotomy. Correction involves complete osteotomy and infracture. Treatment of the high septal deformity is difficult, but the use of Asch tissue forceps to crush the perpendicular plate of the ethmoid allows some success to be achieved. Correction of depressed nasal bones is best achieved with onlay grafting instead of outfracture technique (Fig. 10-1).

Stair-step Deformity

Stair-step deformity is due to a previous osteotomy that was made high on the nasal process of the maxilla, leaving a projection of the maxilla lateral the base of the

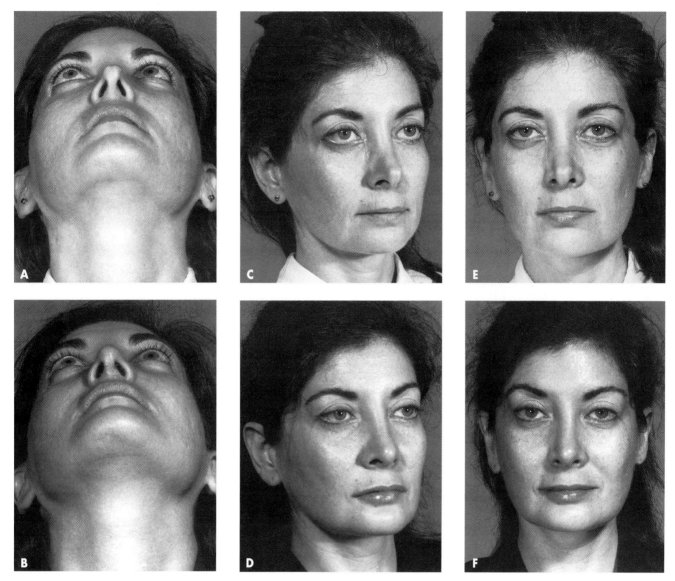

Figure 10-1. Saddle deformity with bilateral alar collapse. The saddle deformity was corrected with a dorsal graft. The alar collapse and bifid tip was corrected with an alar strut and domal unification. **(A, C, E)** Preoperative. **(B, D, F)** Postoperative.

nasal bones. Correction requires reosteotomy at the proper level.

Middle Vault Dorsal Deviation

As with the deviations of the bony dorsum, secondary asymmetries of the middle vault are due to unrecognized high septal deviations. These deformities become apparent after elimination of a dorsal hump, which may have been well centralized. Treatment involves primarily correction of septal deviation. Spreader grafts are ideal for the more recalcitrant septal deformities (Fig. 10–2).

These grafts will provide rigidity to the dorsal septum and symmetry to the middle vault when placed in an asymmetric fashion. Often the correction of the intrinsic septal deviation is incomplete, thus placement of a spreader graft on the affected side is an ideal choice of treatment.

A spreader graft is a cartilage graft placed between the septum and the upper lateral cartilage. This graft is about 2 cm long by 5 mm wide. Its thickness is determined by the nature of the defect, so that in cases of significant collapse of the upper lateral cartilage, multiple grafts are used in parallel. These grafts should be secured

Mid-Vault Deviation

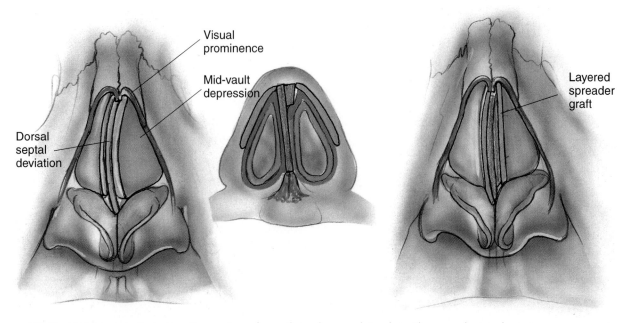

Figure 10–2. Middle vault deviation. Depression of a unilateral upper lateral cartilage or deviated septum can present as a twisted nose or as a bony prominence at the caudal border of the bony vault. Septal spreader grafts correct this deformity.

to the dorsal septum in at least two sites to avoid dorsal displacement of the graft. The placement of the grafts should follow the osteotomies during the surgical procedure to fully appreciate the severity and location of the deficit. When the procedure is performed through an open approach, the pocket for placement of the cartilage should be generous. Grafts are sutured into place against the septum with 6-0 polydioxanone (PDS) suture. However, in the closed approach, the pocket should be limited so that the benefits of the graft are not nullified.

For subtle asymmetries of the middle vault, where the internal nasal valves are not affected and in the absence of nasal airway problems, onlay crushed cartilage placed over the upper lateral cartilage is an acceptable substitute for spreader grafts.

Middle Vault Collapse

Middle vault collapse is a relatively common problem for which secondary rhinoplasty is sought. Patients present with airway problems and the perception that they have a

residual bony prominence at the caudal border of the nasal bones. The predisposing factors for the postsurgical collapse of the middle vault are several. The main one is the presence of short nasal bones (nasal bones that support less than 40% of the nasal dorsum) with thin soft tissue in the middle vault areas. Resection of the dorsal hump in these patients, especially in association with an osteotomy, without reconstruction of the middle vault is likely to affect adversely the relationship between the upper lateral cartilage and the septum. This creates a visible collapse of the middle vault with disruption of the nasal dorsal line and a compromise of the internal nasal valves associated airway obstruction. The work of Sheen has elegantly explained the nature of this problem and provided a predictable solution with the use of spreader grafts.

Supra tip Fullness

Fullness in the region of the septal angle is common and is caused by a variety of factors that are quite diverse. The most common cause is an inadequate lowering of the septal angle (Fig. 10–3A) and is a reflection of the timidity of the surgeon and the fear of causing a saddle nose deformity. One of the key elements in a rhinoplasty, particularly in the closed approach, is judging intraoperatively where the final tip position will eventually be. Because many of the maneuvers of the surgical exposure, particularly in the closed approach, tend to diminish tip projection, forecasting accurately the final projection of the tip requires experience and some guesswork. Misjudging the subsequent loss in projection of the nasal tip would create a setup for future visibility of the septal angle with supratip fullness. These problems should be

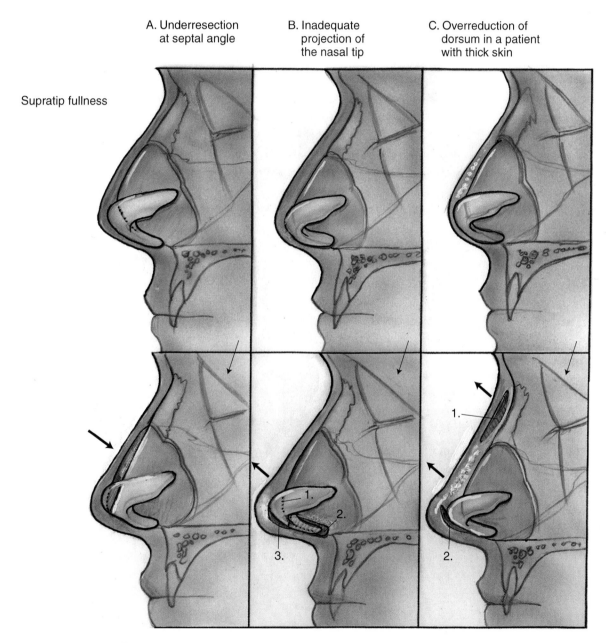

Figure 10–3. Supra tip fullness. **(A)** Underresection of the septal angle is treated by resection of the underresected septum. **(B)** Inadequate projection of the nasal tip is corrected by lateral crural recruitment, columellar strut, tip grafts. **(C)** Overreduction of the dorsum in a patient with thick skin is corrected by radix and tip augmentation.

less common in the open approach because this exposure causes less disturbance in the tip-supporting elements. In addition, the surgeon has the ability to visually assess the adequacy of the relationship between the septal angle and the domes. Approximately 8 mm should separate these two structures to create a visible supratip break.

Another common cause of supratip fullness is the inadequate projection of the nasal tip (Fig. 10–3B), which was present preoperatively and went unrecognized.

In such situations, dorsal reductions will cause further loss of projection in an already deficient tip. Attempts

at creating the proper balance between the dorsum and tip projection are bound to fail because additional lowering of the dorsum is associated with additional loss of tip projection. The correction of this problem entails an enhancement of tip projection with a variety of maneuvers, including tip grafts, columellar struts, or enhancement of the domes with suture techniques.

Finally, the least common cause of supratip fullness is overreduction of the dorsum in a patient with thick skin (Fig. 10–4). The inability of the soft tissue to redrape to a much lowered dorsal height creates the setup for the

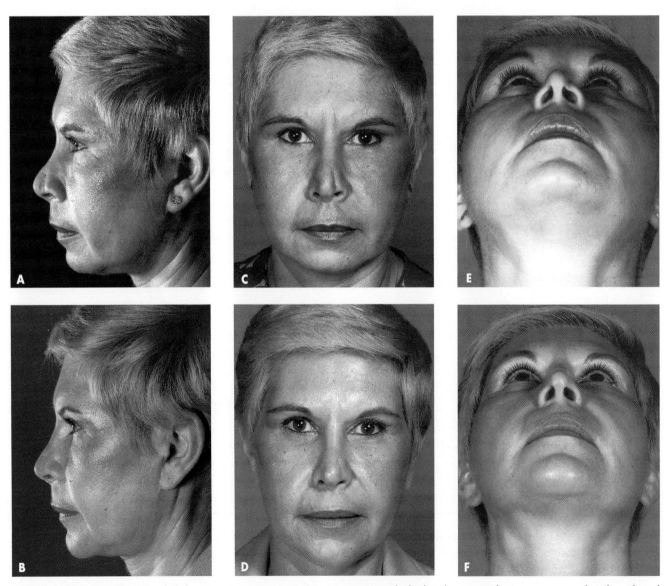

Figure 10–4. Supratip nasal deformity. Supratip scarring in a patient with thick sebaceous skin was corrected with a dorsal augmentation graft and shield tip graft (closed approach). NOTE: chin augmentation was also performed. **(A, C, E)** Preoperative. **(B, D, F)** Postoperative.

creation of dead space and subsequent scar tissue formation in the supratip area. Such problems can be most difficult to treat. Steroid injection in the supratip area can be occasionally helpful in mild-to-moderate deformities, but the recalcitrant situation will require dorsal augmentation with enhancement of tip projection. Thus one is choosing the height of the supratip as the new dorsal height. The ideal treatment for these patents is the combination of tip graft to improve tip projection, with or without dorsal augmentation.

Underprojected Tip

Correction of the underprojected tip can be achieved in several ways, depending on the approached used and the condition of the alar cartilages. Generally, in the closed approach, one relies on the insertion of tip grafts, shield shaped or as onlay with or without unification of the domes. Although potentially beneficial, these grafts can cause tip deformity through misplacement.

In contradistinction, the open approach allows a more productive use of the native cartilage in the tip. Correction of the buckling or weakness of the medial crura is best treated here by the placement of a columellar strut. This is done by creating a pocket between the medial crura and placing a 1.5 to 2-cm by 5-mm cartilage strut into the pocket. The medial crura are then temporarily fixed to the graft with 25-guage needles and then sutured inplace with 4-0 plain gut suture. The placement of a strut long enough to rest on the anterior nasal spine can cause lateral mobility at the nasal base with subsequent tip asymmetry. However, appropriate placement of the columellar strut allows more beneficial recruitment of the lateral crura. Particular attention should be paid to the avoidance of excessive tip projection with overuse of struts and shield grafts.

Tip Asymmetry

Correction of tip asymmetry is best achieved with an open approach because it allows structural modification of the native tip cartilage with the use of sutures or supporting grafts (Fig. 10–5). The use of sutures in tip modification significantly decreases the need for tip grating and the associated undesirable effects of visible grafts. PDS sutures (6-0) are judiciously used to unify the domes and provide the framework for additional grafts, if needed. Colored suture materials (nylon or prolene) should be avoided because of the potential visibility through the overlying skin.

Alar Collapse

The most common cause of alar collapse is overreduction of the lateral crus in the thin-skinned patient. Aggressive attenuation of the lateral crura is most common with the use of the transcartilaginous incision in the closed technique. Another cause of this deformity is the so-called Goldman tip, which involves a willful division of the domes to correct the boxy tip. Lastly, transection of the lateral crus with subsequent collapse can be caused by inadvertent division of the lateral crura because of an unrecognized malpositioned lateral alar cartilage (i.e., parenthesis deformity).

The treatment of alar collapse depends on its cause. In situations where disruption or excessive weakening of the lateral crura is present, the addition of alar struts that are placed between the crural remnants and the underlying mucosa will provide dependable support to the alar rim (Fig. 10–1).

If the deformity is the result of overresection of the cephalic portion of the lateral crura, Gunter suggests either alar strip grafts or alar spreader grafts (Fig. 10–6A). The strip grafts span the dome to overlap the pyriform aperture rims. In contrast, alar spreader grafts use a triangular piece of cartilage to span the supratip and to push the remaining lateral crural strips laterally. We use a variation of the alar spreader graft, which spans the underside of both lower lateral crura (Fig. 10–6B). Fixing one side of the graft and advancing the contralateral side determines the amount of alar flare obtained.

In cases of total domal transection, the correction should entail a domal reconstruction with suture tech-

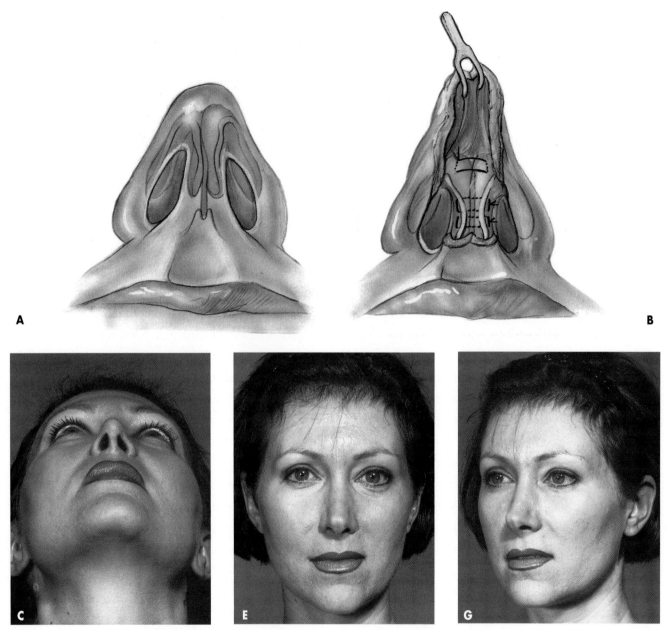

Figure 10–5. Bifid tip. **(A, B)** Knuckling of the dome was corrected with domal unification and a cartilage onlay graft through an open approach. **(C, E, G)** Preoperative.

nique along with onlay grafts. This approach is best suited for the open technique. Total domal reconstruction with a large umbrella graft is a less desirable option.

Alar Retraction

Alar retraction is caused by surgical maneuvers that cause upward movement of the lower lateral cartilages. These forces can be a result of overresection of the cephalic border of the lateral crura or vestibular lining and a poorly placed rim incision, especially in the region of the soft triangle.

Correction of this problem can be achieved by releasing the scar tissue contracture by making an incision in the vestibular skin 2 to 3 mm above the area of the alar rim

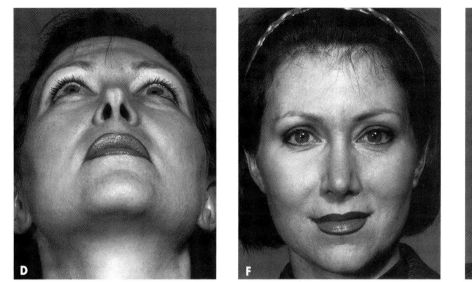
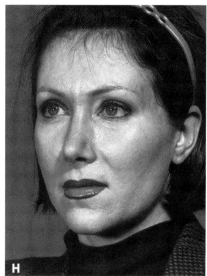

Figure 10–5 *(continued)* **(D, F, H)** Postoperative.

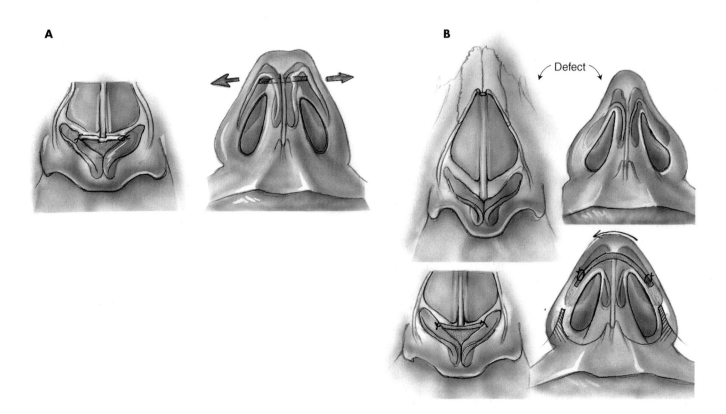

Figure 10–6. Alar collapse as as result of excessive domal resection is corrected by a sliding alar spreader graft.

that is retracted. The scar tissue is undermined, and the alar rim is brought inferiorly to the desired height. The resultant defect in the vestibular lining can be filled with a composite cartilage graft from the ear. Ellenbogen corrects this problem by releasing the scar contracture previously described but then puts a cartilage strip graft in the undermined pocket paralleling the rim. The vestibular skin edge is then sutured in position, resulting in a raw surface above the graft. This location is allowed to granulate.

Short Nose

This is perhaps the most difficult problem in secondary rhinoplasty to correct. Its cause is generally overresection of the caudal septum. Subsequent soft tissue retraction and scarring make any attempt to reverse this deformity tenuous at best. True lengthening of the nose relies on inferior displacement of the tip elements by complete release of the soft tissue and mucoperichondrial lining of the nasal septum along with extended spreader grafts that extend beyond the caudal edge of the septum and act as spacers.

SUMMARY

Secondary rhinoplasty requires careful evaluation of the nasal deformity along with a keen understanding of the patients' desires and expectations. Because each additional nasal procedure adds a degree of scarring and irreversibility to the soft tissue of the nose, every attempt should be made to address adequately all the presenting problems. Structural deficits can be easily surmounted with nasal augmentation. However, soft tissue problems may significantly diminish the positive nature of the potential outcome. Through careful analysis and meticulous execution, many patients seeking correction of the post surgical deformity should expect a modicum of improvement.

PEARLS

- Operative reports should be read with some skepticism because often a discrepancy exists between the procedure therein described and the unfavorable outcome.
- With the exception of small revisions, all secondary nasal surgery should be performed by means of an open approach. The main advantage of this technique is the improved exposures, and its disadvantages are visible scarring and possible tip edema.
- The use of synthetic material in secondary surgery should be avoided.
- Benefits of the closed technique include concealed scars, reduced surgical time, and reduced swelling. However, disadvantages are limited exposure and inability to accurately examine the nasal architecture.

SUGGESTED READINGS

Daniel RK. *Aesthetic Plastic Surgery: Rhinoplasty*. Boston: Little, Brown & Co.; 1993.

Ellenbogen R. Alar rim lowering. *Plast Reconstr Surg*. 1987; 79:50.

Gruber RP. Lengthening the short nose. *Plast Reconstr Surg*. 1993; 91:1252.

Gunter JP, Rohrich RJ. Lengthening the asthetically short nose. 1989; 83:793.

Gunter JP, Rohrich RJ. Correction of the pinched nasal tip with alar spreader grafts. *Plast Reconstr Surg*. 1992; 90:821.

Johnson CM, Toriumi DM. *Open Structure Rhinoplasty*. Philadelphia: W.B. Saunders Co.; 1990.

Peck GC. *Techniques in Aesthetic Rhinoplasty*. Philadelphia: Lippincott; 1990.

Rees TD, LaTrenta G. *Aesthetic Plastic Surgery*. Philadelphia: WB Saunders; 1994.

Sheen JH. Spreader graft: A method of reconstructing the roof of the middle nasal vault following rhinoplasty. *Plast Reonstr Surg*. 1984; 73:230.

Sheen JH. Tip graft: A 20-year retrospective. *Plast Reconstr Surg*. 1993; 91:48.

Tabbal N, Freund RM. Sliding spreader graft for alar collapse. *In press*.

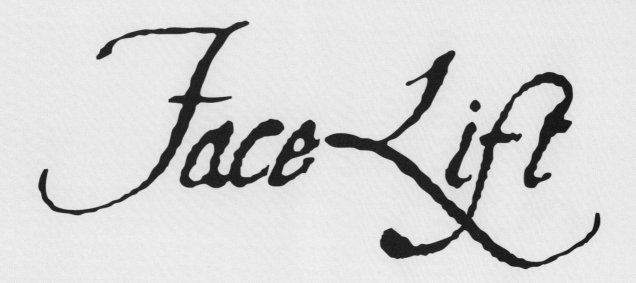

Face Lift

The facelift chapters most embody the entire textbook more than any specific chapter. The technique of facelifting is a window into all the technological and surgical technique evolution that has occurred in the last decade and the chapters by Dr. Ramirez and Dr. Kamer embody that evolution.

Dr. Kamer, a renowned facial surgeon, describes the foundations of facial anatomy and their relation to surgical technique from basic facelifting procedures through deep plane subcutaneous musculosponeurotic system (SMAS)–based procedures and range of extended procedures to enhance facial results.

Dr. Ramirez further expounds and concentrates on the most recent evolution of subperiosteal plane use in the endoscopic technique of facelifting. Both authors recognize that each of the techniques need be individualized to the needs of a given patient, and those needs are dictated by physical findings and frequently the age of the patient. The two chapters complement each other beautifully and virtually represent a textbook within a textbook on facial surgery.

Face Lift

Aesthetic Facial Plastic Surgery, edited by Thomas Romo, III, and Arthur L. Millman, Thieme Medical Publishers, Inc., New York, New York, Copyright © 2000.

CHAPTER 11

A Facial Plastic Surgeon's Perspective

FRANK M. KAMER AND PATRICK G. PIEPER

Rhytidectomy is an operation designed to alleviate signs of aging in the face and neck. With advancing years there is increased laxity and hence redundancy in the cervicofacial skin, atrophy of subcutaneous fat, attenuation of the subcutaneous musculoaponeurotic system, and resorption of alveolar bone. These changes combine to produce an obtuse cervicomental angle, anterior platysmal banding, jowling with loss of inferior mandibular contour, inferior displacement of cheek fat with diminution of the malar eminence and accentuation of the nasolabial fold, and ptosis of the lateral brow. The presence and degree of these deformities must be determined by a careful and detailed preoperative physical examination and correlated with the findings at surgery. Only in this way can the procedure be tailored to the individual patient to ensure an anatomically sound and aesthetically pleasing result.

PATIENT SELECTION

Success in aesthetic facial surgery, more than any other discipline, depends on proper motivation of the patient coupled with reasonable expectation as to the postoperative recovery and ultimate outcome of the procedure. These factors must be determined by the surgeon during the initial consultation. A poorly selected patient or one who is inadequately prepared for surgery is likely to be unhappy even with a technically flawless result.

The ideal patient seeks surgery to bring his or her appearance closer to an appropriate self-image, not to satisfy the demands of others or achieve goals unrelated to the surgical result. The history should also assess the patient's psychological state. It is of interest that "major" psychiatric problems, including depression and anxiety disorders, are less likely to be associated with postoperative dissatisfaction in cosmetic surgery patients than are personality disorders.[1] Studies have shown that patients most likely to be dissatisfied with surgery are found within the following personality types: borderline, obsessive-compulsive, antisocial, schizotypal, and paranoid.

The consultation must also include a complete review of the patient's medical history, with emphasis on any conditions that could present a surgical risk. Hypertension, cardiovascular disease, pulmonary problems, diabetes, and prior anesthetic complications should be identified, as well as any bleeding diathesis. A history of recent aspirin, nonsteroidal anti-inflammatory, or excessive vitamin E ingestion is sought to further avoid perioperative bleeding problems. Tobacco, alcohol, or other substance abuse must be determined and treated before further consideration of surgery. For smokers, complete abstinence for a minimum of 2 weeks before surgery is required. When necessary, particularly with patients older than 50, medical clearance for surgery, which may include a chest x-ray film and electrocardiogram, is obtained from the patient's primary care physician. In all patients the history and physical examination are complemented by a complete blood count and screening for hepatitis B and human immunodeficiency virus.

As the interview continues, the patient is encouraged to indicate the "problem areas" in his or her face and neck for which correction is desired, and possible surgical solutions are discussed. This provides the surgeon with the opportunity to conduct a complete examination, emphasizing those areas of concern and pointing out any problems the patient might not have mentioned or even noticed. Many patients presenting for facelift surgery are primarily concerned with rhytids and signs of chronic sun exposure of the skin. Despite the plethora of options available for ancillary dermatologic treatments, including the burgeoning field of laser resurfacing, both patient and surgeon must understand that extensive facial rhytidosis and actinic damage can present a significant limiting factor to the overall success of rhytidectomy. For patients contemplating revision surgery, the examination should include assessment for hypertrophic scar tissue or other signs of poor wound healing, as well as any iatrogenic surgical deformities such as accentuation of anterior platysmal banding by aggressive liposuction, frank cobra deformity, a witch's chin, distortion of the auricular lobule, and areas of alopecia, or hairline step-off. These findings should be shown to the patient and management options can be discussed.

Finally, the entire surgical process is discussed with the patient in a sequential fashion and in considerable detail. The site and extent of all incisions are carefully demonstrated, as well as the type of wound closure, dressings, and any drains required. It is critical that the patient be counseled as to the degree of postoperative edema, ecchymoses, and discomfort to be expected, as well as restrictions on diet, level of activity, and any special instructions. It is far easier to prevent misunderstanding about these issues before surgery than to cope with a dissatisfied patient postoperatively.

TIMING OF SURGERY

Although facial aging is inevitable and progressive, it is neither linear nor predictable in its rate. As a general guideline, 45 to 55 years can be considered the "golden interval" for consideration of primary rhytidectomy, but this may be modified by such factors as a patient's general health, level of activity, occupation, and lifestyle. Although a trend has occured in recent years toward earlier surgical intervention, the benefit of such procedures for younger patients must be carefully weighed against the risks of surgery. Often, waiting until more is to be achieved by surgery can result in increased patient satisfaction. Conversely, although advanced age alone is not a contraindication for rhytidectomy, patients in their late 60s and beyond are most likely to benefit from surgery if they continue to lead an active lifestyle both physically and socially.

In addition to age, a patient's weight may also influence the timing of surgery. Morbidly obese patients clearly are not surgical candidates. Moreover, patients who need to lose 10 to 20 pounds or more to achieve an "ideal weight" consistent with their lifestyle and motivation should reach this goal and then maintain a stable weight for several months before surgery.

CHOICE OF PROCEDURE

The recent acceleration in the evolution of rhytidectomy as a surgical procedure has provided the surgeon with a number of options in the choice of technique. Historically, rhytidectomy began in the early twentieth century as a very limited procedure involving minimal subcutaneous undermining and excision of redundant skin.[2] The modern concept of facelift surgery began in the early 1970s with Skoog, who pioneered a deeper anatomic plane of dissection: "In addition to tightening and excising superfluous skin, the subcutaneous fat layer with its fascia, as well as the cutaneous muscles of the neck and face, are repositioned."[3]

In Skoog's technique the superficial fascia of the lower cheek, which he called the "buccal fascia," is undermined to the nasolabial fold and advanced posteriorly. The retrodisplaced buccal fascia is then sutured to the masse-

teric fascia. In the neck the platysma muscle is similarly undermined, advanced, and fixed to the mastoid fascia.

The histologic basis of the Skoog technique was soon clarified by the anatomic studies of Mitz and Peyronie, who identified Skoog's "buccal fascia" as part of a single tissue layer continuous with the tempoparietal fascia superiorly and the platysma inferiorly and intimately related to the overlying subcutaneous fat and skin by fibrous attachments.[4] This structure, referred to as the SMAS, was described as superficial to the parotid fascia and shown to invest the mimetic musculature of the face and neck. It was demonstrated that because of these anatomic relationships, traction on the SMAS can affect facial skin, fat, and muscle.

In 1980, Lemmon and Hamra published a variation of the Skoog technique involving a series of 577 patients.[5] Modifications in this study included limiting the sub-SMAS dissection to a line 1.5 to 2.0 cm posterior to the nasolabial fold, complete undermining of the platysma to the midline inferior to the mandible coupled with horizontal transection of this muscle in the manner of Connell,[6] and placement of a double row of sutures to imbricate the superficial fascia. The authors reported fewer contour irregularities in the face and a longer lasting result in the neck with this technique, with no increase in complications.

Owsley also recommended complete transection of the platysma to prevent recurrent banding of the muscle postoperatively.[7] In another large clinical series, he described a sub-SMAS and subplatysmal dissection with superoposterior suspension of the lower face and neck combined with subcutaneous undermining and lateral traction of the mid and upper cheek to produce a "bidirectional" rhytidectomy. A more superiorly directed vector of pull on the lower SMAS and platysma was purported to correct submental deformities without the need for a submental incision and direct approach. Kamer et al. subsequently confirmed the efficacy of the SMAS-platysma lift, finding superior results compared with skin undermining and imbrication alone.[8]

During the next decade, surgeons began to concentrate on aesthetic restoration of the midface, particularly the nasolabial fold region. In the deep plane rhytidectomy the technique of Skoog was extended to include the upper cheek, where the malar fat pad was elevated from the underlying zygomaticus major and minor muscles.[9–10] Adopting techniques from craniofacial surgery, other surgeons began to use subperiosteal forehead and midfacial dissection by means of a coronal incision in which the origins of the muscles of the midface were released and repositioned superiorly.[11–12] By this approach, a preauricular scar was avoided in patients with lower grades of facial aging, whereas those with more extensive rhytidosis still required standard incisions for subcutaneous undermining in the cheek and neck. Hamra reported the composite rhytidectomy as an extension of the deep plane procedure to include exposure of the orbicularis oculi muscle by connecting the facelift dissection with a lower blepharoplasty skin-muscle flap.[13] Excision of an inferior crescent of orbicularis was combined with superomedial resuspension of the muscle to treat malar bags and festoons.

As procedures in the midface became more extensive, surgeons began to move away from more radical techniques in the neck. The early words of caution by Kamer and Halsey[14] were later echoed by Hamra, who abandoned horizontal division of the platysma muscle in the composite rhytidectomy to avoid an angled, "operated" look to the neck over time. Midline suture approximation of the anterior platysmal margins as previously described became the procedure of choice to treat and prevent recurrence of muscle banding.

Although more extensive techniques and deeper planes of dissection have been shown to be safe and effective in skilled, experienced hands, their use has not been universally accepted. Baker has warned of the risk of facial nerve injury,[15] and other surgeons concerned with the technical difficulty and potential morbidity of these complex procedures have suggested a return to more superficial techniques.[16] Our current method, a modification of the Skoog technique, has been reported previously and is

described again here. Ultimately, the choice of technique will depend on the individual surgeon's training, level of experience, degree of skill, and aesthetic judgement.

PREOPERATIVE PREPARATION

The patient is brought to the operating suite, a cardiac monitor and pulse oximeter are placed, and an intravenous line is started. With the patient in a sitting position, the proposed lines of incision are marked (Fig. 11–1), and any platysmal banding is outlined. The temporal incision is marked 4 to 5 cm from the hairline, curving posteriorly and then anteriorly to emerge from the hair along the anterosuperior helical fold in a natural crease posterior to the sideburn. In women a posttragal incision is normally used. It is outlined at a distinct angle, continuing into the intertragal incisure, and then descends just posterior to the tragal prominence to blend into the cheek-lobule crease. In men a pretragal incision is usually indicated to avoid advancing the sideburn onto the ear. This incision courses from the intertragal groove a few millimeters anterior to the tragus, merging with the cheek-lobule crease inferiorly. It then continues superiorly along the posterior attachment of the lobule onto the posterior concha, a few millimeters lateral to the postauricular sulcus. At a level approximating the superior aspect of the external auditory canal, the incision turns posteriorly to curve over the mastoid process and then continues posteroinferiorly into the hair of the occipital scalp. For those patients requiring anterior platysmal band surgery, a 2.0 to 2.5-cm incision is marked in the submental crease (Fig. 11–2).

Although a number of anesthetic techniques can be used successfully, administration of propofol by continuous intravenous infusion provides profound sedation while allowing the patient to continue breathing spontaneously without ventilatory support. The anesthesiologist calculates the rate of infusion from the patient's weight and adjusts the dosage to the clinical response. Local anesthesia and vasoconstriction are accomplished by subcutaneous infiltration of a solution of 0.75%

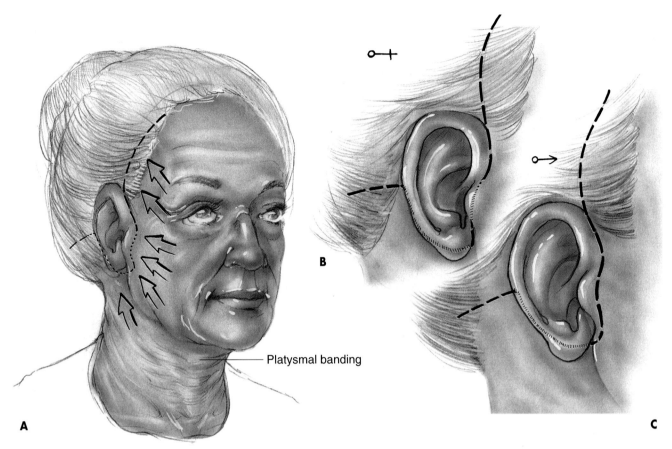

Platysmal banding

Figure 11–1. (A) Preoperative marking of proposed incisions. Note posttragal incision for female patient **(B)** and pretragal incision for male patient **(C)**.

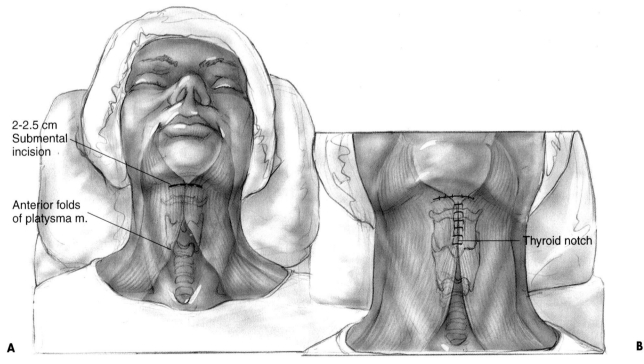

2-2.5 cm Submental incision

Anterior folds of platysma m.

Thyroid notch

Figure 11–2. (A) A 2- to 2.5-cm incision is marked in the submental crease before anterior platysmal banding surgery. **(B)** The platysmal bands are sutured beginning inferiorly at the level of the thyroid.

lidocaine with a 1 : 150,000 dilution of epinephrine along the marked lines of incision and throughout the areas to be undermined. In the more anterior areas of the face, this injection is facilitated by the use of a 22-gauge spinal needle introduced at the inferior junction of the lobule with the cheek.

The hair is then parted along the incision lines and secured with rubber bands. Preparation of the surgical field is completed, and the patient is draped. Using methylene blue and the carved, fine point of a cotton applicator, the periauricular portion of the incision is then drawn.

INTRAOPERATIVE TECHNIQUE

Surgery usually begins with the platysmorrhaphy procedure. The submental incision is made through the skin, and wide subcutaneous scissors dissection in the preplatysmal plane is extended inferiorly to the level of the thyroid cartilage and laterally over the submandibular triangle. Redundant fat lying in the midline between the anterior platysmal bands is excised with scissors. The medial margins of the platysma muscles are identified and sewn together with interrupted 4-0 polyglycolic acid (Dexon) sutures, beginning inferiorly at the level of the thyroid notch and progressing superiorly to the inferior border of the mandible. This creates a complete anterior muscle sling in the upper aspect of the neck. Subplatysmal dissections, myotomies, and myectomies are avoided. Any superfluous fat can be judiciously suctioned or trimmed with scissors to render the platysmal and subcutaneous tissues smooth and free of irregularities. The submental incision is closed with a running subcuticular suture of 5-0 nylon after the facelift is complete.

The remaining marked incisions are carried through the skin and scalp with a No. 15 blade. In the face a subcutaneous dissection is begun over the tragus (Fig. 11–3). Care must be taken not to disturb the tragal perichondrium while incising this thin-skinned area. Dissection is extended approximately 4 to 5 cm toward the cheek anteriorly and continues inferiorly into the neck, below the body of the mandible. Care is taken to avoid entering the

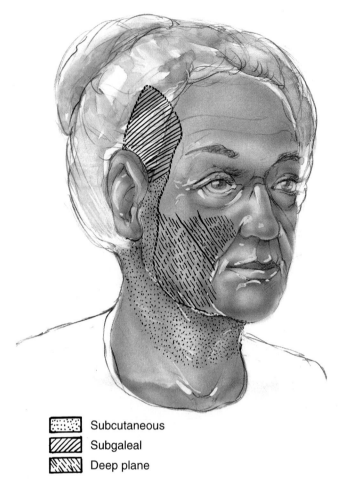

⠿	Subcutaneous
▨	Subgaleal
▧	Deep plane

Figure 11–3. Extent and levels of undermining.

fascia of the sternocleidomastoid muscle inferior to the mastoid process. This preplatysmal plane is widely undermined toward the midline, joining the subcutaneous submental dissection overlying the previously sutured platysmal bands. In the scalp the temporoparietal fascia and galea are separated from the deep temporal fascia in an areolar plane, with care taken not to injure the temporal branch of the facial nerve as the dissection proceeds anteriorly toward the lateral brow. For patients with significant lateral brow ptosis, this dissection can be continued anteriorly with transition to a subperiosteal plane over the superolateral orbital rim. This maneuver provides release of the lateral brow and can be facilitated by use of the endoscope as necessary. From the subgaleal level superiorly, a transition is made to a subcutaneous plane over the zygomatic arch, again to protect the temporal branch, as continuity is achieved with the dissection in the cheek.

Entrance into the sub-SMAS deep plane in the face is facilitated by retracting the skin and subcutaneous tissues, thus tenting the SMAS and platysma laterally. An incision is made through the SMAS beginning in the malar region, approximately 1 cm posterior to the anterior extent of subcutaneous undermining. This will leave a small "tongue" or free edge of SMAS separate from the skin to facilitate later suturing. The incision in the SMAS is carried inferiorly toward the posterior border of the platysma, just inferior to the angle of the mandible (Fig. 11–4). Traction is maintained laterally as the SMAS is dissected from the deeper parotidomasseteric fascia. Dense fibrous attachments between the superficial and deep fasciae exist along the anterior zygomatic arch, overlying the parotid gland, and along the anterior border of the masseter muscle (Fig. 11–5). A less adherent, areolar plane exists between these fascial layers in the lower cheek, directly overlying the masseter mus-

cle, and deep to the platysma. Dissection is facilitated by vertically spreading the scissors directly along the underside of the platysma, peeling the fat and loose areolar tissue off this structure. Sharp dissection is required to transect the parotidocutaneous, masseteric-cutaneous, and zygomatic osteocutaneous ligaments. The sub-SMAS plane is quite avascular except for a perforating branch of the transverse facial artery, which is relatively constant in the cheek.

The extent of anterior dissection depends on the degree of mobilization necessary to attain the required aesthetic result. To influence malar bags, dissection must proceed beneath the inferior border of the orbicularis oculi, transecting the thick osteocutaneous ligaments of the malar pad (McGregor's patch). Likewise, dissection should continue anteriorly within the fibroadipose tissues of the melolabial fold and deep to the SMAS of the jowl to mobilize these structures effectively.

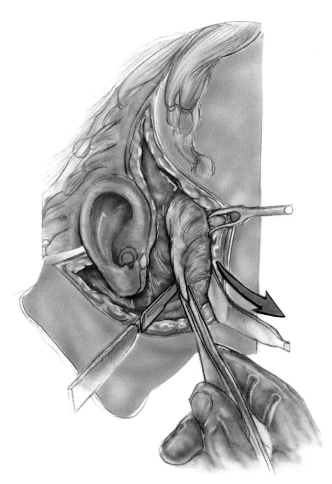

Figure 11–4. Retraction of skin flap tents the SMAS, facilitating the beginning of deep plane dissection.

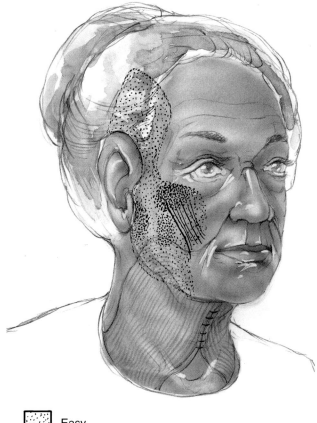

 Easy
Firm

Figure 11–5. Approximate position of facial ligaments and relative ease of dissection.

The nasolabial fold is approached by undermining the fibroadipose layer of the cheek overlying the major and minor zygomatic muscles. Blunt finger dissection easily separates this plane superficial to the mimetic muscles and continues anteriorly toward the nose and upper lip (Fig. 11–6). Because the facial nerve branches innervate these muscles from their deep surfaces, it is important for the surgeon to remain in a plane superficial to the zygomatic muscles. If this area is approached from the inferior subplatysmal dissection, the nerve can become subject to injury because the SMAS envelops these muscles and danger of dissecting beneath them exists. The dissection of the prezygomatic area can be connected with the subplatysmal undermining as the dissection proceeds inferiorly. Fibrous attachments between the two planes are severed, but the confluence of mimetic muscles near the oral commissure (modiolus) is not disturbed.

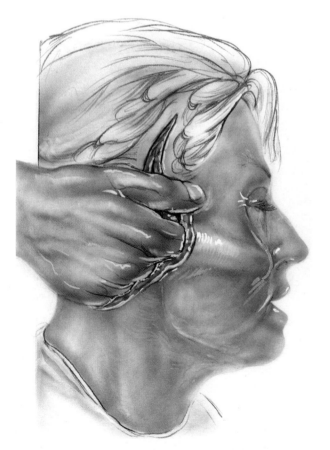

Figure 11–6. The fibroadipose tissue overlying the zygomatic muscles can be safely undermined by blunt finger dissection.

The jowl area is then undermined. An areolar plane exists overlying the masseter muscle, allowing the SMAS to be rapidly elevated by means of a blunt technique from the anterior border of the parotid gland as far forward as the anterior border of the masseter, where the fibrous septae of the masseteric-cutaneous ligaments are encountered. These are severed, and the dissection in the subplatysmal plane is continued anteriorly over the masseter muscle border and inferiorly to the lower border of the mandible, extending anteriorly to where the facial artery crosses. As long as the underlying parotidomasseteric fascia is not violated during this dissection, injury to the marginal mandibular nerve is virtually impossible. Further subplatysmal dissection inferior to the mandible is unnecessary. A subcutaneous plane in the neck has already been created.

Once the flap is adequately mobilized, hemostasis is assured and the resultant widely undermined, multiplane, musculocutaneous flap can be advanced to attain the desired aesthetic effect. Before closure of the deep plane, redundant preauricular subcutaneous tissue is excised to better define the tragus. To facilitate advancement, the SMAS and platysma are freed from the overlying skin for 1 to 2 cm, creating a small strip of SMAS that is used for suturing. The cheek flap is closed by suturing this SMAS tongue to the firm preauricular tissues with 4-0 polyglycolic acid sutures (Fig. 11–7). These sutures, tied under some tension, determine the direction of the vector forces on the mobilized flaps and take some of the tension off the skin before closure. The superior suture advances the cheek in a posterosuperior direction. Three intermediate sutures anchor the flap posteriorly just anterior to the tragus, softening the melolabial fold and jowl while substantially obliterating the subcutaneous preauricular dead space. The inferior suture's vector is almost directly posterior, anchoring the platysmal flap to the dense fascia of the retrolobular area. This helps to eliminate the lower jowl and to delineate the jawline and the upper aspect of the neck. The excess SMAS tongue and any irregular fibroadipose tissue are trimmed and smoothed with scissors. Any areas of dog-ears or

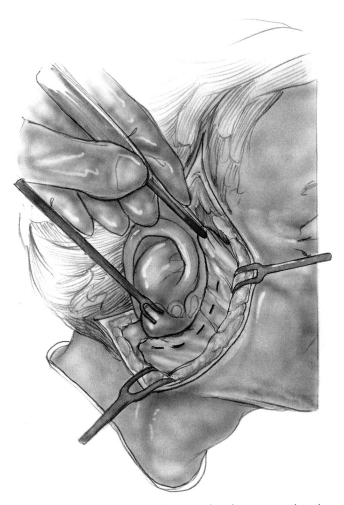

Figure 11-7. The SMAS "tongue" has been sutured to the preauricular tissues and the redundant portion will be excised.

puckering can be dealt with by judicious subcutaneous undermining. To retain the compound flap, however, more extensive undermining between skin and SMAS should be avoided.

The temporal-brow region is then elevated by superoposterior advancement of the subgaleal flap. Excess tissue is excised beginning at the most anterior aspect of the wound. Inappropriate tension to excessively elevate the eyebrow should be avoided, and the incision is closed in sequential fashion[17] with stainless steel staples. As closure proceeds inferiorly in the area of the superior pinna, the sideburn is brought more directly posterior rather than elevated to prevent the temporal tuft of hair and sideburn from being overlifted.

After the skin flaps have been adequately mobilized and advanced, the skin is trimmed and sutured. Excision

and closure again proceed in sequential fashion. To better delineate the tragus, the small flap of skin advanced over it is judiciously defatted and closed without tension with interrupted 6-0 nylon sutures. Cervical skin is likewise excised and closed without tension, making sure that hairline disruptions or step-off deformities do not interrupt the normal individual anatomic configuration of the postauricular and occipital areas. A simple running suture of 5-0 plain gut is used to close the postauricular wound, and stainless steel staples are used for the hair-bearing incisions.

A drain should be considered in any case in which there is a question of persistent or probable postoperative bleeding. It emerges from a separate stab incision in the occipital scalp and is connected to a negative pressure reservoir before the drapes are removed and the dressing is placed. A compressive head dressing is secured with burn netting at the end of the procedure.

POSTOPERATIVE COURSE

Postoperative antibiotics are not given routinely, and patients rarely require more than a mild narcotic orally for analgesia. The dressing and drain are removed the morning after surgery, the incisions are examined, and a lighter, less compressive dressing is applied. This second dressing remains in place for 2 more days, after which the patient can shower and wash his or her hair daily. The sutures and surgical staples are removed after 1 week. The patient is instructed to avoid strenuous activity and is encouraged to rest and eat well during this recovery period. The postsurgical edema and ecchymoses are essentially resolved by 2 to 3 weeks in most cases, and patients are usually able to return to work in 2 to 3 weeks.

COMPLICATIONS AND SEQUELAE

Although the complication rate with the procedure just described is low, problems do occur at times. Because complications cannot be entirely prevented, it is essential that the surgeon be able to recognize and manage any untoward results appropriately. With proper care, most of these problems can be resolved without significant long-term sequelae.

Hematoma is perhaps the most dreaded complication of rhytidectomy because a major episode constitutes a true surgical emergency. Virtually all major hematomas occur within 24 hours of surgery. Rapidly increasing pain, edema, and ecchymoses, particularly when unilateral, should raise suspicion of a hematoma and prompt immediate examination of the patient. If evidence of an expanding hematoma is found, the patient should be taken to the operating room without delay for evacuation of the clot. A few sutures or staples are removed from the area of incision closest to the collection, and the clot is expressed manually and removed by suction. Rapid reaccumulation of blood usually indicates an arterial bleeder, which requires opening of the wound on the affected side for cautery or ligation of the offending vessel. Smaller collections that do not recur after the clot is expressed and the wound is irrigated may be treated by careful observation.

If an unsuspected hematoma is identified on routine examination the morning after surgery or thereafter, it is usually fairly limited and can often be evacuated by suction after removing one or two staples. An option with small collections is to wait several days until clot lysis occurs, at which time the serosanguinous fluid can be readily aspirated with an 18-gauge needle transcutaneously. In such cases the skin should still be relatively insensate, and local anesthesia is seldom needed.

Certainly the best treatment of hematoma is prevention. Several large retrospective studies have shown that the only significant factor that correlates with hematoma formation is perioperative fluctuation in blood pressure.[18–20] Thus skilled administration of anesthesia and careful postoperative monitoring are critical. Most surgeons also agree that men have a higher rate of hematomas, and this concept is supported in the literature.[21] Anecdotal evidence suggests that such measures as prohibiting preoperative aspirin, NSAIDs, and vitamin E ingestion, minimizing patient anxiety, and avoidance of postoperative straining and vomiting may be useful in the prevention of hematomas.

In a compilation of major series of rhytidectomy in the world literature, the incidence of large hematomas varied from 0.9 to 8.0%, with a mean of 3.6%.[22] The rate reported for the deep plane technique presented here is 2.8%. It is of interest that to date no hematomas in the senior author's experience have occurred deep to the SMAS or platysma; they all developed in the subcutaneous plane of dissection.

Other wound complications that have occurred with this technique are infection, hypertrophic scar formation, and hypoesthesia of the skin. Infection is a rare problem and is usually related to some degree of hematoma formation. Appropriate use of oral antibiotics guided by wound culture results has resolved the infection without sequelae in the few cases encountered. Hypertrophy of incisional scars may occur, particularly in the postauricular region, but it usually improves spontaneously. Persistently troublesome scar tissue may be treated cautiously with intralesional triamcinolone acetate injection. It is not unusual for patients to complain of small areas of skin numbness postoperatively, especially in the periauricular region. Reassurance is all that is necessary. Although it may take up to a year in rare cases, sensation gradually returns.

Since beginning to use the deep plane rhytidectomy, the senior author has had no cases of permanent facial nerve paresis or paralysis and no significant skin slough, alopecia, or alteration of the hairline. Some minor contour irregularities persisted for several weeks in the areas of subcutaneous undermining preauricularly and in the neck, but this did not occur in the cheek where the dissection was in the deeper plane.

RESULTS

Improvement in the jawline and jowl area has often been dramatic, and considerable relief of temporal and malar redundancy has been obtained (Fig. 11–8). The nasolabial fold is softened and in many cases substantially effaced. Anterior platysmorraphy combined with a subcutaneous cervical rhytidectomy has achieved optimal aesthetic results in the neck while minimizing the irregularities and scar contractures that can occur with more radical procedures. Wound healing has been uniformly excellent because of

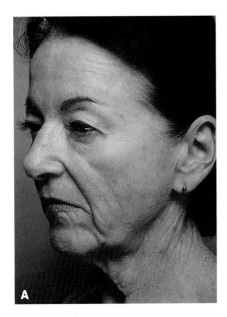
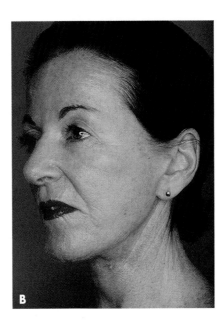

Figure 11–8. Preoperative **(A)** and postoperative **(B)** photographs of a patient demonstrating the results of deep plane rhytidectomy.

the thickness and vascularity of the compound musculocutaneous cheek flap. Signs of cutaneous ischemia, necrosis, and slough, which can plague extensive skin flap procedures, have not been seen. With extended deep dissection, a tendency toward prolonged edema in the cheek has occurred in some patients, but this has not presented a significant problem. In a series of the first 100 patients treated by this technique, 97 were happy with the results. Further experience has revealed a similar rate of patient satisfaction.

CONCLUSION

Regardless of the choice of surgical technique, careful patient selection, proper timing of surgical intervention, and thorough preoperative preparation are paramount if rhytidectomy is to be rewarding for both surgeon and patient. Surgeons must choose a procedure that is suited to the anatomic findings and aesthetic needs of the individual patient, consistent with their training and skill, and with which they can expect to obtain the most reliable, safe, and effective results.

Experience with the deep plane rhytidectomy technique has shown that these goals can be fulfilled in most cases. The aesthetic benefit has increased, particularly with respect to the nasolabial fold and jowl, while wound healing has improved and complications have been few.

Mastery of the procedure, as with any aesthetic surgical technique, requires ongoing, critical evaluation of one's results and continuing modification. Perfection, however elusive, is the goal that inspires excellence.

PEARLS

- Entrance into the sub-SMAS deep plane in the face is facilitated by retracting the skin and subcutaneous tissues, thus tenting the SMAS and platysma laterally.
- Dissection is facilitated by vertically spreading the scissors directly along the underside of the platysma, peeling the fat and loose areolar tissue off this structure.
- As the facial nerve branches innervate these muscles from their deep surfaces, it is important for the surgeon to remain in a plane superficial to the zygomatic muscles.
- As long as the underlying parotidomasseteric fascia is not violated during this dissection, injury to the marginal mandibular nerve is virtually impossible.
- To facilitate advancement, the SMAS and platysma are freed from the overlying skin for 1 to 2 cm, creating a small "tongue" of SMAS that is used for suturing.

REFERENCES

1. Napoleon A. The presentation of personalities in plastic surgery. *Ann Plast Surg.* 1993; 31:193–208.

2. Bettman AG. Plastic and cosmetic surgery of the face. *Northwest Med.* 1922; 21:170.

3. Skoog T. The aging face. In: *Plastic Surgery: New Methods and Refinements.* Philadelphia, PA: WB Saunders Co; 1974: 300–330.

4. Mitz V, Peyronie M. The superficial musculoaponeurotic system (SMAS) in the parotid and cheek area. *Plast Reconstr Surg.* 1976; 58:80–88.

5. Lemmon ML, Hamra ST. Skoog Rhytidectomy: A five-year experience with 577 patients. *Plast Reconstr Surg.* 1980; 63:283–297.

6. Connell BF. Cervical lifts: The value of platysma muscle flaps. *Ann Plast Surg.* 1978; 1:34.

7. Owsley JQ SMAS-platysma facelift. *Clin Plast Surg.* 1983; 10:429–440.

8. Kamer FM, Damiani J, Churukian M. 512 Rhytidectomies: A retrospective study. *Arch Otolaryngol.* 1984; 110:368–371.

9. Hamra ST. The deep-plane rhytidectomy. *Plast Reconstr Surg.* 1990; 86:53–61.

10. Kamer Fk One hundred consecutive deep plane face-lifts. *Arch Otolaryngol Head Neck Surg.* 1996; 122:17–22.

11. Tessier P. Le lifting facial sous-perioste. *Ann Chir Plast Esthet.* 1989; 34:199.

12. Del Campo AF. Face lift without preauricular scars. *Plast Reconstr Surg.* 1993; 90:642–661.

13. Hamra ST. Composite rhytidectomy. *Plast Reconstr Surg.* 1992; 90:1–22.

14. Kamer FM, Halsey W. The two-layer rhytidectomy. *Arch Otolaryngol.* 1981; 107:450–453.

15. Baker DC. Deep dissection rhytidectomy: A plea for caution. *Plast Reconstr Surg.* 1994; 93:1498–1499.

16. Duffy MJ, Friedland JA. The superficial plane rhytidectomy revisited. *Plast Reconstr Surg.* 1994; 93:1392–1403.

17. Kamer FM, Parks M. Sequential rhytidectomy. *Laryngoscope.* 1978; 88:1196–1203.

18. Berner RE, Morain WD, Noe JM. Postoperative hypertension as an etiological factor in hematoma after rhytidectomy. *Plast Reconstr Surg.* 1976; 57:314–319.

19. Straith RE, Raju DR, Hipps CJ. The study of hematomas in 500 consecutive face lifts. *Plast Reconstr Surg.* 1977; 59: 694–698.

20. Rees TD, Barone CM, Valauri FA, Ginsberg GD, Nolan III WB. Hematomas requiring surgical evacuation following face lift surgery. *Plast Reconstr Surg.* 1994; 93:1185–1190.

21. Baker DC, Aston SJ, Guy CL, et al. The male rhytidectomy. *Plast Reconstr Surg.* 1977; 60:512.

22. Baker DC. Complications of cervicofacial rhytidectomy. *Clin Plast Surg.* 1983; 10:543–562.

Face Lift

Aesthetic Facial Plastic Surgery, edited by Thomas Romo, III, and Arthur L. Millman, Thieme Medical Publishers, Inc., New York, New York, Copyright © 2000.

CHAPTER 12

A Plastic Surgeon's Perspective

OSCAR M. RAMIREZ

The surgical treatment of the aging face has been traditionally done by different isolated surgical techniques. The technique used by a particular surgeon was influenced by that person's surgical background, by the preferred surgical school that a particular surgeon follows, and by the aesthetic goals determined by the interrelation during the preoperative consultations between the surgeon and the patient. Many techniques have crossed interspecialty barriers, and the tendency nowadays is to use two or more combinations of techniques in an effort to improve the aesthetic and long-term results that isolated procedures cannot provide.

In the plastic and aesthetic surgery specialty, the following four trends have been developed that have changed the way that we approach facial rejuvenation.

1. Tendency toward a deeper plane of dissection[1-4]
2. The increased use of endoscopic techniques that have either decreased the length of the incisions or minimized to slit incisions[5]
3. Emphasis on the treatment of the central oval of the face[6-9]
4. A more liberal use of ancillary techniques to refine or restore some features not amenable to treatment with traditional methods, for example, lasers for fine facial wrinkles and severely sun-damaged skin, fat grafting for volume restoration, alloplastic implants for skeletal augmentation and support, and the like[10-13]

Although all these trends have not been widely accepted yet, my experience indicates that they will eventually be included in the routine surgical armamentarium because patients demand more and more superior results, and surgeons are realizing that their own isolated traditional techniques may not be sufficient to fulfill those demands. In this chapter, I will explain my personal analysis of facial aesthetics, aging process, and rationality of the surgical techniques I routinely use. I also will describe the surgical techniques most commonly used in my practice for the treatment of the aging face.

AESTHETIC ANALYSIS OF THE FACE AND THE AGING FACE

Traditionally, on the basis of the analysis of Leonardo da Vinci, the face has been divided into thirds: upper, middle, and lower. Although good for cephalometric analysis and craniomaxillofacial surgery, surgical manipulation of the soft tissues on the basis of this division breaks important anatomic units such as the eyelid from the brows, the lips from the nose, the upper lip from the cheek, and so on. The disruption of these aesthetic units will give an

unsightly and operated look. Furthermore, this analysis has made us approach the face from the surgical point of view in a segmental fashion without taking into consideration more comprehensive units that have harmony and important relationships from the anatomic, surgical, and aesthetic points of view.[14] These units are the central oval and the peripheral hemicircle (Fig. 12–1). The central oval is the part of the face in which the facial mimetic and sphincteric muscles of the face are concentrated. The constant contraction and relaxation of these muscles are transmitted to the overlying skin. When the collagen composition in the skin is damaged because of aging, sun exposure, and so forth, these muscle contractions will leave permanent marks that are translated into deep and superficial wrinkles. These wrinkles are located mostly in

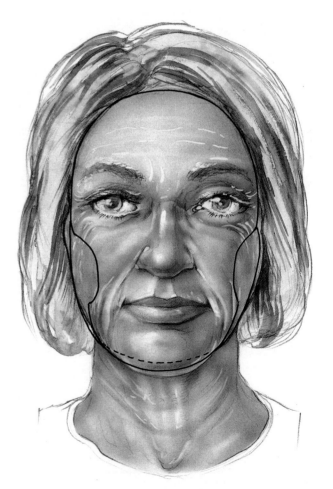

Figure 12–1. The central oval of the face is a definite aesthetic and functional unit that is separate from the peripheral hemicircle. The central oval is more affected by the gravitory forces and by the activity of the facial mimetic muscles.

the central oval. Because of its inherent mobility and relative looseness of the soft tissues in the central oval, gravity affects this area more predominantly than the peripheral hemicircle. For these reasons, the aging process affects the central oval of the face more prematurely and with more severity. The peripheral hemicircle is involved only very late in life. These two aesthetic units are defined by abrupt changes in light shadow going from central to peripheral. Usually the nerves are more prone to be injured at the junction of the central oval with the peripheral hemicircle because it is at this level that the nerves become more superficial. Because of its decreased accessibility, the central oval is more difficult and less reliable to rejuvenate with standard facelift techniques. However, with the advent of endoscopic techniques, a reliable rejuvenation of the central oval of the face can be obtained with minimal risk. Younger and middle-aged patients could have this oval treated without the need to address the peripheral hemicircle. Later in life, this peripheral hemicircle may be addressed, but only as a secondary maneuver to the main area of attention: the central oval.

SUBPERIOSTEAL FACELIFT

Proponents of the traditional and more superficial facelift techniques have questioned the rationality and safety of the subperiosteal facelift. On the basis of more than 500 complete facelift procedures, over a period of 14 years, using the technique outlined in the following, I recommend the subperiosteal facelift for the following reasons.

1. During the aging process, balance among the skeletal framework and the overlying soft tissue envelope is lost. This balance can be restored to some degree with the undermining of the soft tissue at the subperiosteal plane.

2. With aging, the skeleton undergoes an overall reduction of volume and muscle mass elasticity is diminished. This muscle mass elasticity over the smaller framework can be restored at the subperiosteal plane.

3. As one ages, fat migrates by gravitory forces and the deep supportive structures are lost. These deep structures can be tightened with a subperiosteal facelift.

4. This progressive sagging of the soft tissues is more evident in areas with less fibrous connections to the deep structures. This is even worse in patients who have lost dentition, with the consequential loss of skeletal volume and support. This loss of bone support can be restored with alloplastic implants or osteotomies.

5. Some patients have a genetic and racial predisposition to develop soft tissue sagging at an early age, despite a normal volume of facial skeleton. This can be rearranged with a subperiosteal lift.

6. The galea frontalis, corrugator, depressor supercilii, and procerus have strong attachments to the pericranium and the bone. Subperiosteal facelift allows safer manipulation of these structures, close to its origin in the bone. Likewise, modification of the orbicularis oculi and the lateral canthal ligament can be done at the subperiosteal level because strong attachments to the periosteum exist.

7. At the level of the cheek the muscle attachments to the periosteum can be repositioned at a higher level to elevate the position of the modiolus, the upper lip, and the soft tissues of the nose.

8. The deep plane rhytidectomy or the extended subcutaneous musculoaponeurotic system (SMAS) techniques are an attempt to pull the muscle mass of the cheek through its insertion into the SMAS. This is accomplished without detaching the muscle at its point of origin. However, with the subperiosteal facelift, a direct detachment of the origin can be made, and the muscle mass can be redraped directly.

9. The detractors of the technique have pointed out the fact that the periosteum is rigid and nondistensible, therefore difficult to stretch. However, I consider this an advantage in the subperiosteal facelift because it allows me to release and spread the periosteum at key points such as the infrabrow and inframalar/maxillary areas, allowing the overlying structures to be moved en bloc. This requires different anchoring techniques to maintain the elevation.

ENDOSCOPIC FACELIFT

The endoscopic techniques as applied to facial rejuvenation have permitted us to completely replace the bicoronal incision. The rationality, advantages, and disadvantages of the endoforehead compared with the open approach have been fully described in a recent article.[15] In my practice some significant advantages are as follows.

1. Patient acceptance has been significantly high. At present, patients requesting facial rejuvenation and needing forehead/brow lift do not have any reservations with the endoforehead because this can be done with minimal incisions, quicker recovery, and almost no sequela.

2. The endoscope has allowed us to balance facial rejuvenation and significantly improve the results in the entire periorbital area, which cannot be obtained if the surgery is restricted to the lower two thirds of the face. This has in turn decreased the need to perform upper blepharoplasty, which is routinely done in conventional facelift procedures.

3. In regards to the midface, the endoscope has made subperiosteal degloving less traumatic, with almost complete absence of nerve injury and, in some cases, has avoided incisions in the orbicularis oculi muscle for access to perform the vertical lift of the cheek. This has almost eliminated the risk of ectropion and dysfunction of the orbicularis oculi muscle.[16]

4. In some cases during subperiosteal degloving of the chin for mentopexy or treatment of the witch's chin, the endoscope has made possible extensive dissection with minimal trauma. Likewise, a wide subplatysmal dissection under and around the submaxillary salivary gland can easily be performed with the aid of the endoscope.[17]

5. In general, the endoscope has made it possible to remodel and lift the central oval of the face in a manner that would be difficult, dangerous, or impossible with other methods. In this way, the area of the face with early aging can be approached with pure endoscopic techniques without removing skin.[5]

6. In cases of severe aging, the area most severely affected (the central oval) can be dealt with first at the subperiosteal level and with minimal incisions using the endoscope. The skin redraping and excision is done as a secondary maneuver after the central oval is corrected. In this way, a well-balanced rejuvenation can be obtained.

In the past, male patients were reluctant to undergo brow lifting procedures because in most cases, this entailed performing a bicoronal incision. This may not be acceptable, particularly for the patient with male pattern baldness. However, due to the advent of endoscopic techniques, we can perform a complete forehead lift with minimal incisions, which is most acceptable for this group of patients. Furthermore, if the patient does not want any scars in the bald forehead, most of the surgery can be done with the aid of the endoscope through the transblepharoplasty approach. In that way, the incisions are limited to the upper eyelid and to the temporal ports. In terms of the rest of the facelift, the lower blepharoplasty incision is well accepted; however, this can also be eliminated if the intraoral approach is combined with a temporal endoscopic incision. This requires use of CO_2 laser resurfacing for improvement of the redundant skin on the lower eyelid. In terms of the standard facelift component, my preference is still to perform a marginal tragal incision and defat and remove the hair follicles from underneath the flap in the area to be redraped over the tragus and the preauricular section of the face. If this is not satisfactory, the hair can be removed with one of the lasers now available for follicular ablation. I prefer to do the retroauricular component of the incision very high, which follows the hairline of the retroauricular area so this will not cross the mastoid process, which can be visible in patients with short hair.

PATIENT SELECTION, TIMING OF SURGERY, AND CHOICE OF THE PROCEDURE

Patient selection is critical for the techniques described in the following. Each one of the variations has its own limitations and optimal indications that should be applied judiciously to each group of patients.

The full endoscopic facelift without skin excisions is indicated in younger patients, around the late 30s to early 40s.[5] In patients in their late 40s and early 50s, the subperiosteal minimally invasive laser endoscopic (SMILE) rhytidectomy is indicated.[10] This procedure will improve the central oval of the face, remove the fine early wrinkles, and, to some extent, take care of minimal excess skin. CO_2 laser resurfacing can provide a greater degree of skin contracture when the patient has severely damaged skin. However, when the patient has a lot of loose skin and no wrinkles, the laser does very little to improve this condition.

For patients older than 50, the endoscopic-assisted biplanar facelift is indicated.[18] As it will be described, this technique includes subcutaneous cervicofacial rhytidectomy, which helps to improve the jowls, mandibular lines, and the neck. This, in addition to the significant improvement obtained in the central oval of the face with the subperiosteal endoscopic lifting of the forehead and midface, provides significant rejuvenative effect.

For patients in their 60s, the biplanar facelift is combined with a full-face laser resurfacing.[11] These two technologies (facelift and laser) rejuvenate the sagging soft tissues and at the same time, rejuvenate the quality and texture of the skin.

For any group of patients, according to the objectives, we include fat grafting in a very liberal way to either enhance the features that are flat or restore those to a more youthful projection. Patients with a relatively good central oval, whose main concerns are the jowls and the laxity of the neck, will benefit from a standard cervicofacial rhytidectomy alone. In my practice, this is the exception rather than the rule. Obviously, patients who want lesser procedures and limited surgery can choose to have standard techniques, knowing that they will be limited in terms of the areas of correction and the degree of improvement that can be obtained.

The most important portion of the surgical techniques to be described is the subperiosteal dissection of the central oval of the face. These are indicated in the following patients.

1. Those who have significant aging and ptosis of the central oval of the face: brows, eyelid commissure, nasoglabellar soft tissues, nose, nasolabial fold, cheeks, angle of the mouth, and jowls.
2. Those who present a tear trough deformity or deep infraorbital hollow
3. Those who request secondary or tertiary rhytidectomy[19]
4. Those who have frontal bossing or forehead irregularities (Neanderthal forehead)[20]
5. Those who have significant skeletal/soft tissue disproportion requiring manipulation of the skeletal foundation by augmentation or reduction
6. Those who present with excessive scleral show or ectropion (In my view, the lower eyelid and the cheek is one functional and aesthetic unit; therefore the scleral show or ectropion can be corrected better with a subperiosteal dissection of the entire cheek.)
7. Those who have antimongoloid eyelid slant (This can be repositioned to a horizontal or almond-shaped eyelid.)
8. Those who have severe malar bags (These malar bags can be repositioned to a higher level and can fill in the area of the tear trough deformity.)
9. Those who require simultaneous resurfacing of the skin because of aging or actinic damage (In this setting, the deep peel or CO_2 laser resurfacing can be done safely.[11])
10. Those who present with a history of facial fracture (The soft tissues can be repositioned better at the subperiosteal plane. After facial fractures many patients have some degree of ptosis of the soft tissues from the initial injury.)

11. Those who have a history of facial implants that require exchange (It is better to approach this at the subperiosteal plane with removal of the implant and replacement with a new implant in a virgin plane.)

12. Those who require soft tissue augmentation by means of fat grafting because the fat can be injected in the layer that has not been dissected

13. Those who request beautification, in addition to rejuvenation (The soft tissues can be repositioned to a more pleasing level with subperiosteal undermining.)

14. Those who are smokers because the subperiosteal dissection preserves the blood supply of the overlying soft tissues

PREOPERATIVE EVALUATION

Most of the patients coming to our practice for facial rejuvenation are well informed of the modern techniques of facelifting. They are aware of the feasibility of doing part or most of the their facelifting with minimal incisions and the other high-tech interface that is available. The most informed group seems to be the "baby boomers." They have read information in scientific magazines about the different techniques available for facial rejuvenation and are inquisitive about the technical details of each step of the operation. Older patients are not quite as inquisitive about these technical details; however, they are very well aware of the new developments.

Our consultation starts with a complete medical history with special attention to previous eyelid and facial cosmetic surgery, eye wetness, and visual problems. We have the patient hold a mirror in front of his or her face and analyze, step by step, all the features with which the patient is concerned. Nowadays, most patients request a more complete rejuvenation, which goes along with our preference to treat the whole face during one operative procedure to achieve an appropriate balance and avoid a piecemeal operated look. We analyze the patient's face from top to bottom, going down to the neck. We assess their concerns and pinpoint the aesthetic deformities from our point of view. We explain to the patient our philosophical, logical, and practical reasons to approach the larger aesthetic units or the whole face rather than isolated small aesthetic units. On many occasions, patients may have a different perspective in the sense that their expectations from any given surgical procedure may go beyond its feasibility. Sometimes they may not be aware of the limitations of segmental surgery versus a more comprehensive approach. It is up to the surgeon to educate and take the patient through the limitations, indications, contraindications, and different variations and extent of the techniques that can be applied to each particular case. The forehead is analyzed first; we note the degree of brow ptosis and we make vertical measurements from the lateral canthus, mid pupil, and medial canthus to the respective portions of the brow. We then measure the brow-to-hairline distance. We notice the corrugator and procerus activity. The eyes are discussed next with attention to fat bulging, ptosis of the upper eyelid, and excess skin without the brow elevated. Next, after digital elevation of the brow, we determine whether any need exists to resect fat and/or skin from the upper eyelid. If any doubt exists, we prefer to stage the upper eyelid surgery later. With respect to the lower eyelid, we decide to perform either CO_2 laser resurfacing or skin excision with or without fat pad excision. Our approach to excision of the fat pads from the lower eyelids has changed over the years. We perform fat pad excision in a conservative fashion in less than 10% of our patients. Standard fat excisions are reserved only for patients with bulging eyes.

We then analyze the inferior orbital area and examine the presence of a tear trough deformity. We consider the lower eyelid and the cheek as one interrelated cosmetic and functional unit that needs to be approached as such.

The degree of ptosis and nasolabial folding are noticed. We also analyze the skeletal support of the cheek and the fat pad atrophy or excess at each one of the levels of the cheek. If a trial of elevation of the soft tissues with the fingers determines that not enough exists to create volume in the cheek, we suggest the placement of a small cheek implant. The pros and cons of alloplastic material versus fat grafting injection are explained to the patient, and informed consent is obtained.

Men require more fat grafting to the cheeks than women because a tendency for more atrophy of fat exists in men. For this reason, we routinely include fat grafting to the nasolabial folds and to the cheek areas.

The lower face is examined next. We notice the degree of chin ptosis and the amount of laxity of the soft tissues in the perioral area. We also analyze the degree of support of the mandible and the chin. More laterally, the presence of jowls is noticed and again, after a trial of elevation of the cheek, we see how much correction of the jowls can be made. If this does not improve the jowls enough, we then decide to add an additional vector of pull with a periauricular skin excision in addition to direct lipectomy of the jowls. The need for a chin implant is also assessed.

Next we examine the neck. We note the amount of laxity of skin, the presence of supraplatysma and subplatysma fat deposits, ptosis of the submandibular gland, and the presence of platysma bands. According to the findings, we decide to do either an anterior approach cervicoplasty or a bidirectional cervicoplasty. We also determine whether a need exists to remove fat at the subplatysma plane, suspend the submaxillary salivary gland, or both.

The quality and texture of the skin of the face is analyzed next. If the patient has deep creases in the forehead, deep nasolabial sulcus, or marionette lines, we suggest fat injections to this area. Also, if the patient has thin lips, we suggests fat injections if the patient so desires. If the patient has actinic damage of the skin, we suggest a variety of treatment, ranging from a skin-conditioning program to chemical peel to CO_2 laser resurfacing. The CO_2 resurfacing can be done as a staged procedure or at the same operative setting.

After the initial consultation is finished and the office manager has discussed the financial aspects of the surgery, another preoperative visit is scheduled. During the first consultation with the patient, the aspirin and other related medication list and cigarette smoking warnings are given. A specially trained nurse is in charge of educating the patient and taking him or her step by step through the preoperative preparation, explaining what to expect intraoperatively and postoperatively. Patients with well-known medical problems are sent to their physicians for clearance for surgery, which includes an electrocardiogram and a chest x-ray film. If any history of anxiety-related hypertension is present, we pretreat the patient with beta blockers for several days before the surgery.

PREOPERATIVE PREPARATION

The operation is usually done with the patient under general anesthesia. In addition to the standard monitoring, PO_2 and CO_2 monitors are routinely used. A "long distance anesthesia" is used to avoid interference of the anesthesiologist around the operative field.[21] A Foley catheter and thromboembolic stockings with intermittent compression devices are applied. A well-padded operative table is used and the anesthesiologist controls the electric table for mobilization of the patient side to side, rather than trying to hyperextend the patient's neck.

INTRAOPERATIVE TECHNIQUE

The procedure chosen will depend on the patient's age, aesthetic goals, and the degree of rejuvenation requested by the patient. The operation is tailored to fit these conditions. For these reasons, the operation increases in complexity proportional to the increased age, higher aesthetic goals, and the degree of rejuvenation requested by the patient.

ENDOSCOPIC FOREHEAD AND FACELIFT

The endoscopic facelift has several variations. The most common is the combination endoforehead/endomidface. It can be combined with an anterior approach cervicoplasty. The endoforehead is approached by means of four slit incisions. These are done inside the hairline. The incisions are located one on each temporal area and two on the frontal scalp, each one paramedian about 3 cm from the midline. Occasionally, a small port of access is made in the central frontal scalp for introduction of the endoscope only.

Dissection is done in a sequential fashion. For this, we divide the forehead into four zones (Fig. 12–2). Zone 2 and zone 3 can be done without the endoscope; however, zone 1 and zone 4 require the use of the endoscope.

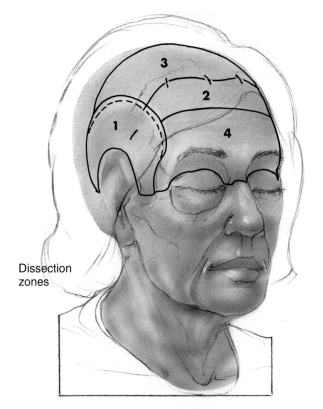

Dissection zones

Figure 12–2. The forehead is divided in four zones. The numbers indicate the sequence of the dissection. Zone 1 and zone 4 need to be done under strict endoscopic control. To allow smooth and complete transition between zones 2, 3, and 4 with zone 1, the periosteum along the temporal line of fusion should be elevated initially with the dissection of zone 1.

Zone 1 is dissected through the temporal slit incision, which is made about 2 to 3 cm inside the temporal scalp. Silastic port protectors are introduced after clearing the margins of the flap. Initially elevator No. 4 is introduced to release the superficial temporal fascia around the port for a few centimeters. The endoscope is then introduced, as is elevator No. 8. The lower limits of the dissection are about 0.5 cm above the superior border of the zygomatic arch posteriorly and up to the zygomatic arch itself on the anterior third. The temporal area contains three communicating veins between the superficial and deep systems; they are called TV1, TV2, and TV3. Of these, the most important is TV2 because this is the largest and should be saved during the dissection. Near TV3 is the zygomaticotemporal nerve, which also should be preserved if feasible. The preservation of TV2 diminishes the swelling and prevents the potential of the superficial arborizations of the venous network in the temporal area to become engorged and visible postoperatively. Dissection around and inferior to the TV2 and zygomaticotemporal nerve is done with elevator No. 0. Medially, dissection proceeds toward the temporal line of fusion. The periosteal insertion at the temporal line of fusion is elevated for about 1 cm in width. This will secure later connection between zones 2 and 3 with zone 1. Dissection is done on the contralateral side in a similar fashion.

Zone 2 is dissected through the two paramedian incisions. The slit incision should include the periosteum and the periosteal flaps are elevated to secure an entire subperiosteal dissection. Zone 2 extends up to about the midforehead level. Using this paramedian port, zone 3 is also dissected posteriorly up to the level of the vertex. The posterior boundaries of the pocket in zone 1 are is connected with zone 3.

Zone 4 is located below the midforehead level, and this dissection should be done under strict endoscopic control. Dissection is done initially toward the lateral aspect of the superior orbital rim and more laterally toward the temporal line of fusion, connecting zone 4 with zone 1.

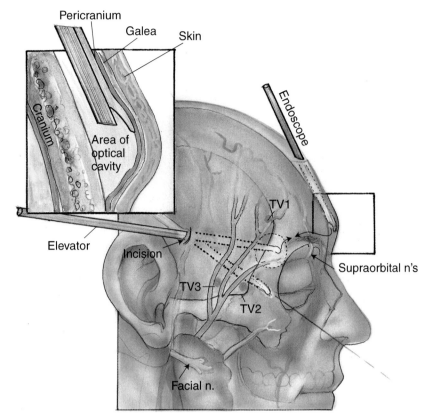

Figure 12-3. The triangulation technique to perform the endoforehead. The cobra tip cannula allows one to lift the soft tissues with less trauma. The angulated and curved elevators can be introduced and manipulated through the temporal ports. The subperiosteal dissection has several advantages, including better light reflection and better orientation of the anatomic landmarks.

Dissection then progresses gradually toward the supraorbital nerve, releasing all the periosteum at the level of the superior orbital rim (Fig. 12–3). This is done either with elevator No. 5 introduced through the temporal pocket or with the arcus marginalis endoscopic scissors. Medial to the supraorbital nerve, dissection is continued to release the periosteum just behind the corrugator muscles. The corrugator muscles are identified at the level of origin. The dissection in the corrugator muscle is done to identify the fascicles of the supratrochlear nerve. An average of three fascicles are found and should be identified before resection of the corrugator muscles is performed. The corrugator muscles are resected at the point of origin, around the fascicles of the supratrochlear nerve and between the supratrochlear nerve and the supraorbital nerves (Fig. 12–4). The segment of corrugator lateral and superficial to the supraorbital nerves is left intact because these are already in a more superficial plane.

Dissection is continued at the level of the nasoglabellar angle with the periosteal elevator No. 5. However, in

men or patients with thick periosteum, the release is done with double-angle endoscopic scissors. After the soft tissues, including the periosteum of the nasoglabellar angle, are elevated, the depressor supercilii muscles are identified, and these are resected with the endoscopic biter. The last maneuver in this area is to resect a small section of the procerus muscle of about 0.5 cm in a horizontal direction, very low at the level of the nasoglabellar angle (nasal radix).

The remaining fibers of the procerus are spread apart with the elevator No. 7. If any small bleeders remain at the level of the procerus muscle, these should be electrocoagulated with a small suction coagulator or with the laser according to the surgeon's preference. I do not think that the laser is quite important for dissection and/or coagulation during endoforehead lift because the methods previously described work very well and very efficiently.

The forehead is suspended after the midface suspension is finished. The initial suspension of the elevated forehead is placed at the level of the temporal ports. At

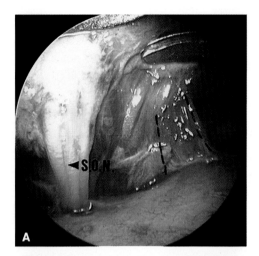
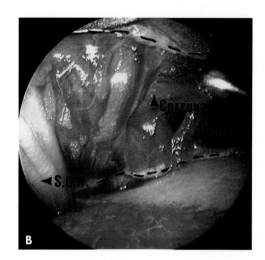
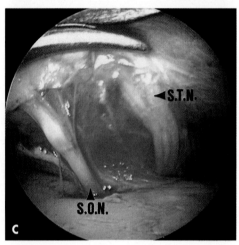

Figure 12–4. This sequence of endoscopic views demonstrates the way that the corrugator muscles are handled. **(A)** The supraorbital nerve (*SON*) is identified, the periosteum is released and spread. The origin of the corrugator muscle is identified medial to this. L; left. **(B)** The corrugator muscle is excised after the fascicles of the supratrochlear nerve are identified. Observe the release of the periosteum in the inferior boundaries of the forehead at the level of the supraorbital rim. L; left. **(C)** After resection of the corrugator muscle, the supraorbital nerve (*SON*) and the supratrochlear nerve (*STN*) are well visualized. Careful dissection and identification of the fascicles of the supratrochlear nerve are mandatory during corrugator resection.

this level, we anchor the superficial temporal fascia underneath the inferior flap of the temporal port toward the temporal fascia proper with two 3-0 polydioxanone (PDS) sutures. This suspension is vertically oriented to lift all the soft tissues on the temporal area. A small butterfly drain is left in the glabella and brought through a separate stab wound incision on the central scalp near the vertex. The paramedian ports are closed in two layers, including the deep layer of galea and periosteum with one or two inverted 3-0 PDS sutures. The skin scalp is closed with skin staples.

A blunt percutaneous hook is applied to the scalp to apply traction according to the desired direction and degree of traction. While the traction is maintained with the hook, a puncture wound with a No. 11 blade is made in the scalp about 2 cm in front of the traction hook. Through the percutaneous puncture wound, a hole is

drilled in the outer cortex using a 1.1-mm bit with a 4-mm stop. A 1.5-mm titanium custom post with a 4-mm stop is placed into the drill hole. The shaft of the post does not have a screw component; it is strong and wide enough to provide traction into the scalp without the need for anchoring the scalp to the post with sutures or staples. In most cases two paramedian posts are applied, one on each side at the level of the projection of the central brow with the direction of the traction toward the vertex. This way we provide a nice gentle curve with more traction toward the lateral brow (the area of the hooding).

The midface is approached by either an intraoral (gingivobuccal) incision or an "orbicularis oculi-window" type of incision. The dissection using either of these approaches is complemented by the slit incision already made in the temporal area for the endoforehead. The intraoral approach avoids incisions around the eyelid. This begins with a mucosal incision of about 2 cm, which is made at the level of the canine tooth.

The "orbicularis oculi window" has three variations: (1) crow's foot incision of about 1.5 cm made on one of the lateral eyelid creases; (2) canthotomy, transconjunctival incision (this is made when simultaneous canthopexy and lipectomy of intraorbital fat pad is planned); and (3) subcutaneous lower eyelid incision with orbicularis oculi spreading of about 1.5 cm. The muscle fibers of the orbicularis oculi are not transected in any of these variations, merely spread open for about 1.5 cm to allow introduction of the endoscope and a small periosteal elevator. This way the integrity of the entire muscle is maintained intact and no risk of total or partial denervation exists, particularly the pretarsal portion, the Horner muscle (muscle responsible for the lacrimal pumping mechanism), or both. We have abandoned the full blepharoplasty incision with a skin/muscle flap originally described by us for accessing the midface because that technique almost always required a canthopexy, particularly in the older patient.[5] Furthermore, in older patients an increased risk of denervation of the orbicularis oculi and/or ectropion was present.

Regardless of the variation used, the dissection is carried out as follows: The arcus marginalis is left intact and the periosteum around the inferior orbital rim for about 0.5 cm is preserved. The periosteum is then entered and a subperiosteal dissection is done toward the upper malar area toward the infraorbital nerve to elevate the orbicularis oculi muscle from the orbital rim periosteum and the levator labii superioris, which is located above the infraorbital nerve. This dissection proceeds for about 1 or 2 cm medial to the infraorbital nerve. More laterally, the dissection continues toward the zygomatic arch, and elevation of the zygomatic arch periosteum up to about $\frac{1}{2}$ or $\frac{2}{3}$ of its length is performed. Superiorly, the external lateral orbital rim is elevated and dissection continues toward the temporal area to separate the deep from the intermediate temporal fascia. Inferiorly, dissection of the periosteum of the zygomatic arch and the malar bone

continues with elevation of the fascia of the masseter muscle for about 2 to 3 cm inferiorly. Dissection continues inferiorly toward Bichat's fat pad and the lower boundaries of the malar and maxillary bones. In these lower boundaries the periosteum is released and the Bichat's fat pad is exposed. Then we proceed with a trial of elevation of the entire cheek to be sure that no restrictive forces are present.

At this point, when we are satisfied with the degree of elevation, we proceed with applying the suspension sutures. Usually we use three suspension points; however, in cases that do not need significant cheek elevation, the suspension points can be decreased to two or even one structure. These suspension points in order of frequency are (1) suborbicularis oculi fat (SOOF)/periosteum; (2) the periosteum of the lower cheek area; and (3) Bichat's fat pad. Mattress sutures are applied to each of the structures. It is important to try to weave the suture to the periosteum of the cheek and to the fascia and fat of Bichat's fat pad to avoid too deep a bite that may catch one of the branches of the facial nerve. Bichat's fat pad suspension is anchored to the arcus marginalis at the level of the inferolateral orbital rim. This is done with 3-0 PDS sutures. The SOOF and the periosteum suspension are anchored to the deep temporal fascia directly through the eyelid approach or to the temporal fascia proper in the temporal fossa. For the latter, we need to obtain a tunnel between the temporal pocket and the midface dissection with incision through the intermediate temporal fascia. This is done in the anterior half of the zygomatic arch and for the most part, we do not need to go on the posterior half. This way, the frontal branch of the facial nerve is duly preserved. The tunneled sutures are then anchored to the temporal fascia proper with Peruvian fisherman's knots. We also use 3-0 PDS sutures for this. As I mentioned, after the midface suspension is performed and only then do we proceed with the suspension of the forehead. The incision at the eyelid is closed accordingly (Fig. 12–5).

If the intraoral incision is used for the midface dissection, the steps of the dissection are reversed. The

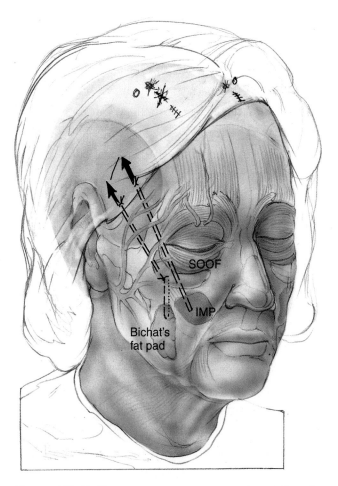

Figure 12–5. The suspension structures at the midface for elevation and improvement of the jowls, nasolabial fold, and effacement of the tear trough deformity are the SOOF, which is suspended to the deep temporal fascia. The inferior malar periosteum (*IMP*) is suspended to the deep temporal fascia, and Bichat's fat (*BF*) pad is suspended to the inferolateral arcus marginalis at the inferior orbital rim. The suspension sutures of the SOOF and the IMP can be alternately guided toward the temporal port and anchored at this level (temporal fascia proper). After the midface has been suspended, the forehead is suspended initially at the temporal area, for which we use the superficial temporal fascia anchored to the deep temporal fascia. The central forehead is suspended to endoscopic posts that are temporarily anchored to the outer cortex (for about 10 days). The paramedian ports are closed independently before to fixation of the forehead in the advanced position.

extent of the dissection is done in a similar fashion. The only variations that we have is that the application of the sutures for suspension are applied initially through the intraoral incision, brought out through the mouth, and then tunneled toward the temporal pocket as explained earlier. The areas of anchoring are exactly the same. When the intraoral incision is used, for the most part,

the way that I handle the lower eyelid skin excess is with CO_2 laser resurfacing of the periocular area or with a lower blepharoplasty type of incision, with separation of the muscles from the skin and skin excision only without transecting the orbicularis oculi muscle. The amount of dissection in the lower eyelid at the subcutaneous level is very limited. During the closure of the lower eyelid skin, it will create some overlapping of orbicularis on the pretarsal area, which is generally desirable to give the youthful look to the lower eyelid. Closure of the intraoral incision is done with interrupted 3-0 chromic catgut sutures.

The neck is approached through a submental incision of about 3 cm just behind the submental crease. Through this incision, initially under direct visualization with the fiber optic light retractor, the skin is separated from the platysma muscle, leaving about a 4-to 5-mm thickness of subcutaneous layer on the skin flap. Any excess fat is removed directly under visualization either with scissors or with a flat cannula. The dissection is extended up to the thyroid cartilage inferiorly and laterally up to the retroauricular areas. If the patient has excessive subplatysma fat in the midline, this is resected. The muscle edges are trimmed, and a modified corset platysmoplasty from the thyroid cartilage to the mentum is performed with interrupted inverted sutures. If no good definition of the cervicomental angle exists, a Guerrerosantos-Giampapa type of suture suspension is applied with interlock 3-0 PDS suture material anchored to the mastoid fascia with a small incision made on the retroauricular skin. The incision is closed in two layers with 5-0 prolene sutures. The forehead and the midface are taped with 1/2-inch Micropore. A circumferential head and neck dressing is applied.

ENDOSCOPIC-ASSISTED BIPLANAR FACELIFT

This is an operation designed for patients in their 50s and older. It can also be applied to younger patients with significant perioral and paracommissural skin excess or jowls. Basically, this combines the operation previously described with a subcutaneous cervicofacial rhytidectomy (Fig. 12–6). The skin incision extends from the area behind the sideburn at the level of the root of the helix to the occipital scalp. I prefer the marginal tragal incision in the front and in the retroauricular sulcus itself rather than in the concha because I find, they are less noticeable, more natural, and less distorting. The subcutaneous dissection extends to the entire parotid region. From here it follows a gentle curvilinear line toward the jowls and the chin. The subcutaneous neck dissection extends from one occipital/retroauricular side to the other. When the anterior cervicoplasty is combined with the posterior approach, placement of the suture suspension is done after the dissection and direct open lipectomy of any excess fat over the platysma is finished. We do not use SMAS flaps or posterior platysma traction. The only use of the SMAS is to tighten the protruding enlarged parotid

gland, which may become more noticeable when the rest of the structures are tighter.

ANCILLARY PROCEDURES

For patients with severely sun-damaged skin with severe wrinkles, ultrapulse CO_2 laser resurfacing can be performed in the same operative setting. The central oval can be treated at standard settings with energy and density similar to any other patient not undergoing facelift (Fig. 12–7). This is feasible because the blood supply after the subperiosteal dissection is excellent and the circulation of the central oval is minimally disturbed. The peripheral hemicircle can be treated with one full pass or with one pass at lesser density to allow blending of the lasered area and avoid visible lines of demarcation (Fig. 12–8). We perform laser resurfacing without the fear of necrosis because the subcutaneous undermining is limited and the blood supply is also better than the very extensive subcutaneous dissection (Fig. 12–9). Laser resurfacing can also be done in men without the fear of necrosis because the skin tends to be thicker and contain more hair follicles. The laser can be extended all the way to the submental

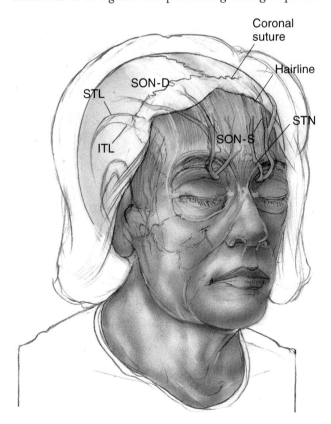

Figure 12–6. The areas of the subperiosteal dissection, as well as the area of the subcutaneous dissection for the so called biplanar facelift. The forehead and the midface are approached by means of endoscopic techniques, and these are suspended and fixed before to the subcutaneous component of the cervicofacial lift.

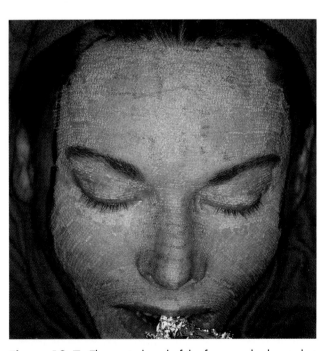

Figure 12–7. The central oval of the face can be lasered at full power in any of the variations of facelifting technique if you use the subperiosteal plane of dissection.

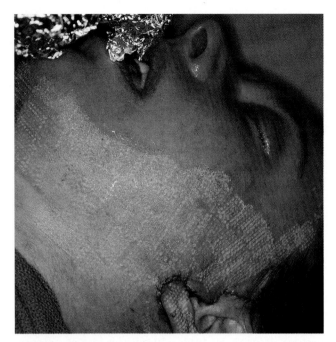

Figure 12–8. The peripheral hemicircle is lasered with one pass at the standard power or at a lesser power or density. This way, no lines of demarcations are visible on the face.

angle. In cases of full endoscopic forehead-midface lift, the entire face can be lasered at full power. This is called the SMILE facelift[10] (Fig.12–10).

With aging, atrophy of facial fat pads occurs. The volumetric restoration of fat can be performed at the intermediate layer, in other words between the subcutaneous and the subperiosteal planes. This can be easily done with this combined technique without the fear of fat migration, particularly in the central oval where only a subperiosteal dissection is done.

POSTOPERATIVE CARE

After the operation is finished, a well-contoured dressing is applied with a bulky dressing around the neck to avoid flexion and tension in the retroauricular skin flaps. The patient is monitored overnight, up to a 23-hr stay, and discharged home under the care of a well-informed relative or a practical nurse to continue his or her postoperative care.

The open subperiosteal approach produces significant swelling of the face, especially during the first 48 to 72 hours. This degree of swelling has been decreased tremendously with the advent of endoscopic techniques. How-

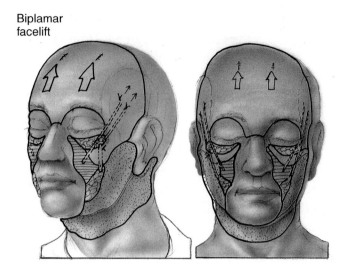

Biplamar facelift

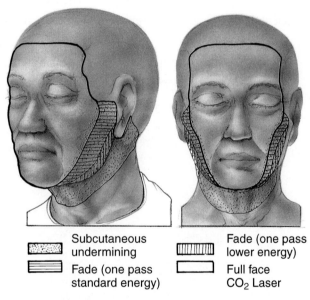

Subcutaneous undermining

Fade (one pass standard energy)

Fade (one pass lower energy)

Full face CO_2 Laser

Figure 12–9. The central oval is lasered at full power. The undermined skin on the lower face and neck are lasered at lesser power or density.

ever, occasionally the patient may still have a relatively high degree of edema, of which the patient should be warned. Patients who require significant remodeling of the soft tissues around the eyes with brow lifting and cheek elevation occasionally may have a slight orientalization of the eyelid raphe. The patient should be warned about this as well. If no detachment of the lateral canthal ligament has been made, the temporary orientalization subsides in about 4 to 6 weeks. We usually leave a small butterfly drain in the

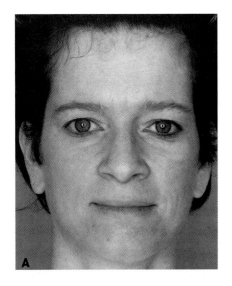
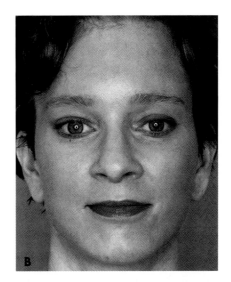
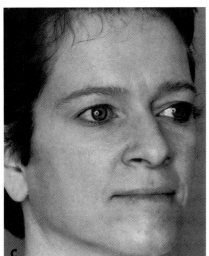
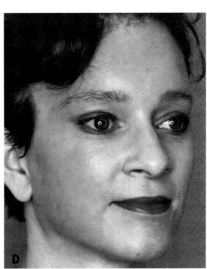
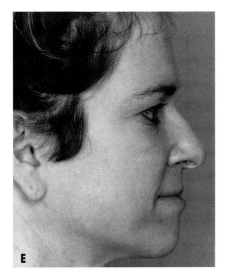
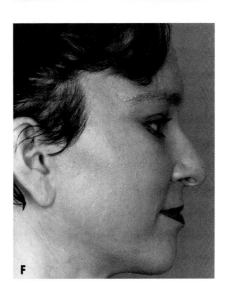

Figure 12–10. (A) The preoperative frontal view of a 39-year-old woman with typical signs of early aging. Note the brow position, forehead rhytides, and generalized cheek laxity. **(B)** Postoperative frontal view after SMILE rhytidectomy (endoforehead, endomidface, and full-face CO_2 laser resurfacing), placement of Medpor malar implants, and fat grafting to the lips. Observe the absence of forehead rhytides and the generalized youthful appearance without the stigmata of facelifting. **(C)** Preoperative three-quarters view. Observe the oblique glabellar creases, periocular rhytides, and cheek laxity. Also observe the tear trough deformity on the nasolabial folds. **(D)** Postoperative three-quarters view. Observe the brow and forehead improvement. Observe the improvement of the tear trough, the cheek mound, and the nasolabial folds. **(E)** Preoperative lateral view. Observe the brow ptosis, hooding of the eyelids, tear trough deformity, cheek laxity, and nasolabial folds. **(F)** Postoperative lateral view. Observe the glabellar and brow position. Note the improvement of the tear trough and the elevation of the cheek position and improvement on the nasolabial fold. (From Ramirez OM, Pozner JN. Subperiosteal minimally invasive laser endoscopic rhytidectomy: the SMILE facelift. *Aesth Plast Surg* 1996; 20:463, with permission.)

central forehead connected to a Vacutainer. We also apply small drains to the cheek area, brought out through the respective side of the scalp, and these are connected to Vacutainer tubing as well. We leave them in for about 48 hours. The amount of edema has been minimized tremendously with the routine use of these drains. In most cases, about 10 to 20 mL of fluid can be collected, which would be translated into edema if this was not done. Compresses 4 × 4 moistened in iced saline are applied to the eyes for the first 24 to 48 hours. A 5-day regimen of antibiotics is given routinely. If laser resurfacing is done, antibiotics are continued until complete re-epithelization is obtained. For CO_2 laser or chemical peel, we use antiviral medication, which is given until epithelization is complete. The use of the CO_2 laser has added another dimension to the postoperative care of the patient. This has been published recently and is beyond the scope of this chapter.[22,23]

If the patient had a full endoscopic facelift without skin excision, the patient can return to work in about 10 days with makeup to cover the residual ecchymosis. If the biplanar technique with full cervicoplasty is performed, then the down time is about 2 weeks. If laser resurfacing or chemical peel is done at the same operative setting, the down time increases to about 3 to 4 weeks. Even at this stage, the patient will still be red, and concealing makeup will be needed. The long-term redness, which lasts about 3 to 4 months, is still a problem with the CO_2 laser resurfacing, although in my experience, male patients have less tendency to have long-term redness develop than female patients.

COMPLICATIONS AND SEQUELAE

One of the most dreaded complications of facelift is facial nerve injury. With modern techniques, particularly with the use of the endoscope, the danger of frontal branch injury with temporary neuropraxia is about 0.4%. I have not seen permanent palsy of the frontalis muscle. In one patient, 0.2% had temporary neuropraxia of the zygomaticus branch. In 0.4% we have seen temporary numbness in the area of the infraorbital nerve. One of the patients had painful neuropathy that required neurolysis

of the infraorbital nerve with complete resolution of her symptoms. This was probably due to a small hematoma around the nerve with subsequent formation of scarring. One patient (0.2%) had a hematoma resulting from a crisis of hypertension about 4 days after surgery. The hematoma was drained, and she recovered uneventfully.

Occasionally, we have seen small areas of necrosis of the skin on the retroauricular area, and these occurred in a patient with a history of smoking, too tight closure of the skin, or both. The incidence was about 0.8%, and this is probably lower than the incidence with standard techniques.

Although most patients desire increase in the volume of the cheeks with upward elevation, one patient was very unsatisfied with the new look (0.2%). She required lipectomy of the Bichat's fat pad through the intraoral approach to decrease the bulkiness of the cheek. This patient also had microgenia. This lower face deficit probably enhanced the increased volume of the cheek. For this reason, any skeletal support deficits should be explained to the patient so that when changes are made postoperatively, this will be an expected event rather than a surprise.

One of the critiques regarding open or endoscopic forehead lift has been the "surprised look." Although on occasion a patient's brow appears higher in photographs, in reality, this seems to be an infrequent occurrence. From more than 600 brow lift cases, only one patient was unsatisfied with the elevation of her brow. However, she did not want another operation to correct this. Two patients (0.4%) required cantholysis to diminish the effect of lateral canthal tendon tightening. Conversely, about 2% of patients required an additional procedure on the lower eyelid to improve the tightening of the same or to correct minor asymmetries and ectropion.

RESULTS

The superiosteal facelift I did 14 years ago is not the same technique that I perform today.[24] Although the basic surgical principles and the basic structural surgical results may have not changed very much, several things have been incorporated into the present surgical procedure that have had a significant impact in the short-term and long-term postoperative evolution and surgical results.

The techniques described in this chapter, which are a significant departure from the original subperiosteal facelift technique include shorter incisions; use of the endoscope; better fixation, particularly of the cheek; less skin excision; more ancillary procedures; and more tendency to treat all layers of the facial structure, starting from the skeletal support and finishing with the outer layers of the skin. Repositioning of Bichat's fat pad for cheek augmentation and treatment of the suprajawl fullness is one of our latest additions.

Use of these techniques has decreased morbidity significantly compared with the old subperiosteal facelift. The surgical results have also been significantly enhanced. Improvements obtained include less facial edema, quicker recovery, less eyelid problems, more direct and effective elevation of the cheeks, better enhancement of the cheek volume, and more balanced facial appearance compared with the standard facelift.

The logical outcome of these improvements has been significant patient satisfaction and more acceptance of the techniques by surgeons and patients. Subsequently, younger and younger patients are requesting early facial rejuvenation. It is also not surprising to see many publications and presentations at national meetings of techniques based on these principles. Among the latest 200 cases done with these latest techniques, the complication rate has been minimal, the rate of patient satisfaction extremely high, and the rate of reoperation negligible.

The operation can be tailored to the patient's age, degree of facial aging, and expectations, as can be seen in the case examples included here. The first case (Fig 12–10) is a patient with early signs of aging for which a SMILE rhytidectomy was performed. The second case (Fig. 12–11) is a patient with a significantly sagging and aging face for her chronological age with severe actinic damage to her skin. This patient had an endoscopic forehead lift, endoscopic-assisted biplanar facelift, and a full cutaneous cervicofacial rhytidectomy. She also had an immediate CO_2 laser resurfacing. The third case (Fig. 12–12) is another patient with less severe aging compared with the previous patient, but she requested the max-

imum improvement. She also underwent endoscopic forehead lift, endoscopic-assisted biplanar facelift, full cervicoplasty, and immediate full-face CO_2 laser resurfacing.

CONCLUSIONS

The subperiosteal facelift is a very versatile operation. Many variations have been designed to fit the specific problems and aesthetic goals of each age group.[25] It can easily and safely incorporate ancillary techniques (1) to restore the skeletal framework; (2) to increase the volume of the intermedial layers of the central oval of the face; and (3) to rejuvenate the sun-damaged and aging skin envelope. This way we can provide a comprehensive approach to the aging face obtaining well-balanced facial features without the stigmata of the traditional facelift techniques. Most importantly, this can be done with minimal morbidity and a very low rate of complications.

PEARLS

- The advanced subperiosteal facelift emphasizes its initial approach to the central oval of the face. Only after the central oval of the face has been rejuvenated and the soft tissues repositioned is the peripheral hemicircle treated. This is usually approached with a standard limited cervicofacial rhytidectomy.
- A key area for the success of the subperiosteal central oval facelift is release of the periosteum at the superior orbital rim for the endoforehead and the submalar/maxillary areas for the midface lift.
- The maintenance of the vertically lifted soft tissues requires suspension of deep structures of the forehead and the cheek.
- The excellent vascularity of the flaps during the subperiosteal facelift allows the liberal use of ancillary procedures such as CO_2 laser and chemical peel.
- Subperiosteal exposure of the bone allows us to remodel the skeletal foundation with reduction or with augmentation by means of alloplastic implants.
- Because the intermediate layer of the soft tissues of the face are not operated on, we can inject fat to those areas for further facial remodeling.

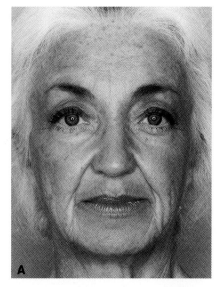
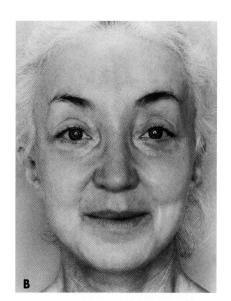
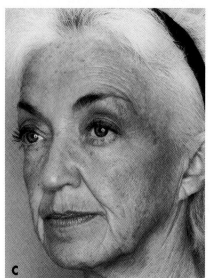
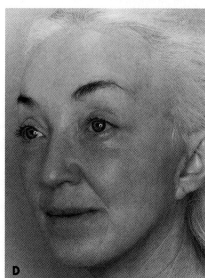
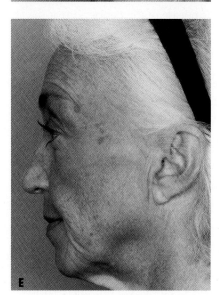
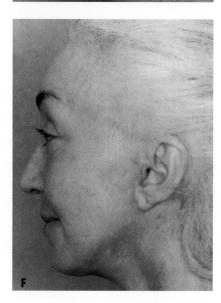

Figure 12–11. **(A)** Preoperative view of 56-year-old woman who has significant sagging of the soft tissues of the face and severe sun-damaged skin. **(B)** Postoperative view after endoscopic forehead lift, endoscopic midface lift, upper and lower blepharoplasty (skin only), cutaneous limited cervicofacial rhytidectomy, fat grafting to the glabellar and lip areas, and full-face CO_2 laser resurfacing.
(C) Preoperative three-quarters view of the same patient showing the significant ptosis of the soft tissues with hyperactivity of the frontalis muscle, corrugator, procerus, tear trough deformity on the lower eyelid, nasolabial fold and crease, atrophy of the fat on the submalar areas, marionette lines, jowls, and significant laxity of the skin on the neck with platysma bands.
(D) Postoperative three-quarters view of the same patient after the procedures described previously.
(E) Lateral view of the same patient showing the significant aging process of the entire face.
(F) Postoperative lateral view showing the beneficial effects of the combined techniques of facelifting, which include endoscopic forehead and midface lift, cutaneous cervicofacial rhytidectomy, and full-face laser resurfacing.

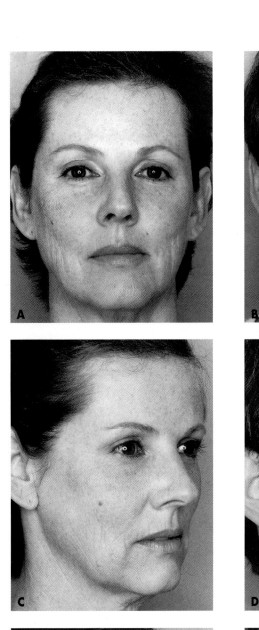
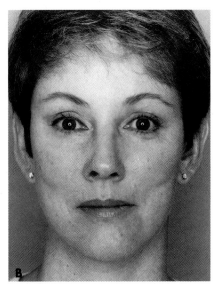
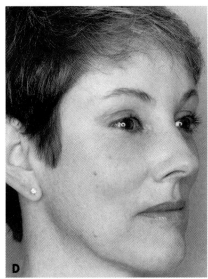
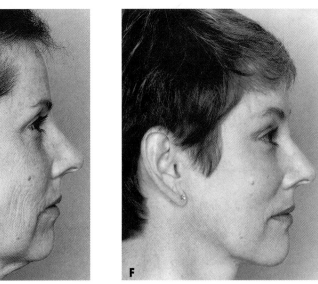

Figure 12–12. (A) Preoperative frontal view: 51-year-old woman. Observe the aging concentrated to the central oval. **(B)** Postoperative frontal view 18 months after endoscopic forehead lift, biplanar facelift (endoscopic midface lift and limited subcutaneous lower facelift), and full-face CO_2 laser resurfacing. No eyelid surgery done. Observe the overall balanced rejuvenation of the face. **(C)** Preoperative three-quarters view. Observe the generalized aging process. **(D)** Postoperative three-quarters view. All the elements of the face are rejuvenated at the same degree after 18 months. **(E)** Preoperative lateral view. Observe the laxity, ptosis, and wrinkles of the central oval of the face. **(F)** Postoperative lateral view. Observe the overall youthful appearance of the face. Observe brow and midface elevation, cheek volume restoration, tear though effacement, and the excellent quality of skin. (From Ramirez OM, Pozner JN. Laser resurfacing as an adjunct to endoforehead lift, endofacelift and biplanar facelift. *Ann Plast Surg.* 1997; 38:315–322, with permission.)

REFERENCES

1. Tessier P. Lifting facial sous-perioste. *Ann Chir Plast Esthet.* 1989; 34:193.

2. Ramirez OM. The subperiosteal rhytidectomy: The third generation face lift. *Ann Plast Surg.* 1992; 28:218.

3. Hamra ST. Composite rhytidectomy. *Plast Reconstr Surg.* 1992; 90:1.

4. Hinderer UT. The sub-SMAS and subperiosteal rhytidectomy of the forehead and middle third of the face: A new approach to the aging face. *Facial Plast Surg.* 1992; 8:18.

5. Ramirez OM. Endoscopic full facelift. *Aesthetic Plast Surg.* 1994; 18:363.

6. Ramirez OM. The subperiosteal approach for the correction of the deep nasolabial fold and the central third of the face. *Clin Plast Surg.* 1995; 22(2):341.

7. Ramirez OM, Pozner JN. Correction of the Infraorbital hollow with direct cheek lift. *Plast Surg Forum.* 1996; XIX:152–153.

8. Owsley JQ. Lifting the malar fat pad for correction of prominent nasolabial folds. *Plast Reconstr Surg.* 1993; 91:463.

9. Barton FE Jr. The SMAS and the nasolabial fold. *Plast Reconstr Surg.* 1992; 89:1054.

10. Ramirez OM, Pozner JN. Subperiosteal minimally invasive laser endoscopic rhytidectomy: The SMILE facelift. *Aesth Plast Surg.* 1996; 20:463.

11. Ramirez OM, Pozner JN. Laser resurfacing as an adjunct to endoforehead lift, endofacelift, and biplanar facelift. *Ann Plast Surg.* 1997; 38:315.

12. Terino EO. Alloplastic facial contouring: Surgery of the fourth plane. *Aesth Plast Surg.* 1992; 16:195.

13. Ramirez OM. High-tech facelift. *Aesth Plast Surg.* 1998; 22:318–328.

14. Ramirez, OM. The central oval of the face: A critical anatomical, surgical and aesthetic unit. In: Ramirez OM, ed. *Subperiosteal Facelift.* New York: Springer-Verlag; in press.

15. Ramirez OM. Why I prefer the endoscopic forehead lift. *Plast Reconstr Surg.* 1997; 100:1033.

16. Ramirez OM. Fourth-generation subperiosteal approach to the midface: The tridimentional functional cheek lift. *Aesth Surg J.* 1998; 18:133–135.

17. Ramirez OM. Cervicoplasty: Non-excisional anterior approach. *Plast Reconstr Surg.* 1997; 99:1576–1585.

18. Ramirez OM. Endoscopic subperiosteal browlift and facelift. *Clin Plast Surg.* 1995; 22:639.

19. Ramirez OM, Pozner JN. Subperiosteal endoscopic techniques in secondary rhytidectomy. *Aesth Surg J.* 1997; 17:22.

20. Ramirez OM. Aesthetic craniofacial surgery. *Clin Plast Surg.* 1994; 21:649–659.

21. Boyd GL, Funderburg BJ, Vasconez LO, Guzman G. Long distance anesthesia. *Anesth Analg.* 1992; 74:467–477.

22. Weinstein C, Pozner JN, Ramirez OM. Complications of carbon dioxide laser resurfacing and their prevention. *Aesth Surg J.* 1997; 17:216.

23. Weinstein C, Ramirez OM, Pozner JN. Post-operative care following CO_2 laser resurfacing: Avoiding pitfalls. *Plast Reconstr Surg.* 1997; 100:1855–1866.

24. Ramirez OM, Maillard GF, Musolas A. The extended subperiosteal facelift: A definitive soft-tissue remodeling for facial rejuvenation. *Plast Reconstr Surg.* 1991; 88:227.

25. Ramirez OM. Classification of facial rejuvenation techniques based on the subperiosteal approach and ancillary procedures. *Plast Reconstr Surg.* 1996; 97:45.

Note: The instrumentation mentioned in this chapter is manufactured by Deknatel-Snowden Percer Inc. Tucker, Georgia, under "Ramirez Endoscopic Periosteal Elevators" and "Ramirez Endoscopic Manipulators."

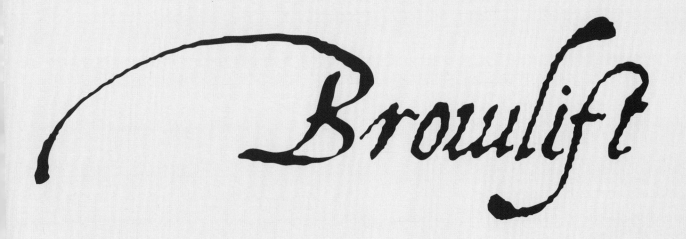

Browlift

The chapters by Drs. Goldberg and Keller are superb descriptions in the management of the brow and upper face. Dr. Goldberg, an oculoplastic surgeon, opens the chapter with a careful description of pre-operative evaluation and philosophy of the intimate relationship of the upper eyelid, brow, and fore-head complex. It can be generalized that blepharoplasty is performed very commonly in concert with endoscopic brow elevation in an oculoplastic practice as opposed to isolated endoscopic brow elevation. This is probably due to a slightly different patient demographic, which we have noted informally, to be present in an oculoplastic practice. The oculoplastic practice is generally made up of a slightly older clientele because of the nature of the referral pattern and specialty. For that reason the presence of senescent changes in the 40- to 50-year-old age groups and beyond generally lead to the combined use of blepharoplasty and brow procedures.

The average facial plastic and plastic surgeons must typically involve younger age demograph-ics, with many patients presenting in the third and fourth decades of life. These younger patients com-monly have little or no dermatochalasia, and their aesthetic concerns in the upper eyelid are more commonly attributable to brow position or fullness of the brow than to the eyelid itself. These findings are more compatible with isolated endoscopic brow lifting. The perspective of each of these surgeons is unique and valuable.

Dr. Goldberg specifically describes his technique as it relates to blepharoplasty and the tech-nique of combined upper lid blepharoplasty and brow elevation with use of the upper lid crease incision to aid in the brow dissection when available.

Dr. Keller, who is a facial plastic surgeon, has marvelous components of extended brow dissec-tion with careful description of endoscopic manipulation of the frontotemporal, zygomatic, and malar areas, which become a segue to the endoscopic facelift chapters of Drs. Kamer and Ramirez.

Because of the introduction and tremendous advancement and evolution of endoscopic surgical technology, the brow lift, which had once been an infrequently performed procedure, has become one of the most commonly performed facial aesthetic procedures, and the descriptions of Drs. Goldberg and Keller encompass it totally.

Brouillet

Aesthetic Facial Plastic Surgery, edited by Thomas Romo, III, and Arthur L. Millman, Thieme Medical Publishers, Inc., New York, New York, Copyright © 2000.

CHAPTER 13

An Oculoplastic Surgeon's Perspective

ROBERT ALAN GOLDBERG

The surgeon performing rehabilitation and rejuvenation of the eyelid complex is at a significant disadvantage if he or she does not perform eyebrow lift. Many patients requesting blepharoplasty to address heavy upper eyelids actually have significant eyebrow ptosis. It is easy to fall into a trap: the patient may maintain their eyebrows above the orbital rim using maximum frontalis muscle compensation, but when skin is taken from the eyelid or eyelid margin ptosis is corrected, the drive for frontalis compensation is reduced and the eyebrow falls to a new resting level (Fig. 13–1).

If the patient is not warned preoperatively of this possibility, he or she may be unhappy with the results of blepharoplasty or ptosis surgery. It is far better to recognize eyebrow problems preoperatively and to discuss with the patient the advisability of eyebrow surgery and if the patient elects to proceed without addressing eyebrow ptosis, the nature of the limitations of surgical results imposed by eyebrow descent.

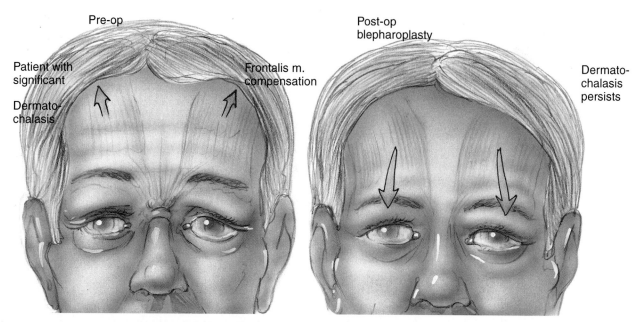

Figure 13–1. Postoperatively after blepharoplasty, the frontalis muscle relaxes because of decreased compensatory drive, and the eyebrow falls. The eyebrow droop "eats up" much of the blepharoplasty results. (Copyright 1996, Regents of the University of California, UCLA. Used with permission Regents UC, UCLA.)

A significant part of the upper eyelid contour is formed from eyebrow tissues, both the deep components (primarily the eyebrow fat pad or retro-orbicularis oculi-fat [ROOF] fat pad) and the cutaneous component of the extended eyebrow complex. Eyebrow surgery is the most effective way to address these tissue components.[6–8] Blepharoplasty alone does not address these tissues well and, in fact, well-meaning surgery of the eyelid performed in an effort to treat problems that are truly eyebrow ptosis can result in complications such as scars in the lateral sub-brow region created in an effort to "chase temporal hooding" and vertical inadequacy of the eyelid skin created by aggressive excision.

PATIENT SELECTION

It is important in preoperative planning to evaluate the role of the various tissues in creating the preoperative eyelid contours and to individualize a plan for each patient that accomplishes an aesthetically pleasing balance of sculpture of the eyebrow and eyelid tissues. The two structures are obviously completely interrelated. I do not buy into the concept that one should perform the eye-

brow surgery first and then remove all the remaining skin from the eyelid. This is not only a rote and nonindividualized approach but also subscribes to the old-fashioned notion that blepharoplasty is about removing skin. In actuality, both functionally and aesthetically, blepharoplasty is about leaving skin. The effect of blepharoplasty and browlift is achieved as much by the sculpture of the deep tissue as it is by surgery on the skin itself. The major complications of surgery result from removing too much skin; particularly if the eyebrows are elevated or stabilized through eyebrow surgery, 20 to 25 mm of skin are required for comfortable eyelid closure. Therefore I think it is valuable to decide preoperatively how much sculpture and skin excision is going to be performed in the eyebrow and the eyelid and to stick to this preoperative plan. For this reason, I do not believe it is necessary to start with the eyebrow, and in fact I begin with the eyelid. First I perform the predetermined amount of skin excision and deep sculpture, and then I inject the brow with local anesthetic before closing the eyelid incision. The last step is to perform the endoscopic forehead lift.

Having said that (and perhaps being overrepetitive regarding our philosophy of the importance of the eyebrow in eyelid surgery), blepharoplasty has a clear role in conjunction with eyebrow elevation. Particularly with age, redundant tissues develop in the eyelid complex that cannot be addressed with browlift alone. In younger patients, I typically excise 1 to 2 mm of skin through an eyelid crease incision and then sculpt the underlying septum and orbital fat to improve the definition of the tarsal plate and to create a lid crease. In older patients, I will often excise as much as 5 to 8 mm of skin and reposition or conservatively remove some of the orbital fat.

The combination of eyebrow sculpting and elevation and upper eyelid blepharoplasty is powerful, and it is important to plan carefully to avoid an overdone or overly sculpted eyelid that is aesthetically displeasing. Overcorrections are much more difficult to revise than undercorrections.

CHOICE OF PROCEDURE

Before endoscopic techniques became available, it was not always easy to convince the patient to agree to eyebrow elevation. We were significantly limited, particularly in men, by the need to somehow hide the incision sites. Long incisions above the brow or in the mid forehead, although they may satisfy some patients, are in my experience unlikely to satisfy the typical critical and sophisticated patient who wants the best possible cosmetic outcome. The open coronal forehead lift is a superb operation that was my mainstay five years ago.[1] It provides excellent access to the orbital rim, glabella, and temporal area, and the incision is hidden in the hair. However, it requires an adequate hairline, which is typically not available in a man who might have undergone or may undergo male pattern balding. Also, because of the long incision, numbness, hair loss, and slow healing were significant problems that decreased patient acceptance. The result of endoscopic eyebrow lift are essentially identical to those of the open coronal lift, but because of the lack of a long ear-to-ear incision, numbness, bruising, hair loss, and recuperation time[2-5] are decreased substantially. Patient acceptance is dramatically

improved, and as a result I now do far more eyebrow surgeries, resulting in a higher surgical volume and happier eyelid surgery patients, without postblepharoplasty eyebrow descent. In male patients endoscopic browlift allows us to offer surgery to a group of patients who had no practical option to hide the scar. For men with male pattern baldness the scars can be hidden in the hair, or, at least, small 2 cm incisions can be used instead of a conspicuous ear-to-ear incision.

Endoscopic forehead and browlift is a significant advancement in cosmetic surgery. However, some minor disadvantages exist with the endoscopic approach. Certainly a learning curve is necessary in mastering endoscopic forehead lift surgery. For the ophthalmologist who has some experience using endoscopes (e.g., in nasal lacrimal surgery) and who is familiar with the open coronal forehead approach, learning should be rapid. On the other hand, if one has to master coronal anatomy and use of the endoscope, a significant commitment to dissection, laboratory training, and perhaps an initial period of performing open forehead lift surgery will likely be necessary to achieve comfort with the anatomy and technique. With experience, surgical time is equivalent to that required for open coronal lift (about 1 hour), but in the learning period surgical time may be significantly increased. The learning curve also includes the operating room staff. The equipment is expensive. The endoscope, video monitoring equipment, and dissection instruments can cost $15,000 to $20,000. However, the endoscopic setup is already available in most operating rooms.

PREOPERATIVE PREPARATION
INCISIONS

The patient must have washed his or her hair thoroughly. The incision sites are marked by parting the scalp (Fig. 13–2). I make the temporal incisions 2 to 3 cm from the hairline in circumferential fashion, 3 to 4 cm long, drawn superiorly based on a line from the oral commissure through the lateral canthus. I then make

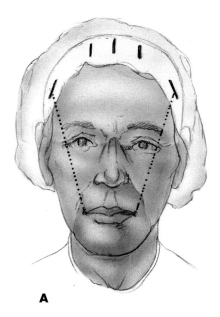

A

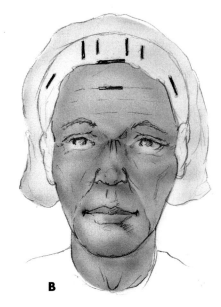

B

Figure 13-2. Location of incisions for endoscopic forehead lift. **(A)** Typical pattern. **(B)** Composite of various options, including pretrichial small incision for patient with high forehead and midforehead incision for patient with male pattern balding.

either three or four radial incisions each 2 to 3 cm long beginning 2 cm behind the hairline. I use four incisions when I want to create more lift at the medial brow: two paramedian incisions are more powerful in this regard than one central incision (Fig. 13–2A). The tail of the brow and the zygomatic tissues are contoured with the temporal incisions. In a man with male pattern balding, the central incisions may not be hidden in the hairline; the surgeon may elect to place a small central incision in a midforehead rhytid (Fig. 13–2B).

ANESTHESIA

Endoscopic browlift is performed with local anesthesia sedation. I use 150 to 200 mL of a dilute lidocaine mixture (0.2% lidocaine with 1:1,000,000 epinephrine) and a supraorbital block with several milliliters of bupivicaine, 0.75%. I find that the most sensitive areas are over the lateral orbital rim and at the lateral canthus, and therefore I am careful to adequately anesthetize these areas. The anesthesia should cover the entire area from zygomatic prominence back to the vertex of the scalp.

If concomitant blepharoplasty is to be performed, I usually start with the eyelid surgery. In this case, during the initial deep sedation I inject the eyelids with lidocaine and epinephrine and block the supraorbital nerves with bupivicaine. Then, later in the case, before

closing the eyelid incisions, the patient is again sedated deeply and dilute lidocaine with epinephrine solution is injected into the brow and orbital rim. In this way, maximal epinephrine-induced vasoconstriction is in place at the time of brow surgery.

TECHNIQUE

Three major phases make up endoscopic brow surgery: dissection of the optical pockets, release of the eyebrow at the orbital rim, and fixation of the flap.

DISSECTION OF OPTICAL POCKETS

The central radial incisions are carried down to the bone, and the temporal incisions are carried down to the shiny white deep temporalis fascia. I begin my dissection of the temporalis fascia by using scissors under direct visualization to carry the pocket down to the hairline. The anatomy of this area is characterized by layers of fascia that must be followed carefully to achieve maximal surgical results and avoid injury to the facial nerve (Fig. 13–3).

As the central and temporal pockets are created, the surgeon encounters a tight adherence along the temporal line, which is known as the conjoined fascia (Fig. 13–3B). This represents an adhesion between the periosteum over the frontal bone and the deep temporalis fascia.

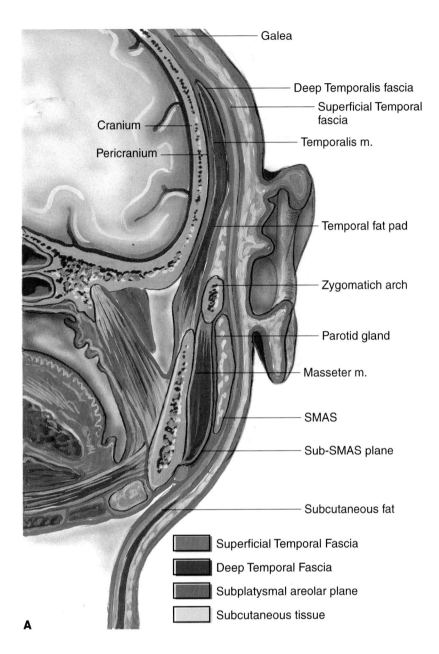

Figure 13–3. (A) Fascial planes in the temporal region: the SMAS and the deep fascia. *(Figure continued on next page)*

The conjoined fascia, as mentioned previously, continues down along the lateral edge of the zygoma to the takeoff of the zygomatic arch, attaching the zygomatic periosteum to the deep temporal fascia. This adhesion must be released by dissecting along the curve of the temporal line down to the superolateral orbital rim. Sometimes some significant vessels lie within this conjoined fascia, and a combination of sharp dissection, endoscopic scissors, and cautery or laser is used.

This part of the dissection incorporates the only real dangerous anatomy in endoscopic brow surgery:[9–14] the frontal branch of the facial nerve runs just superficial to the deep temporal fascia in the area of the lateral orbital rim (Fig. 13–3C). Care must be taken to maintain a deep plane on the temporal fascia to avoid injury to the nerve, which could produce a permanent eyebrow paralysis.

The endoscope is introduced and the dissection is continued along the deep temporal fascia until the lateral bony orbital rim is reached (Fig. 13–4). The sentinel vessel is often identified and cauterized within the deep temporal fat pad (Fig. 13–5) as the dissection between the temporoparietal fascia (subcutaneous muscoloaponeurotic system) and

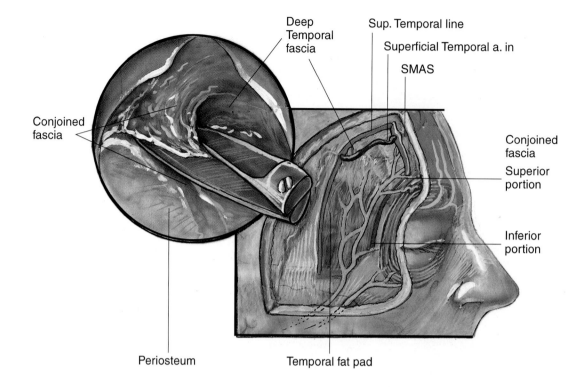

B

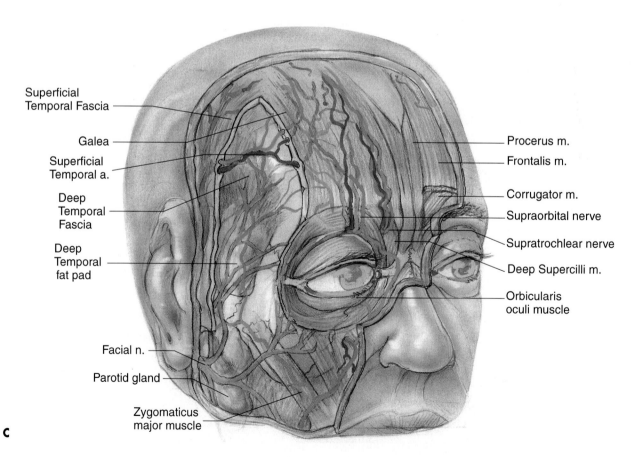

C

Figure 13–3. *(continued)* **(B)** Conjoined tendon (upper segment). **(C)** Facial nerve anatomy.

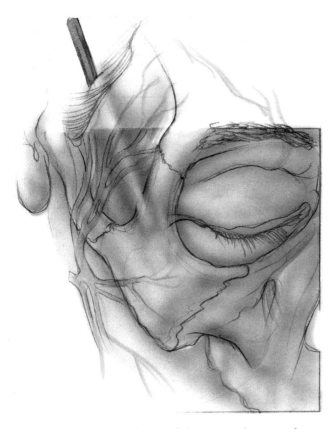

Figure 13–4. External view of dissection: drawing of surgical technique, elevator in "transview" seen through skin. (Copyright 1996, Regents of the University of California, UCLA. Used with permission Regents UC, UCLA.)

the deep temporal fascia continues down toward the takeoff of the zygomatic arch. An important part of the release includes the most inferior part of the conjoined fascia, which follows the lateral surface of the zygoma inferior to the level of the lateral canthus and onto the takeoff of the zygomatic arch; therefore the release should include the takeoff of the arch (Fig. 13–6). The facial nerve crosses the arch midway between the tragus and the canthus and can be damaged as the dissection is carried over the arch, particularly if the dissection is carried lateral to this "danger area" where the nerve crosses (Fig. 13–7). Staying medial to this point and keeping a careful subperiosteal plane should minimize the risk of frontal branch injury here. I often carry the dissection down over the medial third of the zygomatic arch and sometimes even onto the malar eminence to release and lift the lateral canthus and cheek (Fig. 13–8).

I then dissect the central pocket. Again, the initial dissection is carried out without the endoscope. Working

by feel, a subperiosteal dissection is carried down toward the orbital rim, stopping 1 to 2 cm above the rim to avoid injuring the superior orbital neurovascular bundle (Fig. 13–9). Special malleable curved dissectors are used to work beneath the flap. The dissection is also carried posteriorly a few centimeters posterior to the incisions, and all of the incisions are connected in the subperiosteal plane.

The endoscope is then inserted through the central radial incisions and, working within the optical pocket created by the subperiosteal dissection, the superior orbital neurovascular bundle (Fig. 3–10), and the depressor muscles of the glabella including the corrugator, procerus, and supraciliary orbicularis are identified.[15]

RELEASE

After the entire dissection has been completed and the conjoined fascia released on both sides, the surgeon has a view of the entire sub-brow region from the zygoma all the way across the orbital rims. The next part of the surgery is the most important. The surgeon must carefully release the entire brow from the midline to the zygoma. This release is the key to successful endoscopic brow surgery, and any residual attachments that are missed will result in late failure. The periosteum at the arcus marginalis is released and opened across the entire brow. Care is taken to work around the superior neurovascular bundles (supraorbital and supratrochlear), which can emanate from a notch or foramen at the orbital rim.[16] The release can be accomplished with sharp dissection or with CO_2 laser or cautery dissection (Fig. 13–11).

Centrally, the brow is held down actively and passively by the depressor muscles of the glabella, particularly the corrugators and supraciliary orbicularis. These muscles can be clearly visualized with the endoscope, and scissors, cutting cautery, or my preference, the CO_2 laser can be used to interrupt the course of these muscles and variably ablate them (Fig. 13–12). The neurovascular bundle runs through the corregator, and it must be carefully dissected and avoided to minimize postoperative numbness. Because botulinum toxin can be used to chemically denervate these muscles, I am less aggressive

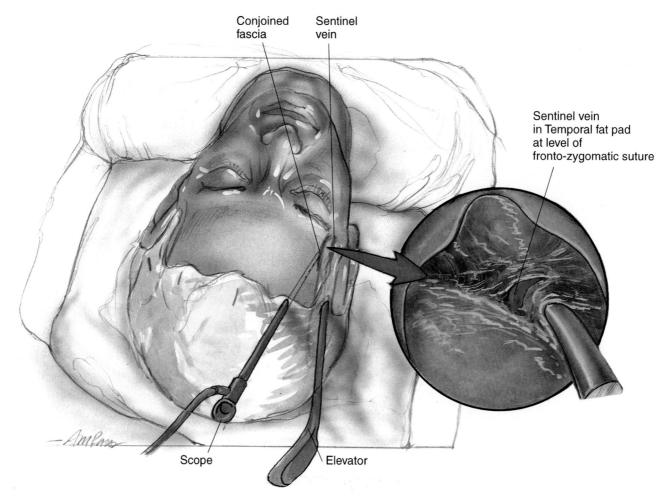

Conjoined fascia   Sentinel vein

Sentinel vein
in Temporal fat pad
at level of
fronto-zygomatic suture

Scope   Elevator

Figure 13–5. Sentinel vein at edge of orbital rim, approximately at the level of the frontozygomatic suture (endoscopic view). (Copyright 1996, Regents of the University of California, UCLA. Used with permission Regents UC, UCLA.)

than I used to be in ablating them: aggressive ablation can create a visible depression in the glabella, and aggressive corrugator weakening can widen the eyebrows.

The lateral adhesions are difficult to visualize for the inexperienced surgeon. It is important to release the arcus marginalis at the orbital rim all the way down to the lateral canthus to achieve lateral brow elevation. This dissection, which can be carried out with sharp dissection or with CO_2 laser, exposes the ROOF fat (which can be sculpted) and exposes the orbital fat as the arcus marginalis is released (Fig. 13–13).

FIXATION

After the brow has been adequately released, attention is turned to fixation. A number of ideas for eyebrow fixation have been proposed, including Y to V advancements, triangular skin excision, various suture techniques, tape

alone, and varied bony fixations. I prefer the use of removable screws, which are rapid, straightforward, and effective. At the posterior end of the radial incisions I drill a 4-mm deep hole with a guarded hand-operated drill. I place a 14 mm × 1.7 mm screw in each 4-mm hole. A nerve hook is then inserted into the radial incision and used to elevate the flap. As the flap is advanced, the radial incision slides backward so that the screw is now near the front of the incision. A surgical staple that had been pre-placed in front of the incision is then lifted over the screw and used to stabilize the flap on the screw, hanging by the staple (Fig. 13–14). Several staples are placed across the radial incision. If eyebrow asymmetry is present 3 to 5 days postoperatively, the flap can be released by lifting the staples over the screw and allowing the flap to gradually fall down. An alternative technique for fixation is to use a heavy suture (such as 2-0 Vicryl) to fixate the screw to

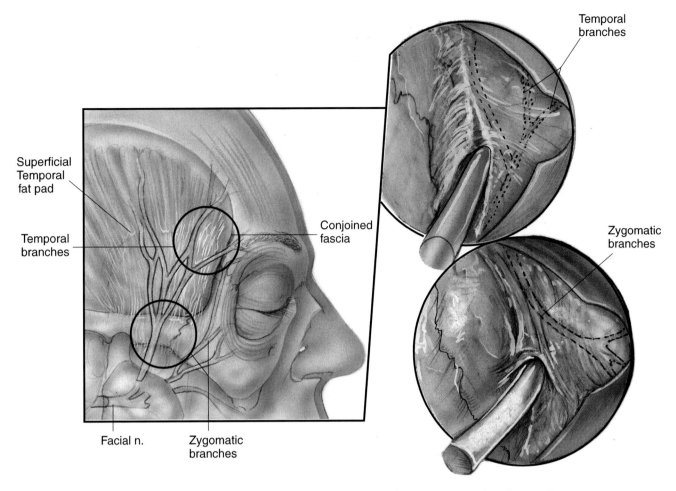

Figure 13–6. Danger area of facial nerve as it crosses the zygomatic arch. (After Larabee.)

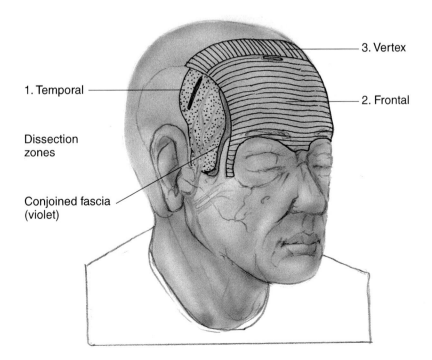

Figure 13–7. Total dissection zone, shaded diagram.

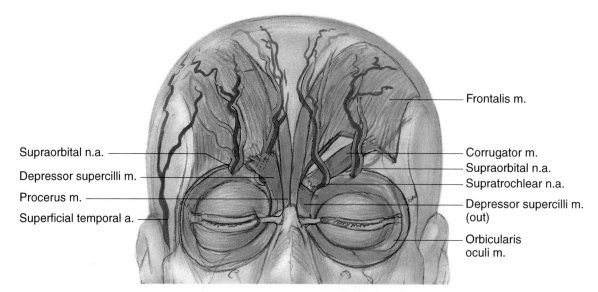

Frontalis m.

Supraorbital n.a.

Depressor supercilli m.

Procerus m.

Superficial temporal a.

Corrugator m.

Supraorbital n.a.

Supratrochlear n.a.

Depressor supercilli m. (out)

Orbicularis oculi m.

Figure 13–8. Overview of supraorbital anatomy.

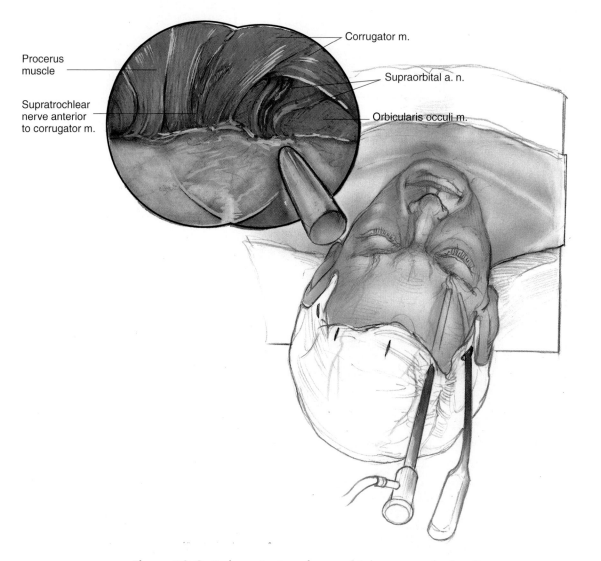

Corrugator m.

Procerus muscle

Supraorbital a. n.

Supratrochlear nerve anterior to corrugator m.

Orbicularis occuli m.

Figure 13–9. Endoscopic view of supraorbital neurovascular bundle.

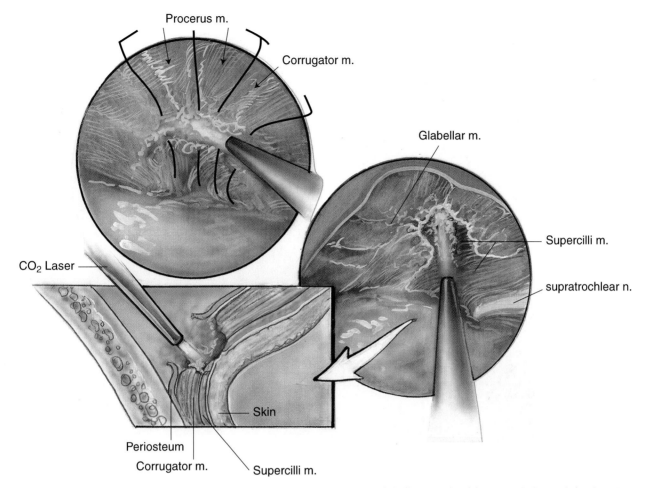

Procerus m.

Corrugator m.

Glabellar m.

Supercilli m.

supratrochlear n.

CO₂ Laser

Skin

Periosteum

Corrugator m.

Supercilli m.

Figure 13–10. Endoscopic view of central release using CO₂ laser and glabellar muscle ablation with the endoforehead tip on the Luxar CO₂ laser.

the subcutaneous tissues of the anterior portion of the radial incision. Several companies make special screws that are unthreaded except for the 4 to 5 mm at the tip because the threads tend to fray and break the sutures. Some surgeons have reported hair loss associated with the strangulation that these sutures may cause, and I do not use them. On the other hand, in non-hair-bearing areas such as in a man with a recessed hairline, I often use a buried absorbable suture fixated to a bony tunnel. The bony tunnel is created with a 3-mm cutting burr (Fig. 13–15).

The temporal flaps are fixated to the underlying deep temporal fascia with 2-0 Vicryl suture. I like to make a SMAS flap by dissecting the superficial temporoparietal fascia from the skin for several cm and suturing this to a cut edge of deep temporal fascia. An ellipse or triangle of skin can be removed from the scalp for even greater temporal fixation.

ASSOCIATED PROCEDURES

Endoscopic eyebrow lift is often performed in conjunction with upper blepharoplasty. Elevating and stabilizing the eyebrow against postblepharoplasty brow descent and elevating the ROOF out of the eyelid space allow conservative blepharoplasty to be effectively performed. Endoscopic dissection can be carried beneath the lateral canthal angle onto the face of the zygoma. In this way, the lateral canthal area and upper cheek can be lifted along with the temporal brow. Lower blepharoplasty and periorbital laser resurfacing can also be combined with endoscopic forehead lift.

POSTOPERATIVE COURSE

The scalp flap is covered with a Kerlex or net dressing after the hair has been cleansed of any blood with warm

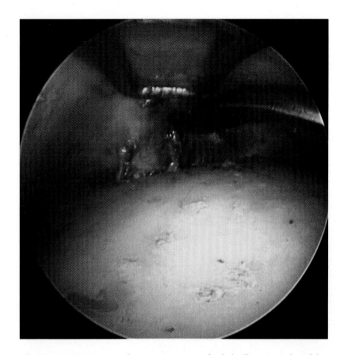

Figure 13–11. Endoscopic view of glabellar muscle ablation with the endoforehead tip on the Luxar CO_2 laser. (Copyright 1996, Regents of the University of California, UCLA. Used with permission Regents UC, UCLA.)

water and baby shampoo. I do not routinely use postoperative antibiotics. The patient removes the dressing on the second postoperative day and takes a gentle warm shampoo. I telephone patients the night after surgery and see them back in the office in 3 to 5 days. The screws (we tell the patients these are "posts" or "screw tacks") are removed at 2 weeks along with the staples. The patient can generally return to work in 1 to 2 weeks. Numbness can persist for 1 to 3 months along with a tingling or crawling sensation and "hair shock" can result in some alopecia around the incision sites lasting for 1 to 2 months. Permanent numbness or hair loss is rare.

COMPLICATIONS AND SEQUELAE

Although damage to the frontal branch of the facial nerve with resulting eyebrow paralysis is a major worry and one that we take great care to prevent, the actual occurrence is rare. In my experience of more than 100 endoscopic browlifts I have had none, nor have I seen any by referral; but I have heard the complication reported and

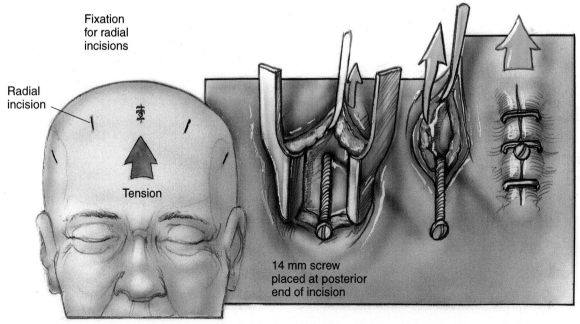

Figure 13–12. (A) 14-mm screw is placed into a 4-mmm deep pilot hole in the skill and preplaced staples are lifted over the head of the screw as poesterior traction is placed on the flap. **(B)** Alternatively, a PDS buried suture can be used to stabilize the flap against the screw.

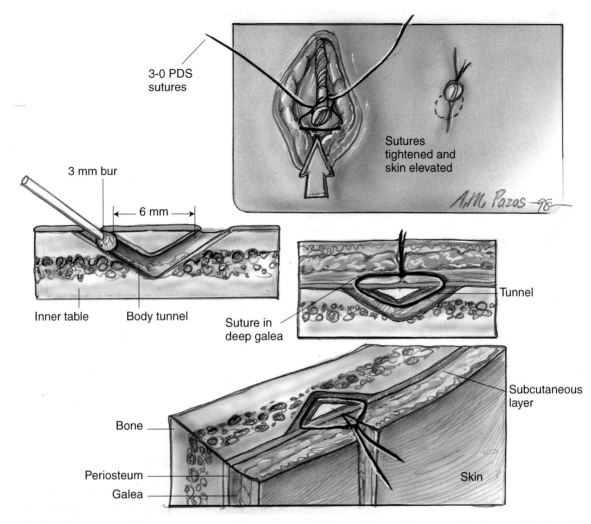

3-0 PDS sutures

Sutures tightened and skin elevated

A.M Pazos -98

3 mm bur

6 mm

Inner table   Body tunnel

Suture in deep galea

Tunnel

Subcutaneous layer

Bone

Periosteum

Galea

Skin

Figure 13–13. Flap supported by suture to burred bony tunnel. **(A)** Two oblique holes are drilled into each other with 3-mm cutting burr. **(B)** Suture through holes and galea.

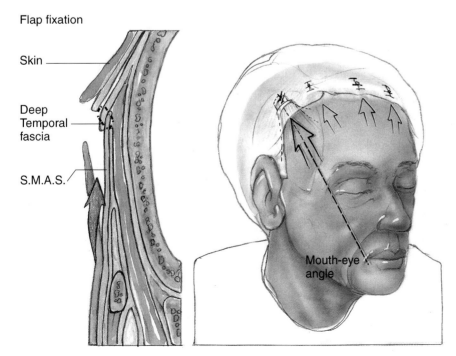

Flap fixation

Skin

Deep Temporal fascia

S.M.A.S.

Mouth-eye angle

Figure 13–14. Temporal flap fixation. A galeal flap is dissected from the skin and sutured through a slit in the deep temporal fascia with an absorbable matress suture.

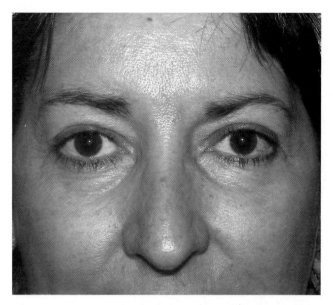

Figure 13–15. Patient 1 year after endoscopic forehead lift combined with blepharoplasty and erbium resurfacing. (Copyright 1996, Regents of the University of California, UCLA. Used with permission Regents UC, UCLA.)

the surgeon should carefully learn the anatomy of the facial nerve and avoid damage to the nerve.

Temporary numbness is common, but permanent numbness or paresthesia rarely occurs. By directly observing and carefully avoiding the main sensory trunk as it exits the superior orbit, this complication can be minimized. Hair loss at the incision sites can rarely occur. The best form of prevention is avoidance of excess cautery at the hair follicles and careful closure with minimal tension on the wound. Hematomas and infections can occur but are not specific to the endoscopic approach.

Aesthetic complications occur, and with all aesthetic surgeries the surgeon should be prepared to reoperate and touch-up unhappy patients. Asymmetric eyebrow position can occur. In the first postoperative week the high side can be adjusted by removing staples over the screw; later, asymmetry is best addressed by re-elevation of the more ptotic side. Depression in the area of the glabella can occur after aggressive resection of muscle; when aggressive resection is performed, considera-

tion should be given to autogenous or alloplastic implants into the glabellar region. If the corrugator is aggressively relaxed, widening of the central brow can occur.

CONCLUSION

Endoscopic forehead elevation represents a significant advancement in oculoplastic surgery. The surgery is effective, well tolerated by the patient, and entirely within the scope of the ophthalmologist who is interested in the eyebrow and willing to learn the regional anatomy and endoscopic techniques. Patient acceptance is very high. It offers a surgical alternative to men with male pattern baldness and to any patient reluctant to have a standard open coronal incision, allowing us to treat patients who previously had no good surgical alternatives.

PEARLS

- It is important in preoperative planning to evaluate the role of the various tissues in creating the preoperative eyelid contours and to individualize a plan for each patient that accomplishes an aesthetically pleasing balance of sculpture of the eyebrow and eyelid tissues.
- Four radial incisions can be used to create more lift at the brow.
- Care must be taken when interrupting or ablating the depressor muscles of the glabella. Aggressive ablation can create a visible depression in the glabella and aggressive corrugator weakening can widen the eyebrows.
- To fixate the eyebrow in a non-hair-bearing area or in a man with a recessed hairline, a buried absorbable suture can be fixated to a bony tunnel.

SUGGESTED READINGS

Baylis HI. The trans-eyelid small incision forehead lift. Presented at the 27th Annual ASOPRS Scientific Symposium; October 26, 1996: Chicago, IL.

Correia P, Zani R. Surgical anatomy of the facial nerve, as related to the ancillary operations and rhytidoplasty. *Plast Reconstr Surg.* 1973; 52:549–552.

Ellenbogen R. Medial brow lift. *Ann Plast Surg.* 1980; 5:151–152.

Ellenbogen R. Transcoronal eyebrow lift with concomitant upper blepharoplasty. *Plast Reconstr Surg.* 1983, 71:490–499.

Furnas DW. Landmarks for the trunk and the temporofacial division of the facial nerve. Br J Surg. 1965; 52:694–696.

Goldberg RA. Endoscopic browlift. In: Romo T, Millman A, eds. *Aesthetic Facial Plastic Surgery: A Multidisciplinary Approach.* Thieme. In press.

Green JP, Goldberg RA, Shorr N. Eyebrow ptosis. In: Kikkawa D, ed. *International Ophthalmology Clinica.* Boston: Little Brown and Co; Vol. 37. 1997:97–122.

Keller G. Endoscopic forehead lift. *West J Med.* 1995; 163(2):157.

Loeb R. Technique for preservation of the temporal branches of the facial nerve during face lift operations. Br J Plast Surg. 1979;23:390–394.

McCord CD, Doxanas MT. Browplasty and browpexy: An adjunct to blepharoplasty. *Plast Reconstr Surg.* 1990; 86:248–254.

Nahai F, Eaves FF, Bostwick J. Forehead lift and glabellar frown lines. In: Bostwick J, Eaves FF, Nahai F, eds. *Endoscopic Plastic Surgery.* St. Louis: Quality Medical Publishing, Inc.; 1995: 165–230.

Pitanguay I, Ramos AS. The frontal branch of the facial nerve: The importance of its variations in face lifting. *Plast Reconstr Surg.* 1966; 38:352–356.

Shorr N, Green JP, Shorr J. Eyebrow ptosis in cosmetic surgery of the eyelid. In: Patipa M, ed. *Seminars in Ophthalmology,* Vol. 11. Philadelphia: Saunders; 1996:138–156.

Steinsapir KD, Shorr N, Hoenig J, Goldberg RA, Baylis H, Morrow D. The endoscopic forehead lift. *Ophthal Plast Reconstr Surg.* 1998; 14(2):107–118.

Stuzin JM, Baker TJ, Gordon HL. The relationship of the superficial and deep facial fascias: Relevance to rhytidectomy and aging. *Plast Reconstr Surg.* 1992; <Nessuno>89:441–452.

Stuzin JS, Wagstom L, Kawamoto HK, Wolfe SA. Anatomy of the frontal branch of the facial nerve: The significance of the temporal fat pad. *Plast Reconstr Surg.* 1989; 83:265–271.

Webster RC, Gaunt JM, Hamdan US, et al. Supraorbital and supratrochlear notches and foramina: Anatomical variations and surgical relevance. *Laryngoscope.* 1986; 96:311–317.

Brouillis

Aesthetic Facial Plastic Surgery, edited by Thomas Romo, III, and Arthur L. Millman, Thieme Medical Publishers, Inc., New York, New York, Copyright © 2000.

CHAPTER 14

A Facial Plastic Surgeon's Perspective

GREGORY S. KELLER AND ROBERT W. HUTCHERSON

Endoscopic techniques for rejuvenation of the aging forehead and brow have received significant attention since their introduction in 1991.[1] The approach was initially viewed as an alternative to the standardized coronal and pretrichial operations, offering less scarring, hair loss, and numbness than these larger incision procedures.[2–5] With accumulated experience and time to critically evaluate postoperative results, we now regard endoscopic forehead and browlifting as the preferred technique to aesthetically modify the upper third of the face.

The primary advantage of these procedures is that they use small, minimally invasive incisions to expose the large anatomic unit of the forehead, temporal region, and lateral orbit. With the endoscope providing visualization, precise modification of the musculature and soft tissue can be obtained. Laser-assisted procedures enhance hemostasis and further reduce postoperative ecchymosis and edema.

PATIENT SELECTION

An array of factors, including exposure history, genetics, overall health, and age, determine the relaxation of the forehead and descent of the brow. As the forehead musculature is affected by these factors, the occipitalis-galea-frontalis sling becomes subservient to the depressor musculature of the mid and medial brow. The corrugator, procerus, depressor supercilii, and orbicularis muscles become dominant over the brow elevator. These muscles pull the brow downward and inward.

The lateral brow descent contributes to drooping of the brow tail that may place it lower than the normal horizontal tangent that exists between the medial and lateral brow. The resultant lateral hooding can extend beyond the lateral canthus and even beyond the lateral orbital rim. Blepharoplasty surgery will not fully correct this pathologic condition, and lifting of the lateral brow becomes necessary to create an aesthetically pleasing eye.

The clinical appearance of a patient with brow ptosis can often be categorized as a "brow elevator" or as a "squinter and frowner."[6] "Brow elevators" will elevate the brow artificially as patients open their eyes, producing characteristic horizontal lines across the forehead. These horizontal lines will be ameliorated when the brows are surgically elevated. However, postoperative brow position in these patients will often appear minimally changed unless the surgeon has taken "eyes closed" preoperative photographs during which the patient is not elevating the brow. In addition, patients who elevate their brows during facial expression should be evaluated preoperatively for levator attenuation and eyelid ptosis, because these particular patients will use brow elevation as a compensatory mechanism for the eyelid ptosis. Endoscopic correction of their brow ptosis can result in worsening of the levator weakness unless it is also corrected.

"Frowners and squinters" usually have prominent vertical glabellar creases that may be present at an early age. Endoscopically, these patients often demonstrate hypertrophy of the medial depressor musculature, and the procerus, corrugator, and depressor supercilii muscles require meticulous attention. Occasionally, this muscle hypertrophy results in a clinically apparent "supraorbital wad" in the glabellar region, which will soften with muscle release and inactivation.

PREOPERATIVE PREPARATION

Preoperative assessment should include evaluation of "frame height"[7] and "brow glide."[8] Frame height is the distance from the mid pupil to the top of the brow centrally. Brow ptosis is present if this measurement is less than 2.5 cm. We also make this measurement from an imaginary line placed horizontally tangent to the mid pupil at the medial margin and tall of the brow. These measurements assist in quantifying preoperative differences in brow symmetry.

Brow glide is measured by lifting the brow and recording maximal excursion of the medial, central, and lateral portions of the brow from the neutral position. The average measurement is 1 to 2 cm. Ethnicity affects brow glide, and patients of Asian, African-American, and Mediterranean descent may have reduced measurements. Patients who demonstrate high glide indices (3 to 4 cm) will not have comparable results with patients who have lower indices.

INSTRUMENTATION

Advances in instrumentation are progressively allowing sharper anatomic imaging and more facile dissection with less tissue trauma. The endoscopic system consists of the light source, the fiberoptic light delivery system, an endoscope, and a camera with a coupling device to send an electronic signal of the imaged anatomy to a central processing unit where the signal is decoded and sent to the monitor. The 4.0-mm endoscope with a 30-degree lens is commonly used for the endoscopic brow lift. In an effort to maximize visibility and minimize instruments being placed through incision ports, a variety of retractor sheaths that fit over the endoscope and assist with dissection are available. These sheaths also support overlying soft tissue and prevent obstruction of the operating field.

In the frontal region, blind undermining can be carried out subperiosteally to the glabellar region. The head of the dissection instrument should be turned downward at a near right angle to the shaft, which should be straight or slightly curved.

The temporal dissection is best performed with a straight or slightly curved freer. Here, a straight or flared endoscope sheath is helpful.

Orbital rim dissection is facilitated by a knuckle elevator, which has a slightly curved shaft and a small, sharply downward angulating head. Orbital dissection sheaths are now available that can obviate the need for other instrumentation in this area. Because of their severe angulation, these sheaths are especially helpful in patients with high foreheads.

We prefer to use the carbon dioxide laser with a flexible, thin waveguide for release of the brow musculature and hemostasis. An insulated endoscopic bipolar suction-cautery is also used for coagulation of bleeders.

PROCEDURE

The endoscopic brow procedure can be divided into four stages. All endoscopic brow procedures use these stages, albeit in different manners. They are (1) placement of small incisions; (2) dissection of the optical cavity; (3) release of periosteum and muscles; and (4) elevation and fixation of the brow. Before the surgical aspects of the procedure, the forehead and temporal regions are infiltrated with a tumescent anesthesia, which may be obtained with a tumescent pump.

STAGE 1: PLACEMENT OF SMALL INCISIONS

The use of small incisions is a distinguishing feature of the endoscopic brow operation. These incisions are difficult for an observer to visualize, do not change the hairline or hairline pattern, and preserve the sensation to the scalp.

Four vertical incisions over the frontal bone are constructed between the hairs (Fig. 14–1). They are placed 1 cm behind the hairline and are 1 cm long. The two medial frontal incisions are placed in the vertical plane of a line drawn tangentially to each medial brow. The two lateral frontal incisions are placed in the vertical plane of a line tangential to the lateral canthus or at the juncture of thick frontal hair and temporal thinning hair

close to the temporal line. An incision is made with a knife in the scalp, extending deep to the hair bulbs. The incision is then carried down to the bone with a laser or Colorado needle.

Two curvilinear temporal incisions are then placed in the temporoparietal scalp 2 to 3 cm posterior to the hairline. The midpoint of these incisions is at the horizontal plane of the bony rim. They may be extended to 2 cm in length if the hair is reasonably thick. The incisions are beveled at an angle to preserve the hair bulbs and are carried downward to the temporoparietal fascia. The temporoparietal fascia is a bluish white–appearing layer that moves with the skin when the skin is pulled backward. The temporoparietal fascia is then incised until the gleaming silver-white deep temporal fascia is seen. The deep temporal fascia does not move when the skin is grasped and pulled.

STAGE 2: DISSECTION OF THE OPTICAL CAVITY

In the forehead no naturally occurring cavities for the placement of an endoscope are present. Consequently, an optical cavity must be created in the forehead and temporal regions. Creation of the optical cavity proceeds in three stages: (1) blind dissection over the frontal and parietal bones; (2) temporal dissection; and (3) joining the frontal and temporal dissections.

Forehead Dissection Over the Frontal and Parietal Bones

Generally, the optical cavity over the frontal bone is created blindly in the superiosteal plane until the glabellar region is reached, whereupon the dissection becomes supraperiosteal (Fig. 14–2). A short elevator, with its tip angled downward at 80 degrees, is placed into the right lateral incision, and the subperiosteal plane is gently uncovered with scraping and prying movements. By use of each of the four frontal incisions, the subperiosteal dissection is carried 2 to 3 cm posteriorly toward the occiput, inferiorly and laterally over the parietal bone, and downward toward the brow. In the central area over

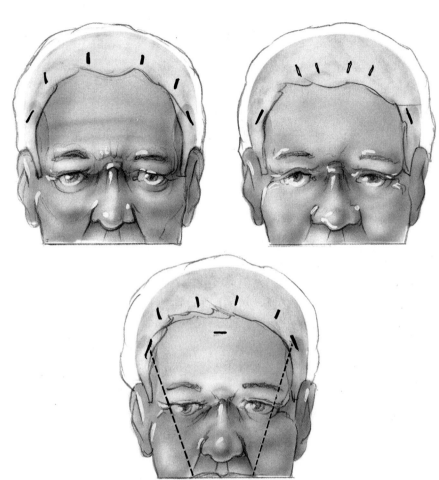

Figure 14–1. Incisions for endoscopic forehead and browlift.

the glabella, a restriction of the elevator's movement will be noted at approximately the level of the brow. This point is at the origin of the corrugator muscles. The elevation is brought superficially at this point and extended supraperiosteally over the nose. The elevator is insinu-

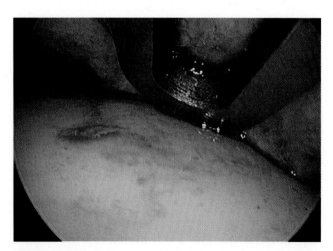

Figure 14–2. Subperiosteal dissection over frontal bone toward orbital rim.

ated between the corrugator muscles' origins with twisting motions until a "pop" is felt in the supraperiosteal plane over the glabella and nose. This supraperiosteal dissection is preferred for exposure of the medial brow depressors. This area is not blindly dissected, in part to avoid shearing off an anomalous supraorbital nerve that emerges from a foramen above the orbital rim in about 20% of the cases.

Temporal Dissection

The temporal dissection creates an optical cavity over the temporalis muscle, the zygomatic process of the frontal bone, the frontal process of the zygomatic bone, and the malar eminence. The posterior edge of the temporal incision edge is grasped and pulled upward. The elevator is then used to lift the areolar tissue (innominate fascia) from the deep temporal fascia posteriorly until bone is felt. The anterior edge of the temporal incision is then

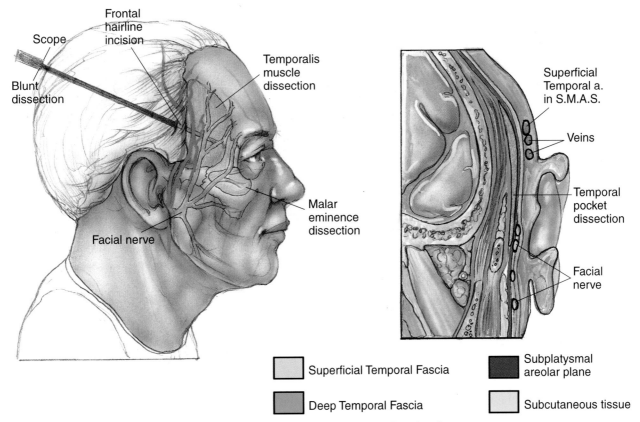

Figure 14-3. Depiction of extent of temporal pocket dissection.

grasped and pulled upward. The innominate fascia is separated from the deep temporal fascia to a point corresponding to the anterior edge of the hairline (Fig. 14–3).

The endoscope and elevator are then placed in the temporal incision and the innominate fascia is dissected and separated form the deep temporal fascia angling toward the malar eminence. Above the dissection, through a fascial layer, is the temporoparietal fat pad, which is yellow. As the dissection extends inferiorly to the level of the brow, a yellowish tinge may be seen beneath the deep temporal fascia. This represents the superficial fat pad, which sits between the superficial and deep layers of the deep temporal fascia.

At the level of the frontozygomatic suture and approximately 1 cm lateral to it, the "sentinel vein" can be seen (Figs. 14–4 and 14–5). This vein is a branch of the zygomaticotemporal vein. As this vein is followed superiorly, a branch is given off approximately 1 cm lateral to the tail of the brow. This vein is a reliable marker for the facial nerve, which is just lateral to it.

The dissection is carried medial and inferiorly to the sentinel vein in the supraperiosteal plane over the frontal process of the zygoma and the malar eminence. Another branch of the zygornaticotemporal vein, accompanied by a sensory nerve, is encountered immediately lateral to the malar eminence. Normally, identification of this second vein marks the inferiormost margin of the dissection.

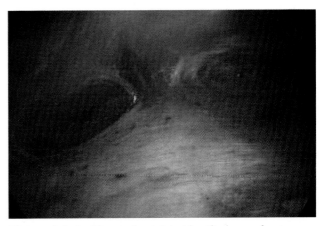

Figure 14-4. "Sentinel vein" is identified near frontozygomatic suture. Innominate fascia dissection is completed. The conjoint tendon is remaining.

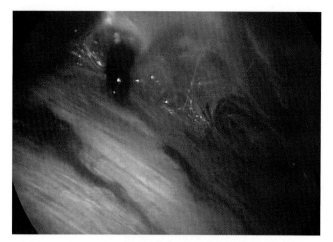

Figure 14–5. "Sentinel vein" with innominate fascia remaining inferiorly.

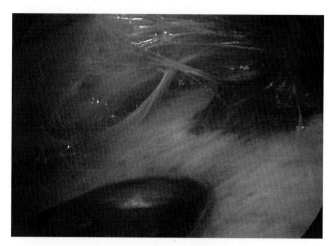

Figure 14–6. Innominate fascia dissection superior to zygomatic arch with small branch of zygomaticotemporal vein.

If the surgeon must free up the temple extensively, dissection extends laterally along the zygomatic arch, where another branch of the zygornaticotemporal vein can be identified (Fig. 14–6). By gently pushing upward with the elevator along the vein, a nerve ascending in a diagonal direction over the zygomatic arch is identified. This is the frontal branch of the facial nerve. Proceeding medial to the vein over the malar bone, the zygomaticus muscle can be identified.

The dissection over the deep temporalis fascia is developed to the frontal bone by pushing upward through the innominate fascia until the frontal bone can be palpated beneath the elevator. This dissection is relatively avascular.

Joining the Frontal and Temporal Optical Cavities

The fusion of the galea and the temporoparietal fascia is termed the "conjoint fascia." The conjoint fascia is pushed upward and the elevator is leveled onto the bone at a point approximately 7 cm above the brow. By initially elevating the periosteum at this point, the facial nerve is avoided.

The periosteum is then sharply elevated from the frontal bone at the temporal line, connecting the frontal and temporal cavities. The periosteal dissection is carried inferiorly along the temporal line until resistance to further

dissection is felt at about the level of the brow. This thickening of the periosteum is termed the *conjoint tendon*, and it often contains a communicating vein, which is cauterized with the bipolar cautery. About 1 cm lateral to this vein, a branch of the frontal nerve may be reliably identified in, or immediately beneath, the temporoparietal fat pad.

The conjoint tendon is then incised sharply over the bone with the elevator or scissors (Fig. 14–7). This maneuver connects the supraperiosteal dissection over the zygomatic process of the frontal bone with the subperiosteal dissection over the remainder of the frontal bone. An adequate release of the conjoint tendon is an essential part of the release of the tail of the brow.

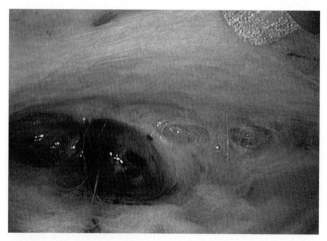

Figure 14–7. Right "sentinel vein" with suction-cautery tip in dissection pocket.

STAGE 3: RELEASE OF PERIOSTEUM AND DEPRESSOR MUSCULATURE

Failure to thoroughly release the periosteum and depressor muscles is probably the most common reason that endoscopic forehead and brow procedures fail. The tail of the brow, in particular, can only be elevated when a complete release is performed.

The release of the periosteum and depressor muscles can be reviewed in three parts: (1) periosteal release with exposure of the supraorbital nerve; (2) release of the central musculature medial to the supraorbital nerve; and (3) release of the orbicularis occuli muscle lateral to the supraorbital nerve.

Periosteal Release With Exposure of the Supraorbital Nerve

The periosteum is dissected to the orbital rim. If a dissecting sheath and a one-handed technique are used, the endoscope is placed into the lateral frontal incision. In the two-handed technique the endoscope with a visualization sheath is placed in the central frontal incision, and the dissecting instruments are placed in the lateral frontal incision. As the rim is approached in the midpupillary line, supraorbital nerves are visualized. These may all emerge from a single large foramen, or a smaller lateral branch may emerge from a foramen and the larger medial branch may exit from a prominent notch below the orbital rim (Fig. 14–8). All supraorbital branches are preserved whether they emerge from a foramen or a notch.

The periosteal dissection must be continued over the lateral orbital rim. The dissector is then used to pry the arcus marginalis upward, thus exposing roof fat. By continuing in this plane medially, the supraorbital nerves that emerge from a notch below the rim are identified.

Medial to the supraorbital nerve, the periosteum is swept under the corrugator muscle with the elevator. The corrugator is identified as it attaches to the frontal bone between the brows. In this area the subperiosteal dissection has transitioned to a supraperiosteal one and extends over the nose (Fig. 14–9). Thus the procerus muscle is already separated from the periosteum.

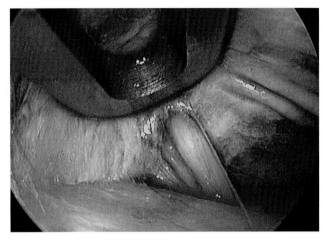

Figure 14–8. Left supraorbital nerve with subperiosteal dissection not yet completed over orbital rim lateral to nerve.

Two sets of veins can be identified at this point. The most medial veins are branches of the facial and lateral nasal veins. The more lateral veins are branches of the supraorbital and supratrochlear veins. Cauterizing these veins as they are exposed can avoid a great deal of troublesome bleeding. They can be cauterized with bipolar cautery or the flexible laser wavelength guide, because a significant amount of muscle mass is present between the veins and skin.

Release of the Central Musculature Medial to the Supraorbital Nerve

These muscles are incised. We do not remove muscle with grasping forceps to avoid resultant depressions from the absence of muscle mass. The muscle incisons may be performed either with endoscopic scissors or with a laser. If a laser with an endoscopic handpiece is available, its use will result in less patient bruising.

The procerus muscle is incised horizontally. The incision is placed low on the muscle at a point corresponding to the nasion. This avoids a retraction of a thick procerus into the nasion, which could produce blunting of the nasofrontal angle. Correspondingly, if a nasal hump or a nasofrontal angle that is too deep is present, the horizontal procerus incision may be placed high, thus allowing the muscle to retract into the nasion, blunting the angle or filling in the nasion above the nasal hump, thereby diminishing it.

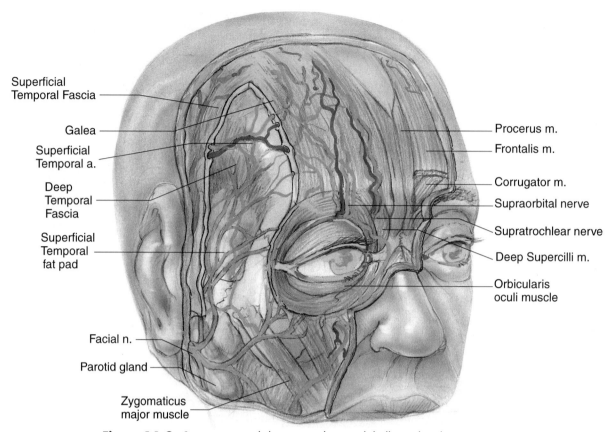

Superficial Temporal Fascia

Galea

Superficial Temporal a.

Deep Temporal Fascia

Superficial Temporal fat pad

Facial n.

Parotid gland

Zygomaticus major muscle

Procerus m.

Frontalis m.

Corrugator m.

Supraorbital nerve

Supratrochlear nerve

Deep Supercilli m.

Orbicularis oculi muscle

Figure 14–9. Supraperiosteal dissection planes: glabella and malar eminence.

The corrugator muscle is next incised. The supratrochlear nerves are identified behind the corrugator muscle and in front of the depressor supercilii muscle (Fig. 14–10). These nerves can branch in many different ways, although two distribution patterns are the most common: if the surgeon sees a prominent stalk emerging and then branching, the supratrochlear nerve is usually exiting from its own foramen or notch; if multiple branches of the supratrochlear nerve are noted, the nerve is usually emerging from the same notch as the supraorbital nerve and branches are given off in all directions. It is desirable to preserve all branches of the nerve.

The corrugator muscle is in front of the supratrochlear nerves (Fig. 14–11). Muscle that is behind the

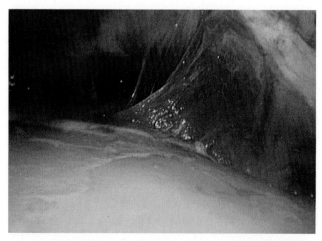

Figure 14–10. Left supercilii muscle with supratrochlear nerve fibers and thicker branch of supraorbital nerve.

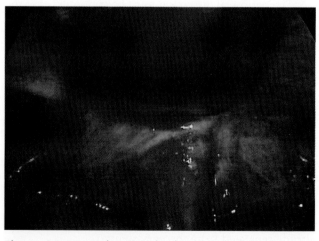

Figure 14–11. Right supraorbital nerve with bluish-appearing corrugator muscle extending medially.

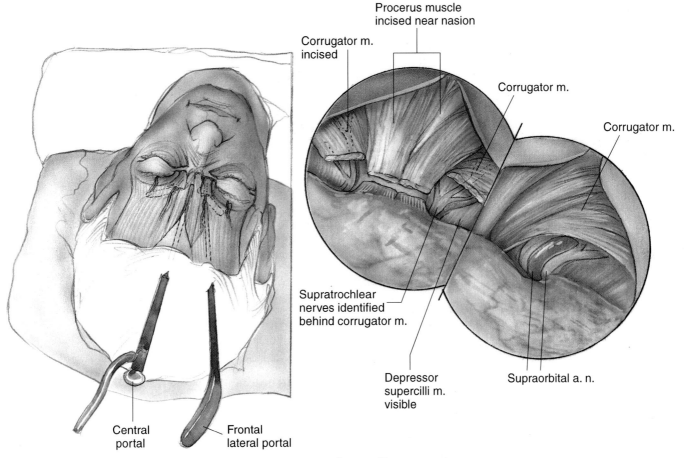

Figure 14-12. Surgical view of brow musculature.

supratrochlear nerve is depressor supercillii muscle. Muscle that is between the supratrochlear nerve and the supraorbital nerve is corrugator (Fig. 14–12). Incision and release of both of these muscles are completed medial to the supraorbital nerve and below the orbital rim. If the incision of these muscles is incomplete, "stumps" of muscle contraction may form, resulting in visible soft tissue irregularity.

If prominent glabellar rhytids are present, the musculature surrounding them is often hypertrophic, and cross-hatching must be done to weaken it. Nerve dissection is accomplished vertically through the muscle, starting superiorly. Horizontal incision of the muscles, with direct visualization of the nerves, can then be completed.

Release of the Orbicularis Muscle Lateral to the Supraorbital Nerve

At this point in the procedure, if the forehead is retracted upward from the lateral hairline, the tall of the brow will still be tethered to some degree. When the orbicularis muscle is incised, the tall of the brow will retract freely.

Lateral to the supraorbital nerve, a horizontal incision below the bony rim is made in the orbicularis. This incision is carried along the curve of the rim and becomes more vertical at the lateral aspect of the rim. At the lower portion of the rim, a horizontal incision is made onto the malar eminence. This incision completes the release of the lateral orbicularis, which can then retract upward. The release frees the tail of the brow for upward fixation.

STAGE 4: ELEVATION AND FIXATION OF THE BROW

After release of the depressor muscle and periosteum, the brows are free for fixation. Although many methods of fixation exist, we prefer screw fixation, which was originally described by Isse.

A screw is placed into the outer table of the frontal bone at a predetermined distance (usually 5 to 15 mm) from the anterior margin of the lateral frontal incision. The incision is pulled backward with a skin hook, and a staple bridging the incision is placed posterior to the screw. This secures the upward fixation.

The placement of the screw in the lateral frontal incision provides the maximum upward pull at the level of the tail of the brow. This is important because the tail of the brow is the portion of the brow that is not pulled upward by the frontalis muscle, and therefore, it requires the most support.

At the temporal incision, additional fixation is provided. The temporoparietal fascia at the anterior margin of the incision is pulled backward and is sutured to the deep temporal fascia in the posterior margin of the incision. This maneuver fixates the temporal region and lateral brow position.

Patients who have an unstable tail of the brow (older patients with an extreme brow glide) may be treated with a suspension suture placed in the brow tail. This suture is not used to elevate the brow but is useful for stabilization of a brow tail that has a high probability of descent in the postoperative period.[9] These patients are among the most difficult to achieve a satisfactory result and should be appropriately counseled before surgery.

POSTOPERATIVE COURSE

Postoperative care is straightforward. A bulky pressure dressing is removed after 24 hours, and if drains are used, they are removed at that time. The patient sleeps in a semi-Fowler's position for 72 hours and wears a headband to minimize swelling. Postoperative pain is usually minimal. Strenuous activity is restricted for 3 weeks, although patients are able to return to work in a short time.

COMPLICATIONS AND SEQUELAE

Despite better patient tolerance to endoscopic procedures, potential complications exist. Numbness, seroma, ecchymosis, suture abscess, neuropraxia of the temporal branch of the facial nerve, cautery-related burns of the skin, localized alopecia, relapse of brow ptosis, and asymmetric brows must be listed as potential problems. In addition, a learning curve to these procedures is significant and extends beyond instructional courses.

Nevertheless, endoscopic-related complications appear to be fewer and of less severity than those of larger incision procedures owing to minimal wound tension and lack of hair-bearing scalp resection. Overall results and patient satisfaction warrant that the aesthetic surgeon be familiar with the techniques.

CONCLUSION

The endoscopic browlift has replaced standard coronal and pretrichial techniques in our practices. We believe that endoscopic techniques allow us to aesthetically modify brow and forehead anatomy without disproportionately changing facial anatomic relationships. The 10x magnification provided by the endoscope creates unsurpassed ability to precisely alter brow and forehead musculature. Improvement of endoscopic instrumentation has facilitated dissection and accessability of difficult-to-reach areas.

PEARLS

- Patients who elevate their brows during facial expression should be evaluated preoperatively for levator attenuation and eyelid ptosis because these patients will use brow elevation as a compensatory mechanism for the eyelid ptosis.
- The use of small incisions in the endoscopic browlift, which are not noticeable, do not change the hairline or hairline pattern, and preserve sensation to the scalp, distinguishes this procedure from other methods of browlift.
- The sentinel vein is a reliable marker for the facial nerve, which lies just lateral to it.
- Failure to thoroughly release the periosteum and depressor muscles is probably the most common reason that endoscopic forehead and browlifts fail.

REFERENCES

1. Keller GS. Endolaser excision of glabellar frown lines and forehead rhytids. American Academy of Facial Plastic Surgery and Reconstructive Surgery, February 1, 1992; Los Angeles, CA.
2. Gore GB, Vasconez LO, Askren C, Yamamoto Y, Gamboa M. Coronal face-lift with endoscopic techniques. *Plast Surg Forum* 1992; XV227–228.
3. Keller GS, Razum N, et al. Small incision laser lift for forehead creases and glabellar furrows. *Arch Otolaryngol Head Neck Surg.* 1993; 119:632–635.
4. Isse NG. Endoscopic facial rejuvenation: Endoforehead, the functional lift. *Aesth Plast Surg.* 1994; 18:2.
5. Ramirez OM. Endoscopic options in facial rejuvenation: An overview. *Aesth Plast Surg.* 1994; 18:141–147.
6. Ellis DA, Masai H. The effect of facial animation on the aging upper half of the face. *Arch Otolaryngol Head Neck Surg.* 1989; 1155:710–713.
7. McKinney P, Mossie RD, Zubrows ML. Criteria for the forehead lift. *Aesth Plast Surg.* 1991; 15:141.
8. Sasaki G. Brow ptosis. In Sasaki G, ed. *Endoscopic, Aesthetic, and Reconstructive Surgery.* Philadelphia: Lippincott-Raven Publishers; 1996; 19–28.
9. Keller, GS, Hutcherson RW. Endoscopic forehead and brow lift. In Keller GS, ed. *Endoscopic Facial Plastic Surgery.* St. Louis: Mosby; 1997: 46–70.

Blepharoplasty

The chapters on blepharoplasty have been written by preeminent leaders in their field with thousands of surgeries of case experience. The chapter by Dr. Perkins, a prominent facial plastic surgeon, describes an excellent approach to blepharoplasty that uses skin and skin muscle flap techniques.

He carefully uses the technique with meticulous attention to detail and description of exact surgical landmarks and measurements.

The second portion of the chapter, written by Drs. Putterman and Millman, brings an oculoplastic viewpoint with their "bread-and-butter" technique of blepharoplasty. This chapter emphasizes the use of a retractor-based blepharoplasty technique that uses levator aponeurosis isolation in the upper lid and lower lid retraction or capsulopalpebral fascia manipulation and lateral tendon surgery as common component of blepharoplasty. The deeper functional structures are naturally integrated into the blepharoplasty technique for a slightly more complicated technique, with the advantage of slightly increased control over many factors of both functional and aesthetic goals.

Both authors address the incorporation of new technologies, specifically laser-assisted technology, in blepharoplasty and the common use of skin resurfacing. Dr. Millman presents his technique for an all laser-based blepharoplasty with CO_2, erbium: YAG, and combined erbium/CO_2 technologies to complement surgical technique.

Blepharoplasty

Aesthetic Facial Plastic Surgery, edited by Thomas Romo, III, and Arthur L. Millman, Thieme Medical Publishers, Inc., New York, New York, Copyright © 2000.

CHAPTER 15

An Oculoplastic Surgeon's Perspective

ALLEN M. PUTTERMAN AND ARTHUR L. MILLMAN

Blepharoplasty is the definition and anatomic substrate that defines the "youthful form" that cosmetic surgeons must attain aesthetically and artistically. The technique of blepharoplasty, or the aesthetic rejuvenation of the eyelids, is centuries old. Historically, whether by mechanical clamping and pinching of the skin[1] or modern-day laser resection and resurfacing of the skin, it has always involved an attempt at rejuvenating the eyelids, with the goal of restoring the eyelid and periorbital area to a more youthful form. That goal is then mated with a surgical technique that will yield the most consistent and safe result while maintaining or improving form and function of the eyelid anatomy. In blepharoplasty, today more than ever, the facial surgeon must consider not only the anatomy of the eyelids but also the anatomy of the periorbita, forehead, and midface in totality to determine the best direction of aesthetic rejuvenation.

PATIENT SELECTION

Patients presenting for blepharoplasty fall into two groups, which are mainly defined by age and the corresponding anatomic involutional changes. The first group consists of patients who are usually less than 40 years old, some as young as their teens, whose main concern is herniated orbital fat of the lower lid. Little cheek or midface descent is present at this time and the lower lid rejuvenation generally involves contouring the herniated orbital fat or baggy lower lid. The two methods described in this chapter address two basic methods to improve lower lid and midface function in the younger patient.

The first method is the most classic: excision of herniated orbital fat, which is described as a transconjunctival technique[2-4] and necessitates no disturbance of the anterior myocutaneous lamella. The carbon dioxide laser–based technique described in the following is state of the art and has the lowest possible morbidity rate.

Adjuncts to blepharoplasty include a significant evolution of thought originally described by Hamra,[5] in which, rather than excising orbital fat, herniated orbital fat is prolapsed redraped over the orbital rim, and fixated to a cheek or subperiosteal flap. This technique, which is sometimes done in combination with cheek and midface lift, is a progression toward the concept that a fullness of the midface and its continuity to the lower lid is desirable. More importantly, the long-term effect of blepharoplasty conventionally has been the removal of fat pads, which is, ironically, the last effect of the involutional changes of the eyelid or the senescent atrophy of orbital fat in the elderly.

Thus preservation of the fat pads must be considered if the orbital rim and its flow to the midface must be contoured (also see Chapter 16) and if any midface descent is present.

In patients in their upper 40s, usually a small element of dermatochalasia is present in the upper lids that is involutional and usually a hereditary-based brow position is present. A decision must be made whether the cause of a lower brow position is a "full" upper lid, in which case endoscopic brow elevation should be used, or true dermatochalasia or excess of the upper lid skin, in which case conventional upper lid blepharoplasty or excision of upper lid skin would be most useful. Nasal and central herniated orbital fat usually must be contoured as needed, depending on fullness of the medial fossa and supratrochlear area.

In the second group of patients, those who are older than 40 years of age, decision making depends more on evaluation of the full face to determine the requirements for rejuvenation of the periorbital area. As with the previous patient group, in this group we start with lower periorbital rejuvenation. In this area, lower lid laxity, lower lid position vertically to the globe, exclusion of pre-existing thyroid disease, and anatomic physiologic abnormalities are critical. In addition, careful evaluation of the midface and cheek is necessary to determine whether blepharoplasty should be limited to the eyelid or should extend to the midface. The "teardrop" deformity, which occurs at a later age, usually in the 40s and 50s, and is caused by descent of the malar fat pad, exposes the inferior orbital rim and creates a demarcation between midface and eyelid. It is critical that the surgeon determine whether conventional blepharoplasty with removal of herniated orbital fat will create a deep lower sulcus and accentuate teardrop cheek deformity. This determination divides patients into two groups: those who are amenable to simple fat excision and those who should be considered for fat pad advancement over the orbital rim in combination with midface and cheeklift.[5] In the upper lid and periorbita, the complex relationship between the forehead, brow, and eyelid must be defined and an assessment of dermatochalasia alone versus dermatochalasia with brow ptosis and the patient's aesthetic goals regarding forehead rejuvenation must be discussed.

Very general rules of thumb regarding anatomic landmarks include: the eyelid crease should be approximately 8 to 10 mm above the eyelid lash line, and the brow should be at the orbital rim centrally and above the orbital rim temporally with an aesthetic arch, and it should measure a minimum of 10 mm superior to the upper lid crease. If brow ptosis is present, it must be addressed to obtain satisfactory upper lid blepharoplasty results in this age group, and whether the technique involves internal brow suspension, endoscopic, or coronal technique, it is important that it is done either before or simultaneously with blepharoplasty.

In conclusion, any surgical result can only be successful with an accurate and focused evaluation of the underlying anatomy and its relation to the cause and effect of aesthetic surgical goals. Proper evaluation and an expertly executed surgical plan with successful blepharoplasty will yield tremendous satisfaction to patient and surgeon alike.

LASER BLEPHAROPLASTY

Laser blepharoplasty is intimately connected with the conventional surgical blepharoplasty technique presented in Chapter 18, and, its success relies on the depth of experience the surgeon has with these techniques. I will separate the quad or four-lid surgical technique into the upper and lower lids. All of the cosmetic lid and facial techniques included in this volume can be incorporated and frequently aided by carbon dioxide (CO_2) laser–assisted technique. Modifying previous techniques is a challenge to the surgeon, but well worth it. Since 1995 laser-assisted procedures have become a routine and successful part of our aesthetic facial surgical technique. We have found significant reduction of postoperative morbidity, with patients returning to work in as little as 4 to 5 days, and a distinct reduction of edema and ecchymosis. No serious additional complications have occurred.

LASER SURGICAL SETUP

To ensure laser efficacy and safety during oculoplastic surgery with the CO_2 laser, a number of special instruments and precautions in the setup of the surgical field are required. These include the use of protective eye wear for all members of the surgical team. Contact lenses or eye shields, preferably made of metallic surgical steel, are

necessary for the patient. The internal surface of the steel contact lenses should be smooth and the external surface sandblasted for antireflective properties. Topical tetracaine and ophthalmic ointment are usually used on the inner surface of the shield for patient comfort. All surgical personnel should wear wavelength-appropriate eye wear, including eye goggles, surgical loupes, or simple eyeglasses. Sandblasting the surface of all metallic instruments used in the surgical procedure is recommended. Desmarre retractors and any broad metallic surfaces should be sandblasted. This antireflective status will prevent the inadvertent reflection of the CO_2 laser beam in unwanted areas or tissue.

The surgical field should include wet towels and dressings that are soaked in sterile water or saline to surround the face or surgical area (Fig. 15–1). (Some surgeons use aluminum foil, although we find it cumbersome and do not recommend it.) A smoke or laser plume evacuator is mandatory (Fig. 15–2). Improper laser plume evacuation will result in chronic pharyngitis for the surgeon. Furthermore, biologic and viral particles have been recovered in and are transmissible by the laser plume. Standard operating room suction will not suffice. If general anesthesia is being administered, anesthetics should be nonflammable and endotracheal tubes must be

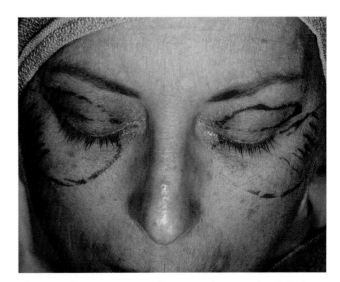

Figure 15–1. Damp towels surround patient for CO_2 laser blepharoplasty. Upper lid skin excision and lower lid area for laser CSR is marked.

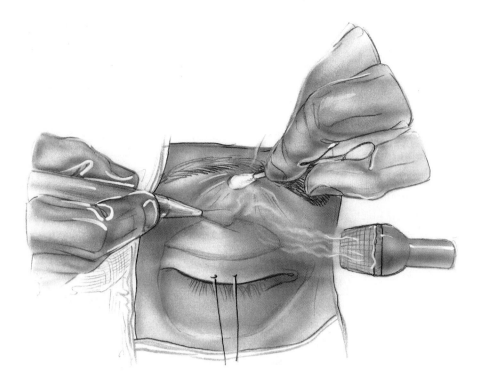

Figure 15–2. Laser handpiece and plume evacuator.

wavelength appropriate and have a metallic or antireflective coating. A large basin of water should be within or near the surgical field for lavage should a fire start and a UL-approved fire extinguisher should be present in the surgical suite.

THE CO$_2$ SURGICAL LASER

A number of CO$_2$ lasers are available for plastic surgery. The technology and equipment available for this modality change rapidly and frequently. We have extensive experience with the Coherent Ultrapulse, the Luxar Novapulse, and Sharplans Silk Touch, and Feather Touch system. Although new instruments and companies are continually entering the market, instrumentation is basically divided into two groups. The first group includes lasers that are superpulse lasers, which are defined as lasers used for incisional and resurfacing surgery and are capable of delivering CO$_2$ laser energy in very short ($<1/500$ μs) bursts, so as to maximize tissue ablation and minimize thermal damage or heat capacitance within the tissue to be treated. The second group of lasers (i.e., Sharplans Silk Touch and Feather Touch) are continuous wave lasers, which are defined as lasers that deliver

energy in a continuous mode and are frequently introduced to the skin's surface by means of a mechanical mirror-reflecting system that moves the laser energy spot in a spill or dot matrix pattern to perform resurfacing as a stationary spot for incisional surgery. Use of the superpulse laser for some incisional and all resurfacing surgery is ideal and recommended. The user should understand the basic laser physics principles that guide laser setting in the practice of laser surgery.[12]

For incisional surgery a small spot size will deliver a more precise cutting incision width and more power per unit area. Fluence, however, will have decreased thermal or hemostatic effect. In general, a 0.2- to 0.4-mm spot size is ideal for cutting at 7 to 8 mm watts of power in a standard continuous wave mode. The surgeon can accurately modify the amount of energy delivery by focusing and defocusing the laser spot, which is done by positioning the laser handpiece. Laser energy is delivered at a maximum energy level at the exact focal point of the given laser. (The working distance, or focal point, of each unit is determined by the manufacturer and the given model and is usually delineated by a footplate attached to the handpiece that reminds the surgeon of the working distance, which usually measures approximately 1 to 1.5 inches in the Coherent and Sharplans models. The exception is the Luxar Novapulse unit, which works on a hollow fiber delivery system and in a near contact mode; its focal point is simply adjacent by 2 to 3 mm to the tip of the laser handpiece.) By working at the exact focal point or working distance of the given laser, the surgeon can deliver maximum energy and maximum vaporization or cutting with a minimum of thermal or peripheral damage to the surgical tissue. Conversely, the surgeon can defocus by withdrawing or increasing the distance of the handpiece to the tissue, thus decreasing power delivered, which decreases the ability to cut and maximizes the thermal or coagulative ability of the laser (Fig. 15–3). This is useful for hemostasis and for contouring or ablating tissue.

Cutting can also be done in a superpulse mode (i.e., Novapulse and Coherent Ultrapulse), with laser delivery set at 25 µs and 30 Hz program settings with power levels of 7 to 8 watts. This ultrapulse cutting mode increases the depth of the incision by approximately 1 to 20% and, most importantly, decreases the charring or thermal component by 20 to 30%. Histopathologic evaluation of continuous-wave and superpulse cutting modes has demonstrated that the zone of necrosis (the area of peripheral damage surrounding the actual incision) is reduced by almost 30% in the superpulse mode, which provides a cleaner incision with significant reduction of postoperative inflammation, scarring, and contracture of tissue. Histopathologic samples show an average peripheral zone of necrosis of 130 µm at 7 watts of continuous wave energy as opposed to a peripheral zone of necrosis of 100 µm in the superpulse mode at the same 7-watt power level.[12]

SURGICAL TECHNIQUE
LASER QUAD BLEPHAROPLASTY
Upper Lid Laser Blepharoplasty

The upper lid blepharoplasty is begun with surgical prepping and draping; saline-soaked cloth towels are placed around the patient's face and the surgical field to help prevent fire damage. Also required are smoke evacuators and carefully manufactured surgical instruments whose surfaces have been sandblasted to eliminate reflective surfaces from the surgical field. Specific instruments, including the David-Baker clamp for lid stabilization, can be used at the surgeon's preference. Anesthetics should be nonflammable, and if endotracheal tubes are used, they should be wavelength appropriate.

The technique begins with identification of an upper lid crease, usually found 8 to 10 mm above the lid margin, which is marked and brought out to the lateral canthus with a slight upward angulation. A pinch technique can be used to judge excess upper lid skin, which is generally between 10 and 20 mm, until slight lash and lid margin eversion is noted. This is then marked nasally, centrally, and temporally, and the redundant skin ellipse is marked continuous (Fig. 15–4). The length of the upper skin resection line and its relation to the upper brow and the upper side and symmetry should then be evaluated. In general, a minimum of 10 to 15 mm from

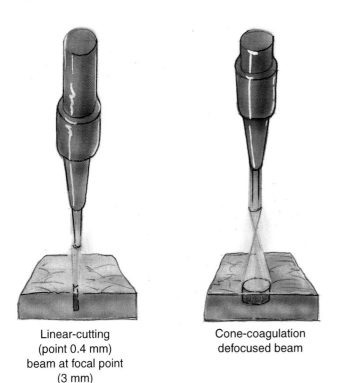

Linear-cutting
(point 0.4 mm)
beam at focal point
(3 mm)

Cone-coagulation
defocused beam

Figure 15–3. Laser handpiece illustration demonstrates focusing (cutting) and defocusing (coagulation).

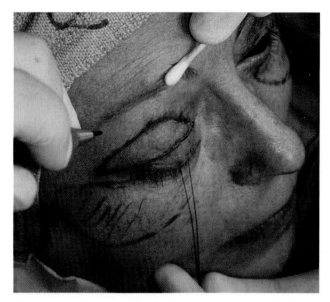

Figure 15–4. See text for details.

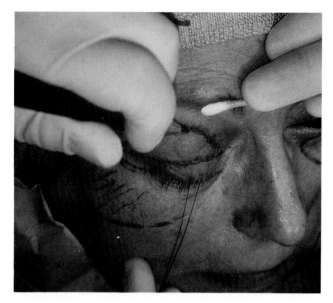

Figure 15–5. See text for details.

the upper brow must be maintained to allow for proper lid excursion and closure.

At this point infiltration of a 2% lidocaine and 1:200,000 epinephrine dilution, with or without Wydase, is delivered as a supraorbital-frontal retrobulbar nerve block. Five to ten minutes is allotted to allow for maximum chemical tourniquet. The laser is then set on continuous wave with a 0.2- to 0.4-mm spot and approximately 7 to 8 watts of power. A *careful tempo* is necessary; the incision should not be rushed. Marking the incision too rapidly results in only superficial cutting. An overly slow progression of incision prevents significant depth of cutting and buildup of thermal capacitance and may cause charring and scarring. Cutting can also be done in a superpulsed mode, with the laser set at 25 ms and 30 Hz with power levels of 7 to 10 watts. This increases the depth of incision and significantly decreases charring or thermal component. However, there can be some decrease in hemostasis. At the proper lid rate, the incision is first made along the upper lid crease, and then along the superior aspect of the resection line. In general, the assistant should allow for a taut upper lid and tension on all skin wounds to allow for separation. Use of 4–0 silk traction sutures is recommended. With the upper lid skin incision complete, dissection is begun from the lateral aspect of the wound, where in a slightly defocused

mode the handpiece is used to elevate the skin flap. Either a skin-only flap can be elevated (Fig. 15–5) or a skin-muscle flap can be elevated in an en bloc method. When a skin muscle flap is created, a general hemostasis is automatic because the laser seals all blood vessels as it goes. If a breakthrough bleeding vessel is noted, the handpiece should be slightly withdrawn and "defocused" to allow for instant cauterization of all vessels. Again, a proper tempo is necessary to avoid charring and increased thermal ablation and contracture of tissue. With the skin flap elevated as the dissection is brought to the medial canthus, care should be taken to avoid inadvertent burn when severing the skin flap. The medial canthus is frequently protected with a moist gauze pad.

At this point an incision is made either through the remaining orbicularis or, in the case of the skin muscle flap, through the remaining orbital septum to prolapse both nasal and septal orbital fat pads. The central pad is approached first. An incision is made and the fat pad prolapsed. A combination of direct cutting or defocused coagulation of the orbital fat pad can be used. The lack of clamps and minimum manipulation of the fat pad necessary with the laser handpiece allows for increased patient comfort, and gentle retropulsion of the globe allows for easy prolapse of the orbital fat pads and laser ablation. (The Luxar Novapulse with 0.4-mm cutting tip is

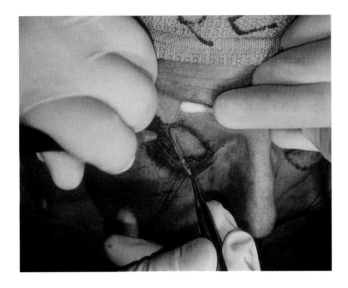
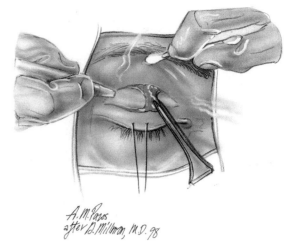

A. M. Pazos
after D. Millman, M.D. 98

Figure 15-6. See text for details.

demonstrated in all photos in this section.) The nasal fat pad has a more whitish color than the yellowish appearance of the central fat pad and can be easily differentiated (Figs. 15–6 and 15–7). A Demarre retractor with a sandblasted surface is used for retraction of the septum and for easy exposure of the fat pads. With the fat pads ablated the skin can either be closed directly with a 6–0 nylon suture and a more advanced technique (e.g., supratarsal levator fixation) can be used for eyelid crease reconstruction.

Supratarsal levator fixation for eyelid crease reconstruction, is the recommended method. This is modified for laser technique by used a defocused beam along the supratarsal orbicularis to allow for levator aponeurosis-orbicularis "fusion contraction" of this tissue (Figs. 15–8 and 15–9). The leading edge of the levator aponeurosis is identified (Fig. 15–8) and formed into a sharp continuous edge with 6–0 nylon sutures to the levator aponeurosis (Fig. 15–10). The leading edge is attached to the pretarsal orbicularis and skin surface approximately four or five positions nasally, centrally, and temporally (Fig. 15–9). The patient is instructed to look in upgaze to confirm lid crease formation. Nylon closure (6–0) is completed as before.

If it is necessary to perform ptosis surgery in conjunction with blepharoplasty to normalize lid levels, the levator can be advanced at this point in the procedure and fixated nasally, centrally, and temporally with either permanent Mersilene suturing or temporary Vicryl sutur-

ing. If a posterior "tarsoconjunctival resection" ptosis Mueller muscle (Fasanella or Putterman) technique is planned, it should be done before skin blepharoplasty incision of the upper lid to prevent full-thickness lid injury. With the upper lid now closed, attention can be directed to the lower lid blepharoplasty.

Lower Lid Transconjunctival CO_2 Laser Blepharoplasty

The basic anatomy and technique are similar to that of conventional transconjunctival blepharoplasty as described in Chapter 20. However, certain laser techniques allow for greater ease and decreased morbidity and recuperative time. Gentle retropulsion on the contact lens allows for prolapse of the inferior fornix, and a temporal-to-nasal direction incision is made at the midfornix approximately 5 mm below the inferior tarsal border. A 4–0 silk suture is used to retract the lower lid (Fig. 15–11). Again, a *proper tempo* for depth of incision must be used so that the conjunctiva and lower lid retractor or capsulopalpebral fascia are incised in one pass. The same 0.2- to 0.4-mm spot at 7 to 8 watts, either in continuous wave or superpulse mode, is used.

At this point, a toothed forceps is used to further separate the tissue and a sandblasted Desmarre retractor is used to retract the lower lid inferiorly. A 4-0 silk suture is passed through the lid retractor flap, and the flap is

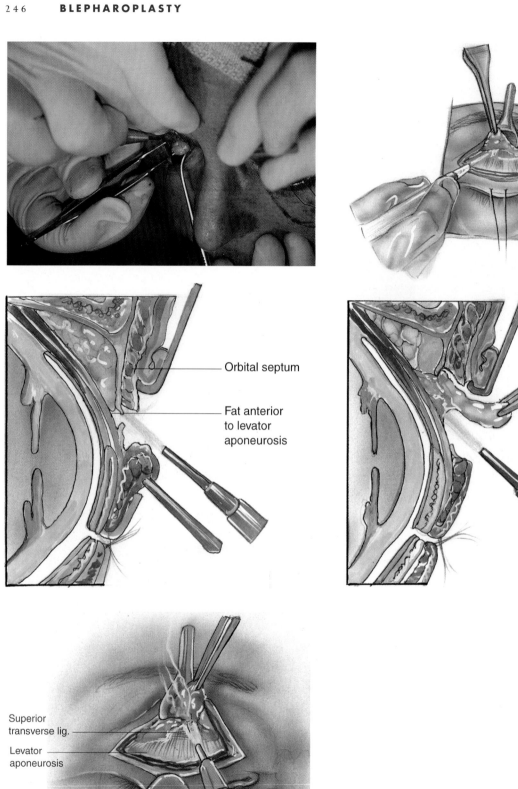

Orbital septum

Fat anterior
to levator
aponeurosis

Superior
transverse lig.

Levator
aponeurosis

Figure 15-7. See text for details.

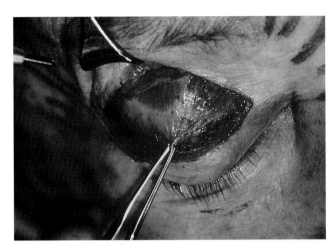

Figure 15–8. See text for details.

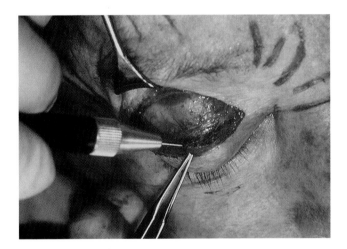

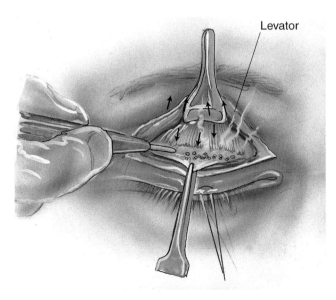

Figure 15–9. See text for details.

retracted superiorly. This exposes the orbital septum, which is incised with the laser handpiece, and the temporal fat pad is exposed first with intermittent gentle retropulsion of the contact lens and globe (Fig. 15–12). The fat pad is then incised and removed. It is amputated to the base of the fat pad by a laser incision with a focused beam. With removal of the fat pad and simultaneous coagulation of all vessels and maintenance of hemostasis, a defocused handpiece is used for any additional coagulation necessary and for vaporizing the remnants or contouring the shape of the fat pad to the orbital rim. The fat pad can actually be beautifully sculpted and shaped by the laser, so that a natural and aesthetically acceptable contour from the cheek, orbital rim, and eyelid can be established.

It is important to note that the least movement of the laser cutting beam should be used for safety and inadvertent laser delivery. Therefore the fat pad is moved to and free of a stationary laser cutting tip (Figs. 15–11 and 15–12). With movement of the fat pad back and forth across the laser beam, it is then carefully coagulated, incised, and removed simultaneously. Further contouring of the nasal fat pad can be used with direct application of the laser in a defocused mode to vaporize the fat pad until a smooth continuity from the orbital rim to the lid margin can be achieved. With the lid reapposed at various points during fat excision the surgeon ascertains the proper amount of fat pad removal and lid contouring and sculpting.

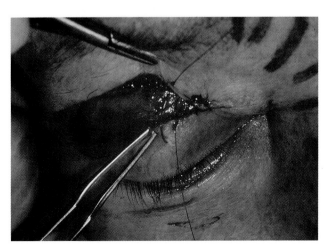

Figure 15–10. See text for details.

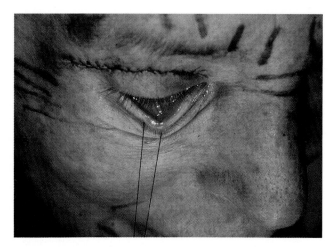

Figure 15–11. See text for details.

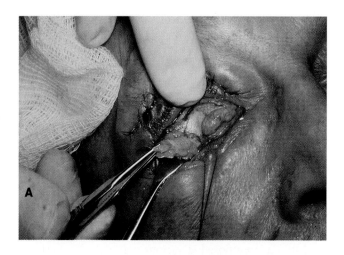

A

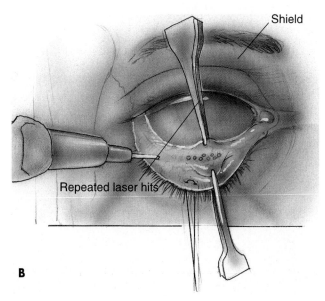

Shield

Repeated laser hits

B

Figure 15–12 See text for details.

With the temporal fat pad removed, attention is directed to the central pad. At this point, the *inferior oblique* muscle will come into view nasal to the central pad and separating the nasal and central orbital fat pads (Fig. 15–14B). The central septum is incised and retropulsion is used to prolapse the fat pad. Central and temporal pads are yellowish in color and the nasal pad is a more whitish color because of its fibrovascular histologic character. The surgeon should take care to protect the inferior oblique, which should always be identified. The surgeon uses moistened Q-tips or Demarre retraction of the oblique muscle, and then incises the nasal fat pad, keeping the laser cutting tip stationary and moving the fat pad back and forth. Figure 15–15 demonstrates completion of all herniated orbital fat pads.

At this point attention is directed to the nasal fat pad, which is prolapsed with gentle retropulsion on the globe. Care is taken to retract the inferior oblique temporally to protect inadvertent damage to the muscle. The nasal pad is prolapsed and incised in a similar manner. It should be noted that the nasal pad in both the upper and lower lids has specific large-caliber blood vessels. These can be coagulated and contracted with a defocused laser handpiece in advance of cutting. The nasal fat pads are then removed directly in the same manner described, completing lower fat pad excision. The conjunctiva and lid retractor can be apposed with a 5–0 plain suture or allowed to heal spontaneously. The lid is then reposited and attention directed

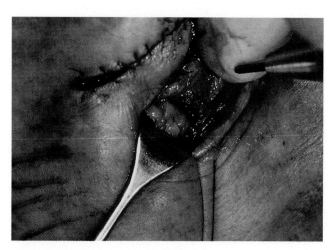

Figure 15–13. See text for details.

to the amount of lid laxity at this point. If a positive "snap" test is noted, attention should be directed to ectropion and lateral canthal tendon suspension[6–9] or horizontal shortening of the lower lid to prevent ectropion. This can be accomplished with a 4–0 prolene suture to the lateral tarsal strip or tendon attached to the lateral orbital rim and periosteum nasal and posterior to the rim to allow for normal positioning of the lower and lateral canthus.

An integrated lower lid transconjunctival blepharoplasty and simultaneous septomyocutaneous flap can be used to eliminate large amounts of excess lower lid skin and laxity. This technique takes advantage of the already dissected transconjunctival-developed postseptal plane. A lateral canthal crease incision is made with the laser, and the postseptal cavity (now free of orbital fat) is easily entered (Fig. 15–16A,B). The septomyocutaneous advancement flap technique[10] simultaneously complements transconjunctival blepharoplasty for excision of herniated orbital fat and directly addresses skin laxity and orbicularis defects. It also provides access for correcting lateral tarsoligamentous laxity in selected patients. Anatomic defects of the anterior lamella, posterior lamella, and lateral canthal angle are managed on the basis of a thorough preoperative evaluation, thus allowing lower eyelid blepharoplasty to be performed safely with an emphasis on functional restoration and preservation of lower eyelid function of almost any patient.

Transconjunctival lower lid blepharoplasty[2] allows removal of herniated orbital fat without violating the anterior skin-muscle lamella. It does not improve folds, redundancy, poor lateral canthal tendon support, or hypertrophic orbicularis muscle. It also does not significantly alter the appearance of fine or deep wrinkles in the lower lid region. Skin and skin-muscle flap blepharoplasty techniques improve these problems but do not address the lateral canthal angle and predispose to anterior lamella cicatrization, lid retraction, lagophthalmos, and ectropion. When carefully assessed, clinically intermittent ectropion and lower lid laxity are common in patients older than 50 and should be properly addressed during primary blepharoplasty. Patients of this age are at increased risk for cosmetic and functional complications if these defects remain uncorrected during the procedure. Developing an en bloc septomyocutaneous flap, with wide undermining of the postseptal plane, combined with lateral flap rotation and resection of skin and muscle of the lateral lid successfully addresses the anterior lamellar defects. The technique also affords direct access to the lateral canthus region so that any necessary lid tightening procedures can be performed.

In patients with skin laxity or orbicularis hypertrophy, as is commonly encountered after the fifth decade of life, a lateral canthal infraciliary incision, which typically includes the lateral third of the lid and extends to

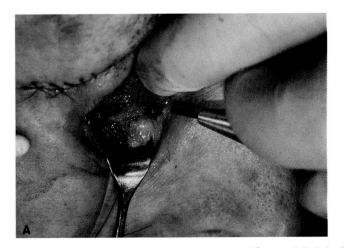
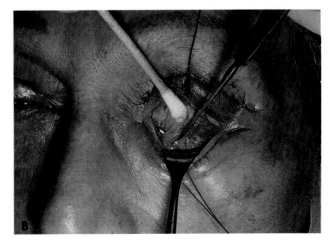

Figure 15–14. See text for details.

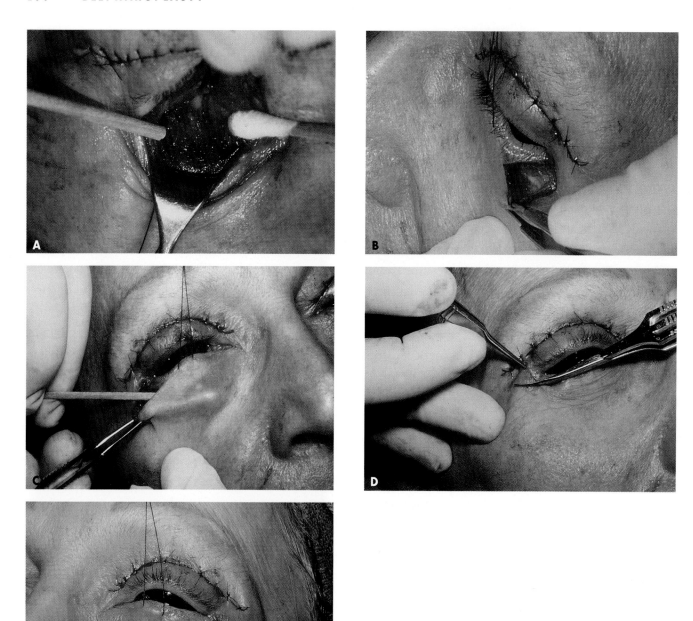

Figure 15–15. (A) Fully removed lower lid nasal, central, and temporal fat pads. Inferior oblique shown. **(B)** Lateral canthal crease incision after transconjunctival blepharoplasty to create a "septomyocutaneous flap." **(C)** Creation of a septomyocutaneous flap. **(D)** PostLateral skin excision. **(E)** Fully contoured lower lid.

the orbital rim, is made. A septomyocutaneous flap is developed en bloc along a postseptal plane past the orbital bony margin and across the horizontal length of the lid (Fig. 15–16A). This flap takes advantage of the plane already created by the transconjunctival lower lid retractor dissection (Fig. 15–16B). To aid in resuspen-

sion of the lower lid structures, the flap, which includes skin, orbicularis muscle, and orbital septum, is advanced full thickness to skin and deeper tissues before closure (Fig. 15–16). In this fashion, the skin-muscle flap is redraped superiorly and laterally, and excess tissue is then excised in two triangles (Fig. 15–16A). The septal-

Extent of septal-myocutaneous flap

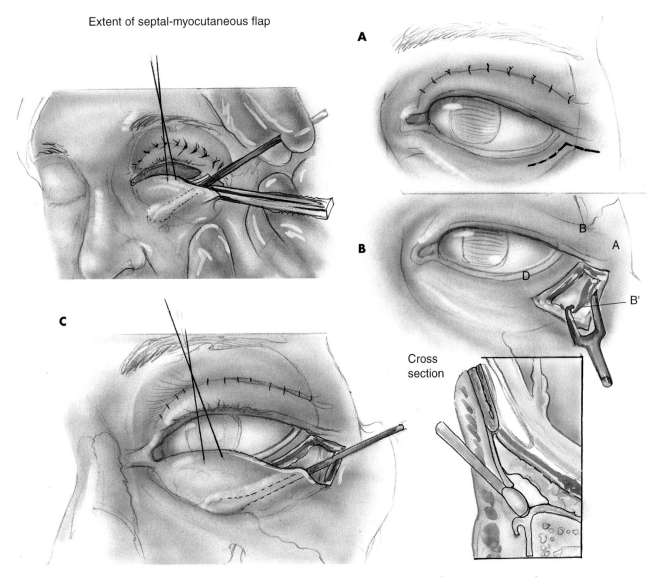

Figure 15–16. (A-H) The septomyocutaneuos flap procedure demonstrated. *(Figure continued on next page)*

orbicularis to fascial plane is resuspended to the lateral canthus by 6–0 Vicryl sutures (Fig. 15–16C). The skin is closed with a series of interrupted 6–0 nylon sutures (Fig. 15–16D). The whole anterior septal-orbicularis-cutaneous plane is then rotated laterally and superiorly and suspended (Fig. 15–16E,F). This is ideal for patients older than 55 to 60 years of age with maximal skin and lid laxity.

Lower blepharoplasty also can be used in combination, and done simultaneously with laser skin resurfacing.[12]

EYELID RESURFACING

Incisional blepharoplasty should always be completed before resurfacing. Proper laser safety must be used at all times, including the previously dictated methods of wet surgical packs surrounding all surgical laser fields. Proper caution and protection to the eye with a contact lens is imperative. The eyelid area can be broken down into anatomic regions corresponding to pretarsal, preseptal, and orbital orbicularis regions.

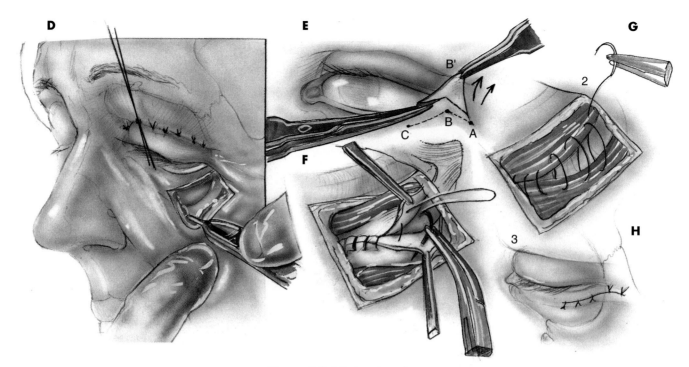

Figure 15–16 *(continued)*

Each of the skin surfaces associated with these regions varies in thickness, with skin in the pretarsal region being the thinnest, increasing to the orbital region and the cheek. It is rare to use more than two passes, and the inexperienced surgeon is advised to begin with slower repetition programs and lower laser power settings. In the periorbital and orbital regions and adnexal areas, including the cheek, lateral canthus, and temple, deeper penetration can be used. The medial third, or peripunctal area, should be avoided to prevent punctal ectropion. Advanced techniques include pretreatment of specific wrinkles, scars, or acne pits, and treatment of the "shoulders" of deep kinetic and static wrinkles. Ideally, the shoulders are treated first (Fig. 15–17A), with removal of ablated debris, and then uniform passes over the entire area are done in layers to resurface. After each pass of laser resurfacing, the skin should be kept taut for homogeneous application of the laser so that the pattern is

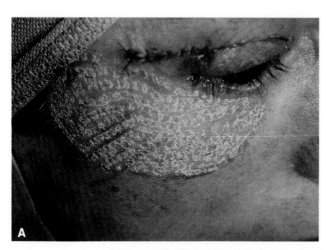

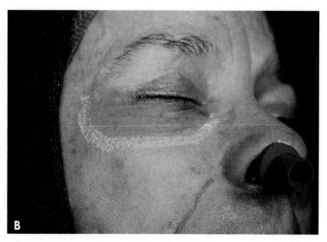

Figure 15–17 (A,B) Lower lid laser CSR with peripheral area of "feathering" to cheek.

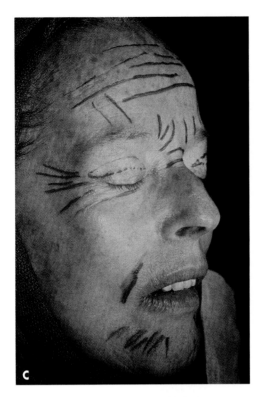 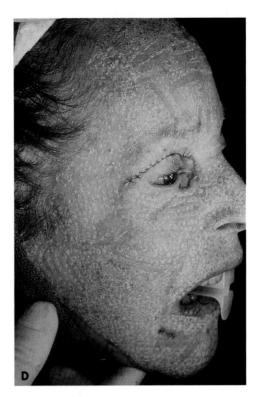

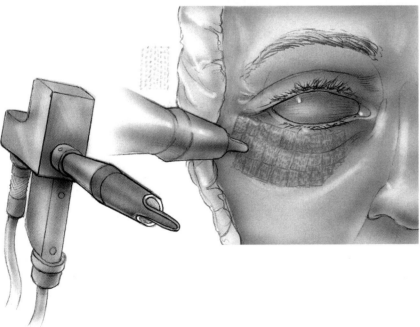

Figure 15–17. *(continued)* **(C)** Forehead and face marked for focal, deep wrinkle ablation. **(D)** The forehead shows areas treated focally surrounded by broad confluent laser passes.

reproducible in each patient. We call this the "2 and half" technique: Previously identified areas of deep rhytids, creases, or scars are treated focally as the first "half" pass and then two broad confluent passes are made over the entire area to be treated. Figure 15–18 shows where deep forehead horizontal rhytids have been focally treated, followed by two additional broad confluent passes. It should be noted that overlap of each burn should be avoided

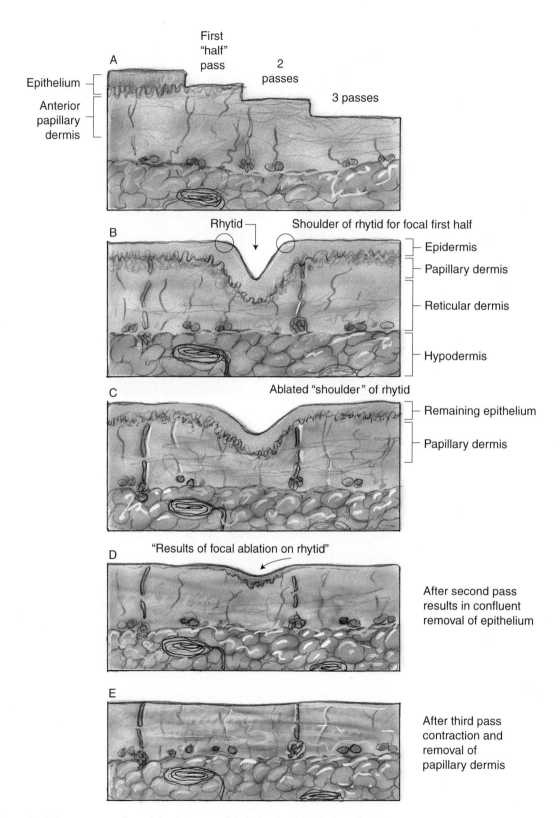

Figure 15–18. (A) First, second, and third passes of the CO_2 laser. **(B)** Shoulder of rhytid for focal first half. **(C)** Ablated shoulder of the rhytid. **(D)** Result of focal ablation on rhytid. Epithelium is removed after second pass. **(E)** After third pass, papillary dermis is contracted and removed.

because any overlap of superpulsed lasing results in significant uncontrolled application of energy; the ablated debris acts as a "heat sink" and delivers a much higher degree of thermal energy and, therefore, tissue damage than would be expected. It is important to wipe away all ablated debris between each pass of the laser. This should be done vigorously with a saline-soaked gauze pad until a clean, clear skin surface remains.

Judging the depth of penetration is aided by tissue color differentiation. In general, a first pass allows for complete removal of epithelium and a pink, erythematous appearance to the skin. Ideally, each pass will remove 60 to 80 mm of tissue. A second pass allows for entry into the papillary dermis and the skin takes on an orange-like tinge that begins to border on yellow-orange (Fig. 15–19). High-power second or medium-power third passes allow for entrance into the reticular layer of the dermis and begin to bring out a "chamois" yellow and white appearance. This should be a definite end point to skin resurfacing because further penetration into deeper dermis and a white and grayish appearance to the resurfaced area may result in coagulative necrosis. This stimulates healing by secondary intention and granulation tissue and, of course, subsequent scarring may occur. The

inexperienced surgeon should be advised to be very conservative in initial treatments and to use lower power settings and slower program settings. When laser resurfacing is completed, fine tuning and feathering can be done (Figs. 15–17 and 15–18). This is generally best done at lower power levels in a layered technique; that is, in decreasing amounts of penetration and ablation, which allows for a transition zone between the area to be resurfaced and the untreated area (see Figs. 15–17 and 15–19). The peripheral border of ablated tissue should show a clear stepdown from normal epithelium to very superficial papillary dermis then to deeper papillary dermis.

COMPLICATIONS AND SEQUELAE

From 1995 to 1997 we used CO_2 CSR exclusively, with good results. Patients were troubled mainly with lengthy postoperative recovery because of persistent erythema, which lasted as long as 6 to 12 weeks. From 1997 to 1999 we developed and published a technique that uses a new modality of erbium-YAG laser resurfacing.[15] The erbium-YAG produces little thermal damage and erythema and is used to remove layers from the epithelium to the dermis (substituting for the first pass of the CO_2 laser). It uses a single pass of 300 mJ CO_2 pulsed laser to contract and smooth the papillary dermis. This combined erbium/CO_2 laser decreased recovery time to less than 2 weeks with excellent results (Figs. 15–20 to 15–22).

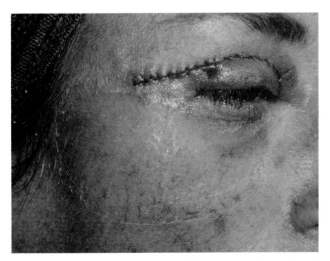

Figure 15–19. Finished lower lid laser CSR with peripheral feathering—all debris wiped away. Note peripheral "stepdown" and change of color where feathered.

POSTOPERATIVE COURSE

Postoperatively, the treated surface is irrigated with cop salin. The surface is then towel dried gently. The use of a very cool-low temperature hair drying gun can then be used to further dry the treated area. An occlusive dressing, such as Flexzan, is applied directly to accomplish "dry dressing" technique.

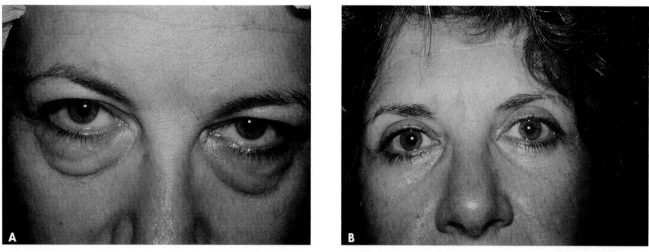

Figure 15–20. (A,B) Final results. A usual laser blepharoplasty with laser resurfacing and septomyocutaneous lateral flap.

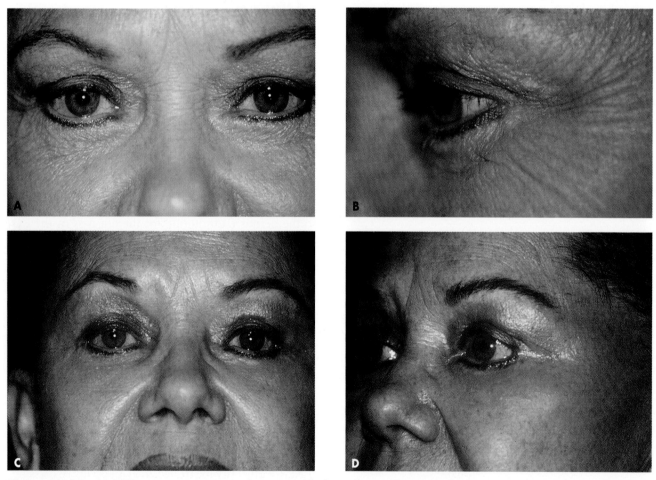

Figure 15–21. (A,B) Preoperative (patient with previous blepharoplasty and ectropion repair and residual rhytides). **(C,D)** Post-operative erbium-CO_2 combo laser technique.

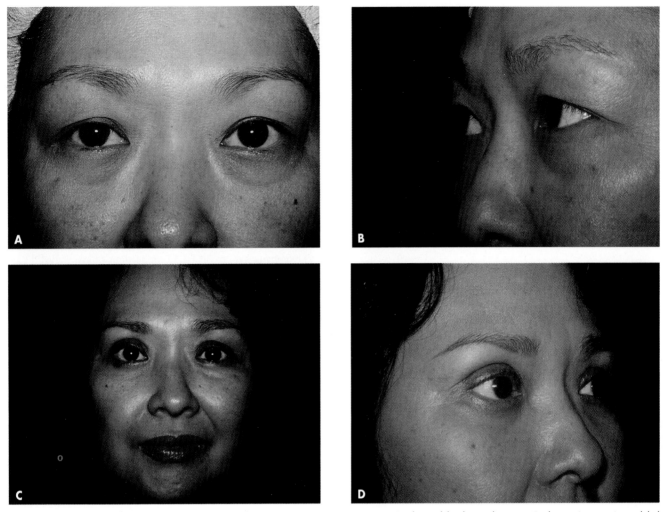

Figure 15–22. (A,B) Preoperative Asian woman. **(C,D)** Postoperative CO_2 laser blepharoplasty at 8 days. A supratarsal lid crease reconstruction was performed.

Epithelialization of combined erbium-CO_2 laser surface generally occurs in 4 to 7 days. Dry Flexzan dressing can be left in place initially for 3 to 4 days. This appears to act as a scaffold for epithelialization and may accelerate healing and decrease erythema.

CONCLUSIONS

The decision whether to perform fat excision alone, fat excision with laser skin resurfacing, or the combined integrated technique just described must be evaluated individually. The quality of skin, thickness, color, wrinkling, and amount of laxity are all factors. The addition of CO_2 laser incisional and erbium-CO_2 resurfacing technique adds many "colors" to the surgical palette.

Careful preoperative examination combined with discussion of the patient's concerns is the best guide to determining the best surgical approach. It is also critical to not evaluate blepharoplasty in a vacuum. The eyebrow and cheek should be assessed carefully to determine whether adjunctive procedures such as endoscopic brow elevation (see Chapters 13 and 14) or midface cheek lift should be considered and involved (see Chapter 17) for an ideal facial result.

PEARLS

- Evaluate brow and cheek carefully as to their contribution to eyelid abnormalities for ideal aesthetic result.
- Procedures that minimize skin excision yield the safest and most aesthetically natural results.
- Upper lid crease formation is the key to upper lid aesthetics.
- The creation of a continuous contour from the lower eyelid margin to the cheek and midface is the key to lower lid aesthetic success.
- At the end of blepharoplasty, the result that you see on the table is most typically the result that you will see in the final postoperative evaluation. It must, therefore, be perfect on the table.

REFERENCES

1. Bourquet. Les hernies graisseuses de l'orbite. Notre traitement chirurgical. *Bull Acad Med (Paris)*. 1924; 92(3 ser);1270–1272.
2. Baylis HI, Long JA, Groth MJ. Transconjunctival lower eyelid blepharoplasty. Techniques and complications. *Ophthalmology*. 1989; 96:1027–1032.
3. Tomlinson FB, Hovey LM. Transconjunctival lower lid blepharoplasty for removal of fat. *Plast Reconstr Surg*. 1975; 56:314–318.
4. Schwartz F, Randall P. Conjunctival incision for herniated orbital fat. *Ophthalmol Surg*. 1980; 11:276–279.
5. Hester TR, Codner MA, et al. Transorbital lower lid and mid face rejuvenation. *Op Tech Plast Reconstr Surg*. 1998; 5:163–185.
6. Edgerton MT Jr. Causes and prevention of lower lid ectropion following blepharoplasty. *Plast Reconstr Surg*. 1972; 49:367–373.
7. Neuhaus RW, Baylis HI. Complications of lower eyelid blepharoplasty. In: Putterman AM, ed. *Cosmetic Oculoplasty Surgery*. New York: Grune & Stratton, 1982:276–306.
8. Rees TD, Jelks GW. Blepharoplasty and the dry eye syndrome. *Plast Reconstr Surg*. 1981; 99:249–254.
9. Anderson RL, Gurdy DD. The tarsal strip procedure. *Arch Ophthalmol*. 1979; 97:2192–2196
10. Millman A, et al. The septal-myocutaneous flap in blepharoplasty. *Ophthalmol Plast Reconstr Surg*. 1997; 13:2.
11. Kamer FM, Mikaelian AJ. Pre-excision blepharoplasty. *Arch Otolaryngol Head Neck Surg*. 1991; 117:995–999.
12. Millman A, et al. Cosmetic blepharoplasty. In: Putterman, ed. *Cosmetic Oculoplastic Surgery*. Philadelphia: W. B. Saunders, 1998.
13. Thomas JR, Davis WE. Pinch-technique blepharoplasty for the upper eyelid. *ENT J*. 1977; 65:40–42.
14. Weber PJ, Popp JC, Wulc AE. Simultaneous lateral, anterior n posterior lower lid blepharoplasty. *Ophthalmol Surg*. 1992; 4:260–264.
15. Millman AL. Histology of convalescent combined erbium-YAG and CO_2 laser skin resurfacing. *Am J Ophthalmol* Feb, 1999.

Blepharoplasty

CHAPTER 16

A Facial Plastic Surgeon's Perspective

STEPHEN W. PERKINS AND RANDALL C. LATORRE

Aesthetic Facial Plastic Surgery, edited by Thomas Romo, III, and Arthur L. Millman, Thieme Medical Publishers, Inc., New York, New York, Copyright © 2000.

In 1818 Von Graefe coined the word *blepharoplasty* (Greek, *blepharon* = eyelid; *plastos* = formed) to describe an eyelid reconstruction he had performed. Today, blepharoplasty denotes excision of redundant skin, with or without the excision of orbital fat, for functional or cosmetic indications. Excess eyelid skin, orbicularis oculi hypertrophy, pseudoherniation of orbital fat, and increased lateral scleral show convey an aged and tired appearance.

Cosmetic improvement of the upper and lower eyelids will be discussed beginning with preoperative assessment. In addition, various surgical techniques, complications, and adjunctive procedures will be addressed.

PATIENT SELECTION
PREOPERATIVE EVALUATION

Blepharoplasty, compared with other facial cosmetic procedures, is a relatively easy experience for both patient and surgeon. During the consultation, the surgeon must determine three important points: (1) does the patient have realistic expectations; (2) is the patient's desire cosmetic or functional; and (3) does the appropriate pathologic condition exist. A thorough history and physical examination, including photographic examples and computer imaging, facilitates the patient's understanding of results that are achievable. Once appropriate patient expectations are established, the facial plastic surgeon must define whether the procedure sought by the patient is for cosmetic or functional reasons. Redundancy of upper eyelid skin can be significant, interfering with a person's peripheral vision (Fig. 16–1). If obstructed visual fields are apparent, it is absolutely necessary to consult an ophthalmologist for proper documentation of visual field deficit. Differentiation between functional and cosmetic will facilitate the discussion on the patient's financial responsibilities.

Does a pathologic condition exist that can be corrected by blepharoplasty? Systemic diseases, such as Grave's disease, Sjogren's syndrome, collagen vascular diseases (systemic lupus erythematosus, panarteritis

nodosa, and scleroderma), Wegener's granulomatosis, ocular pemphigoid, and Stephens-Johnson syndrome can predispose the patient to xerophthalmia, a complication following blepharoplasty, especially of the upper eyelid. Patient's with Grave's disease may have upper lid retraction, exophthalmos, lower lid retraction, and history of exposure keratitis. Therefore it is important to check thyroid function studies. The myxedematous state of hypothyroidism may mimic dermatochalasis, and pseudoherniation of orbital fat must be evaluated before surgical intervention.

A baseline ocular examination, including visual acuity, visual fields, extraocular movements, and corneal reflexes, should be performed on all patients. If any indication exists from the history that the patient may have dry eye syndrome, he or she should be evaluated with Schirmer's test to quantitate tear output and tear film breakup times. This can be done by the surgeon by placing several drops of topical anesthetic to the inferior fornix of each eye. Excess fluid is blotted from the lower lid palpebral conjunctiva with tissue paper. Schirmer's strip is then bent and tucked into the lower lid inferior temporal fornix. The patient is then instructed to look upward. After approximately 5 minutes, the strip is removed and measured from the notch to the wet end. The tear film should measure between 10 and 15 mm. A history of dry eye syndrome alerts the surgeon to advise

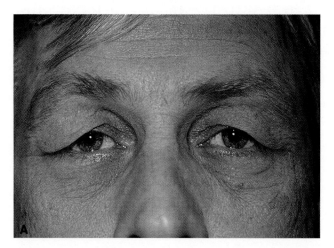 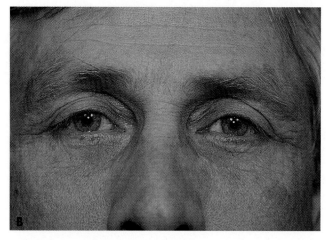

Figure 16–1. (A) A 56-year-old man demonstrating marked lateral dermatochalasis obstructing his peripheral vision. **(B)** A 56-year-old man after functional upper lid blepharoplasty.

the patient of the likely need of postoperative lubrication. More severe cases of dry eye syndrome require documentation of the tear film and consultation with an ophthalmologist.

However, if the patient reports any unusual history, such as glaucoma, optic neuritis, iritis, retinal detachment, vitreous tears, or cataracts, the surgeon should at least obtain clearance by an ophthalmologist if not a complete preoperative ocular examination.

Finally, appropriate candidates for surgery are placed on preoperative antibiotics and antiviral agents as indicated.

PHYSICAL EXAMINATION

Examination of the eyelids begins with the general appearance, taking into account the patient's skin: pigmented versus nonpigmented, dry versus oily, thick versus thin. In upper lid blepharoplasty, the redundancy of upper eyelid skin can be so significant that it can interfere with a person's peripheral vision. Upper lid blepharoplasty will directly and immediately correct this visual field defect. The aging process and gravity work together, along with the inherent loss of elasticity that occurs within the skin to create crepiness and excess eyelid skin, called dermatochalasis. Relaxation of the orbital septum allows pseudoherniation of fat to cause a bulging fold of the ptotic eyelid skin. The increased crepiness of the upper eyelid skin, in turn, interferes with application of cosmetics, such as eye shadow or makeup. The lateral hooding that can occur presents a tired look to the eyelid region. Redundancy of the skin and weakening of the orbital septum initially occurs in the third decade and becomes increasingly visible over the ensuing decades. Therefore the most common motivation for upper lid blepharoplasty is the patient's desire to achieve a much younger and refreshed look rather than to change or gain a different appearance. Blepharochalasis, a rare and hereditary condition associated with repeated swelling and edema of the eyelids, results in blepharedema and stretching of the lid skin and fat prolapse. This is associated with true

ptosis of the lid that is a result of stretching of the levator aponeurosis or dehiscence of the levator aponeurosis from the tarsus.

Examination of the eye includes the shape and positioning of the upper and lower lid margins in relation to the globe. Both upper and lower eyelids should be measured for symmetry, with measurement of the palpebral fissure height and length. Positioning of the upper lid and lower lid margin should be at the level of the superior and inferior limbus of the globe, respectively. In addition, the presence of ptosis is important, and the patient must be advised that repair of the ptotic lid may be the indicated procedure rather than excision of lid skin (Fig. 16–2). A referral to a surgeon skilled in such repair should be scheduled for the patient. Special note should be taken for any abnormal pigmentation or discoloration, (i.e., venous stasis that will not be changed with blepharoplasty). Crow's feet at the lateral periorbital area should be addressed, and it should be conveyed to the patient that adjunctive procedures can be incorporated to manage these signs of aging not associated with the procedure.

Along with the eyelid skin, proper evaluation of the muscularis orbicularis oculi must be addressed. Often, patients present with hypertrophy of this muscle, which is exaggerated on smiling or squinting. Simply removing orbital fat and skin will not address this problem but

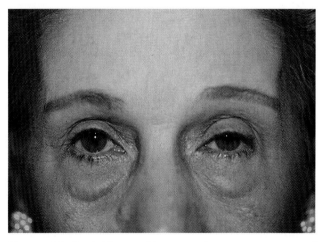

Figure 16–2. A 60-year-old woman demonstrating ptosis of the left upper eyelid.

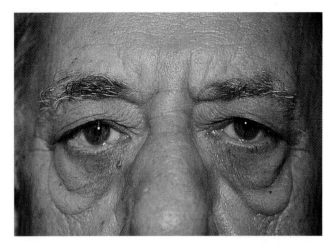

Figure 16–3. A 63-year-old man with significant malar festoons.

rather accentuate this preoperative condition. Treatment should include orbicularis oculi muscle stripping or debulking. Orbital festoons or "malar bags" develop with age and are manifested by a ptotic and attenuated inferior portion of the orbicularis oculi muscle resting on the malar eminence (Fig. 16–3). Understanding the cause of the festoon is important because standard lower lid blepharoplasty does not address this problem.[1] Small et al. describe the extended blepharoplasty, which we perform as described in the following.

Assessment of Herniated Orbital Fat

The orbital fat is compartmentalized into a smaller lateral, central, and medial pocket of the upper and lower eyelids.

Controversy exists as to whether a true lateral fat pad exists in the upper eyelid. It is imperative to identify the infraorbital rim because aggressive resection of orbital fat can create a sunken or cadaveric appearance. Pseudoherniation of orbital fat can be demonstrated on the direction of the patient's gaze. Gaze in the superior direction will accentuate the lower central and medial fat pockets, whereas superior gaze in the contralateral direction will accentuate the lateral compartment (Fig. 16–4). Further evaluation of orbital fat pseudoherniation can be accomplished by applying gentle pressure on the globe and observing protrusion of the fat from the respective pockets.

Evaluation of Lower Lid Laxity

It is important for the surgeon to determine the amount of lower lid laxity and tarsal strength and resilience. Attention to the lower lid strength can help avoid the complication of ectropion, leading to the aggravation or development of dry eye syndrome (Fig. 16–5).

Two clinical tests used to evaluate the lower lid are the lid snap back test and the lid distraction test. The lid snap back test assesses orbicularis and tarsal function, as well as medial and lateral canthal tendon stability (Fig. 16–6A). This is performed by displacing the lower lid toward the orbital rim and releasing the eyelid. It is important to note the pattern and rate of return of the lid

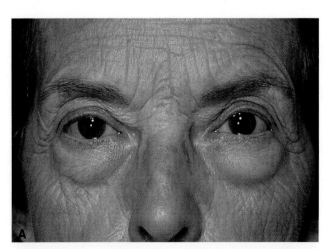
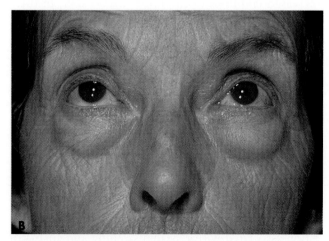

Figure 16–4. (A,B) A 71-year-old woman demonstrating lower lid pseudoherniation of orbital fat in straight and superiorly directed gaze.

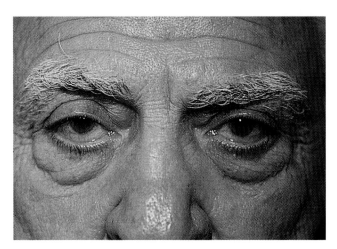

Figure 16–5. Demonstration of decreased lower lid tone with senile ectropion and inferior scleral show.

to the resting position. The slow return of the lid or evidence of inferior scleral show reveal poor lid tone and eyelid support. The results of this test help the surgeon determine how much skin and muscle to resect and whether the patient would benefit from a lid shortening, canthoplasty, or orbicularis muscle suspension.

The lid distraction test is performed by grasping the mid lower eyelid between the thumb and index finger (Fig. 16–6B). Movement of the lid margin greater than 10 mm is an indication of poor lower lid support. Quick release of the eyelid and evidence of a slow return or apposition to the globe signifies potential risk for ectropion, epiphora, and exposure keratitis. These findings

should alert the surgeon that a lid-tightening procedure may be warranted.[2,3]

ANATOMY

The eyelids are composed of two lamellae: the anterior lamella consists of the skin and orbicularis oculi muscle. The posterior lamella consists of the tarsus and conjunctiva. Skin is connected to the underlying orbicularis muscle by fine fibrous septae with essentially no subcutaneous fat layer.

The orbicularis oculi muscle can be subdivided into an orbital and palpebral portion. The palpebral portion is divided into pretarsal and preseptal musculature. The pretarsal musculature condenses medially and attaches to the anterior and posterior lacrimal crest, forming the medial canthal tendon. Lateral condensations attach to the orbital tubercle, forming the lateral canthal tendon. The preseptal muscle, which overlies the orbital septum and attaches to the medial orbital wall, fans out laterally to interdigitate with the soft tissue, creating what is known as crow's feet.

The orbital septum is an extension of the periosteum of the orbital rim. It originates at the arcus marginalis and fuses to the capsulopalpebral fascia posteriorly and continues on as the levator aponeurosis. The levator aponeurosis then attaches to the anterior

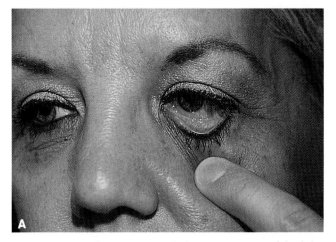
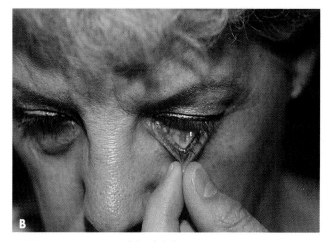

Figure 16–6. (A) Demonstration of the lid snap test. **(B)** Demonstration of the lid distraction test.

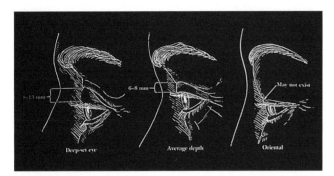

Figure 16–7. Comparison of the supratarsal crease of the Occidental and Asian upper eyelid.

face of the tarsus and interdigitates with the anterior lamellae. Definition of the superior lid crease is defined at the point where the orbital septum attaches to the levator aponeurosis. Differences in the point of attachment of the septum to the aponeurosis are manifested by lack of development of the superior lid crease as in the Asian upper eyelid (Fig. 16–7).

In the lower lid the orbital septum attaches to the capsulopalpebral fascia, which is the anterior extension of dense fibrous connective tissue. The capsulopalpebral fascia then attaches to the inferior border of the inferior tarsus and may extend through orbital fat, contributing to compartment formation. It extends through the preseptal musculature and attaches subcutaneously to the skin, contributing to the lower lid creases.

PREOPERATIVE PREPARATION

Upper and lower lid blepharoplasty can easily and generally be performed with local anesthesia while the patient is mildly sedated with intravenous anesthetics and analgesics. We have found adequate preoperative sedation by using 10 to 20 mg of diazepam, 50 mg of prochlorperazine, and 10 mg of metoclopramide orally approximately $1\frac{1}{2}$ hours before the surgery. The upper and lower lids are degreased thoroughly with a light pass of an alcohol pad to prevent blurring of the ink.

After marking the patient, an intravenous line is started and before local anesthetic injection, 0.5 to 1.0 mg of hydromorphone HCl and 2 to 5 mg of midazolam HCl is administered. An alternative intravenous anesthetic

solution propofol (Diprivan) can be administered. The dose of propofol is 40 to 60 mg/kg/min.

Once adequate anesthesia and sedation have been administered, 1 to 2% xylocaine with 1 : 100,000 units of epinephrine is infiltrated in the immediate subcutaneous layer of the upper lid. To prevent postoperative bruising, care is taken not to injure any vessels immediately below the overlying skin and in the orbicularis muscle. The anesthetic solution is administered with a 27-gauge needle in advance, creating a bleb of fluid that dissects the plane above the muscle. The only additional anesthetic required is a small amount of local anesthetic injected directly into the protruding central and nasal orbital fat pockets just before bipolar cauterization and removal.

OPERATIVE TECHNIQUE
UPPER LID BLEPHAROPLASTY

It is imperative to use a fine tip marker to create a thin line because differences of 1 to 3 mm from one eyelid to the next can create asymmetries that are otherwise not planned. The use of small calipers in upper lid blepharoplasty is imperative for measuring the distance between the superior lid crease and lid margin (Fig. 16–8). One can account for asymmetries and excess of redundant

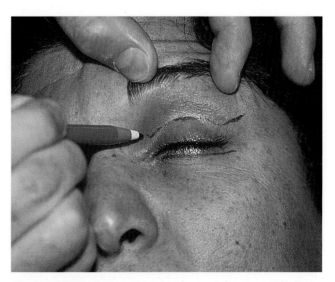

Figure 16–8. Preoperative marking of the upper blepharoplasty inferior limb.

eyelid skin, but generally equal amounts of skin are removed on both upper lids.

The initial skin marking must denote the supratarsal fold at an appropriate measured level above the ciliary margin. This is most commonly along the natural lid crease, but not always. It is important to maintain a minimum of 8 mm above the lid margin, but no higher than 12 mm. On average, for a woman 10 to 11 mm and for a man 8 to 9 mm is measured at the center of the palpebral margin.[4] The skin markings should curve medially to within 1 to 2 mm of the punctum and laterally to the lateral canthus, curving gently and paralleling the lid margins in both directions. Laterally, the incision should sweep diagonally upward to the level of the orbital rim. If the incision is carried along the curve of the lid crease lateral to the lateral canthus, the final closure scar line will bring the upper lid tissue downward, resulting in a hooded or a saddened appearance. Positioning of the incision between the lateral canthus and lateral eyebrow margin will eliminate the lateral hooding by pulling the tissue upward. This modification of the lateral incision makes it easy for women to camouflage with makeup (Fig. 16–9). In a man the lateral upper eyelid incision should end within 1 to 2 mm of the lateral canthus. Medially, one must be certain not to cross the nasal-orbital depression to avoid creating a webbed scar. The upper limb of the lazy fusiform marking is determined by the extent of the redundant skin and partially by the distance remaining between the eyebrow itself and the true crepy upper eyelid skin. A smooth forceps is used to "pinch" the excess amount of skin gathered

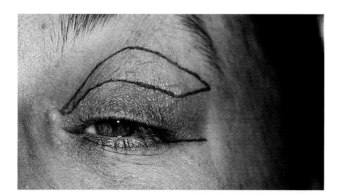

Figure 16–9. Completion of the upper lid blepharoplasty skin markings demonstrating the diagonal sweep lateral to the canthus.

gently so as to roll the lashes upward or slightly open from a comfortably closed lid.[5] The upper and lower limbs of the skin marking meet laterally and medially at approximately a 30-degree angle. If a large pseudoherniation of medial fat pad exists, it is crucial to avoid overresection of medial lid skin. Even a large amount of fat requires adequate skin to redrape over the defect. The resection of the skin can result in tenting medially, with a resultant thickened scar or lagophthalmos. Some degree of initial temporary lagophthalmos is common after suture closure of the upper lid. Much of this lagophthalmos will resolve by the next morning or when the local anesthetic diminishes. With the diminution of swelling, 3 to 4 mm of lagophthalmos will usually resolve. If significant lagophthalmos occurs (up to 6 mm centrally or anything greater than 1 to 2 mm medially), the surgeon should replace some of the excised lid skin immediately as a full-thickness skin graft. Saving the excised skin overnight is a wise and safe precaution, especially if a skin graft be necessary the next day.

Stabilization of the skin in the eyelid is paramount to making the "skin-only" incision of the upper eyelid. The help of an assistant is required to place tension on the skin, while the inferior limb of the preplanned incision is made in the lid crease. The incision is made with a small blade (a 15 Bard Parker or 6700 Beaver blade). The belly of the blade is used to create an incision through the depth of the thin upper lid skin. The incision begins medially and extends laterally with a single graceful sweep upward. A round-handled scalpel is ideal for making the upper limb of the incision as it curves and rolls from medial to lateral. The skin is then sharply dissected with either a blade or dissecting beveled scissors. The scissors are advanced, spreading and completely undermining the skin, allowing easy trimming of the incised edges. Some surgeons prefer an intentional "pinch" to judge the appropriate amount of skin to excise by lightly crushing the capillaries of the dermal edge. Trimming the "pinched" portion is then accomplished with the scissors.

At this time, evaluation of the orbicularis oculi muscle is done to determine possible excision of a muscle strip. The muscle to be removed is the preseptal portion of the orbicularis oculi muscle. Normally, only a very thin strip of the muscle is excised medially, exposing the fat compartments unless the muscle is very thin and atrophic.[4] For thicker, heavier lids more orbicularis can be excised along the entire lateral to medial length of the lid to improve the contour of the lid itself, especially laterally. Care is taken to lift the strip of muscle away from the orbital septum to avoid inadvertent trimming. Meticulous hemostasis is achieved with either a bipolar cautery or a thin-tipped monopolar unit during each step of the procedure.

Attention is then directed to the pseudoherniation of orbital fat. Most of this involves the central and medial compartments. The medial fat pad is almost always pale compared with the more yellow central and lateral fat pads. Generally, a small opening is made in the orbital septum overlying each fat pad rather than a long incision of the orbital septum. Gentle pressure on the globe can demonstrate the fat pads that need to be reduced and excised.[5] A Griffiths-Brown, fine multitooth forceps is used to hold the herniated fat away from the orbital septum. Lidocaine (Xylocaine) (2%) is then injected directly into the fat pad. A bipolar cautery is then used to meticulously cauterize the fat pad before excision with small trimming scissors (Fig. 16–10). Previous preoperative local infiltration was made superficial to the orbicularis

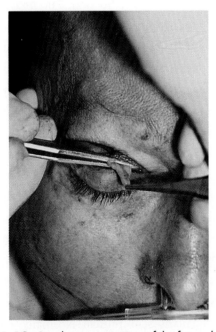

Figure 16–10. Bipolar cauterization of the fat pad stalk.

and orbital septum. Therefore patients will experience deep pain sensation with cauterization of the fat pad, especially in the nasal pocket. By first infiltrating a small amount of local anesthetic, the surgeon can minimize any discomfort or sensation felt by the patient.

Less commonly, a lateral fat pad is bulging and creating a very full or heavy eyelid appearance. When the aesthetic decision is made preoperatively to contour and deepen the eyelid laterally toward the orbital rim, the surgeon must carefully identify the lateral fat pad. Specific care is taken to differentiate between a pseudoherniation of the lateral fat and a prolapsing or partially prolapsed lacrimal gland.[6] Often, the lacrimal gland may lie behind yellow herniated temporal fat. The gland is much grayer in appearance and firmer in texture. Very rarely does one need to resuspend the gland. If suspension is required, the gland can be suspended with one or two double-arm sutures of 5-0 polypropylene to the leading edge of the gland, which is then tacked to the periosteum of the superior orbital rim. When these sutures are tied, the gland should return to the lacrimal gland fossa.[7]

The nasal or most medial fat compartment can be most difficult to identify and remains the most common residual aesthetic complication of upper lid blepharoplasty. Underestimation of the amount of fat to be removed or difficulty finding the fat pad is common because the pad retracts into the orbit when the patient is in the supine position. The superior oblique muscle and tendon lie deep in this area between the central and medial fat compartments. Direct visualization of the fat stalk before cauterization excision is imperative.

Skin Closure

The wound can then be closed with several different choices of suture. A polypropylene suture has been shown to be the least reactive. A simple running suture of 7-0 polypropylene or a running 6-0 polypropylene subcuticular suture are the two most commonly used[4] (Fig. 16–11). A 6-0 mild chromic or a fast-absorbing gut suture can create an inflammatory response and ultimately produce suture tracts, tunnels, or milia. A 7-0 size rarely produces milia. The surgeon should use very fine

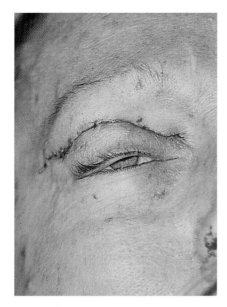

Figure 16–11. Skin closure of the upper blepharoplasty incision using a 6-0 polypropylene suture in a subcuticular fashion.

0.3-mm single-tooth forceps and a delicate Castroviejo needle holder for precise finger touch control when approximating the wound edges. The lateral aspect of the wound lateral to the lateral canthus is closed first with an interrupted suture so as to closely approximate a 30-degree triangle and not create redundancy of tissue. This is the point of maximum tension. Once the halving principle has been used to line up the unequal length of the superior and inferior limbs, the wound is closed medial to lateral with the running subcuticular suture (Figs. 16–12 and 16–13).

LOWER LID BLEPHAROPLASTY

Several techniques of lower lid blepharoplasty have been developed to address particular clinical findings of the

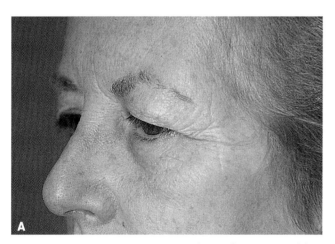
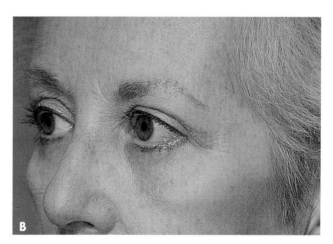

Figure 16–12. (A) Preoperative photo of a 53-year-old woman demonstrating marked dermatochalasis and excessive lateral hooding. **(B)** A 53-year-old woman after an upper lid blepharoplasty. Note the creation of a supratarsal crease that extends but does not go beyond the lateral canthus.

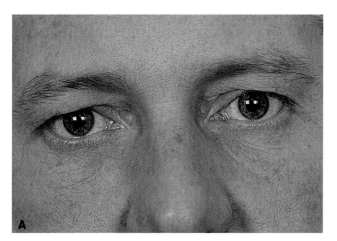
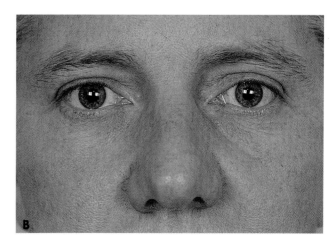

Figure 16–13. (A) A man demonstrating redundancy of the upper eyelid skin. Note the greater redundancy of the right versus left upper lid. **(B)** Postoperative picture of the patient in Figure 16–13A after upper lid blepharoplasty.

lower lid. Such characteristics, including dermatochalasis, orbicularis oculi hypertrophy, pseudoherniation of orbital fat, poor lid support based on the lid snap back test and lid distraction test, "festooning," and blepharochalasis, will determine the surgical approach to the lower lid.

The following procedures will be discussed: skin-muscle flap technique, extended lower lid blepharoplasty, skin flap technique, and transconjunctival approach. Adjunctive procedures include lateral cantholysis with lateral lower lid shortening and suspension, transconjunctival lower lid blepharoplasty (TCB) with skin pinch technique, TCB with simultaneous chemical peel or CO_2 laser resurfacing, and micropigmentation of the eyelids.

The skin-muscle flap technique is the most commonly used. The indications are the presence of pseudoherniation of orbital fat and excess lid skin. The advantages of this technique is that elevation occurs in an avascular, submuscular plane, preventing the likelihood of hematoma, infection, lymphadema, and prolonged lower lid ecchymosis (Fig. 16–14).

A fine-tipped skin marker is used to mark the incision, beginning at the lower punctum medially and running 2 mm inferior to the lower lid margin toward the lateral canthus. At the lateral canthus, the incision takes a more horizontal position and is extended lateral to the canthus approximately 4 to 8 mm. Extension of this incision minimizes the potential for rounding the canthal

angle and lateral scleral show.[8] If upper blepharoplasty is performed in conjunction with a skin-muscle or skin-flap technique, care must be taken to maintain a ridge of tissue between the lateral extensions of the upper and lower blepharoplasty incisions that measures at least 6 mm, preferably 10 mm. Before prepping the skin, 1 or 2% lidocaine with 1 : 100,000 units of epinephrine is infiltrated along the incision line beneath the orbicularis within the potential space superficial to the orbital septum.

After adequate anesthetic time, a No. 15 Bard Parker scalpel is used to incise the skin from the medial extent of the incision to the lateral canthus. Lateral to the canthus, the incision is made through skin and muscle. At this point, a fine curved scissors is placed into the lateral portion of the incision and blunt, spreading motions are used to dissect onto the lateral orbital rim. A blunt-tipped, outwardly beveled scissors is used to elevate and separate the muscle from the orbital septum along the avascular plane to the level of the inferior orbital rim inferiorly and the incision superiorly. Further elevation of the skin muscle flap can be accomplished if malar extension and suspension of the inferior orbicularis oculi muscle are required (Fig. 16–15). The subciliary incision is then completed using the scissors, with placement of one tip beneath the orbicularis muscle and the other above the incision. The cut is then made in a beveled fashion to preserve the muscular sling of the

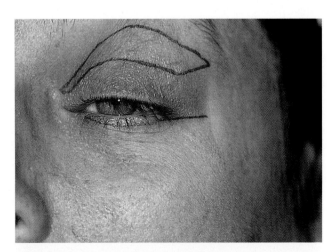

Figure 16–14. Demonstration of the subciliary incision in preparation for the skin-muscle flap technique. Observe that the lateral extension from the canthus is at a slightly higher position than the subciliary incision.

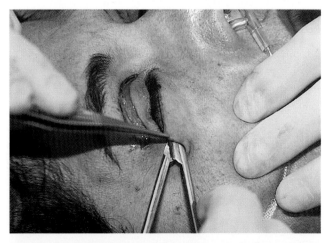

Figure 16–15. Elevation of the skin-muscle flap working from a lateral to medial direction.

lower lid. The cotton-tipped applicator can then be used to dissect the remaining strands of muscle from the underlying orbital septum. A double ball retractor is then used to expose the pocket, and hemostasis can be achieved with the bipolar cautery[9] (Fig. 16–16). If pseudoherniation of fat was recognized preoperatively, access to the fat compartments can be made by creating selected openings over each fat compartment. Demonstration of orbital fat can be done with gentle palpation of the globe and observation for proptosis of orbital fat. The lateral fat pocket is addressed first because the amount of fat is difficult to assess after removal of fat from the central compartment. A fine, multitoothed Griffiths-Brown forceps is used to hold the herniated fat away from the orbital septum, and a bipolar cautery is used to meticulously cauterize the fat pad before excision with small trimming scissors. Just before cauterization, it is necessary to inject a small amount of local anesthetic, usually 2% lidocaine, directly into the fat pad stalk. This avoids the pain associated with bipolar cauterization of the fat pad stalk because prior local anesthetic was applied superficial to the orbital septum. Further hemostasis is achieved with the bipolar cautery. Reassessment of orbital fat in the compartment can be done with gentle retropulsion of the globe. If excess fat remains, this can be removed in a similar fashion. A conservative approach to fat resection should be maintained to avoid the creation of a sunken appearance. With the infraorbital rim as a limit for fat resection, remaining blebs of fat may be cauterized to the level of the infraorbital rim. The goal is to create a smooth transition from lower eyelid skin to malar skin.

The central and medial fat compartments are addressed in a similar fashion. Extreme care must be taken to avoid iatrogenic trauma to the inferior oblique muscle, which separates these fat compartments (Fig. 16–17). Access to the medial compartment may be hindered by the subciliary incision. Therefore the fat should be brought into the incision rather than extending the subciliary incision.

On completion of fat resection, the skin-muscle flap is then redraped over the lower lid margin until the appropriate amount of tension of the lower eyelid skin is achieved. If the patient is awake, he or she is asked to open the jaws widely and gaze superiorly, which creates maximal separation of the wound edges, thereby allowing conservative resection of skin and muscle. If the patient is completely sedated, single-finger pressure at the inferomedial portion of the melolabial mound just above the nasoalar groove will create the same maximal stretch effect.

At the level of the lateral canthus, the amount of skin overlap is judged by making a segmental vertical cut

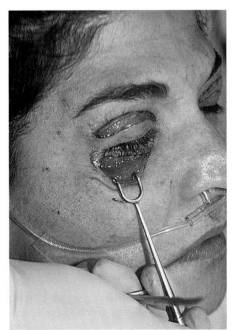

Figure 16–16. Photograph displaying retraction with the double ball retractor to gain access to the orbital septum.

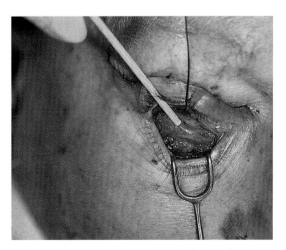

Figure 16–17. Demonstration of the inferior oblique muscle separating the medial and central fat compartments.

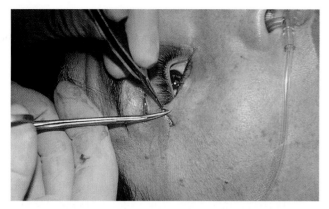

Figure 16–18. While the patient is asked to open his jaws widely, an inferiorly directed segmental cut is made to determine a conservative and appropriate amount of skin to be excised.

inferiorly (Fig. 16–18). A tacking stitch of 7-0 blue polypropylene is placed to maintain the position of the skin-muscle flap. At this point, eyelid scissors are used to excise the overlapping skin beginning laterally to medially, with care to bevel the incision so as to allow for 1 to 2-mm strip resection of the orbicularis oculi muscle. If the orbicularis is truly thick and hypertrophied, this cut prevents ridge formation with closure of the subciliary incision. Conservative skin-muscle resection is warranted to prevent the complications of postoperative ectropion and epiphora. Lateral orbicularis oculi muscle suspension is useful in correcting orbicularis muscle laxity without evidence of festoon formation. Hemostasis is achieved

and the orbicularis is suspended to the medial aspect of the lateral orbital rim with 5-0 clear polydioxanone (PDS) suture. This supports the lid and is useful in correcting mild laxity.

The skin edges are reapproximated using either 7-0 blue polypropylene suture in selected areas along the subciliary incision or the tissue adhesive Histoacryl (Braun Melsungun, Germany). The incision lateral to the lateral canthus is then closed using interrupted 7-0 blue polypropylene suture.

After completion of skin closure, antibiotic ophthalmic ointment can be placed over the incision site. In addition, a 1/4-inch Steri Strip can be placed on the temporal portion of the incision for added support (Figs. 16–19 and 16–20).

EXTENDED LOWER LID BLEPHAROPLASTY

The extended lower lid blepharoplasty is a modification of the standard subciliary skin-muscle flap blepharoplasty, which addresses the malar bags or festoons. Festoons are a redundancy of the inferior border of the orbicularis oculi muscle that drapes over the malar eminence. Small[1] first described the extended lower lid blepharoplasty. A subciliary incision is created and extended 1 cm beyond

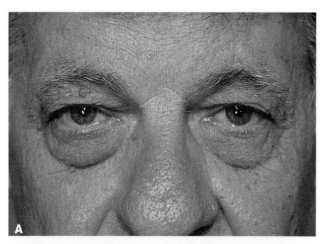
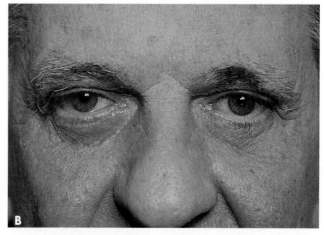

Figure 16–19. (A) A 62-year-old white man demonstrating significant dermatochalasis and pseudoherniation of orbital fat. **(B)** Postoperative photograph of the same male patient after skin-muscle flap technique, removal of pseudoherniated orbital fat, and lateral orbicularis oculi suspension.

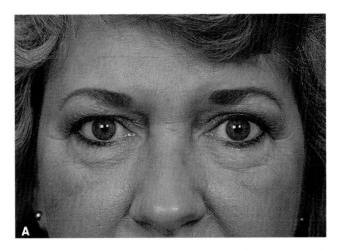 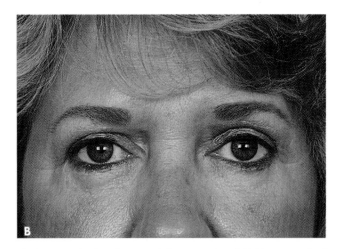

Figure 16–20. (A) A 47-year-old woman demonstrating dermatochalasis and orbicularis oculi hypertrophy. **(B)** Photograph of the same patient in A after lower blepharoplasty skin-muscle flap technique.

the lateral canthus. A skin-muscle flap is then elevated well below the inferior orbital rim. At this time, a 1-cm oval is excised from the superior lateral flap. A full-thickness wedge excision of the lateral lid is then carried out. The dermis of the skin-muscle flap is then suspended to the lateral orbital periosteum with permanent sutures.

We perform a modification on Small's extended lower lid blepharoplasty similar to that described by Becker and Deutsch.[10]

The procedure begins with the standard subciliary incision made 2 mm from the lower eyelid margin. It is carried at least 1 to 2 cm lateral to the lateral canthus in a skin crease. A skin-muscle flap is elevated in the usual fashion but carried below the infraorbital rim to include the most dependent roll of redundant orbicularis oculi muscle. The redundant muscle roll is excised and hemostasis is achieved. The muscle is then suspended as described in the skin-muscle flap technique (Figs. 16–21).

Skin Flap Approach

The uncommonly used technique of the skin flap approach allows independent modifications to the skin and underlying orbicularis oculi muscle. Indications for the skin flap technique are in those patients with

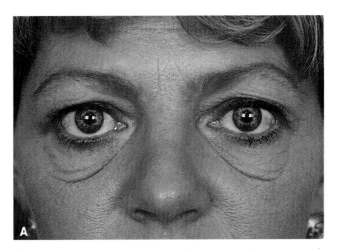 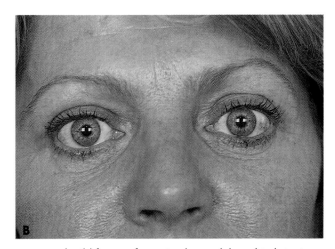

Figure 16–21. (A) A 45-year-old woman with excessive skin crepiness and mild festoon formation beyond the orbital rim is an example of a good candidate for extended lower lid blepharoplasty. **(B)** The patient after extended lower lid blepharoplasty.

excessive amount of lower eyelid skin with significant crepiness without redundancy of orbicularis muscle, an unusual situation. The challenges involved with this technique are a more difficult dissection with a potential for more trauma to the overlying skin, an increased risk of hematoma formation, and development of vertical eyelid retraction.[11,12] For these reasons and with the combined use of transconjunctival lower lid blepharoplasty with simultaneous resurfacing techniques to remove wrinkles, the skin-only flap technique is uncommonly used.

Lower Lid Skin Flap Approach

A small curved scissors is used to develop a supramuscular dissection. It is important to have an assistant apply medial lower lid countertraction. A single hook or a Griffiths-Brown forceps is used to pull the lateral portion of the skin flap in a superior lateral direction. The curved scissors are then used, with the tips up, to create a skin flap over the underlying orbicularis oculi muscle. The flap is extended variably medially as far as the punctum depending on the skin redundancy present. After elevation of the skin flap, the remaining portion of the subciliary incision is performed with the scissors. Hemostasis is then achieved with the bipolar cautery.

If skin redundancy is the main problem, the surgeon can redrape and excise the necessary amount of skin in a similar fashion as that seen in the skin-muscle flap procedure. If the patient has pseudoherniation of orbital fat, access is achieved by creating incisions within the orbicularis oculi muscle over each respective compartment approximately 3 to 4 mm below the initial skin incision. The orbital septum is thereby incised and the orbital fat removed in a similar fashion as previously described in other techniques. No need exists to repair the incisions of the orbicularis oculi.

The question of muscle hypertrophy and festoon formation is critical in the preoperative assessment because each will be treated in a different fashion. If evidence of hypertrophy of the muscle existed in the pre-operative evaluation, the surgeon should perform a skin-muscle flap as described.

TRANSCONJUNCTIVAL BLEPHAROPLASTY OF THE LOWER LID

The transconjunctival blepharoplasty was introduced by Bourquet in 1923.[13] In 1987, Jackson and colleagues presented their experience with 200 patients using the transconjunctival approach for open reduction and internal fixation of orbital floor fractures without incidence of postoperative lid retraction or ectropion.[14] Shore in 1987 and Bayless and coworkers in 1989, all of whom are ophthalmic plastic surgeons, reported on their experience with the transconjunctival-inferior fornix direct approach to correction of the pseudoherniation of lower lid fat, suggesting that the technique was successful and appropriate.[15,16] Most recently, Perkins and Dyer in 1990 reported on their experience with the transconjunctival approach in 300 patients with minimal complications and incidents of lower eyelid malposition. The approach used differed from that of the deep inferior fornix approach in that the initial incision was made just inferior to the tarsus. This allowed a more anterior to posterior access to the fat compartments.[17]

Indications in Patient Selection

It is important to define which patients will benefit and which will not from the transconjunctival approach. Patients without lower lid laxity, true lower lid skin vertical excess, or orbicularis muscle hypertrophy are ideal candidates (Fig. 16–22). Often the patient presents with pseudoherniation of orbital fat causing a dark circle look or tired look to the lower eyelid (Fig. 16–23). If a patient presents with evidence of photoaging and dermatochalasis, he or she can be treated with adjunctive procedures, such as chemical peel and CO_2 laser resurfacing of the lower eyelid skin in addition to transconjunctival ble-

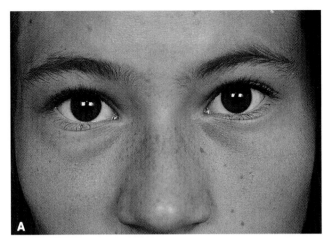
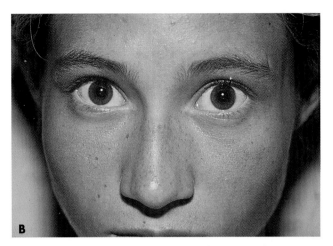

Figure 16–22. (A) A 14-year-old female demonstrating hereditary lower lid pseudoherniation of orbital fat. Given the patient's age and clinical presentation she is a good candidate for transconjunctival blepharoplasty. **(B)** The same patient in A after transconjunctival blepharoplasty.

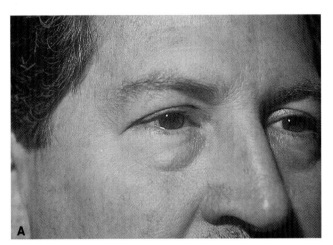
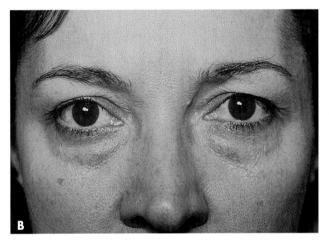

Figure 16–23. (A) An oblique view of a 51-year-old man demonstrating pseudoherniation of lower lid orbital fat without excess skin or muscle. **(B)** Brazilian woman, Fitzpatrick IV, with pseudoherniation of the lower lid orbital fat and dyschromia.

pharoplasty. For those patients presenting with true vertical excess lid skin, a transconjunctival blepharoplasty will fail to achieve a satisfactory result.[18]

An ideal patient for transconjunctival blepharoplasty is the patient who has had a previous blepharoplasty and now presents with recurrent or residual pseudoherniation of orbital fat coexistent with an already tight and elastic lower lid, which may even manifest mild rounding or lateral scleral show. Because the transconjunctival blepharoplasty can correct the pseudoherniation of fat but does not worsen or aggravate the already malpositioned lower lid, it is the procedure of choice.

The transconjunctival approach is also beneficial for those patients who do not desire an external incision or those patients with Fitzpatrick skin types of IV or greater where hypopigmentation of the scar line may be noticeable.

TRANSCONJUNCTIVAL BLEPHAROPLASTY

The patient is anesthetized initially with topical 2% ophthalmic tetracaine HCl, 0.5% (CIBA VISION, ophthalmics, Atlanta, GA), which is placed into the inferior fornix of each eye. With a 30-gauge needle, 2% lidocaine with

TRANSCONJUNCTIVAL APPROACH TO BLEPHAROPLASTY

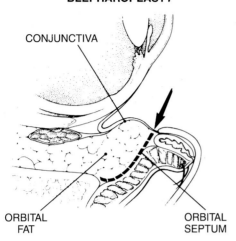

Figure 16–24. Schematic of the transconjunctival approach. Note the position of the incision, which differs from the direct inferior fornix approach.

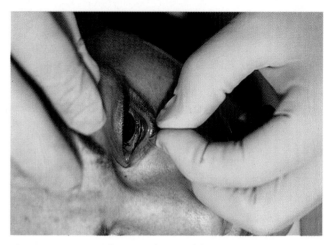

Figure 16–25. After completion of the transconjunctival blepharoplasty, the lower lid skin is picked up, raised, and snapped into position over the lower limbus.

1 : 100,000 units of epinephrine is infiltrated into the subconjunctival plane only. After adequate anesthesia time, a sharp double hook retractor is placed just inside the lid margin and retracted inferiorly. A bipolar cautery is then used to cauterize the central portion of the conjunctiva approximately 1 to 2 mm below the inferior border of the tarsus. The pocket is then elevated laterally and medially, and precauterization is performed using the bipolar. The conjunctiva is opened laterally and medially and the inferior lid retractors are transected sharply with a small curved scissors. The orbicularis oculi muscle is then separated from the orbital septum inferiorly. This allows the surgeon to approach the fat from a *preseptal* direction versus a direct approach throught the inferior fornix (Fig. 16–24). The conjunctiva and inferior retractor muscles are reflected with a single 5-0 silk suture superiorly over the cornea providing protection.

At this junction, Westcott scissors are used to incise the orbital septum. The sharp double prong retractor is replaced by a double ball retractor. Herniated fat is demonstrated by a light retropulsion of the globe, which is then carefully teased up and injected with 2% lidocaine with 1 : 100,000 units of epinephrine. The stalk is then carefully cauterized with the bipolar cautery and excised. Removal of individual herniations of fat is performed in this same fashion for any standard blepharoplasty. Con-

servative resection of fat is done, using the infraorbital rim as a guide. After completion of the fat resection, the lower eyelid skin is redraped in its anatomic position, and evaluation for any residual bulging or irregularity is noted. After symmetry is ensured, the silk suture is removed and the skin flap is picked up, raised, and snapped into position up over the lower limbus (Fig. 16–25). Sutures are not applied to the transconjunctival incision, thus avoiding possible corneal abrasion and irritation (Figs. 16–26 and 16–27).

POSTOPERATIVE COURSE

The upper and lower eyelid wounds are closed and an antibiotic/steroid ophthalmic ointment is applied to the suture lines. Cold compresses are immediately applied postoperatively. Typically, a cold damp washcloth or 4 × 4 gauze squares are used because they are not heavy and easily conform to the eyelid orbital area. A basin of ice water is used to soak the compresses, and they are applied damp every 20 minutes to maintain a cool eyelid. The cold compresses are imperative for the first 24 to 36 hours. The patient and caregiver are instructed to keep the patient's head elevated for the first week. Swelling increases for 1 to 2 days and subsides rapidly by days 5 to 7. However, complete resolution of the swelling of the

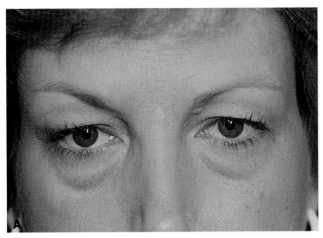 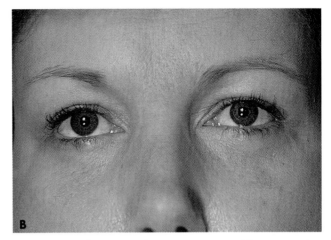

Figure 16–26. (A) A 50-year-old woman before transconjunctival blepharoplasty. **(B)** The same 50-year-old woman after transconjunctival lower blepharoplasty.

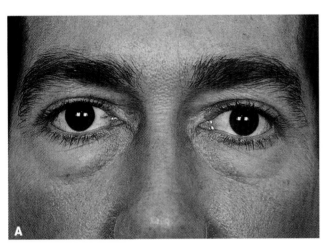 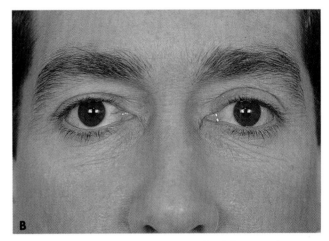

Figure 16–27. (A) A 42-year-old male patient with pre-existing rounding and pseudoherniation of orbital fat. **(B)** The same male patient who underwent a transconjunctival blepharoplasty with maintenance of the preoperative lid position.

lids may take 6 to 8 weeks. The patient is instructed on how to cleanse the suture line four times a day with a peroxide-moistened cotton-tipped applicator and to reapply the ointment to keep the wound continually moist and sealed.

The patient is instructed to restrain from any physical activity for the first 24 to 36 hours. Most patients are comfortable with returning to daily activities by the seventh postoperative day. They are encouraged to avoid any form of straining or heavy lifting for a minimum of 10 days to 2 weeks postoperatively.

A phone call is made to the patient the evening of the surgical procedure and the patient is seen the first morning postoperatively in the office. Any asymmetric

swelling or marked discoloration of one lid must be examined immediately to rule out the possibilities of preseptal or even retrobulbar hematoma. Vision and extraocular movements are confirmed and lid closure is assured. If any degree of lagophthalmos is present, the patient is instructed to put the ophthalmic lubricant in the eye while sleeping and to use artificial normal saline tears frequently during the day.

Between 5 and 7 days the skin sutures are removed. Occasionally, the lateral aspect of the upper lid suture line is reinforced with Steri-Strips for 3 more days. Makeup and cosmetic camouflage can begin at 8 days postoperatively. Makeup consultation is provided to allow the patient to return to normal social and occupational activities as soon as possible. Follow-up office visits are scheduled at 3 to 6 weeks, 3 months, 6 months, and 1 year. Occasionally, a small milia must be excised and drained for the patient along the suture line. Rarely, a slight hypertrophy can occur along the incision line requiring small amounts of intraincisional steroid to soften the scar. The aesthetic result is assessed and in the unusual circumstance that any revision needs to be made, such as further skin tightening or removal of medial fat, these are planned no earlier than 6 months postoperatively. Finally, the satisfaction of each patient is assured before release from care.

COMPLICATIONS OF BLEPHAROPLASTY
GENERAL COMPLICATIONS

Complications that can arise during upper or lower lid blepharoplasty include dry eyes, epiphora, hematoma, blindness, globe injury, infection, and suture line and wound healing complications.

Dry Eyes

A very common complaint of patients after blepharoplasty is the dry or scratchy sensation of the eye, termed dry eye syndrome. The postoperative edema interferes with normal tear production and tear flow. This is usually self-limited and resolves on resolution of edema. Persistent patient complaint of a dry eye should alert the surgeon to search for the cause to avoid problems of exposure keratitis.

It is important to rule out in the preoperative evaluation the possibility of pre-existing dry eye syndrome that can be associated with such medical systemic diseases as Sjogren's syndrome, Wegener's granulomatosis, collagen vascular diseases, and Stevens-Johnsons syndrome. This condition can be ruled out using Shirmer's test as previously described.

During the dry eye period, patients are instructed to use artificial tears several times a day and ophthalmic lubricants at night (e.g., Puralube ophthalmic ointment; E. Foougert & Co. Melville, NY).

It is imperative to rule out the possibility of damage to the lacrimal gland. The gland consists of an inner palpebral lobe and an outer orbital lobe. All tears produced in the orbital lobe must flow through the palpebral lobe before they are released to the globe. Therefore even slight injury to the inner portion of the gland may result in a poor tear film with increased dry eye symptoms.[19]

Epiphora

Assuming that the patient does not have preoperative dry eye syndrome, epiphora may be caused by either a hyperfunctioning gland caused by a reflex hypersecretion from coexisting lagophthalmos, increased vertical retraction of the lower lid, or a dysfunctional lacrimal collecting system. The latter is the most common cause and is usually self-limited. The cause of lacrimal system dysfunction can be due to such things as: (1) punctal eversion with distortion of the lacrimal system from edema; (2) impairment of the lacrimal pumping system caused by increased pressures or atony of the orbicularis oculi sling; and (3) a temporary ectropion. Damage to the lacrimal system can be prevented by keeping the transconjunctival incision lateral to the punctum. If laceration occurs, immediate repair over a Silastic stent should be performed. If punctal eversion is evident and persists, this can be managed by cauterization or diamond excision of the conjunctival surface below the canaliculus.[20]

Hematoma

Hematomas after upper or lower lid blepharoplasty can vary from small collections beneath the suture line that are self-limiting to moderate or large expanding hematomas that may extend into the retrobulbar space and lead to blindness (Fig. 16–28). Hematoma can be prevented by maintaining a normotensive pressure during the surgery and with atraumatic handling of the soft tissue and meticulous cauterization with the bipolar

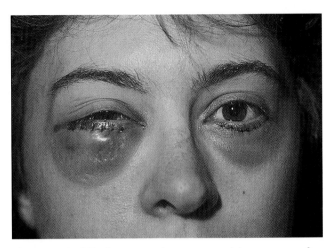

Figure 16-28. Patient with a preseptal hematoma after skin-muscle flap lower lid blepharoplasty.

cautery. Postoperatively, cold compress application to the eyes, elevation of the head, prevention of straining, and adequate pain control can prevent hematoma formation.

If a small collection is noted, this can be aspirated with a large-bore needle. Organization of the hematoma can occur beneath the skin presenting as an indurated mass. Injection of steroid (Kenalog 10) may aid with the healing process.

Retrobulbar hemorrhage is an emergency because it may result in blindness. Blindness arises because of increasing intraorbital or intraocular pressure causing central retinal artery occlusion or ischemic optic neuropathy.[21] Should a retrobulbar hemorrhage arise, immediate head elevation and orbital massage should be performed. Intravenous diuretics, mannitol, or both should be administered. Occasionally, lateral canthotomy with inferior cantholysis should be performed immediately with subsequent intraoperative exploration of the wound. Ophthalmologic consultation should be requested.

Blindness

Moser et al. have reported a 0.04% of sudden blindness after blepharoplasty.[22] Blindness usually occurs within the first 24 hours after surgery and is associated with resection of orbital fat and subsequent bleeding into the

retrobulbar space. The most common site of origin for bleeding is the lower lid medial fat pad. Cautions, such as delaying intraoperative closure, avoiding occlusive pressure–type dressings over the eyes, and extending the recovery period, facilitate early recognition of hematoma. It is imperative that an ophthalmologic consultation be obtained, as well as the emergency measures performed as previously discussed.

Globe Injury

Globe injury is an uncommon complication from eyelid surgery and is one that can be most easily avoided. Avoiding passing instruments over the eyes is the first step in preventing corneal or globe injury. The use of corneal protectors, keeping the eyelid in a closed position during upper blepharoplasty, and performing transconjunctival blepharoplasty using a 5-0 silk suture to retract the posterior lamella over the cornea are methods of preventing iatrogenic injury.

Mydriasis can be caused by inadvertent direct injection of local anesthetic into the globe or spread of the anesthetic into the sub-conjunctival space during transconjunctival anesthetic injection. This is self-limiting as the anesthetic dissipates.

With the advent of lasers and sophisticated handpiece delivery systems, blepharoplasty can be performed by use of the laser with inadvertent injury to the globe. Such injuries can be avoided through the use of anodized corneal protectors and Jaeger plates.

Infection

Infection of the upper or lower eyelid can result in a periorbital cellulitis manifested by fever, eyelid edema, chemosis, and pain. It is imperative that the patient begin an antibiotic regimen to adequately cover more common bacteria such as *Staphylococcus* and *Streptococcus*. Administration of IV antibiotics may be necessary if the patient has debilitating disease or is immunocompromised.[19]

An even rarer complication is orbital abscess as reported by Rees et al.[23] The manifestations can include proptosis, chemosis, diplopia, frozen globe, and eventually blindness. Immediate exploration and drainage of the abscess should be performed, and the patient should be placed on IV antibiotics.

Suture Line and Wound Healing Complications

Milia can occur along the incision line as a result of occlusion of epithelial debris under healed skin. Often times this is associated with simple or running cuticular sutures. The treatment is simple marsupialization of the milia and removal of the sac. Prevention consists of removing sutures 3 to 5 days postoperatively and use of subcuticular closure.

Wound healing complications can occur because of early removal of sutures or poor placement of incision lines, resulting in standing cones or webs. In addition, an adequate tissue bridge should be maintained between the lateral extensions of the upper and lower blepharoplasty incisions. Early wound dehiscence can be treated with taping, especially along the lateral portions of the incision.

COMPLICATIONS OF UPPER LID BLEPHAROPLASTY

Fortunately, complications from upper lid blepharoplasty are very rare. Complications that do occur range from minor to more serious.

Minor Complications and Expected Postoperative Occurrences

Some minor complications and expected postoperative occurrences are the following.

1. Hypertrophy of the incisional scar: Treat with intraincisional steroid and massage.
2. Indentation and visibility of the lateral aspect of the scar: No treatment or re-excise and suture.
3. Residual redundancy or asymmetry of upper lid skin: Treat with skin excision revision or evaluate predisposing factors such as asymmetry of the orbits and/or brow ptosis.
4. Recurrent or persistent nasal fat pad pseudoherniation—uncommon: Treat with an open medial incision and remove fat pad directly.
5. Webbing of the scar medially: Treat with intraincisional steroid and occasionally a Z-plasty scar revision.
6. Persistent or prolonged lid edema: No treatment other than reassurance.

More Serious Complications or Unexpected Sequela

More serious complications or unexpected sequela are the following.

1. Lagophthalmos lasting longer than 3 weeks—unusual: Treat with massage. It may resolve within 6 weeks. Corneal protection is imperative. Lubrication, eyedrops, and taping of the lid, as well as sealing the orbit at night with a Saran/Vaseline–type dressing.
2. Lagophthalmos—permanent—extremely rare: May require scar release and skin grafting.
3. Prolonged significant dry eye syndrome: Besides the treatment as for mild dry eye syndrome, one can add punctum or tear duct lugs (occlusion) and ophthalmic consultation. Most likely will resolve within 6 months.[24]
4. Ptosis (blepharoptosis): Most upper lid ptosis that seems to be caused by upper lid blepharoplasty was actually present preoperatively but unrecognized or not seen because of brow or significant excess lid skin ptosis. Ptosis of the lid present after blepharoplasty can occur from temporary stretching of the levator aponeurosis and will likely resolve within 6 weeks. True iatrogenic ptosis resulting from interruption of the levator aponeurosis is rare and would require operative repair. Involutional and senile ptosis may

require repair if exacerbated by the upper lid blepharoplasty and will not resolve within 6 to 8 weeks.[25]

5. Overresection of fat: This is most common in the central compartment and can lead to asymmetry, retraction, or too much of a deep-set appearance to the eye. Treatment with fat grafting is usually successful, variable in terms of fat graft survival.

6. Diplopia—extremely rare: Damage to the superior oblique muscle during medial fat pocket removal could potentially occur. Most occurrences are temporary from cauterization and will resolve spontaneously. Permanent diplopia can be treated with strabismus surgery.

COMPLICATIONS OF LOWER EYELID BLEPHAROPLASTY

Lower Eyelid Malposition

It is important to identify the patient who has potential for lower lid malposition in the preoperative consultation. The presence of inferior scleral show, rounding of the lateral lower lid, and a poor lid snap back and lid distraction test should alert the surgeon to the potential for postoperative ectropion (Fig. 16–29). With the addition of the lateral orbicularis suspension, the surgeon re-establishes the muscular sling preventing these complications.

With the popularity of the transconjunctival blepharoplasty, the incidence of ectropion is decreasing. The preservation of the muscular sling and the decrease in the amount of scar contracture associated with transconjunctival blepharoplasty has led to lower incidence of lower eyelid malposition.

Malposition of the lower eyelid is based on the grading system developed by McGraw and Adamson.[26] The grading is as follows: grade 0 is normal eyelid position; grade 1 is lateral rounding of the eyelid without scleral show; grade 2 is lateral rounding with central retraction with exposure of sclera below the lower limbus; grade 3 is lower eyelid eversion and pooling of tears in the inferior fornix; and grade 4 is frank ectropion with eversion of the lower eyelid and exposure of the palpebral conjunctiva. Repair of malpositioned lower eyelids is based on grade. Low-grade asymptomatic retraction will usually resolve with time and postoperative massage. If resolution of the everted eyelid does not occur within 9 to 12 months, surgical intervention should be entertained. If severe malposition occurs and is seen in the early postoperative period, it is recommended that the patient return to the operating room for skin grafting. The upper eyelid skin is a perfect donor site provided an upper blepharoplasty has not been performed. Other potential graft sites are the preauricular and postauricular areas.

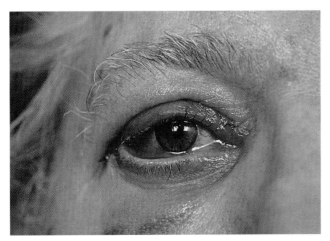

Figure 16–29. A 65-year-old male presenting with postoperative ectropion and epiphora.

Diplopia

Diplopia can occur after lower lid blepharoplasty caused by injury to the inferior oblique muscle. The diplopia usually occurs on upward lateral gaze. Recall, the muscle divides the medial and central compartments of the lower lid. If the muscle has been overly traumatized or affected by the aforementioned causes, the diplopia should resolve over time. Gentle massage may expedite the return of normal vision. Of note, the second muscle most injured during blepharoplasty is the superior oblique muscle, leading to the inability of the globe to depress and adduct.

ADJUNCTIVE PROCEDURES
LATERAL CANTHOLYSIS AND LATERAL LOWER LID SHORTENING AND SUSPENSION

During preoperative evaluation, if lower lid laxity, rounding of the lateral canthal angle, inferior scleral show, or punctal eversion exist, a lid-tightening procedure is indicated. The lower lid is further mobilized by performing a lateral canthotomy and inferior cantholysis. The lateral portion of the lower lid is then divided into an anterior musculocutaneous layer and a posterior tarsal-conjunctival layer. A tarsal strip is then created by removing conjunctiva from the posterior aspect of the tarsus and skin and muscle anteriorly. The lid itself is shortened approximately 2 mm. The tarsal strip is then attached using permanent sutures to the posterior-medial orbital periosteum approximately 2 mm inside the orbital rim just above the level of attachment of the superior limb of the lateral canthal tendon. This tightening is done in slight overcorrection.

Further sculpturing can be done by excising excess musculocutaneous tissue from the anterior surface of the strip. The standard fat removal with subsequent removal of excess skin and muscle follows the standard blepharoplasty procedure.

PINCH EXCISION TECHNIQUE

The pinch technique has been used in conjunction with transconjunctival blepharoplasty and was first described by Parkes and Bassilios and Kamer and Mikaelian.[27,28] We describe a modification to the pinch excision technique.

After completion of the transconjunctival blepharoplasty, the lower eyelid is replaced, and approximately 1 mL of 1% lidocaine with 1 : 100,000 units of epinephrine mixed with hyaluronidase (Wydase, 15 U/mL) is infiltrated subcutaneously. This is injected with a 30-gauge needle across the entire extent of lower eyelid skin and pretarsal orbicularis. Incorporation of Wydase is used to change the normal jellylike consistency of Hyaluronic acid to a liquefied form. This change in hyaluronic acid facilitates the pinching of the skin along the ciliary margin. A small nontoothed forceps is then used to tent the skin up

and a small hemostat used to pinch a strip of skin approximately 1 to 2 mm below the ciliary margin. Pinching of the excess skin is done from the lateral to medial fashion. This method allows the surgeon to visualize the amount of skin to be excised in determining whether it will result in malpositioning of the lower lid. After the pinch, if malposition occurs, the surgeon can make fine adjustments. A small scissors is then used to excise the skin ridge slightly above the level of the eyelid, being careful not to separate the cut edges. The wound can then be closed with 7-0 blue polypropylene sutures in an interrupted fashion or with the tissue adhesive Histoacryl.

CHEMICAL PEEL AND CO_2 LASER RESURFACING OF THE LOWER EYELID

Upper and lower lid blepharoplasty (transconjunctival or percutaneous) cannot effect cutaneous rhytids. Therefore periorbital rhytids can be managed with either chemical peel or CO_2 laser resurfacing.

Chemical peeling or CO_2 laser resurfacing of the lower eyelid can be performed during transconjunctival blepharoplasty. If a percutaneous method is performed, it is advisable to wait 3 months after surgery. This waiting period will help reduce vertical contracture as a result of scarring of the lower lid, thus leading to malposition. However, the surgeon should realize that significant lid skin tightening occurs after resurfacing by chemical peel or laser and that a mild ectropion can result. Therefore it is important that the patient possess good lid support before these procedures.

With Fitzpatrick's classifications of skin types as a guide, patients with skin types I to III are ideal candidates for either chemical peel or CO_2 laser resurfacing. Pigmentation abnormalities increase in patients with skin types IV to VI. In addition, Glogau's classification of photoaging is helpful in deciding the type of peel to be used. Types I and II generally show excellent improvement with medium-depth peels, whereas types III and IV are best treated with medium depth or deep peels.[29]

Classification of peeling agents is based on the depth of injury produced. Medium depth and deep peels are commonly used for the lower eyelids that demonstrate moderate actinic damage, rhytidosis, and for those patients who have contraindications for phenol peels. The changes associated with actinic damage occur at the levels of the epidermis and papillary dermis, making medium-depth peels attractive. The depth of peeling when using medium peels is directly related to the amount of solution applied, the concentration of the agents, and the preoperative skin preparation.

Application of medium-depth peels are most effectively performed by applying two superficial wounding agents to the skin. The area is initially treated with a keratolytic compound, such as Jessner's solution, before application of a 35% trichloroacetic acid. This enhances penetration and the overall result while retaining a margin of safety for the depth of injury. Postoperatively, dermal collagen deposition causes overall skin tightening and a reduction of apparent skin excess.

Deep peels are most commonly performed with phenol-based suspension, first described by Baker and Gordon in the 1960s.[30] The final concentration of phenol used is 50%, which causes injury to the deep papillary and superficial reticular dermis layers. If water is inadvertently added to the solution (i.e., tears), the solution will penetrate deeper and can cause a full-thickness injury. The phenol peel produces the greatest change in skin pigmentation and resolution of rhytids causing the greatest amount of skin tightening by subepidermal collagen deposition (Fig. 16–30).

CO$_2$ LASER RESURFACING OF THE LOWER EYELID

Cutaneous laser exfoliation is gaining widespread acceptance in many specialties involved with skin care. The advent of the CO$_2$ laser has begun to replace the chemical peel and dermabrasion because of the ability for increased precision, variable depth, and consistency. Although not completely replacing these former modalities of skin resurfacing, the laser has taken what used to be millimeter surgery to micrometer surgery. The goal of laser resurfacing is to create a clear vaporization of tissue without thermal damage beyond the impact site. The goal of the laser system is to deliver a high peak power over a short pulse duration (microseconds). Therefore creating a laser system that can deliver a high amount of energy over a time less than the thermal relaxation time for skin (695 to 950 μs) limits the thermal conduction to surrounding tissue.

Our experience is with the Ultrapulse CO$_2$ laser system (Coherent Medical Systems, Palo Alto, California) for resurfacing of the facial skin (pulse duration 600 μs).

It must be noted that the eyelid skin is the thinnest skin of the body with a thickness range of 483 to 1371 μm with the epidermis comprising 63.5 μm on average.[31] Before resurfacing of the lower eyelid, the patient's eyes are protected with a Jaeger plate or an anodized corneal shield that is inserted under the eyelids. Before corneal protection, the

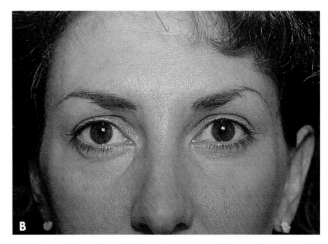

Figure 16–30. (A) A preoperative photograph of a 36-year-old woman with a minimal amount of orbital fat proptosis of the lower lids but with increased pigmentation. **(B)** A 36-year-old woman after transconjunctival lower lid blepharoplasty with an adjunctive lower eyelid Baker's solution chemical peel.

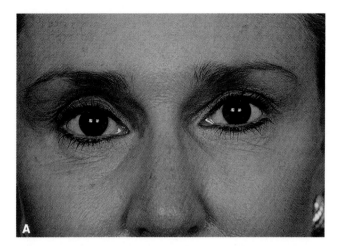 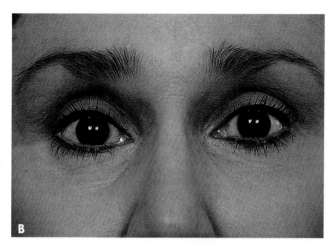

Figure 16–31. (A) A 49-year-old woman displaying fine rhytids, photo damage to the lower lid skin. **(B)** The same 49-year-old woman after transconjunctival lower lid blepharoplasty and adjunctive CO_2 laser resurfacing of the lower eyelid. Note how the dyschromia has been removed with the laser.

cornea is topically anesthetized with 0.5% tetracaine ophthalmic drops. Next, the lower eyelid skin is localized with 1 to 2% lidocaine with 1 : 100,000 units of epinephrine using a 27-gauge needle. Injections should be directed away from the globe and be as atraumatic as possible.

After adequate anesthetic time, the Ultrapulse CO_2 laser with the 2.25-mm computer pattern generator handpiece is brought into the operative field. All personnel are required to wear protective laser eyewear. Before laser use, it is imperative that a vacuum system is in place to handle the laser plume. The lower eyelid skin is divided into a thinner pretarsal and thicker preseptal skin. The laser is first set to treat the pretarsal skin. Before lasering on the patient's eyelid, the laser is first tested on a wet tongue blade to make sure it is in line with the helium-neon aiming beam. The recommended settings for laser exfoliation of the pretarsal skin is 200 mJ, a density of 4 (10% overlap), pattern 3 (square), size of 4. One pass is done over the pretarsal skin. The preseptal skin is then treated with 250 to 300 mJ, density of 5 (20% overlap), pattern of 3 (square), size of 5. On completion of the first pass over both pretarsal and preseptal skin, wet gauze pads are used to carefully remove desiccated skin. Gentle wiping of this area should be done because this is usually performed after transconjunctival blepharoplasty.

A second pass to the preseptal skin may be performed, but this would depend on the appearance of the lasered site after the first pass. After completion of laser

resurfacing, the wound is then dressed with Flexzan (Dow B. Hickman, Sugerland, Texas). This allows the wounded tissue to heal in a moist environment, facilitating reepithelialization from underlying adnexal structures. The Flexzan dressing will be removed in 4 days, at which point the patient will begin application of a topical ointment consisting of Aquaphor (Beiersdorf Inc., Norfold, CT) or Vaseline (Chesebrough-Ponds Co. USA, Greenwich, CT).

Postoperative care will consist of having the patient routinely clean the lasered sites with deionized/bottled water and cotton-tipped applicators or cotton balls. Between each cleaning, the patient will then apply the ointment. Erythema will gradually decrease over a period of 5 to 10 days. Persistent erythema is often seen in patients of Fitzpatrick's groups IV to VI. The erythema can be treated with topical steroid creams (Figs. 16–31 and 16–32).

EYELID MICROPIGMENTATION

Micropigmentation is a technique for dermal tattooing of the eyelash. The procedure is ideally performed with the patient under local anesthesia with intravenous sedation. Before the procedure, it is important that a cosmetic consult be placed to determine the appropriate color selection and desired position of the dye.

The micropigmentation must be done before blepharoplasty. Otherwise, stray pigment will stain any incision line, suture hole, or even needle stick site.

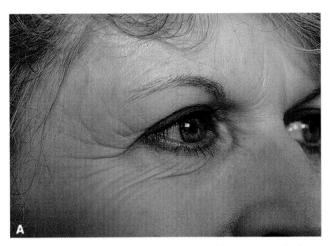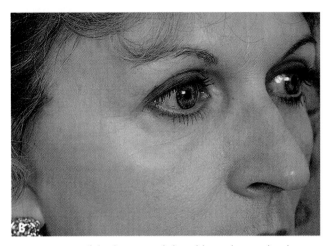

Figure 16–32. (A) This is a 52-year-old woman with deep expression creases of the lower eyelid and lateral periorbital area. In addition, a moderate amount of upper lid dermatochalasis and lateral skin hooding is present. **(B)** The same patient after a transconjunctival blepharoplasty, upper lid blepharoplasty, and adjunctive lateral and lower eyelid CO_2 laser resurfacing.

An oscillating handpiece with tapered needles (1 to 3) is used to apply the pigment. The needles are dipped into the pigment and the excess is removed. A Jaeger plate is placed into the fornix of the lower eyelid to maintain tension of the eyelid and to protect the globe. Oscillation at a high rate is needed to drive the pigment into the dermis. This procedure is repeated until dye deposition is satisfactory (Fig. 16–33).

The most common early postoperative complication is that of uneven application. Another disappointing complication is the fact that micropigmentation is not permanent. We have found that the pigment may fade or disappear within 3 to 6 years. Overall, this is a very valu-able adjunctive procedure for cosmetic enhancement of blepharoplasty.[32,33]

CONCLUSION

Upper and lower blepharoplasty can be an ideal primary surgical procedure for many patients who present for upper face rejuvenation. It is imperative that the surgeon understand the indications, as well as contraindications, of each particular operative technique. It is important to listen to the patient's desires during the preoperative consultation. Equally important is the

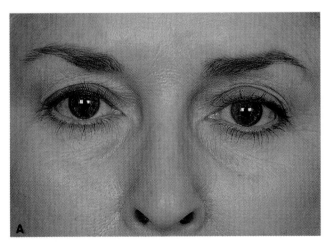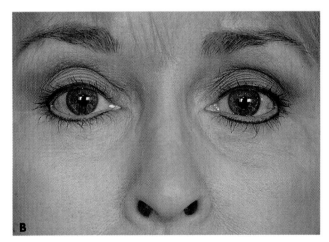

Figure 16–33. (A) A preoperative photo of a woman desiring permanent upper and lower eyeliner and rejuvenation of the upper face. **(B)** The same patient after micropigmentation of the upper and lower eyelids. The patient had an upper and transconjunctival lower lid blepharoplasty after micropigmentation.

surgeon's ability to convey to the patient what is realistic and achievable. The surgical techniques presented provide the surgeon an armamentarium to safely correct the defects of dermatochalasis, pseudoherniation of orbital fat, orbicularis muscular hypertrophy and festooning, actinic damage and dyschromia of the eyelid skin, and malposition of the eyelids. A firm grasp of the upper and lower eyelid anatomy is important to avoid complications and to arrive at a result that is aesthetically pleasing and natural. In addition, the surgeon must recognize the complications from each surgical technique. Early recognition can prevent the long-term sequela of scarring, malposition of the eyelids, and vision loss.

Adjunctive procedures have been presented to further enhance and complement the blepharoplasty procedure.

PEARLS

- During physical examination, quick release of the eyelid and evidence of a slow return or apposition to the globe signifies potential risk for ectropion, epiphora, and exposure keratitis, which may warrant a lid-tightening procedure.
- If upper blepharoplasty is performed in conjunction with a skin-muscle or skin flap technique, the surgeon must maintain a ridge of tissue between the lateral extensions of the upper and lower blepharoplasties that measures at least 6 mm, preferably 10 mm.
- To avoid postoperative dry eye syndrome, preexisting conditions that cause this syndrome (e.g., Sjogren's syndrome, Wegener's granulomatosis, collagen vascular diseases, Stevens-Johnson syndrome) must be ruled out in the preoperative evaluation.

REFERENCES

1. Small RE. Extended lower lid blepharoplasty. *Arch Ophthalmol.* 1981; 99:1402–1405.
2. Holt JE, Holt JR. Blepharoplasty: Indications and preoperative assessment. *Arch Otolaryngol.* 1985; 111:394.
3. Beekhuis GJ. Blepharoplasty. *Otolaryngol Clin North Am.* 1982; 15:179–193.
4. Pastorek N. Upper lid blepharoplasty. *Facial Plast Clin North Am.* 1995:143–157.
5. Putterman A. *Surgical Treatment of the Upper Eyelid Dermatochalasis and Orbital Fat.* 1993:94–116.
6. Smith B, Petrelli R. Surgical repair of prolapsed lacrimal gland. *Arch Ophthalmol.* 1978; 96:113–114.
7. Leone CR. Treatment of a prolapsed lacrimal gland. *Cosmetic Oculoplast Surg.* 1993:186–195.
8. Crumley RL, Arden RL. Lower lid blepharoplasty. *Facial Plast Reconstr Surg.* 1992; 19:169–178.
9. Smullen SM, Mangat DS. Cosmetic lower eyelid surgery: Transcutaneous approach. *Facial Plast Surg Clin North Am.* 1995; 3:167–174.
10. Becker FF, Deutsch BD. Extended lower lid blepharoplasty. *Facial Plast Surg Clin North Am.* 1995; 3:189–194.
11. McCullough EG, English JL. Blepharoplasty: Avoiding plastic eyelids. *Arch Otolaryngol Head Neck Surg.* 1998; 114:645.
12. Wolfey DE. Blepharoplasty: The ophthalmologist's view. *Otolaryngol Clin North Am.* 1980; 13:237.
13. Bourquet J. Les hernies grasseuses de l'orbite: Notre traitment. *Chir Bull Acad Natl Med (Pano).* 1924; 92:1270–1272.
14. Jackson I, Schielz V, et al. The conjunctival approach to orbital floor and maxilla: Advantages and disadvantages. *Ann Plast Surg.* 1987; 19:45–48.
15. Shore JW. The fornix approach to the interior orbit. *Adv Ophthalmic Plast Reconstr Surg.* 1987; 6:377–385.
16. Bayless HI, Long JA, Groth JF. Transconjunctival lower eyelid blepharoplasty, technique and complications. *Ophthalmology.* 1989; 96:1027–1032.
17. Perkins SW, Dyer WK, Simo F. Transconjunctival approach to lower eyelid blepharoplasty: Experience, indications, and techniques in 300 patients. *Arch Otolaryngol.* 1994; 120:172.
18. Palmer FR, Rice DH, Churukian MD. Transconjunctival blepharoplasty complications and their avoidance. A retrospective analysis and review of literature. *Arch Otolaryngol Head Neck Surg.* 1993; 119:993–999.
19. Adamson PA, Constantinides MS. Complications of blepharoplasty. *Facial Plast Surg Clin North Am.* 1995; 3:211–221.
20. Arden RL, Crumley RL. Lower lid blepharoplasty. *Facial Plast Reconstr Surgery.* 1992; 19:169–177.
21. Hartley JH, Lester JC, Schatten WE. Acute retrobulbar hemorrhage during elective blepharoplasty. *Plast Reconstr Surg.* 1993; 52:8–15.
22. Moser MH, Dipirro E, McCoy FJ. Sudden blindness following blepharoplasty. Report of seven cases. *Plast Reconstr Surg.* 1973; 51:364.
23. Rees PD, Craig SM, Fisher Y. Orbital abscess following blepharoplasty. *Plast Reconstr Surg.* 1984; 73:126–127.
24. Becker BB. Punctal occlusion patients with dry eye syndrome. *Arch Otolaryngol Head Neck Surg.* 1991; 117:789–791.
25. Millay DJ, Larrabee WF. Ptosis and blepharoplasty. *Arch Otolaryngol Head Neck Surg.* 1989; 115:198–201.
26. McGraw BL, Adamso, PA. Post blepharoplasty ectropion. *Arch Otolaryngol Head Neck Surg.* 1991; 117:852–856.

27. Parkes MI, Bassilios MI. Experience with the pinch technique in blepharoplasty. *Laryngoscope.* 1978; 88:364–366.

28. Kamer FM, Mikaelian AJ. Pre-excision blepharoplasty. *Arch Otolaryngol Head Neck Surg.* 1991; 117:995–999.

29. Brody HJ. *Chemical peeling.* St. Louis: C.V. Mosby/Yearbook; 1992.

30. Baker TJ, Gordon HL. The ablation of rhytids by chemical means in a preliminary report. *J Fla Med Assoc.* 1961; 48: 451.

31. Oyama MM, Schoenrock LD Transconjunctival blepharoplasty with simultaneous laser resurfacing, operative techniques. *Otolaryngol Head Neck Surg.* 1997; 8:37–42.

32. Angres GG. The Angres Permalid-liner method to enhance the result of cosmetic blepharoplasty. *Ann Ophthalmol.* 1985; 17:176–177.

33. Wilkes TD I. The complications of dermal tattooing. *Ophthalmic Plast Reconstr Surg.* 1986; 2:16.

Revision Blepharoplasty

The section on revision blepharoplasty, written by Drs. Millman and Silver, represents an excellent amalgam of approaches to surgery that has not achieved its desired objective. It should be stressed that both authors easily recognize that it is preoperative evaluation and surgical planning that are probably the most important factors in avoiding the need for revision of blepharoplasty or any surgical procedure.

Dr. Silver, a facial plastic surgeon, presents excellent techniques that are accessible to surgeons of all specialties. He uses an analytic method of correcting various lid malpositions that could result from blepharoplasty and addresses the more subtle aspects of aesthetic insufficiencies and their corresponding corrections.

Dr. Millman, an oculoplastic surgeon, complements Dr. Silver's chapter with addition of a number of oculoplastic reconstructive techniques that have their roots and foundations in functional problems such as the reconstruction of eyelids that have been lost to cancer or trauma and the adjustment of eyelids distorted by physiologic diseases such as thyroid lid retraction and senescent lid malpositions. These procedures are based on deep anatomic structures such as the periosteum, canthal retractors (i.e., levator aponeurosis and lid retractors), and the use of composite grafts to accomplish the desired results.

The true definition of a successful aesthetic blepharoplasty is the achievement of an improvement of both form and function.

Revision Blepharoplasty

Aesthetic Facial Plastic Surgery, edited by Thomas Romo, III, and Arthur L. Millman, Thieme Medical Publishers, Inc., New York, New York, Copyright © 2000.

CHAPTER 17

An Oculoplastic Surgeon's Perspective

ARTHUR L. MILLMAN

Cosmetic blepharoplasty is, of course, a procedure to enhance the appearance and function of the eyelids and the adnexa or surrounding anatomy of the eyelids. Revision blepharoplasty is frequently done for two main reasons: (1) insufficient cosmetic result or (2) functional complication. The goal of revision blepharoplasty is, in essence, the same that of primary blepharoplasty: to provide the patient with an ideal aesthetic result while maintaining or improving ideal functional performance of the eyelid in its role as the protector of the ocular surface and its interaction with the surrounding adnexa (i.e., the brow, canthus, cheek, and midfacial area).

Cosmetic complications generally can be attributed to undercorrection and overcorrection or blepharoplasty that has not taken into account other findings in the adnexa of the brow, canthus, and midface. In my experience the most common aesthetic complaint in an unhappy or unsatisfactory blepharoplasty patient is the presence of residual temporal hooding caused by the presence of brow ptosis, residual herniated orbital fat caused by undercorrection, asymmetric lid levels caused by either undiagnosed pre-existing or subsequent changes in lid levels, postoperative ptosis, ectropion, or entropion.

The anatomy in blepharoplasty is naturally divided into upper and lower lid components. We will begin with the upper lid. I must emphasize that accurate and meticulous preoperative evaluation is imperative. Insuffi-cient initial evaluation and surgical planning often result in the need for revision of an unacceptable result.

UPPER LID

The most common upper lid finding that presents for revision is residual dermatochalasia or temporal hooding. This is most commonly due not to undercorrection of the upper lid skin resection but to the presence of pre-existing and previously undiagnosed, or purposefully untreated, brow ptosis. An endoscopic brow elevation is certainly the procedure of choice to complete the blepharoplasty and improve lid contour, lid crease, and relieve temporal hooding while improving brow position (Figs. 17–1 and 17–2). The procedure is ideally done with a permanent

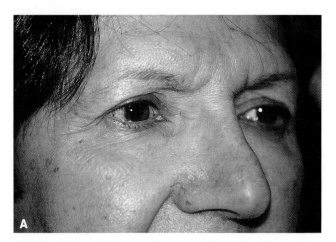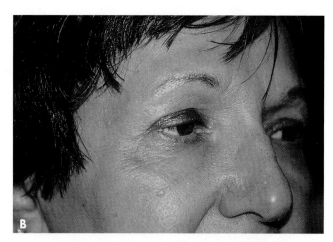

Figure 17–1. (A) Status after upper lid blepharoplasty with persistent temporal hooding as a result of brow ptosis. **(B)** Endoscopic browlift relieves brow ptosis.

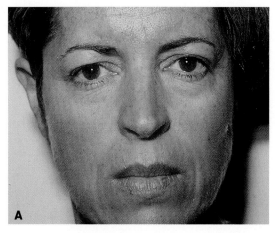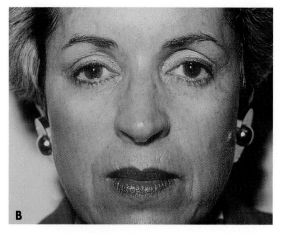

Figure 17–2. Lateral canthoplasty procedure demonstrated (also see Fig. 17–15).

fixation technique with pericranial tunnels or titanium tacks (see Chapters 13 and 14).

On the other side of that coin is overcorrection, where the surgeon overcorrects or overresects the dermatochalasia, removing too much skin from the upper lid, which, ironically, is usually due to the same initial judgment error, the presence of pre-existing brow ptosis. A good blepharoplasty rule of thumb is that a minimum of approximately 20 mm of upper eyelid skin, specifically 10 mm from lid margin to lid crease and 10 mm from the lid crease to the eyebrow, should be present. The pre-existing brow ptosis gives the appearance of exuberant upper lid skin, and overresection is performed in an attempt to resolve this, without treating the primary problem, brow ptosis. In these patients the revision surgeon is left with the dilemma of a lid lag or a tethered lid in down gaze (see Fig. 17–5). Frequently, lagophthalmos, or the inability to close the eyelid, further results in exposure keratopathy and a dry eye syndrome.[1,3] Treatments for the surface of the eye that will increase the available tear secretion and improve ocular lubrication should be considered first. Punctal occlusion and topical artificial eyedrop therapy and lubricants both during the day and at night are the first step in medical management. (Botox to the frontalis to induce brow ptosis and increase eyelid closure is a temporary fix during the first 3 to 6 postoperative months.) Surgical management can take the form of canthoplasty, in which the lateral canthus can be either closed by small tarsorrhaphy or elevated to improve lower lid position to meet the upper lid (Fig. 17–3). In severe cases an upper lid skin graft may be necessary. The graft usually is taken from a retroauricular donor site and placed between the lid lash line and the new upper lid crease positions (Fig. 17–4). This is frequently cosmetically unacceptable because the graft is typically visible. Finally, a brow release can be performed by release of the arcus marginalis and brow fixation, either endoscopically or transcutaneously through the lid crease, to purposefully increase brow ptosis and brow mobilization. The eyelid-orbital septum should be lysed or extirpated (see Fig. 17–5). This will increase the amount of available skin to the upper lid and allow the lid

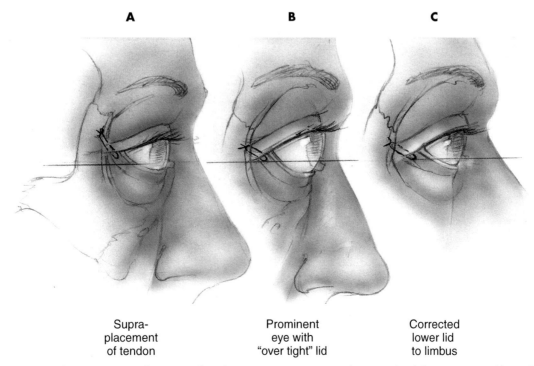

| A | B | C |
| Supra-placement of tendon | Prominent eye with "over tight" lid | Corrected lower lid to limbus |

Figure 17–3. Canthoplasty. **(A)** Supraplacement of tendon. **(B)** Prominent eye with "overtight" lid. **(C)** Corrected lower lid to limbus.

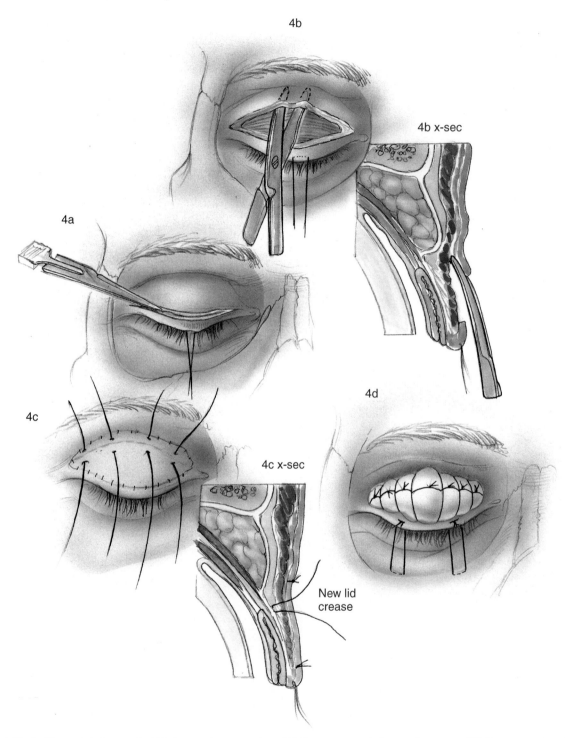

Figure 17–4. Upper lid skin graft. **(A)** Supraciliary incision. **(B)** Free retracted skin and septum. **(C)** Retroauricular donor skin graft. **(D)** Cotton bolster sewn in.

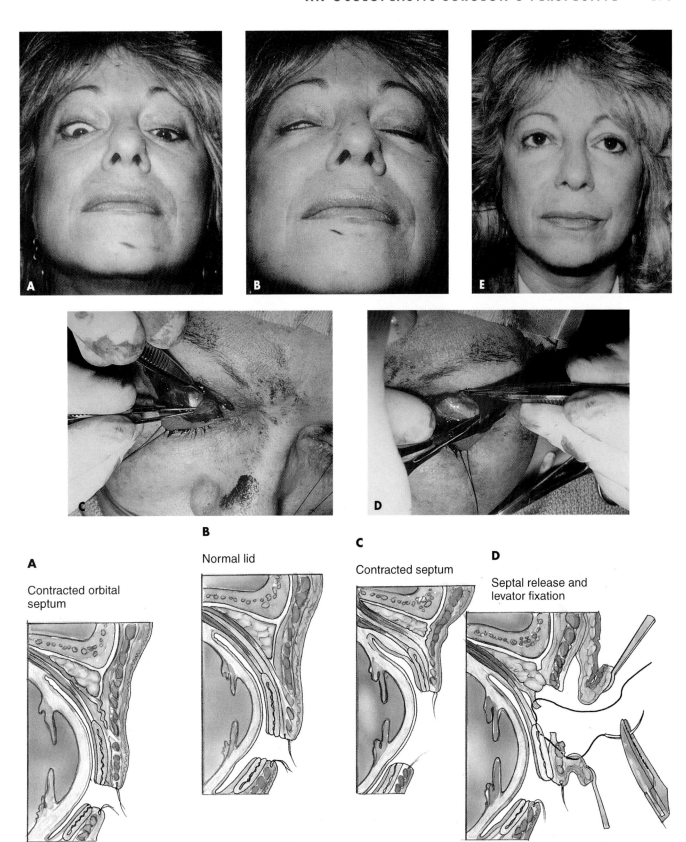

Figure 17–5. (A) After blepharoplasty with contracted orbital septum and skin shortage causing lid lag and **(B)** lagophthalmos, which was intraoperatively corrected by **(C)** isolating the orbital septum (the levator is the white aponeurotic tissue posterior to the septum in the forceps) and **(D)** completely disinserting and extirpating the septum. **(E)** This corrected lid lag, lid retraction, and lagophthalmos in this patient without use of skin grafting.

to close and reduce tethering; however, a side effect may be worsening of the brow ptosis, yielding a good functional but diminished aesthetic result. The last method to approach the tethered and overcorrected upper lid is actually to turn to the lower lid and improve its position.

LOWER LID

Lagophthalmos, or the inability to close the eye, is the most unwanted complication of blepharoplasty, both functionally and aesthetically.[4] In general, I approach the lower lid first in an attempt to both aesthetically and functionally improve the patient's situation. Again, medical management with tear duct closure and lubricants must be tried first. Next, vertical elevation of the lower lid can be used to compensate for a tethered upper lid or lid lag. A shortage of lower lid skin caused by overresection is classically treated by replacement or a lower lid skin grafting technique (see Fig. 17–6). A

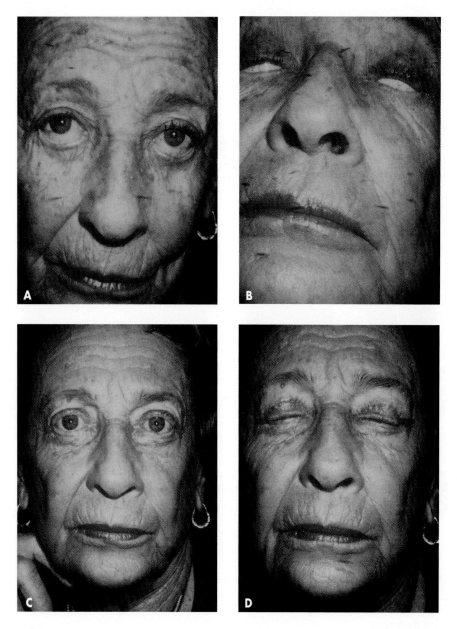

Figure 17–6. After blepharoplasty with lower lid skin shortage— overcorrection. **(A)** Lower lid retraction and ectropion are seen as is **(B)** lagophthalmos. **(C)** Postoperative lower lid skin graft corrects lower lid position and **(D)** upper lid closure.

skin graft frequently can be avoided. By placing a vertical spacer as an infratarsal transconjunctival graft, which can be made from hard palate mucoperichondrium, eye bank scleral graft, or auricular cartilage, the lower lid can be vertically elevated (Figs. 17–7 and 17–8). This procedure can be combined with lateral canthopexy, the septomyocutaneous flap, or the subperiosteal midface lift.

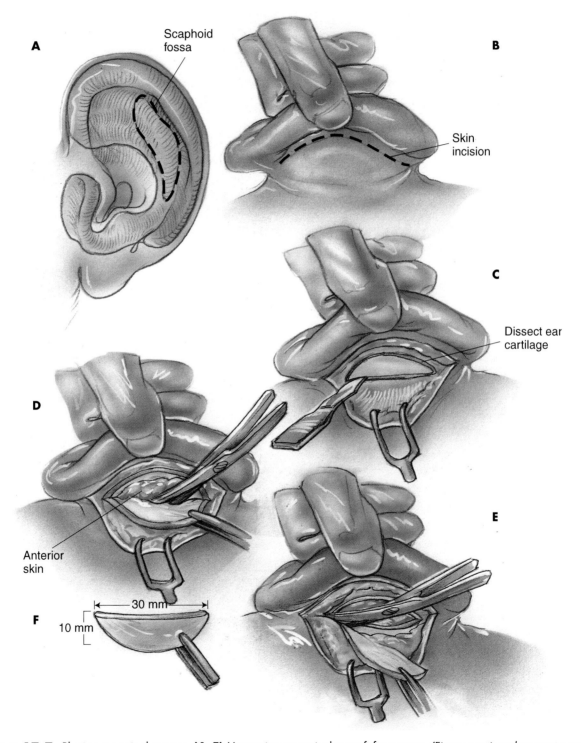

Figure 17–7. Placing a vertical spacer. **(A–F)** Harvesting or auricular graft for spacer. *(Figure continued on next page)*

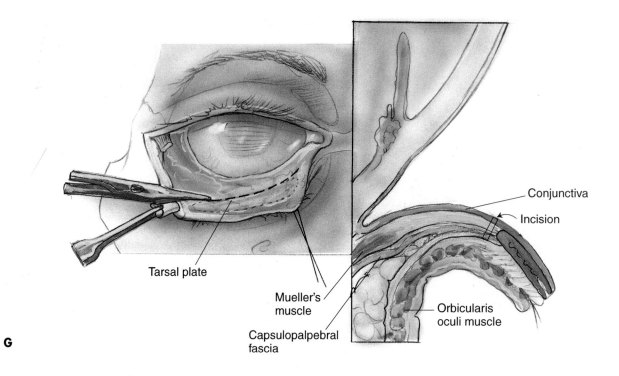

Conjunctiva

Incision

Tarsal plate

Mueller's muscle

Orbicularis oculi muscle

Capsulopalpebral fascia

G

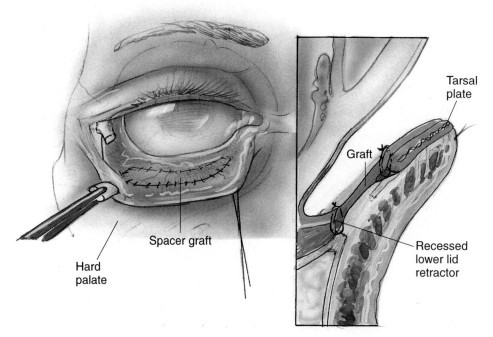

Tarsal plate

Graft

Spacer graft

Hard palate

Recessed lower lid retractor

H

Figure 17–7. *(continued)* **(G–H)** Surgical placement of hard palate or auricular cartilage graft at inferior tarsal border.

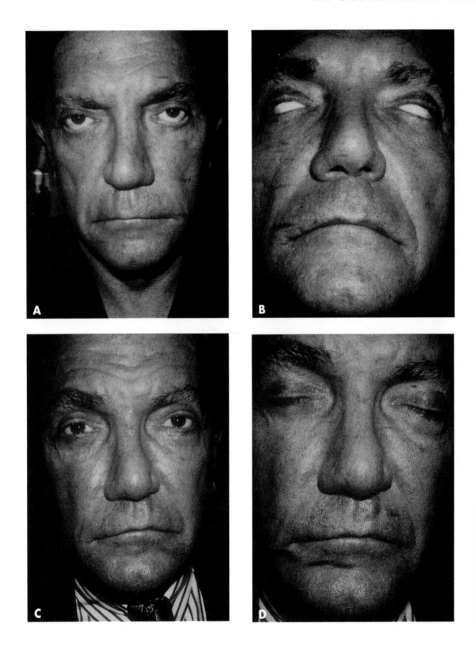

Figure 17–8. (A) Lower blepharoplasty with skin shortage and lid retraction and **(B)** severe lagophthalmos. **(C)** Postoperatively, lower lid hard palate grafts or auricular cartilage posterior spacers correct lid levels and **(D)** normalize closure (without use of skin grafts).

An integrated composite approach to the lower lid that integrates all the preceding techniques, including a vertical spacer to vertically level the lid and augmentation of the lower lid skin and lateral canthus by skin grafting or midface lifting to further enhance lower lid contour and lower lid level (Fig. 17–9).[5,7] This allows the lids to meet and improve corneal or ocular protection.

Last, the septomyocutaneous flap[9] is an ideal method for improving lower lid position and improving skin contour without resorting to grafting techniques. In Figure 17–10A, B, it is demonstrated that this approach improves lid level, tension, and function, as well as skin tone. This can be combined with lower lid skin resurfacing with either the carbon dioxide or erbium: YAG technique or combined laser technique[10] (Fig. 17–10C, D).

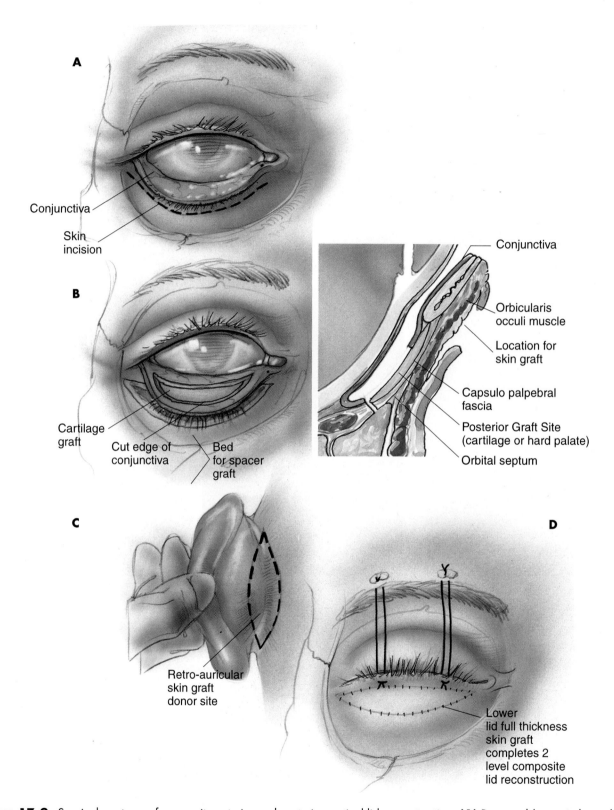

Figure 17-9. Surgical anatomy of composite anterior and posterior vertical lid reconstruction. **(A)** Retracted/ectropic lower lid. **(B)** Recession of lower lid retraction at inferior tarsal border creates bed for auricular cartilage or hard palate posterior spacer graft. **(C)** Harvesting of full skin size for anterior lamellar expansion **(D)** at infraciliary edge.

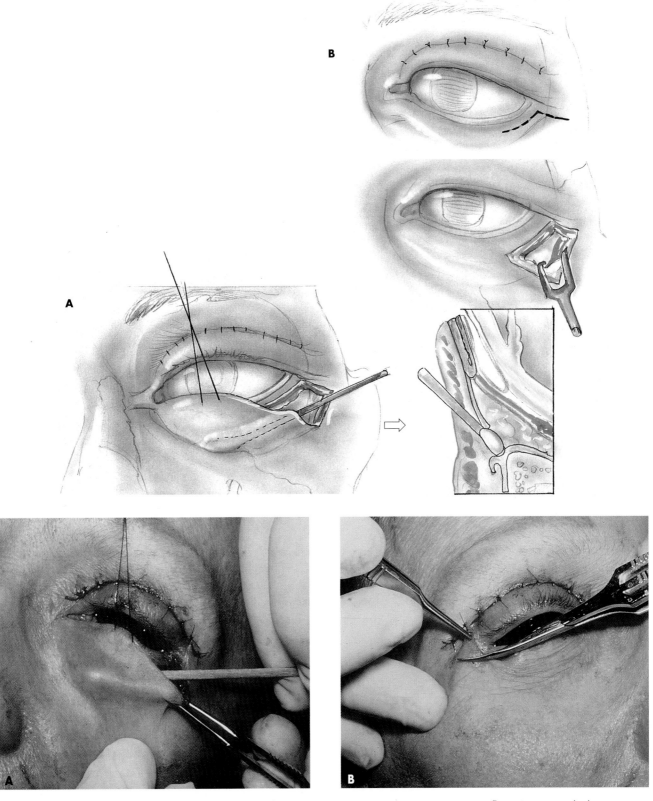

Figure 17-10. Anatomy of the septomyocutaneous flap. **(A)** Intraoperative septomyocutaneous flap. Cotton swab demonstrates retroseptal space and septomyocutaneous flap. **(B-G)** Intraoperative removal of lower lid skin is all lateral to the edge. Preoperative **(H)** and postoperative **(I)** views of lower lid septomyocutaneous flap with laser CSR. *(Figure continued on next page)*

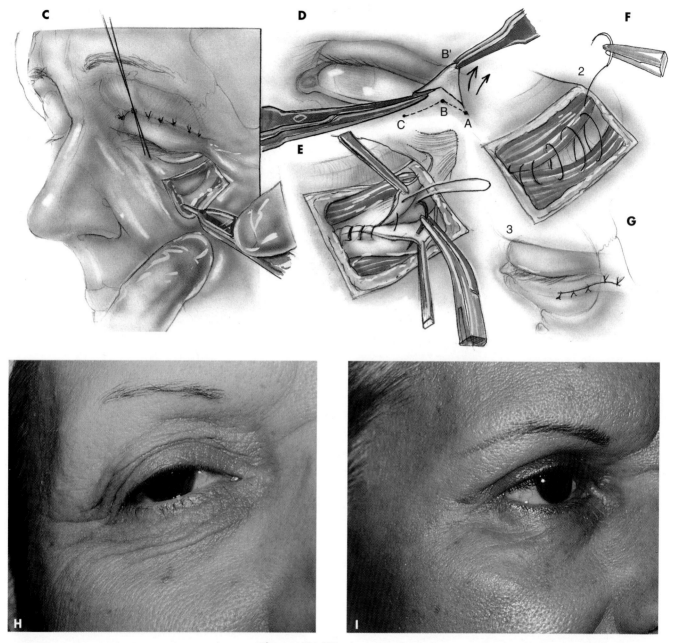

Figure 17–10. *(continued)*

Finally, the surgeon must certainly identify qualitative versus quantitative aspects to the aesthetic surgery evaluation and determine whether quantitative problems, such as removal of anatomic substrate of skin and fat is necessary, or qualitative problems, such as texture, skin tone, wrinkling, and rhytides, should be

improved by means of laser skin resurfacing techniques (Fig. 17–11).

Finally, just as attention to the brow is critical to upper lid evaluation, attention to the midface and cheek is critical to the lower lid evaluation. The presence of malar festoons must be elucidated because they

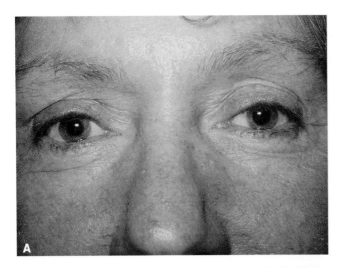

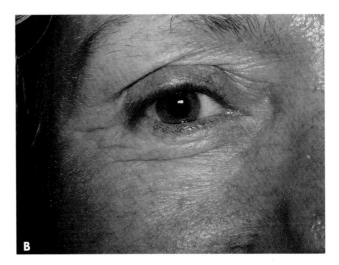

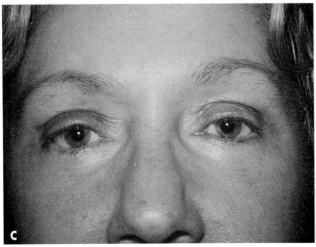

Figure 17–11. (A) After upper lid blepharoplasty with residual "qualitative" findings of eyelid rhytides.
(B) Close-up: Note upper lid skin texture and upper lid crease-fold complex. **(C)** Six months postoperatively, laser resurfacing only (*no* skin incisional surgery) of all four upper lids. Note improved skin texture and reformed upper lid crease.

will not be improved by conventional blepharoplasty. Festoons should be treated separately by either midface lifting or combined septomyocutaneous flap, as previously described, with or without aggressive lower lid skin resurfacing. I prefer to use a septomyocutaneous flap with CO_2/erbium: YAG laser resurfacing. I have had many patients come in with a successful blepharoplasty pointing to their malar festoons as the cause of their concern and if these were treated initially patient satisfaction would have been achieved (Fig. 17–12).

Last, the use of the midface lift to subperiosteally lift the entire midface and cheek complex allows for the cre-

ation of additional excess skin, which can relieve overcorrection of vertical skin resection in the lower lid transcutaneous blepharoplasty. It is clear in this day and age that skin excision in standard blepharoplasty is almost unnecessary with transconjunctival technique and the use of either lateral septomyocutaneous flaps or skin shortening by cosmetic laser skin resurfacing. However, when lower lid lag and retraction is produced by overresection of skin, a midface lift can be used to create excess skin, relieve the lid position and tethering, and create an overall improved aesthetic result.

Lower lid skin shortage has traditionally been treated by skin grafts (Fig. 17–6). The subperiosteal

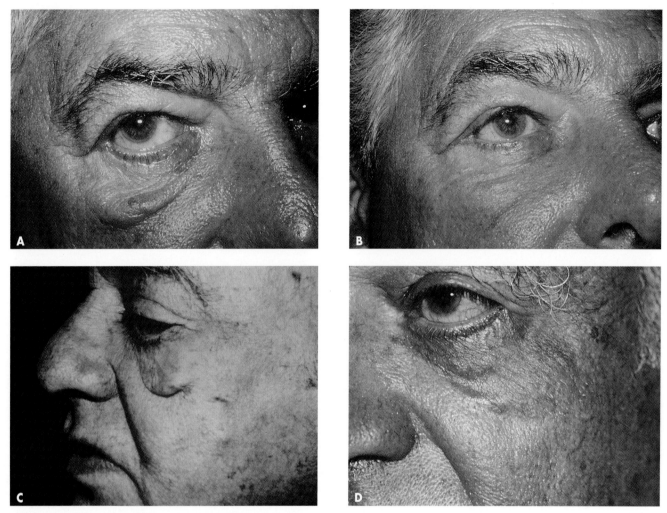

Figure 17–12. (A,C) Preoperative and **(B,D)** postoperative views of malar festoons in two patients who had previous standard blepharoplasties without improvement. After septomyocutaneous flap with laser CSR.

midface lift as described by McCord and Hester[5,6] is such a powerful method to elevate the cheek and lower lid as a composite flap that the need to consider free skin grafting in the lower lid is rarely, if ever, needed. This technique, shown in Figure 17–13A–C, uses an infraciliary incision to isolate the lower lid retractors and sever the orbital septum completely. A subperiosteal flap is then started at the inferior orbital rim and developed across the entire face of the maxilla, sparing the infraorbital nerve and canal. It is critical to completely release and sever the periosteum (as in endoscopic brow technique) to allow for directly vertically upward mobi-

lization of the midface. This creates an enormous amount of residual lower lid skin and allows relief of lid retraction (Figs. 17–14 to 17–18).

An additional fine point can added here for the relief of overcorrected lower lid fat pad resection. A prominent inferior orbital rim, hollowness of the lower lid and orbit, or apparent descent of the malar fat pad can be addressed simultaneously with the midface lift. The lift elevates and repositions the malar cheek pad over the rim. Alone or in combination, the surgeon can release the residual orbital fat on a vascular pedicle and drape it anteriorly over the inferior orbital rim.[8] This recreates a

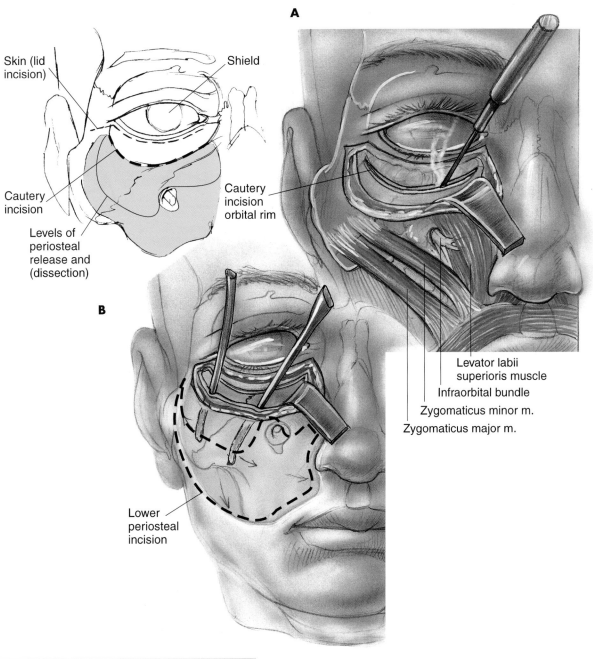

Skin (lid incision)

Shield

Cautery incision

Cautery incision orbital rim

Levels of periosteal release and (dissection)

B

Lower periosteal incision

Levator labii superioris muscle

Infraorbital bundle

Zygomaticus minor m.

Zygomaticus major m.

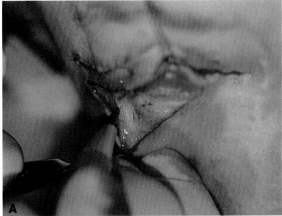

Figure 17–13. Midface cheeklift. **(A)** CO_2 cutting laser approaches midface transpalpebrally. *(Figure continued on next page)*

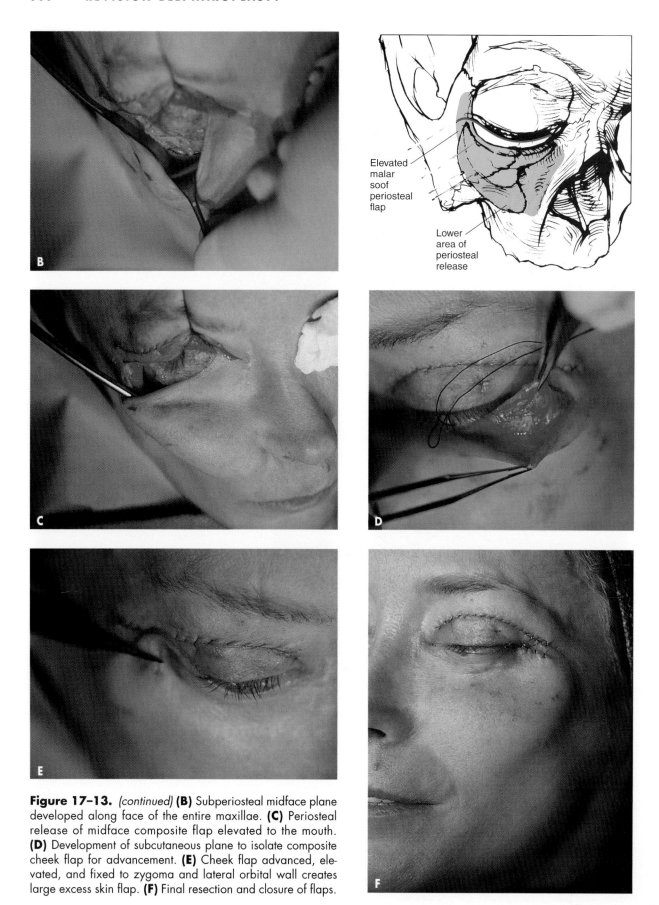

Elevated
malar
soof
periosteal
flap

Lower
area of
periosteal
release

Figure 17–13. *(continued)* **(B)** Subperiosteal midface plane developed along face of the entire maxillae. **(C)** Periosteal release of midface composite flap elevated to the mouth. **(D)** Development of subcutaneous plane to isolate composite cheek flap for advancement. **(E)** Cheek flap advanced, elevated, and fixed to zygoma and lateral orbital wall creates large excess skin flap. **(F)** Final resection and closure of flaps.

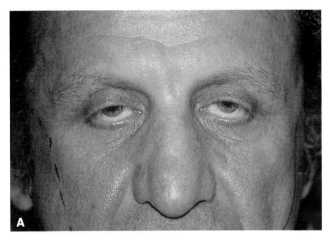
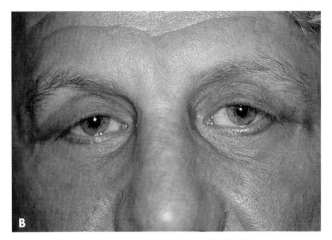

Figure 17–14. (A) Preoperative and **(B)** postoperative views of the subperiosteal midfacelift with relief of lid retraction and improved lid and malar contour.

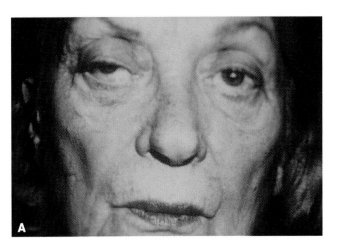
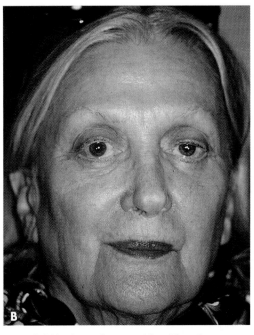

Figure 17–15. (A) Preoperative view shows patient 6 years after upper lid blepharoplasty and facelift with asymmetric upper lid level and herniated fat nasally. Bilateral lower lid retraction, midface ptosis, and tear trough deformity. **(B)** After revision blepharoplasty and subperiosteal midfacelift with laser CSR.

smooth flow from ocular surface to lid margin to the orbital rim and cheek (Figs. 17–15 and 17–18).

The surgical strategy for the lower lid and cheek, be it primary or revision, is thus critically based on the patient's individual anatomic and aesthetic findings.

Finally, lid malpositions as a complication of cosmetic blepharoplasty (Fig. 17–16), such as ectropion, entropion, or lid retraction, need be addressed. Postop-

erative ectropion repairs have been well described in the literature and generally correspond to lower eyelid laxity and failure of the surgeon to recognize and correct laxity horizontally lateral lid tension by means of a lateral canthal suspension (see Fig. 17–15). Postoperative entropion, which is usually due to disinsertion of the lower lid retractor or capsulopalpebral fascia dressing transconjunctival or transcutaneous lower lid blepharoplasty tech-

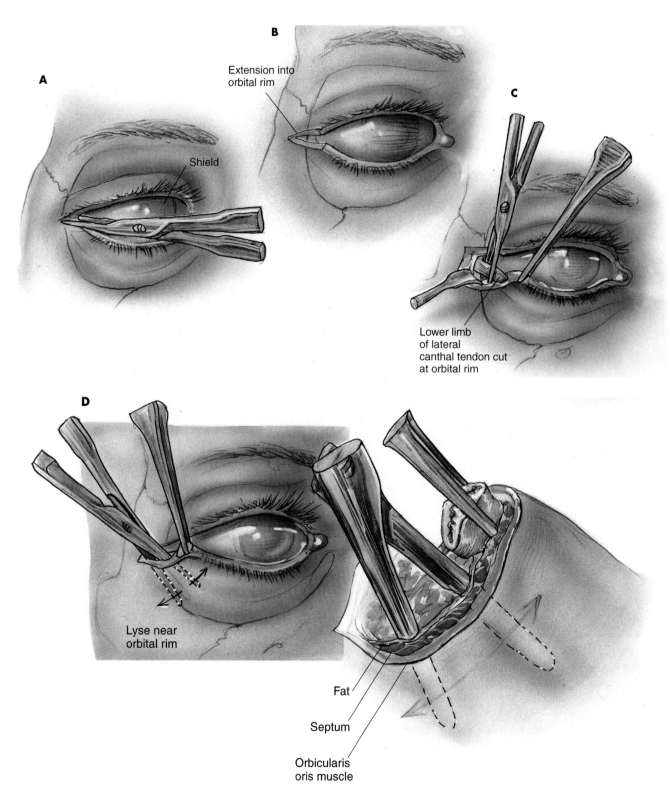

Figure 17–16. Surgical technique showing horizontal lid shortening by lateral canthal suspension. **(A,B)** Canthotomy. **(C–E)** Lateral tendon-inferior crus lysed and lid mobilized. **(F–H)** Formation of lateral tarsal strip. **(I–N)** Permanent fixation and suspension of tarsal strip to lateral orbital rim. *(Figure continued on next page)*

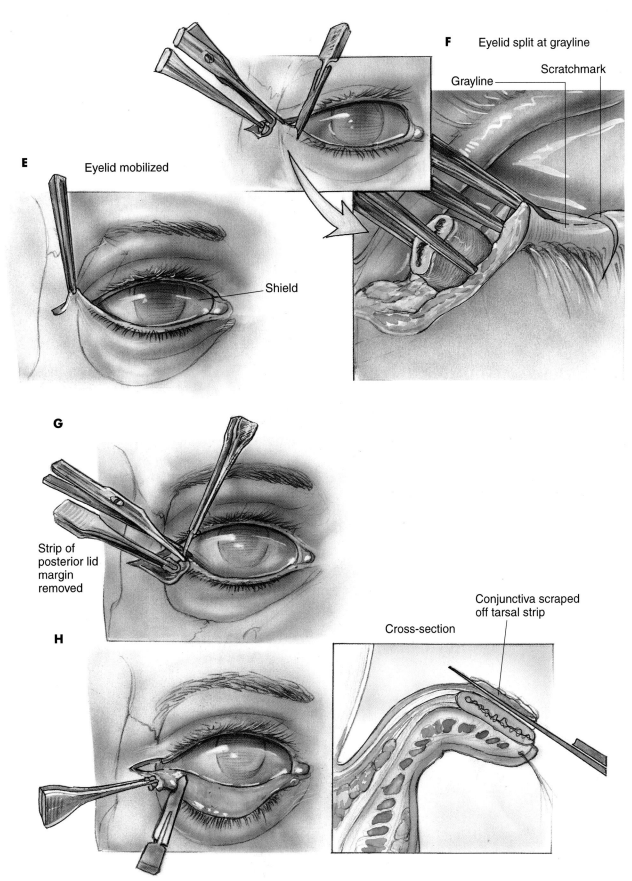

F Eyelid split at grayline

Grayline — Scratchmark

E Eyelid mobilized

Shield

G

Strip of posterior lid margin removed

H

Cross-section

Conjunctiva scraped off tarsal strip

Figure 17–16. *(Figure continued on next page)*

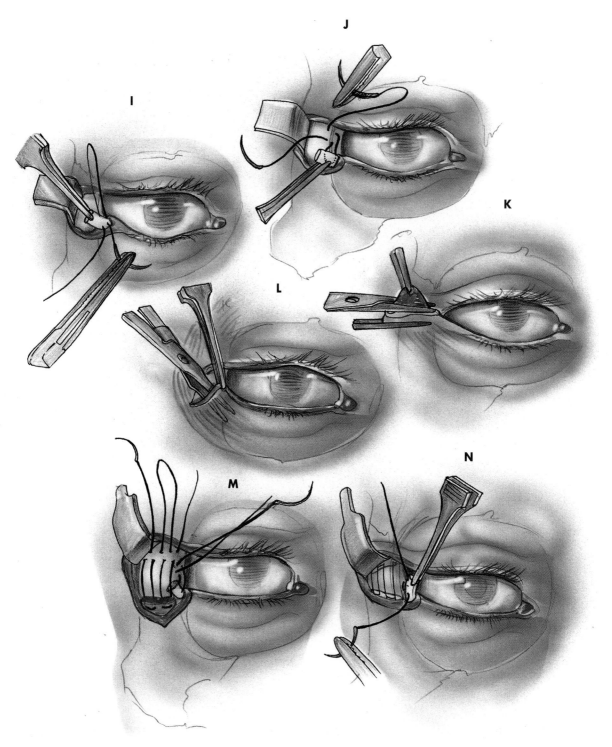

Figure 17–16. *(continued)*

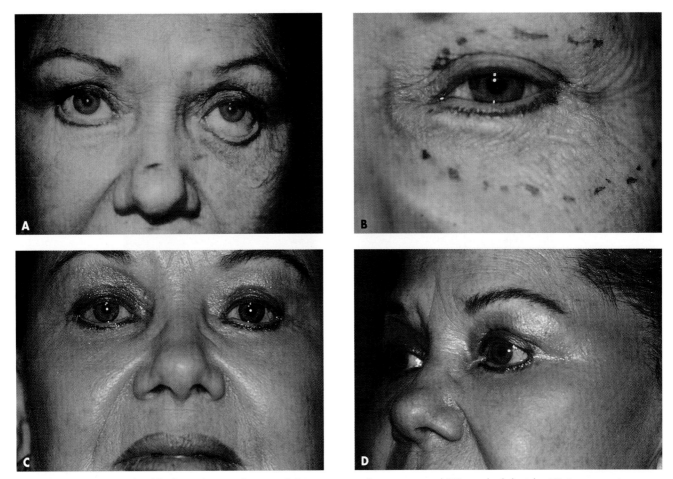

Figure 17–17. (A) After blepharoplasty with severe lid retraction and ectropion and **(B)** residual rhytids. **(C)** Postoperative ectropion repair by canthopexy and **(D)** laser CSR.

nique, requires reconnection and attachment of the lower lid retractor to the inferior tarsal border. This is usually combined with horizontal shortening, such as a lateral canthal suspension as previously described (see Fig. 17–16). Canthopexy can be combined with laser skin CSR for enhanced skin tone (Fig. 17–17).

CONCLUSION

It is clear that in revision blepharoplasty, as with any revision aesthetic procedure, the most important factor for success is a detailed and exacting initial evaluation that yields an initial surgical plan to encompass all aspects of the aesthetic facial patient. For blepharoplasty, this particularly focuses on the evaluation and impact of the surrounding anatomic adnexa of brow position, midfacial and malar findings, and lateral canthal findings (Figs. 17–13 to 17–18). Failing initial successful surgery, revision surgery must take into account those findings that were not addressed at primary surgery and correct them secondarily.

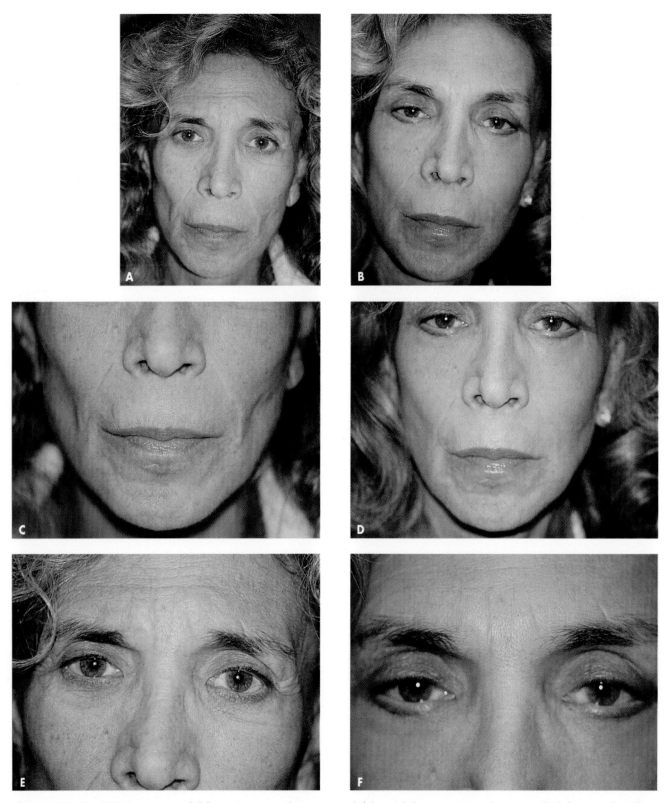

Figure 17–18. (A) Preoperative full-face view. Note brow ptosis, left lower lid retraction, and tear trough deformity of midface ptosis. Previous blepharoplasty caused nasolabial folds. **(B)** Postoperative full-face view. Note resolved brow, cheek, and lid ptosis and improved nasolabial folds. **(C)** Preoperative and **(D)** postoperative close-ups of the midface of the same patient show nasolabial fold elevation. **(E)** Preoperative and **(F)** postoperative close-ups of the lower lid of the same patient show orbital rim and cheek trough deformity resolved.

PEARLS

- Identify the error in either surgical judgment, pre-operative evaluation, or operative technique that was responsible for the complication or patient dissatisfaction.

- Determine the least amount of surgery and least aggressive technique to improve, even if not completely eradicate, the surgical complication.

- Do not hesitate to consult with colleagues or sub-specialists in related fields for help after a surgical complication.

- Using best judgment, if it is clear that a result is becoming undesirable. I find in aesthetic patients it is best to act more promptly than less promptly. This is quite the opposite in functional surgery patients because usually a greater amount of time and understanding on the patient's part, is available to allow surgeries to heal completely.

- Most lower lid complications are due to inadequate evaluation and treatment of horizontal laxity and tension. Correct placement of the lateral canthal tendon and good eyelid tension is usually the best method of repair.

- Most upper eyelid abnormalities are related to crease asymmetry or inadequate eyelid crease formation, and success is generally based on the ability to create a symmetric and properly formed eyelid crease by levator supratarsal fixation to the skin-muscle flap.

REFERENCES

1. Baylis HI, Sutcliff T, Fett DR. Levator injury during blepharoplasty. *Arch Ophthalmol.* 1984; 102:570–571.
2. Smith B, Nesi FA. The complications of cosmetic blepharoplasty. *Ophthalmology.* 1978; 85:726.
3. Levine MR, Boynton J, Tenzel RR, et al. Complications of blepharoplasty. *Ophthalmic Surg.* 1975; 6:53–57.
4. Nelson E, Baylis HI, Goldberg RA. Lower lid eyelid retraction following blepharoplasy. *Ophthalmic Plast Reconstr Surg.* 1992; 8:170–175.
5. Hester TR, Codner MA, McCord CD. Subperiosteal malar cheek lift with lower blepharoplasty. In: McCord CD, Codner MA, eds. *Eyelid Surgery. Principles and Techniques.* Philadelphia: Lippincott-Raven; 1995.
6. Hester TR, Codner M, McCord CD. The "centrofacial" approach for correction of facial aging using the transblepharoplasty subperiosteal cheek lift. *Aesthetic Surg Q.* 1996; 16:51.
7. Shorr N, Fallor MK. "Madame Butterfly" procedure combined with cheek and lateral canthal suspension procedure for post blepharoplatsy "round eye" and lower lid retraction. *Ophthalmol Plast Reconstr Surg.* 1985; 1:229.
8. Hamra ST. Arcus marginalis release and orbital fat preservation in mid–face rejuvination. *Plast Reconstr Surg.* 1995; 96:354.
9. Millman AL, et al. The septomyocutaneous flap in lower lid blepharoplasty. *Ophthalmol Plast Reconst Surg.* 1997; 13:2–6.
10. Millman AL, et al. Convalsescent histopathology of combined erbium: YAG and carbon dioxide cosmetic laser skin resurfacing. *Am J Ophtholmol.* April-May 1999.

Revision Blepharoplasty

Aesthetic Facial Plastic Surgery, edited by Thomas Romo, III, and Arthur L. Millman, Thieme Medical Publishers, Inc., New York, New York, Copyright © 2000.

CHAPTER 18

A Facial Plastic Surgeon's Perspective

WILLIAM E. SILVER, DAVID A. KIEFF, AND ALI SAJJADIAN

When a patient presents for revision blepharoplasty, either for cosmetic reasons or to correct a functional complication, the goals are the same as that of the primary blepharoplasty.

In the upper lids, the ideal result, consists of (1) good space between eyebrow and upper lashes; (2) no residual excess skin; (3) minimally visible, healed incision in supratarsal crease, 10 to 14 mm above the lash line; (4) clear view of the skin over tarsus; (5) no residual fat pad bulging; (6) no ptosis; (7) no lid lag. In the lower lids, the ideal results include (1) minimal residual rhytids, (2) no rounding or scleral show, (3) no residual fat pad bulging, and (4) an imperceptible, healed incision within a subciliary crease.

With these criteria in mind as goals, it is important to understand that failure to meet all of them does necessarily represent a complication. This chapter will focus on how revision surgery can help to achieve the preceding goals. Complications of blepharoplasty are reviewed in Chapters 15 and 16.

Right brow
ptosis

Left brow
normal

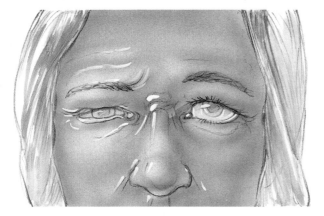

Figure 18–1. Schematic diagram of concomitant excess upper eyelid skin and brow ptosis greater on the right than the left.

INDICATIONS FOR REVISION UPPER EYELID BLEPHAROPLASTY

BROW PTOSIS

If the inferior margin of the eyebrows is close to the upper lashes preoperatively, a full forehead lift or direct browlift may be indicated. If the browlift is indicated and not performed with the blepharoplasty, postoperative revision may become necessary (Fig. 18–1). If the brow ptosis is minor, a browpexy may be adequate.[1] Care must be taken that the eyelid skin is not overresected when a forehead lift (endoscopic or coronal) or a direct browlift and the upper lid blepharoplasty are concomitantly performed. Failure to preserve adequate skin can lead to lagophthalmos (Fig. 18–2).

SCARS

The upper lid incisional scar should optimally fall within the upper lid crease (at the level of the superior margin of the tarsal plate). An exception is if the goal is to raise the level of the crease, as is sometimes done in an Asian eyelid, when a supratarsal fixation is planned. This is usually accomplished by making the incision 10 to 12 mm above the lash line and placing a supratarsal fixation suture[2] (Fig. 18–3).

Superiorly Displaced Scars

A difficult problem arises when the incisional scar falls above the supratarsal crease (Fig. 18–4). Superior displacement of the incisional scar may occur from overresection of minimally excessive skin when removing large fat pads. The incision may heal in a more superior position than intended in such instances when the bulging fat is removed. This results from "excess" skin being needed to fill in the concavity left by the fat resection. The only treatment for such scar malposition is to make a secondary lower incision and resect the skin and primary incisional scar above the secondary incision, thereby moving the final crease/scar down to the site of the secondary, lower incision. The crease can then be fixed to the lower position with supratarsal fixation sutures.[2] Extreme caution must be taken preoperatively to ensure that adequate redundant skin is present to perform this maneuver. If necessary skin is not present, the procedure should not be performed.

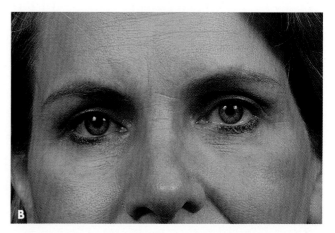

Figure 18–2. (A) Patient with excess upper eyelid skin and brow ptosis greater on the right than on the left. **(B)** Postoperative results after bilateral upper lid blepharoplasty and endoscopic forehead lift with greater elevation of the right brow.

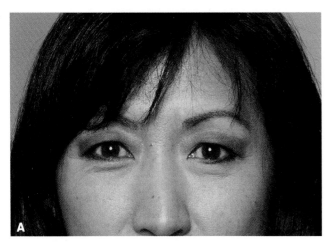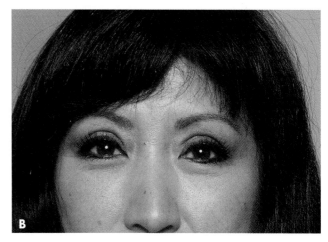

Figure 18–3. (A) Preoperative Oriental eyelid with a very low supratarsal crease. **(B)** Postoperative photographs after correction with repositioning and fixating the supratarsal crease superiorly.

Inferiorly Displaced Scars

If the upper lid incision heals more inferiorly than intended (i.e., less than 10 mm above the lash line), a new incision at 10 to 14 mm above the lash line can be made (Fig. 18–5). Supratarsal fixation sutures can be placed to reposition the crease superiorly.

Widened Scars

Widened scars can be treated in much the same manner as a superiorly displaced scar. A secondary incision with scar resection and subsequent closure may be indicated. Five milligrams of Aristocort may be injected after the closure (i.e., 0.5 ml of 10 mg/mL suspension). Laterally widened scars are much easier to correct than centrally or medially widened scars. In all cases of scar revision, accurate closure

with fine (6.0 nonreactive) mattress sutures and Steri-strips is necessary to prevent further widening from occurring. If the scar is irregular, it can also be excised as in the preceding.

RESIDUAL UPPER LID SKIN

The most common reason for performing revised cosmetic blepharoplasty is residual upper lid skin. The two most frequent causes of residual upper lid skin are inadequate primary resection and primary brow ptosis.

Inadequate Resection

In the case of inadequate primary resection, the excess residual skin can be excised with the patient under local anesthetic. Standard closure follows (Fig. 18–6).

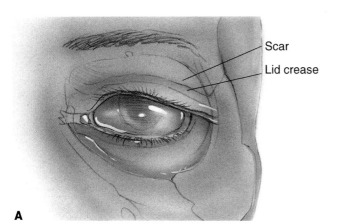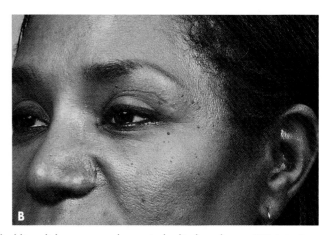

Scar

Lid crease

Figure 18–4. (A) Schematic diagram of the relative position of lashline, lid crease, and superiorly displaced scar. **(B)** A patient with a superiorly displaced scar after upper lid blepharoplasty. The patient was referred for correction, but elected not to undergo the procedure.

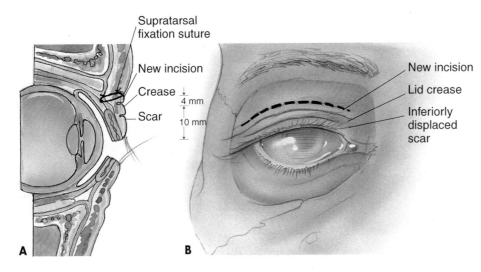

Figure 18–5. (A) Lateral view correction of inferiorly displaced scar using supratarsal fixation technique. Note that the lid crease should be between 10 to 14 mm superior to the lash line. In this technique the levator aponeurosis is sutured to subdermis and orbicularis oculi muscle. This will allow for the crease to be repositioned superiorly in a more natural position. This technique is similar to the one used for correction of an Oriental eyelid. **(B)** Frontal view, note the relative position of inferiorly displaced scar lid crease and the new incision.

Primary Brow Ptosis

Brow ptosis may cause residual skin to become apparent (Fig. 18–7). Brow ptosis is more common in men than women. After healing takes place, the supratarsal fold may fall over the pretarsal skin. This is due to the brow being too close to the lashes primarily. Such patients may be chronic browlifters to compensate for their marked blepharochalasis. After their primary blepharoplasty, these patients will tend to relax the frontalis muscles, leading to a reappearance of brow ptosis and blepharochalasis.

In these cases an endoscopic forehead lift or a direct browlift may be a solution. A supratarsal fixation can also prevent this problem. An endoscopic forehead lift is the technique that we prefer for treatment of brow ptosis. It has minimal morbidity and predictable results in trained hands. The scars are small and can often be hidden in the hairline. Excessive browlifting can cause lid lag and should be avoided.

A direct browlift is the most accurate, long-lasting, and predictable technique to correct brow ptosis. However, it does leave a visible scar.[3] A direct browlift is either performed with an asymmetric brow incision or an incision at the upper margin of the brow. Care is taken to bevel the incision to preserve the brow's follicles. Then an ellipse of skin is removed above the brow, and the incision is fastidiously closed.

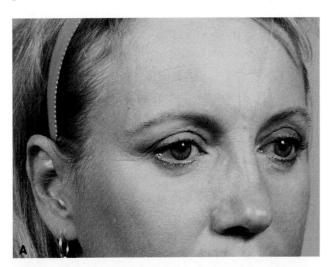
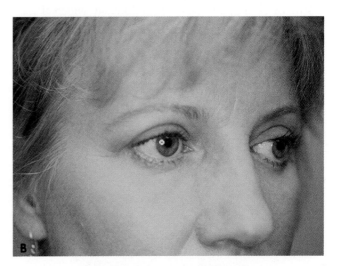

Figure 18–6. (A) Preoperative view of inadequate excision of upper eyelid skin after blepharoplasty. **(B)** Postoperative view of removal of an additional amount of upper eyelid skin.

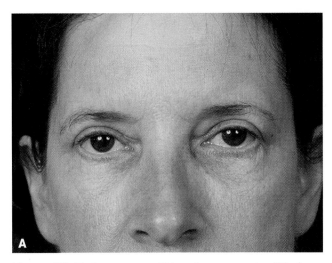
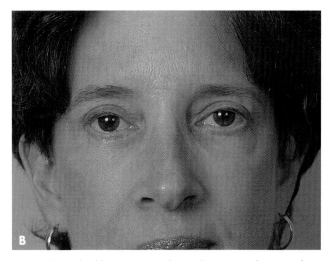

Figure 18–7. Preoperative **(A)** and postoperative **(B)** photos of patient with marked brow ptosis who underwent endoscopic fore-head lift and upper lid blepharoplasty. If the endoscopic forehead lift had not been performed, residual upper eyelid skin would have been present.

A browpexy is the easiest way to treat brow ptosis. Its effect is limited by the small amount that the brow can be elevated. The browpexy is performed through the upper eyelid incision.[1] (Fig. 18–8).

RESIDUAL FAT PAD BULGING

Bulging residual fat is probably the second most frequent reason to perform revision blepharoplasty. Bulging resid-ual fat may occur for two reasons. First, opening the sep-tum to resect fat during primary blepharoplasty may allow orbital fat to migrate forward as the eyelid heals. Second, a small pocket of fat may have been overlooked during the primary blepharoplasty. It may then become visible as healing takes place.

In the upper eyelid the most common site to find resid-ual fat pad bulging is medially (Fig. 18–9). The fat can be resected with a small incision in the previous scar (Fig. 18–10). Minimal to no sedation is necessary. Local anesthesia is all that is required in a cooperative patient. After the skin is incised, the dissection is primarily performed by spreading. The residual septal tissue covering the pad is opened. Fat that prolapses out is removed in the usual man-ner. The small incision is closed with a subcuticular suture.

POSTOPERATIVE UPPER LID PTOSIS

Some cases of mild unilateral upper lid ptosis may not be recognized until after the blepharoplasty has healed. At that stage, mild ptosis that was unnoticed preopera-tively may become more apparent because the upper lid hooding has now been removed from the ptotic eyelid. This is probably the most common "cause" of unilateral mild ptosis after blepharoplasty. To avoid this ptosis post-operatively, careful preoperative evaluation must be per-formed and accurate photos taken. Evaluating the patient preoperatively at different times of the day may also help to reveal mild ptosis. Ptosis that is due to upper lid pto-sis is distinct from ptosis resulting from levator aponeu-rosis disruption. Ptosis from levator disruption is a true complication of blepharoplasty and is considered in Chapter 15 and 16.

If ptosis exists before blepharoplasty, it should be corrected by shortening the levator aponeurosis (Fig. 18–11). To get the necessary intraoperative cooperation from the patient to make an accurate ptosis repair, the patient must be minimally sedated. If the ptosis is recog-nized preoperatively, the blepharoplasty and ptosis repair

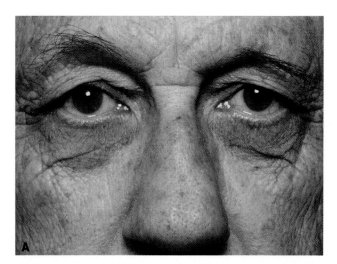
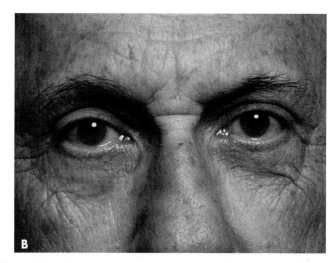

Figure 18-8. Preoperative **(A)** and postoperative **(B)** photos of a patient who underwent revision bilateral upper lid blepharoplasty with browpexy.

can be addressed simultaneously. When performing a blepharoplasty, we prefer a direct approach to the levator aponeurosis. Imbricating the aponeurosis to the tarsal plate or reattaching the aponeurosis to the tarsal plate can repair the dehiscent levator (Fig. 18–12). If correction is performed secondarily, either the Fasanella-Servat procedure or Mueller muscle-conjunctiva resection are the procedures of choice[4,5] (Fig. 18–13).

INDICATIONS FOR REVISION LOWER EYELID BLEPHAROPLASTY

RESIDUAL LID RHYTIDS

The most common indication for lower lid revision blepharoplasty is persistent lower lid rhytids. It is extremely important to explain preoperatively that

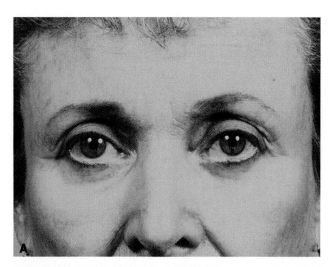
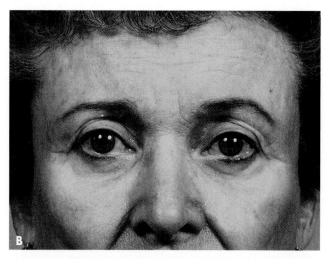

Figure 18-9. (A) Postoperative blepharoplasty with residual medial fat pad. **(B)** Revision upper lid blepharoplasty with removal of medial upper lid fat compartment.

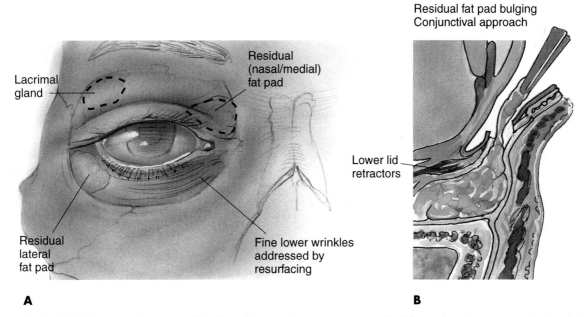

Figure 18–10. (A) Schematic diagram of the frontal view of postoperative residual fat pad in the upper medial and the lower lateral compartments and also some fine residual rhytids in the lower eyelid skin. **(B)** Saggital view of correction of the residual lower lid fat compartments through a transconjunctival approach with rhytids corrected with CO_2 laser resurfacing.

lower lid blepharoplasty may not remove all fine lower lid rhytids. Patients may develop an unrealistic expectation that lower lid blepharoplasty alone will remove the fine wrinkles of the lower eyelid skin. If fine lid rhytids are a major concern, skin resurfacing with a CO_2 laser or chemical peel should be part of the primary procedure (Figs. 18–10 and 18–14). If skin resurfacing is to be part of the primary procedure, we recommend a transconjunctival approach for the blepharoplasty.

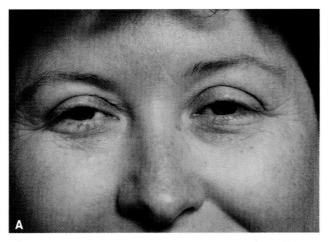
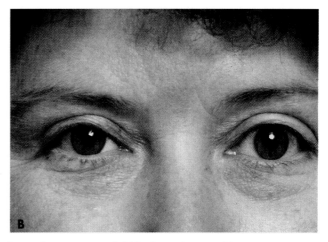

Figure 18–11. Preoperative **(A)** and postoperative **(B)** patient who underwent upper lid blepharoplasty and levator aponeurosis imbrication to tarsal plate to correct bilateral upper lid ptosis.

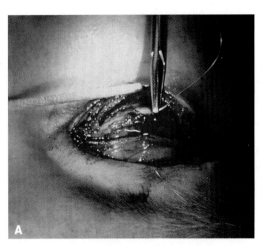
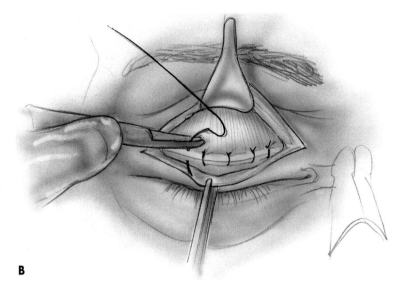

Figure 18–12. (A) Intraoperative photo of aponeurosis being sutured to the superior margin of the tarsal plate to correct upper lid ptosis. **(B)** Schematic diagram showing suturing of tarsal plate to levator aponeurosis.

If a CO_2 laser is to be used for resurfacing the lower lids, the following points should be observed.

1. One pass is sufficient.
2. With the Ultra Pulse CO_2 laser, the settings should be 250 mJ at 30% overlap.
3. For thicker skin or deep rhytids, the power may be increased to 350 mJ. (Because more lasering can be performed later, always err on undertreating.)
4. Crow's feet can be treated up to 400 mJ with two passes or 450 mJ at one pass.
5. If the lower lid blepharoplasty is performed through a subciliary approach, resurfacing should be delayed 12 weeks. Resurfacing lower lids without a delay after a subciliary approach can lead to an ectropion from cicatrix formation.
6. A snap back test should be performed before primary or secondary resurfacing of lower lids to ensure that the lids are strong enough to prevent ectropion formation.

If chemical peel is used instead of the CO_2 laser, we prefer a Jessner 45% triabloroacetic acid (TCA) solution. The Baker's phenol peel is too strong and we do not rec-

ommend its use as a peel in conjunction with blepharoplasty because of the risk of an ectropion.

RESIDUAL BULGING FAT PADS

Residual fat is the second most common reason for revision lower lid blepharoplasty. Residual fat most often is seen in the lateral compartment (Fig. 18–10). The incidence of this problem can be reduced if the blepharo-

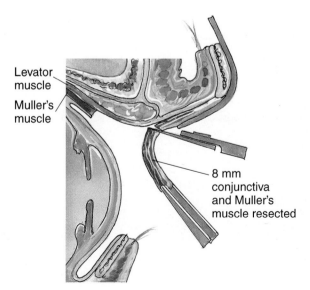

Figure 18–13. Schematic diagram of Mueller's muscle resection for correction of upper lid ptosis.

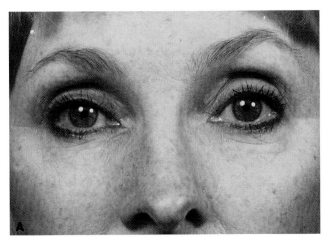 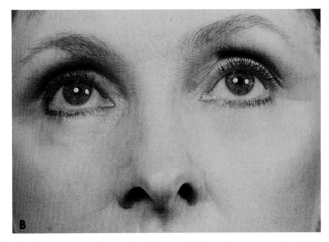

Figure 18–14. Preoperative **(A)** and postoperative **(B)** lower lid blepharoplasty with residual lower lid rhytids treated with CO_2

plasty is performed under minimal sedation. The lateral fat pad can be accentuated by having the patient gaze right when the left pad is being addressed and vice versa. Another maneuver is to re-examine the lateral compartment before completing the lower lid blepharoplasty. If a residual fat pad is noted after healing is complete, revision is best performed through a transconjunctival approach. Revision surgery should be delayed at least 6 months to minimize the scarring that is encountered.

LOWER LID RETRACTION

Lid retraction can appear early or late in the healing process (Fig. 18–15). When it occurs early (as in 1 to 2 weeks), the problem may be solved by injecting dilute (10 mg/mL) triamcinolone into the lid's soft tissues followed by upward taping for 7 days. If retraction persists or occurs late in the healing process (i.e., greater than 4 weeks), revision surgery may be warranted. It is important to review the patient's preoperative photos before revision surgery to determine whether scleral show was present preoperatively, because it may have been unrecognized.

Lower lid retraction is more common after blepharoplasty performed by a subciliary rather than transconjunctival approach. If the lower lid is noted to be lax before surgery, a lid shortening procedure should be considered as an adjunct to the lower lid blepharoplasty.

Revision surgery for lower lid retraction typically involves shortening and elevating the lateral portion of the lower lid. This requires a lateral canthotomy, exposure of the tarsal tendon after removal of the excess skin and conjunctiva laterally, and repositioning of the tendon laterally and superiorly[6,7] (Fig. 18–16).

HYPERTROPHIC SCAR

Hypertrophic incisional scarring may occur after a subciliary approach. This may result if the incision is made too close to the ciliary margin and not in a pre-existing crease. A tendency also exixts for a scar to form if the lateral limb of the incision is closed under tension.

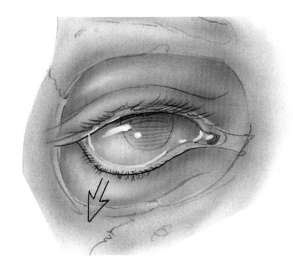

Figure 18–15. Lower lid retraction, frontal view showing the retraction of the lower lid away from the globe.

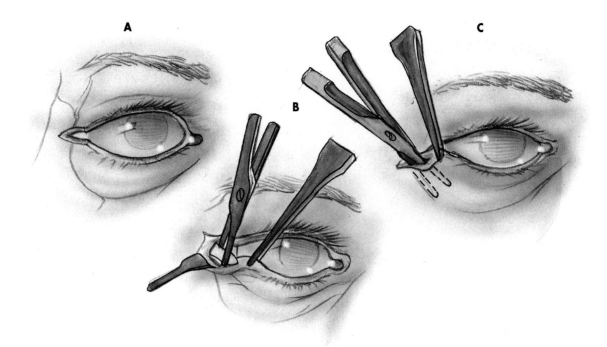

Figure 18–16. Surgical treatment of lower eyelid retraction after blepharoplasty.

Hypertrophic scarring can be treated with steroid injections (0.5 ml of 10 mg/mL dilute triamcinolone suspension) or with CO_2 laser resurfacing. If scar excision is necessary, the presence of adequate skin for closure must be ensured. Adding hyaluronidase to the local anesthetic (Wydase, 75 units in 10 mL of local) will help separate the skin from the muscle so that the scar can be more readily resected and the margins reapproximated. Precise closure is important. Taping the lateral portion of the incision for 7 to 10 days will optimize the resulting scar.

CONCLUSION

Blepharoplasty is one of the most satisfying cosmetic procedures for both the patient and the surgeon. Serious complications may occur but are rare. Minor problems do occur that may warrant revision treatment. It is important to differentiate serious complications from minor problems that indicate revision surgery. Careful preoper-

ative assessment will always help prevent postoperative problems. Minimal, precisely targeted intervention is often the best approach to correct suboptimal results of primary blepharoplasty.

PEARLS

- Endoscopic forehead lift is best to correct brow ptosis because is has minimal morbidity and its results are predictable when performed by a skilled surgeon.
- If skin resurfacing is being performed as part of primary blepharoplasty to avoid lid rhytids, a transconjunctival approach should be used.
- To avoid risk of ectropion, Baker's phenol peel should not be used in conjunction with blepharoplasty.

D

E

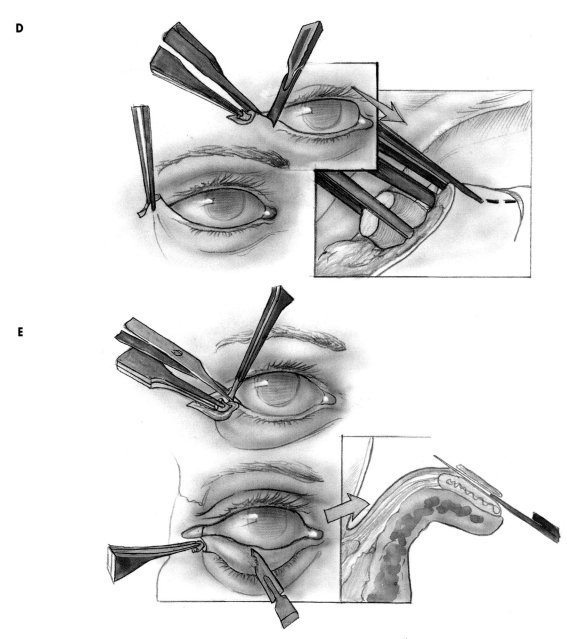

Figure 18–16. *(continued)*

REFERENCES

1. McCord C. Browplasty and browpexy: An adjunct to blepharoplasty. *Plast Reconstr Surg.* 1990; 6:00–00.
2. Sheen JH. Supratarsal fixation in upper blepharoplasty. *Symposium on Surgery of the Aging Face* 1978; 19.
3. Cook TA. The versatile midforehead browlift. *Arch Otolaryngol Head Neck Surg.* 1989; 115:00–00.
4. Beard C. *Ptosis.* 3rd ed. St. Louis: CV Mosby; 1981:151–153.
5. Putterman AM, Urist MJ. Mueller muscle-conjunctiva resection—Technique for treatment of blepharoptosis. *Arch Ophthalmol.* 1975; 93:619–623.
6. Bick MW. Surgical management of orbital tarsal disparity. *Arch Ophthalmol.* 1966; 75:386.
7. Tenzel RR, Buffam FV, Miller GR. The use of the "lateral canthal sling" in ectropion repair. *Can J Ophthalmol.* 1977; 12:199–202.

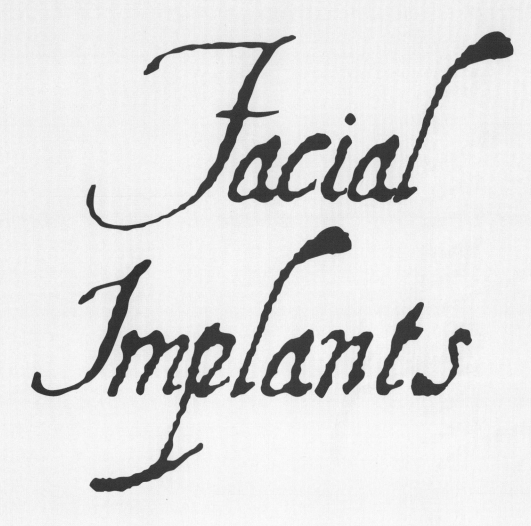

Facial Implants

The chapters on facial implants are presented by two authors who have extensive experience in facial contouring with different implants materials. Dr. Glasgold, a facial plastic surgeon, reviews his treatment of facial contouring with emphasis on Silastic implants. Regional facial augmentation emphasizing malar and mentum augmentation is reviewed. Evaluation and patient selection criteria are established. A custom contouring technique of the mentum with an extension wafer is illustrated. Soft tissue augmentation with Gortex is also reviewed.

Dr. Wellisz, a plastic surgeon, reviews multiple types of facial implants, including autogenous and alloplastic implants. Dr. Wellisz has extensive experience in the use of porous high-density polyethylene implants. In his chapter he reviews his techniques and results with this unique implant material. Together these chapters provide the reader with an understanding of the key types of facial implants and their use in facial plastic surgery.

Facial Implants

Aesthetic Facial Plastic Surgery, edited by Thomas Romo, III, and Arthur L. Millman, Thieme Medical Publishers, Inc., New York, New York, Copyright © 2000.

CHAPTER 19

A Facial Plastic Surgeon's Perspective

ALVIN I. GLASGOLD AND MARK J. GLASGOLD

Facial Silastic implants have been in use for more than 30 years.[1] Preformed implants for mentoplasty date to the mid 1960s[2] and malar implants[3] were introduced somewhat later. Preformed Silastic chin and cheek implants are universally accepted because they have stood the test of time.[4–7] These implants produce minimal host reaction, have a low complication rate, and are easy to insert and remove. They contour well, can be trimmed, and are soft enough for suture fixation, yet when implanted over bone, they assume the firm consistency of the underlying bone. They are flexible, which makes insertion through limited incisions easy. They are readily available and are reasonably priced. The Silastic nasal implants have a higher rate of complication probably because of the thinner nasal skin covering and the nasal prominence, which is susceptible to trauma.[8] We have avoided using preformed Silastic nasal implants and have favored cartilage autographs[9] and, more recently, Gortex for dorsal nasal augmentation. Gortex polytetrafluoroethylene (PTFE) sheeting or strands have proven to be relatively safe for other areas of soft tissue augmentation of the face such as the nasolabial fold, glabellar lines, lips, and dorsal nasal augmentation.[10–12]

MALAR AUGMENTATION

Malar augmentation plays a significant role in facial contouring. Patient awareness of this modality is increasing. As surgeons become comfortable with the evaluation of the midface and the technique of malar augmentation, this will become a more popular procedure.[13–15]

PATIENT EVALUATION

A rather simple but useful approach to evaluating the midface is to divide it into three areas. The upper area represents the suborbital area and the zygomatic arch. The lower portion is the submalar region. The central area between the two is the transition zone. We then analyze where a deficiency exists and what area or how much of the midface we wish to augment. The patient who has a deficiency of zygomatic arch prominence or who requests the appearance of "high cheekbones" will benefit from high implant placement. The thin patient, who has lost submalar fat, requires a low placement to fill in this area. Many patients have a cheek mound just lateral to the nasolabial groove and then a deficiency lateral to this, and they fall into the group that needs augmentation of the central or transition zone. Those patients who present with a generally flat appearance of the entire midface will benefit from augmentation of the entire region.

IMPLANT SELECTION

We have had great success with the Binder submalar implant not only in the submalar area but also when we place the implant high across the zygomatic arch. Its shape contours this region nicely. When the implant will overlap upper and lower zones of the midface, we use the submalar II, which has a larger superior inferior dimension; occasionally we use a Terrino Shell. Implant selection is based on the area to be augmented and the degree of augmentation necessary. Facial symmetry and irregularities should be noted because these will be more noticeable to the patient after implant placement. It is only on rare occasions when such a marked asymmetry exists that we attempt to correct the asymmetry with a different size or shape implant on each side.

PREOPERATIVE PREPARATION AND INTRAOPERATIVE TECHNIQUE

Malar augmentation is an ambulatory procedure done with local anesthesia alone or supplemented with intravenous sedation. The area to be augmented is generally outlined on the face preoperatively and may be shown to the patient. Often a mound of tissue runs along the lateral aspect of the nasolabial groove. This produces the nasolabial mound or prominence. Implant placement should not further accentuate this mound so that the medial position of the implant should be marked at the lateral aspect of the nasolabial prominence. The infraorbital nerve is blocked and then the gingival sulcus and the malar region are locally anesthetized with a modest amount of anesthesia so as not to distort the region. The oral cavity is washed with povidone-iodine (Betadine), 1 g of cephalexin is injected intravenously, and the patient is maintained on oral cephalexin for one week. Exposing the right and left canine fossae, the medial aspect of the incision is marked with cautery on both sides for symmetry. Using a blend cut cautery with a needlepoint, an incision of approximately 1.5 cm is made in the gingival-buccal sulcus and advanced slightly superiorly to the bone. The dissection continues with a Joseph elevator. If a Terrino Shell is used, a very wide elevation must be accomplished. In most instances, we use a Binder Submalar I or II. We like to insert the tail of the implant in a narrow pocket over the lateral aspect of the zygomatic arch or just below it, depending on whether we wish to accentuate the arch. Positioning the implant tail in this pocket firmly fixes the implant. In elevating the pocket for submalar or low placement, we will proceed vertically up from the incision to the desired height of placement, taking care to avoid the infraorbital nerve, and then extend laterally either over the zygomatic arch or just below the arch, depending on where we want the lateral aspect of the implant to sit.

We create a narrow lateral pocket to accept the tail of the implant. The implant is then inserted with a clamp to feed the tail into the lateral pocket. An Aufricht or a long converse retractor assists in visualizing this area and making sure the tail does not fold on itself. Pullout guide sutures on a long Keith needle can be used, if desired. The tail can be shortened or trimmed with scissors as needed. The implant should fit securely in the pocket, and the body of the implant should fill the desired space. We generally leave a little soft tissue on the bone just above the buccal incision so we can use one or two tacking sutures to keep the implant slightly above the mucosal closure.

COMPLICATIONS AND SEQUELAE

Complications of malar augmentation are minimal. They include injury to the infraorbital nerve with a numbness of the cheek and lip and infection, which usually responds to antibiotics. If the implant does not adhere to the underlying bone and remains unstable, it may have to be removed and reinserted. The possibility of asymmetric placement of the implant should be discussed with the patient, and facial asymmetry that would accentuate this should be noted.

RESULTS

The results of midface augmentation in the appropriate patient has been very gratifying. It can produce a nice contour to a flat or poorly defined face (Fig. 19–1). It provides facial balance and, very much like the effect of mentoplasty, will reduce the apparent nasal prominence (Fig. 19–2). It can elevate the check prominence and fill in a deficit in the submalar area, producing a more youthful appearance. It can also slightly exaggerate the contour of the cheek bone producing the effect of a high cheekbone. This midface elevation can either enhance or mimic the effect of facelift (Fig. 19–3).

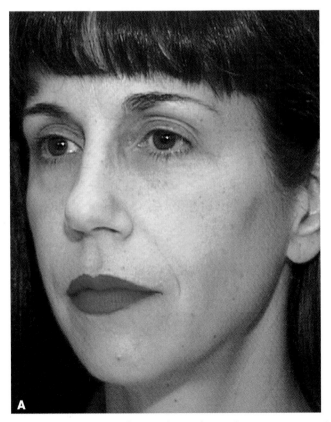 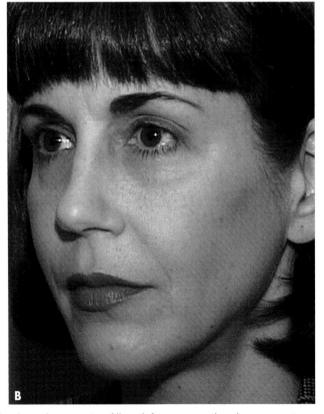

Figure 19–1. (A) Before and **(B)** after malar augmentation (mid to low placement) to fill in deficiency in submalar region. In addition, mentoplasty was performed. Note the significant aesthetic facial improvement with these two contouring procedures.

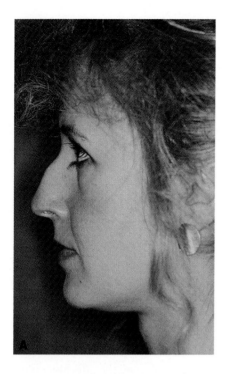
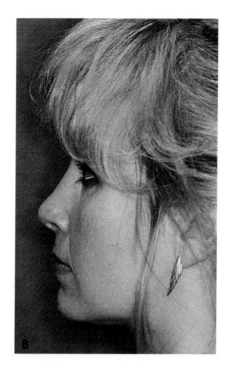

Figure 19–2. (A) Preoperative and **(B)** postoperative malar augmentation combined with rhinoplasty. Malar augmentation improves facial contour and reduces the distance between the cheek and nasal dorsum.

CONTOURING OF THE CHIN AND JAWLINE

Any surgeon dealing with facial cosmetic changes should be comfortable with all the nuances of alloplastic contouring of the mandible.[16] This procedure, when understood completely, is the safest, easiest, most cost-effective cosmetic operation of the face. An appreciation of the benefits of mandibular contouring beyond profile correction will expand the surgeon's use of this procedure.[17] The use of a simplified technique, which should prevent most complications, will further increase the surgeon's comfort in recommending mentoplasty. Mandibular contouring is a procedure that in most cases is recommended by the surgeon as an adjunct to other procedures requested by patients such as rhinoplasty and blepharoplasty.

The benefits of mandibular contouring are facial balance, aesthetic improvement, and facial rejuvenation. Profile analysis of the retrognathic patient indicates that the apparent nasal projection is increased by a receding chin. In some instances patients present for rhinoplasty when the nasal projection is appropriate and the profile problem is purely related to a receding chin (Fig. 19–4). The retrognathic individual generally has an oblique submental-hyoid angle that produces an unattractive neckline and an aging appearance (Fig. 19–5). An unattractive protruding lower lip is commonly associated with retrognathia and improves with chin angmentation (Fig. 19–6). In addition, retrognathic patients frequently have an exaggerated prejowl sulcus that accentuates the jowls and prematurely ages the face. This can be corrected with an appropriately placed and sized extended implant (Fig. 19–5C,D). In the patient undergoing facelift, filling this deficit and establishing a strong jawline will enhance the effect of the facelift on the jowl area, as well as help in contouring the neck.

PATIENT EVALUATION

In evaluating the patient a decision is initially made as to approximately how much projection is desired. The implant will generally not increase the vertical dimension of the chin. The implant produces some contour to the chin, which serves to reduce its apparent length.

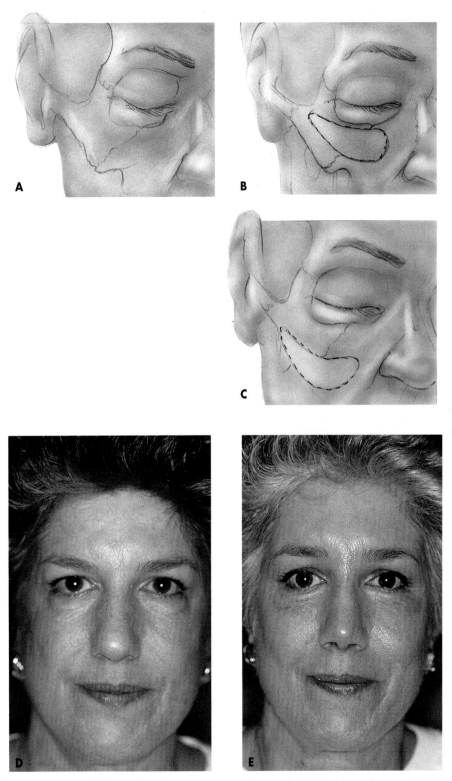

Figure 19–3. (A) Preoperative and **(B)** position of malar augmentation with high implant placement. **(C)** Position of submalar augmentation placed mid to low to fill in submalar deficit operative. **(D)** Preoperative and **(E)** postoperative malar augmentation with high implant placement accentuates cheek bone and makes face look more youthful.

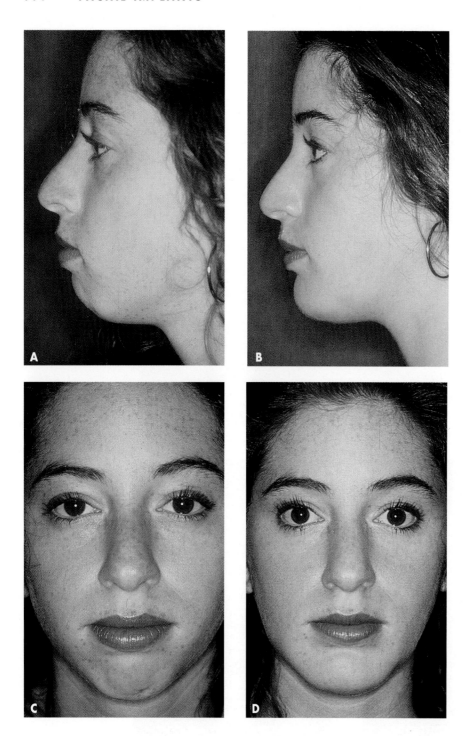

Figure 19–4. (A) Preoperative and **(B)** postoperative mentoplasty. Marked improvement in profile alignment. Patient's nose appears smaller even though it was not done. **(C)** Preoperative and **(D)** postoperative mentoplasty. Note significant improvement in jawline and lower third of face after mentoplasty.

The patient who has a short vertical dimension may benefit from a Flowers mandibular glove implant,[18] which can increase the vertical dimension of the chin somewhat. The Mittleman Chin Jowl implant may be useful in the patient with a very deep prejowl sulcus. The 2-mm Glasgold Extension Wafer can be used to extend the anteroposterior projection of a positioned implant.

Smiling increases chin projection in some people, and it is important to note this when deciding on the size of the implant. In addition asymmetry and any apparent facial nerve weakness must be noted.

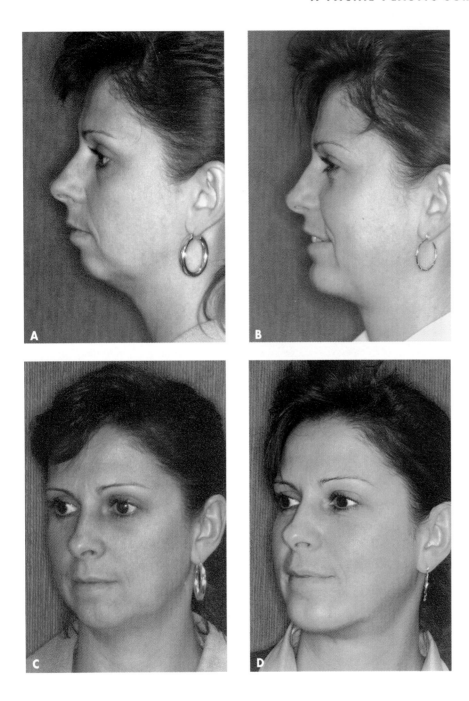

Figure 19–5. (A) Preoperative and **(B)** postoperative mentoplasty and submental liposuction. **(C)** Preoperative and **(D)** postoperative three quarters view mentoplasty and submental liposuction. Note the marked improvement and more youthful appearance of the neckline and jawline with elimination of jowls.

Lip protrusion and irregularities of the surface of the chin should also be noted. We generally wish to increase the anterior projection of the chin no further than the lower lip. In women 1 to 2 mm of underprojection is acceptable. Slight overprojection is more acceptable in men. Occasionally, a woman with a round face can benefit from a very slight overprojection to produce a more oval and thinner appearance to the frontal view of the face.

IMPLANT SELECTION

We have used preformed Silastic implants since 1965. The major improvement in implants over this period of time has been the recognition of the anatomic shape of the mandible and the advantage of extending the implant laterally to contour the entire jawline. These extended or anatomic-shaped implants come in sizes that produce

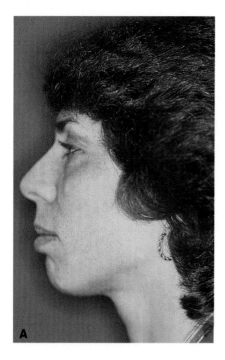
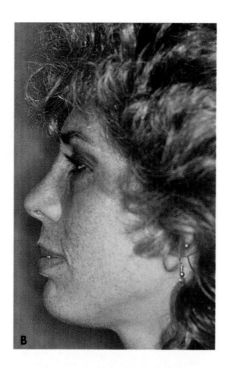

Figure 19–6. (A) Preoperative and **(B)** postoperative mentoplasty and rhinoplasty; improved facial balance and reduction in appearance of protruding lip.

anterior projections of 5 to 12 mm. The overall bulk and the lateral extension increases with the size of the implants. Larger implants can be customized. We measured 100 consecutive patients who presented for mentoplasty and found their deficiency ranged between 3 and 14 mm. It is impractical to insert an implant greater than 12 mm because of the bulk and creation of almost a shelf like projection of the chin. If necessary, the implant can be extended with a Silastic wafer, as described in the following.

TECHNIQUE

We perform all our mentoplasties through the submental approach. This allows for easier implant insertion, more accurate positioning, and suture fixation of the implant to the inferior border of the mandible, which prevents implant shifting.

Creating the Implant Pocket

A horizontal incision is made in a natural submental crease. Dissection proceeds directly to the mandible

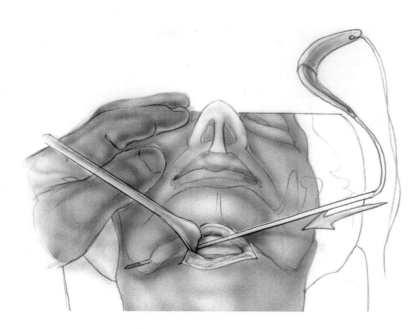

Figure 19–7. Guided suture placement of implant.

through soft tissue and muscle by use of electrocautery with cutting current. The incision is directed to the anterior surface of the mandible, leaving periosteum and soft tissue attached to the undersurface of the mandible. A generous subbperiosteal pocket is elevated superiorly. If the mental sulcus is deep, this area can be released by undermining and even augmenting. Dissectionis then continued laterally with a Joseph elevator, hugging the inferior border of the mandible. After the pocket is adequately developed on both sides, an Aufricht retractor is inserted, which exposes and stretches the pocket.

Implant Insertion

The extended implant is attached to a large Keith needle with a pull-out suture. The guide suture allows for accurate positioning of the lateral tail of the implant and prevents the thin lateral tail from curling up on itself or rotating superiorly (Fig. 19–8). The second guide suture is passed through the pocket on the second side, and the other half of the implant is inserted. The first suture is now used as a traction suture, preventing the first side of the implant from popping out while the second side is inserted (Fig. 19–9). The implant is accurately positioned by lining up a central mark on the implant. Palpation along the lateral extent of the implant will ensure that the implant is properly positioned and that it has not curled on itself.

Implant Fixation

Suture fixation of the implant will prevent it from riding up on the mandible, rotating, or shifting laterally. The implant is sutured to the periosteum and soft tissue, which has been left attached to the underface of the mandible with two 4–0 polydioxanone (PDS) sutures. This also fixes the inferior edge of the implant in continuity with the inferior edge of the mandible (Fig. 19-10).

CUSTOM CONTOURING WITH THE EXTENSION WAFER

Intraoperative implant customization with extension wafers allows a more accurate profile correction in some patients. Intraoperative extension wafers combined with accurate preoperative determination of the appropriate implant size and style can reduce the added manipulation and trauma associated with the use of sizers, implant changes, and pocket enlargements that result from standard trial-and-error sizing. If uncertainty exists during the

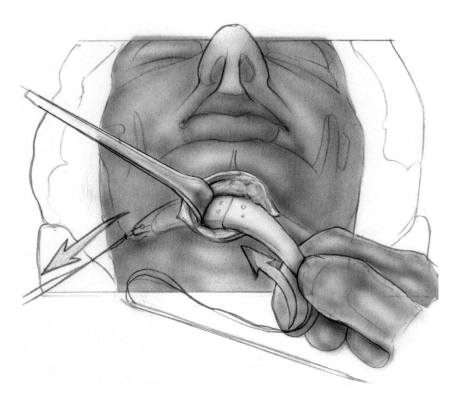

Figure 19–8. Accurate positioning of tail of implant on right side.

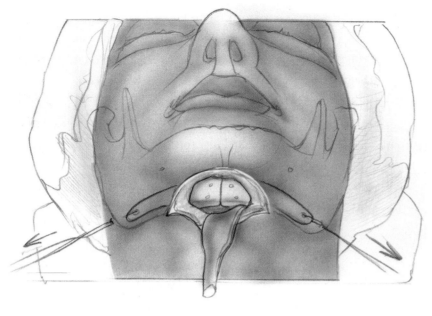

Figure 19–9. Positioning of tail of left side of implant while suture holds right side in place.

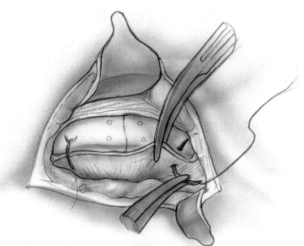

Figure 19–10. Suture fixation of implant to mandibular periosteum.

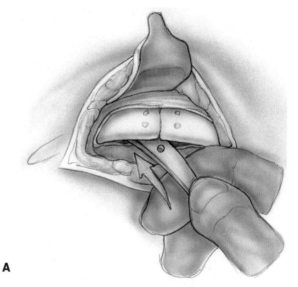

A

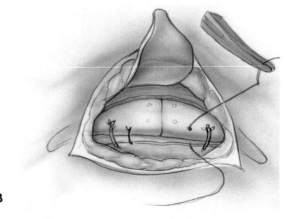

B

Figure 19–11. (A) Insertion of Glasgold wafer under implant. **(B)** Suture fixation of wafer to implant and suture fixation of wafer and implant to periosteum.

preoperative evaluation as to which size chin implant will provide appropriate anterior projection, the smaller size is inserted, and if this is not sufficient, a wafer is inserted to increase projection rather than changing implants.

Extension wafers are used when we wish greater projection than allowed by the largest size implant. The extension wafer is inserted before suturing the implant to the periosteum. It is inserted under the implant and two 4–0 nonresorbable sutures fix the wafer to the implant (Fig. 19–10A). The wafer-implant complex is then sutured, as previously described, to the periosteum of the mandible. A two-layer closure is used (Fig. 19–10B).

Extension wafers are also useful when postoperative evaluation indicates that additional augmentation is desirable. The original incision is opened, and the implant is elevated off the underlying bone. The wafer is then inserted under the original implant and sutured to it as described previously.

ePTFEFACIAL IMPLANTS

Correction of soft tissue facial defects has been greatly enhanced by the introduction of ePTFEGortex™ is presently available in sheets of 1- and 2-mm thickness and in small blocks of 4-mm thickness and thin strands. SoftForm™ comes in hollow tubes of 3.2- and 2.4-mm diameter.

Our early experience with this material was in 1988 to 1989 when we reported a preliminary study correcting the deep nasolabial groove in 30 patients. The results at that time were generally quite satisfactory; however, we had a high incidence of infection associated with the implant. We believe this was related to the method we used, which was to introduce a large triangular piece of Gortex into a preformed pocket. Our goal was to fill the whole defect rather than just improve it. We are now using narrower strands cut from a 2-mm thickness Gortex patch or preformed Gortex fibers. These are threaded through the groove to be filled, leaving significant distance between the implant and the entry and exit points. We are also ensuring that we are in the subcutaneous plane and not staying superficial with our implant. For large defects we will layer the Gortex strands with multiple passes. In addition to the nasolabial groove, Gortex is also used in the marionette lines, glabella, and lips. We have a recent experience with SoftForm in the lips and nasolabial grooves, which provides results comparable to Gortex.

The technique is relatively simple. After measuring and preparing the appropriate length implant and cleansing the area of the face, stab wounds are made with a no. 11 blade at the entry and exit portholes. A 14-gauge intracath is passed subcutaneously. The Gortex strand with a 2–0 black silk pull-out thread on a Keith needle is pulled through the area to be filled ensuring a moderate distance between the implant and the entry and exit points. SoftForm comes in a very easy-to-use trocar kit. We do not soak the implant in antibiotic solution. We do use systemic antibiotic for 1 week (Fig. 19–11).

Gortex is also successfully used to deface defects in the face and nose with appropriately cut 1- or 2-mm thickness implants. It has been effective in postparotidectomy defects and as a treatment for Frey's syndrome. In the nose 1-mm

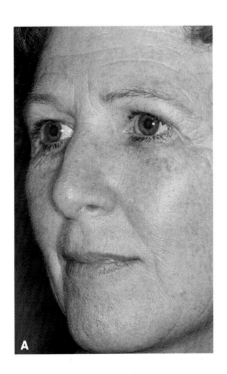 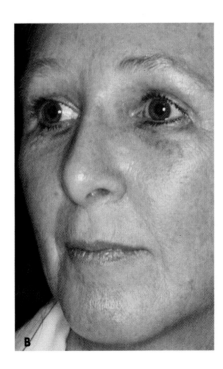

Figure 19–12. Example of **(A)** preoperative and **(B)** postoperative Gortex augmentation of nasolabial groove.

thick Gortex sheets can be used to cover persistent bone irregularities, particularly in thinned-skin individuals, 2-mm thickness sheets can cover mild depressions. For significant dorsal depressions, saddle nose deformities or the platyrhine patient who needs dorsal enhancement, 4-mm thick onlay grafts are used. These sometimes will be augmented by an additional 2-mm patch, which will be sutured to the 4-mm implant. In these patients, a tendency exists for the Gortex to be compressed, so sufficient correction is necessary. We generally prefer to introduce Gortex nasal onlay grafts through an external approach.

CONCLUSION

Facial contouring with implants adds an exciting dimension to improvement in appearance and rejuvenation of the aging face. When used appropriately, it will significantly enhance the results of surgery.

PEARLS

- The use of the Binder Submalar I and II implants to augment the malar and submalar areas.
- Far superior results achieved with extended anatomic implants in contouring the jawline.
- Needle and suture guide of implant tail and suture fixation of the chin implant produces accurate placement and prevents curling of tail and rotation of implant.
- Custom contouring with the extension wafer is easily performed and produces more accurate results.

REFERENCES

1. Perrett DI, May KA, Yoshikawa S. Facial shape and judgements of female attractiveness. *Nature.* 1994; 368:239.
2. Safian J. Progress in nasal and chin augmentation. *Plast Reconstr Surg.* 1966; 37:522.
3. Hinderer U. Maler implants for improvement of facial appearance. *Plast Reconstr Surg.* 1975; 56:157.
4. Glasgold AI, Silver FH. The long-term effect of facial implants. *Am J Cosm Surg.* 1995; 12:133.
5. Silver FH, Glasgold AG, Silicone facial inplants are they safe? *J Long-Term Effects Medical Implants.* 1993; 3:313.
6. Silver FH, Glasgold AI. Performance standards of medical device approval. *Arch Otolaryngol Head Neck Surg.* 1995; 121:719–721.
7. Scaccia FJ. Allphin AL, Stephnick, DW. Complications of agumentation mentoplasty. *Int J Aesthet Restor Surg.* 1993; 1:3.
8. Mackay IS, Boll TR. The fate of silastic implants in the management of saddle nose deformity. *J Laryngol Otolaryngol.* 1983; 97:43.
9. Glasgold AI, Glasgold MJ. Cartilage Autografts in Facial Plastic Surgery. *Applications of Biomaterials in Facial Plastic Surgery.* New York: CRC Press; 1991.
10. Walter C. The Use of Gore-Tex™ In Facial Augmentation. *Applications of Biomaterials in Facial Plastic Surgery.* New York: CRC Press; 1991.
11. Sclajani AP, Thomas JR, Cox HJ, Cooper MH. Clincial and histologic response of subcutaneous expanded polytetra floor ethylene. *Arch Otolaryngol Head Neck Surg.* 1997; 123:328.
12. Conrad K, Reifen E. Gore-Tex™ implant and tissue filler in cheek-lip groove rejuvenation. *J Otolaryngol.* 1992; 21:218.
13. Binder WJ. Submalar augmentation, an alternative to face lift surgery. *Arch Otolaryngol Head Neck Surg.* 1989; 15:797.
14. Terino EO. Alloplastic facial contouring: Surgery of the fourth plane. *Aesthet Plast Surg.* 1992; 16:195.
15. Binder WJ, Schoenrock LD, Terino EO. Augmentation of the Malar. *Submalar Midface Facial Plast Surg Clin North Am.* 1995; 2:265.
16. Glasgold AI, Glasgold MJ. Mentoplasty. *Facial Plast Surg Clin North Am.* 1995; 2:285.
17. Glasgold MJ, Glasgold AI. Augmentation mentoplasty: An approach for increased sophistication and better accuracy. *Am J Cosm Surg.* 1993; 10:29.
18. Glasgold AI, Glasgold MJ. Intra-operative custom contouring of the mandible. *Arch Otolaryngol Head Neck Surg.* 1994; 120:180.

Facial Implants

Aesthetic Facial Plastic Surgery, edited by Thomas Romo, III, and Arthur L. Millman, Thieme Medical Publishers, Inc., New York, New York, Copyright © 2000.

CHAPTER 20

A Plastic Surgeon's Perspective

TADEUSZ WELLISZ AND PAUL SABINI

Facial implants are used extensively in aesthetic plastic surgery of the face. They modify the facial skeleton on which the soft tissue envelope of the face is draped. The aim of the modification can be the augmentation of the facial skeleton, the suspension of the soft tissue envelope, or both.

The goals of the patient and surgeon are shaped by both cultural perceptions of beauty and established norms. Extensive information regarding ideal facial proportions is available. However, analysis of anthropometric studies of the population have shown us that the cannons established in the Renaissance are not the same as those most frequently observed in the general population.[1] Moreover, exaggerated facial features, especially of the facial skeleton, are often associated with great beauty.[2] Facial implants provide the surgeon with a reliable means of reconstructing the facial skeleton in accordance with the perceived and established norms of beauty.

Facial implantation can be achieved with either autogenous tissue or one of a number of synthetic materials currently available. Alloplasts are an attractive alternative to autogenous tissue because (1) no donor site morbidity occurs; (2) total operating time is reduced because of the absence of graft harvest; (3) many alloplasts are available in preformed anatomic shapes; (4) bone and cartilage has the potential to resorb or warp over time; and (5) the amount of autogenous material is limited and can be insufficient for a given procedure.

AUTOGENOUS FACIAL IMPLANTS

Autogenous tissue used for skeletal augmentation includes cartilage and bone. Cartilage can be harvested from the nasal septum, the ear, or the rib. Cartilage grafts are used most commonly for nasal tip augmentation, and they will be covered in greater depth in Chapters 7 and 8. Septal cartilage, when available, can yield an ample piece of material that is harvested using the same operative site used for the rhinoplasty. The ear is also an excellent source of cartilage, although the cartilage is curved and becomes brittle as the age of the patient increases. Most often the conchal cartilage can be harvested from the ear from an incision in the posterior aspect of the ear without leaving an appreciable donor site deformity. Cartilage is often morcellized to soften the appearance of graft;[3] however, this may serve to increase the incidence of resorption.

Rib cartilage, although abundant in the younger patient, is not used frequently as an implant material. Rib cartilage tends to calcify as a patient matures, and this process appears to occur even when the cartilage is used as an implant. The most problematic issue with the use of rib cartilage is the change of shape that occurs after the implant has been cut. This phenomenon is due to the system of locked stresses within the cartilage.[4] Rib grafts also have an unacceptably high resorption rate.

Bone harvested from the outer table of the cranium is a far better choice than rib grafts because it undergoes significantly less remodeling and resorption. Unfortunately, serious complications such as intracranial bleeding after the harvesting of these grafts limit their usefulness in aesthetic facial surgery.[5,6] Thus because of donor site

morbidity, difficulty of use, and late changes of the implant, alloplasts are the most commonly used materials for aesthetic facial surgery.

ALLOPLASTIC FACIAL IMPLANTS
SILICONE

Silicone has been used since the 1950s and remains the most widely used facial implant material.[7] The popularity of silicone rests with (1) its low tissue reactivity, (2) ease of insertion caused by its smooth surface and ability to be deformed, and (3) its ability to be manufactured in a variety of consistencies ranging from a liquid to a soft or hard rubber. Silicone rubber is an organosilicone polymer. The subunits are linked together producing polydioxsone. The chain length and amount of branching determines the firmness of the implant. The final mixture is amorphous and contains a range of sizes, ranging from short-chained to long-chained polymers. A hard implant will have a short chain oil component.[8] Hard silicone rubbers are also fragile and may shed tiny shards of silicone into the tissue surrounding the implant.[9]

Silicone implants work best in areas of good soft tissue coverage. The classic teaching is that silicone rubber, which is nonwettable, repelling blood and fluid, has a low tissue toxicity.[7] In response to implantation the body lays down a thin but tough fibrous capsule consisting primarily of collagen, contractile elements, and sparse inflammatory cells.

Recent media attention and litigation surrounding silicone breast implants have created fear about using any form of silicone among patients, physicians, and medical manufacturers. Although no direct evidence exists in humans of a cause-and-effect autoimmune response occurring as a result of silicone, the issue has not been put to rest in the eyes of the public and the judicial system.[10]

The three well-known complications of silicone implants are infection, soft tissue thinning, and bone resorption. Infection can occur early in the postoperative phase and late after implantation. The risk of early postoperative infection can be reduced with the administration of perioperative antibiotics and the use of a no-touch technique. The risk of late infection is reduced when good soft tissue coverage is achieved around the implant. Soft tissue thinning, which is most commonly observed with silicone implants in the nose, can be reduced by avoiding any tension on the skin overlying the implant. When applied topically to the skin, silicone appears to have the beneficial effect of thinning hypertrophic scars.[11] Bone resorption has been well documented with silicone chin implants.[12,13] In the past, bone resorption had been attributed to mechanical pressure and the active capsule that forms around all silicones.[14] More recent animal studies demonstrate that silicone causes a degree of bone resorption not seen with more rigid materials.[15,16] In the rabbit mandible, silicone implants caused significantly more bone resorption than porous polyethylene and solid methylmethacrylate.[15] Because of these issues, a trend exists toward the use of materials that may not handle as easily as silicone but may exhibit more acceptable long-term results.

POROUS POLYETHYLENE

Porous polyethylene has become an important facial reconstructive material that serves both as a bone and cartilage substitute and as an alternative to silicone. Porous polyethylene is marketed as Medpor Biomaterial (Porex Surgical, College Park, GA) for use in non-load-bearing regions of the craniofacial skeleton (Fig. 20–1) The implant is easy to shape, strong yet somewhat flexible, and highly stable. Most importantly, it exhibits tissue ingrowth into its pores. The tissue ingrowth results in collagen deposition within the pores that forms a highly stable complex, which is resistant to infection, exposure, and deformation by contractile forces.[17–19] Porous polyethylene is now widely used for mandible and malar augmentation, nasal surgery, orbital reconstruction, ear reconstruction, and a variety of craniofacial applications.

The advantage of using a porous material, such as porous polyethylene, is that the body's own healing process fills the pores of the implant with tissue that stabilizes the implant. For a porous compound to be effective as an implant material, it must fulfill four criteria:

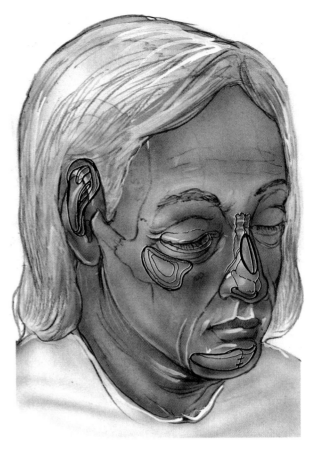

Figure 20–1. Applications for porous polyethylene implants include the chin, malar complex, nasal dorsum, columella, orbital floor, and ear framework.

(1) it must be biocompatible; (2) the pores must be large enough to allow for tissue ingrowth; (3) the pores must interconnect; and (4) the structure of the implant must be both stable and rigid enough to maintain the porous framework under the conditions encountered at the implanted site. To be useful, the material must also be sufficiently easy to use in a clinical setting.

Solid polyethylene, the structural component of porous polyethylene, is a highly inert material with numerous applications in the medical field. High-density polyethylenes are used commonly in orthopedic appliances and have been a standard reference material for biocompatibility testing.[20] Solid polyethylene has been used in the craniofacial skeleton and more than 30 years of patient follow-up have been reported.[21] Porous polyethylene has now been used as an implant material for more than 20 years.[19] Medical grade porous polyethylene is formulated to ensure that more than 50% of the pores

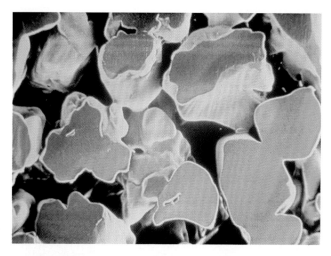

Figure 20–2. A scanning electron micrograph of porous polyethylene reveals the contiguous, large-pore structure of the implant (magnification × 53).

are larger than 150 μm, an ample size for fibrovascular ingrowth.[19] These pores interconnect in multiple dimensions to form an open-pore network of open spaces (Fig. 20–2).

Porous polyethylene has not been shown to cause the bone resorption[22] that has long been known to occur with silicone implants[12,13] and certain formulations of polytetrafluoroethylene (PTFE).[23]

Excellent results with the use of porous polyethylene for facial burn reconstruction have been reported.[24] These results were obtained despite the poor characteristics of the soft tissue, including decreased vascularity, poor compliance, strong contractile forces, and unstable skin coverage. The high rate of success in reconstructing difficult areas such as the burned ear sparked widespread interest in the material for a variety of facial reconstructive and aesthetic applications.[25,26] Once the material had been shown to be effective in facial burns, its use for less demanding applications increased. To date there have been few documented cases of exposures of implants adequately covered with soft tissue.[27] The reported exposures occurred predominantly in burn patients.[28] Animal studies have shown that once implants are vascularized, they become highly resistant to infection.[29–31] The large negative surface charge of polyethylene[32] and the low level of adhesion to its surface[33] have been postulated as con-

tributing factors. When implant exposures do occur, they are remarkably benign.[30,34] Porous polyethylene appears to behave much like osteointegratable titanium implants in this respect. Reports describe the salvage of exposures without removal of the implant.[9,35] In one report an exposed ear framework was allowed to granulate, and the subsequently vascularized implant was effectively salvaged with a split-thickness skin graft placed directly on the exposed portion of the implant.[25] In instances where porous polyethylene implants do need to be removed or revised, the soft tissue surrounding the implant can be lifted off the implant with an elevator, much the way periosteum is lifted off bone.

Porous polyethylene is available in sterile packs in a variety of anatomic shapes and sizes. The material itself can be sculpted with a scalpel or scissors. The edges can be feathered to a fine edge by placing the material on a lint-free surface such as a nylon cutting board and carving it with a sharp scalpel blade. Although a burr may be used to form a rough contour, this will seal the implant's pores, and the final shape needs to be carved using a scalpel. The surface should be free of contour irregularities to ensure that no edges will be felt after surgery. Porous polyethylene can also be molded to some degree. This is done by heating the implant in sterile saline brought to its boiling point. The softened material can be bent into a new shape that is maintained after cooling. Excessive bending of the material after it has cooled will cause it to crack and weaken the implant.

The implant should be soaked in an antibiotic solution containing a cephalosporin before insertion. Because the implant has an open-pore structure and the surface of the polyethylene is charged, capillary action readily disperses the fluid into the interstices of the implant. Placement of the implant within a tissue pocket requires practice. The implant adheres to tissue, much like a piece of Velcro, and will not slide along a tissue surface. When positioning the implant, the tissue should be lifted to allow the implant to be advanced within the tissue pocket. Implants generally do not need to be fixed if they are secure within their pockets at the time of surgery. Implant fixation is necessary when potential for muscle fiber ingrowth exists that may cause subsequent implant movement. Examples include implants placed under the temporalis muscle and mandibular angle implants placed under the masseter muscle. The implants can be stabilized with sutures, K-wires, or screws. If reoperation becomes necessary, implants can either be removed or modified in situ. A small elevator is a useful instrument for this purpose. Lifting the tissue from an implant is much like elevating periosteum from a bony surface.

HYDROXYAPATITE

Hydroxyapatite (HA) is a polycrystalline ceramic that is similar in composition to bone. Porous HA is derived from the porous skeletons of reef-building corals. Porous HA has generated significant interest because of its similar composition to human bone and because of the degree of bone ingrowth into the implant.[36] HA, however, can be difficult to use. Its brittle nature has led some surgeons to caution against its use in areas likely to sustain trauma;[19] whereas others have warned about fracture during attempts at fixation.[37] Although a significant amount of tissue ingrowth may occur into an extremely rigid implant, the surface of the implant may become abrasive when shear forces are applied at the tissue interface. In clinical trials, granular HA mixed with microfibrillar collagen has been effective in malar augmentation.[38]

POLYTETRAFLUOROETHYLENE

PTFE is a polymer containing a carbon atom bonded to four fluorine side groups (Teflon fluorocarbon polymer). These bonds are very stable and resistant to degradation. To be useful to the surgeon, PTFE needs to be formulated into an implantable material. Gore-Tex and Proplast are two preparations with which the facial surgeon should be familiar.

Gore-Tex (W.L. Gore & Associates, Flagstaff, AZ) is a polymer sheet of tightly cross-linked PTFE fibrils. Each fibril measures 5 to 10 μm in diameter and has a length of 22 μm. When expanded, Gore-Tex develops small pores measuring 10 to 30 μm. Gore-Tex has been used extensively for vascular prostheses and for abdominal wall reconstruction. The experience for facial augmenta-

tion has been more limited. Our experience with the use of Gore-Tex in the nose is similar to published reports of the implants occasionally chinking with time and a small incidence of transient inflammatory reactions.[39] Although current reports of significant adverse effects of Gore-Tex implants in the human exist,[40] Gore-Tex was found to cause bone resorption in the orbit in an animal model.[16]

PROPLAST

Proplast (a registered trademark of NovaMed, Inc., Houston, TX), which was removed from the market in the United States in 1990, should be discussed because of the lessons that can be learned from its use. Proplast was made of PTFE combined with a fiber and manufactured as a firm but compressible porous sponge. The pore sizes ranged from 80 to 400 μm. Soft implants, however, such as those made from PTFE may not maintain an open pore structure, and their pores collapse when pressure is applied or as a result of the normal contracture of the regenerating tissue.[23,41,42] When used in load-bearing applications, such as in the temporomandibular joint, Proplast implants became fragmented, causing a severe inflammatory reaction.

METHYLMETHACRYLATE

Methylmethacrylate (acrylic) is used commonly in orthopedic surgery to cement joint prostheses, and occasionally in neurosurgery, but it is not a material used commonly by aesthetic surgeons. Methylmethacrylate is formed by the polymerization of methacrylic acid esters, and it is manufactured in one of two ways. The first is a heat-cured rigid preformed implant. The second is a cold-curing mixture that can be molded as it hardens. Implants can either be formed before surgery and heat sterilized, or the methylmethacrylate can be mixed just before use and an implant can be formed in situ. Powdered polymer granules are mixed with a liquid monomer at room temperature. The exothermic reaction can reach temperatures up to 70°C, so care must be taken to cool the implant as it hardens if it is directly exposed to the tissue.[9] Because the powdered material never becomes completely fused, the resulting implant remains slightly porous.[7] Mixing time is critical, both to ensure the consistency and because of the toxicity of the liquid monomer. Although rare, the monomer has been responsible for allergic reactions, hypotension, dysrhythmia, and cardiac arrest.

A large-pore, open structure form of methylmethacrylate is available as hard tissue replacement (HTR) polymer (HTR polymer is a registered trademark of the United States Surgical Corporation, Norwalk, CT). HTR is manufactured by sintering beads of methylmethacrylate together and coating them with polyhydroxyethyl methacrylate gel and calcium hydroxide to improve the surface characteristics of the implant.[43] Although its physical structure makes this material well suited for facial implantation with excellent biocompatibility and tissue ingrowth, the difficulty in carving or altering the shape of this rigid material makes it somewhat cumbersome to use.

CHIN IMPLANTS
PATIENT SELECTION

Chin augmentation is the most commonly performed implant procedure in facial aesthetic surgery. The procedure is easy to perform and the complication rate is low. The amount of forward projection of the chin is an important feature that determines both the facial harmony of an individual and, to some extent, the way that individual is viewed by others: some believe that a "weak" chin implies a lack of character or resolve.

Although most dentofacial abnormalities are best treated with orthognathic surgery, alloplastic implants are often added to these procedures. Classically, alloplastic implants are used to gain anterior projection of the deficient chin. In some cases a mandible that appears excessively large may be tall in the horizontal dimension with a receding chin. In these patients alloplastic enhancement may give the illusion of shortening the vertical height of the anterior mandible. Patients that appear to need 15 mm or more of augmentation should certainly be considered for an osteotomy or orthognathic treatment.

During the preoperative assessment, the patient needs to be either seated or standing erect because poor posture alone can distort the relationship of the chin to the rest of the face. To determine the appropriate projection of the chin, the entire facial profile must be considered. This includes the forehead, actual or planned projection of the nose, the relationship of the lips, and the projection of the lips. The lower lip should rest slightly posterior to the upper lip. The maximum projection of the chin should not exceed a point that is 1 to 2 mm posterior to the lower lip projection.

Chin implants have undergone an evolution over the past two decades. Originally, chin implants were provided as discrete buttons that added anterior projection in the central area of the chin only, often producing an unnatural round, central protuberance. A sulcus between the central chin and the lateral mandibular elements may become accentuated by the normal process of aging with the development of laxity in the area of the jowls. This sulcus has been referred to as the "marionette groove" or the anterior mandibular sulcus.[44] Most implants in use today extend into this region to minimize this potential deformity. Implants are also available that extend further laterally onto the body of the mandible. Many of the newer implant designs also extend inferiorly and wrap around the inferior border of the mandible. The trend has become to use extended implants and to achieve less of an anterior augmentation. Most manufacturers provide implants that have a rounded anterior projection, which give the chin a feminine look, as well as implants that have a square anterior projection, which masculinize the chin. In the male patient a cleft or chin dimple may be created by suturing the dermis to the implant.

Ethnic considerations also play an important role in choosing the appropriate projection of the chin. The Asian face characteristically has less forward projection than the Caucasian face. The characteristic face of an ethnic Chinese is a receding chin.[45] Another important ethnic consideration is the relationship of the nose and the chin.[46] It is well known that the nose can appear excessively prominent when the chin lacks projection. What can be overlooked, however, is that in the Asian face, for example, chin augmentation could well accentuate a relatively flat nose and may accentuate the presence of a midface retrusion. Similarly, if a nasal enhancement is planned, the effect on the chin should be considered.

PREOPERATIVE PREPARATION

The preoperative evaluation of a patient in whom a facial implant is a consideration includes an extensive discussion of autogenous versus alloplastic materials. When autogenous tissue is unavailable or entails a risk deemed unacceptable, patients are counseled on the use of alloplast implants. Patients who wish to proceed are cautioned about both acute and delayed infection and extrusion of alloplasts. The presence of a chronic infec-

tion such as osteomyelitis and chronic sinusitis is a contraindication to the use of an alloplast. The aforementioned infections must be eradicated before the aesthetic surgery. A history of an autoimmune disease is a relative contraindication to the use of an alloplast implant. Patients are informed that no scientific data exist that causally link alloplastic materials with autoimmune diseases. Nevertheless, the patient's perception of the issue must be ascertained and should factor into the decision to proceed.

SURGICAL TECHNIQUE

Chin implants can be inserted either through an intraoral or an extraoral approach (Fig. 20–3). An intraoral approach is used most commonly with primary chin

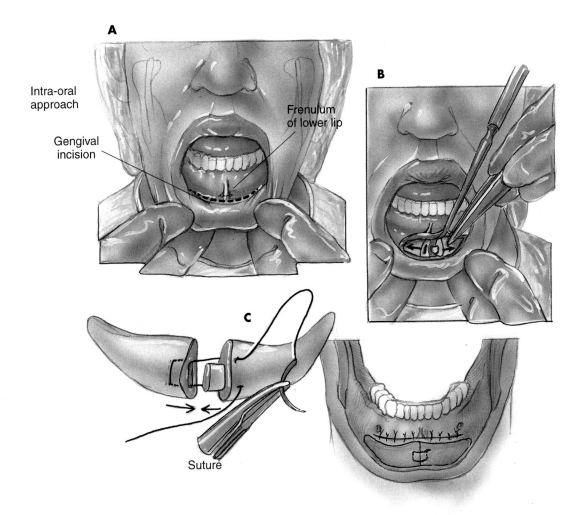

Figure 20–3. A two-piece porous polyethylene chin implant can be placed through an intraoral incision. **(A)** The incision is made ensuring that an adequate cuff of tissue remains on the posterior aspect to allow for subsequent closure over the implant. **(B)** The two halves of the implant are placed into the pocket. **(C)** The suture is tied securing the two pieces of the implant.

augmentation. The planned surgical pocket is infiltrated with lidocaine and epinephrine. The incision should be about 1 cm above the vestibular sulcus, up on the labial mucosa. The dissection is carried down at an angle leaving a generous bulk of soft tissue, including a portion of the mentalis muscle. This is important because it will ensure that a watertight closure will be achievable after insertion of the implant. The size of the pocket will be determined by the type of implant that will be used. With silicone implants, small mucosal incisions (about 1.5 cm long) and rather tight implant pockets are used. A larger pocket needs to be made for porous implants. Whatever the type of implant used, the dissection should extend slightly below the lower border of the mandible to allow the implant to lie along the lower border of the mandible and not to ride up above the border. The lateral dissection of the pocket needs to be performed along the inferior border of the mandible. Care must be taken not to damage the mental nerve. The nerve itself should not be visualized because exposure of the nerve could result either in intraoperative injury or late injury if the implant should ride up and put pressure on the nerve. This is a significant potential when extended chin implants are used. Once an appropriate pocket is created, the implant is inserted. Silicone implants are flexible enough so that a one-piece implant can be inserted through a relatively small incision. In such cases, it is helpful to mark the midpoint of the implant to ensure symmetric placement.

Because porous polyethylene implants are less flexible than silicone, their use requires some modification in surgical technique. Porous polyethylene chin implants are available in a number of styles and sizes, including shapes that wrap around the inferior border of the mandible to minimize upward displacement. Chin implants are available as two pieces that fit together, so as to make insertion through a small incision easier. Both the central and lateral aspect of the implant can be modified with a scalpel to achieve a precise contour alignment to a wide variety of mandibular shapes. Presuturing the two halves of the implant before insertion and then tying the sutures down once the implant is in position facilitate the procedure (Figs. 20–3 and 20–4).

The correction or prevention of the occurrence of a ptotic chin pad and witch's chin deformity is an important use of porous chin implants.[26] The soft tissue envelope of the chin and the chin pad adhere to the implant and remain attached in their normal anatomic position in relation to the bony contour of the mandible. A thin porous implant can be used for suspension of the chin pad, and vertical correction of the chin contour can be achieved without excessive horizontal projection. If an operation is to be performed for chin-pad ptosis after the use of a smooth implant, it is necessary to release the capsule of the old implant completely and to expose the fat of the chin pad, so as to allow it to become adherent to the porous implant. If necessary, several small sutures can be used to secure the released soft tissue to the implant. The fixation of the chin pad is performed frequently in facial burn patients and patients with neck scars that exert downward forces on the face.[24] A porous chin implant placed in a patient with a neck scar contracture restores the normal position of the chin pad and limits the effect of the scar contracture on the face.

Porous implants can also be used to lengthen the vertical dimension of the mandible. To do this, the lower edge of the implant is placed below the lower border of the mandible and is secured to the bone. Whenever the vertical dimension of the chin is modified or downward displacement of the implant is anticipated, it is recommended that the implant be fixed to the mandible with several small screws or K-wires. Self-tapping screws allow implant fixation without the need for power equipment.

MANDIBULAR ANGLE

In the ideal situation the prominence of the mandibular angle should be in concert with the remainder of the face.[47] With an increasing emphasis on bony contouring and alloplastic augmentation for aesthetic purposes, the area of the mandibular angle has become a target for change.[48] Mandibular angles and inferior mandibular borders can be augmented either for aesthetic or reconstructive purposes. Because Whitaker's experience with onlay bone grafts and with sagittal splitting of the lateral

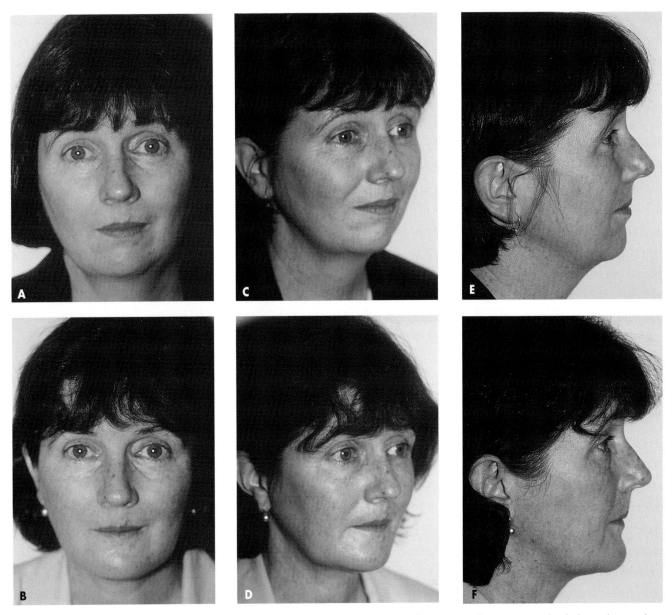

Figure 20–4. Preoperative **(A,C,E)** and 1-year postoperative **(B,D,F)** views of a patient after porous polyethylene chin implant and submental liposuction.

cortex of the mandibular ramus has been unsatisfactory, he advocates the use of implants for this purpose.[49] Epker, believing that proper definition and a well-defined mandibular border are the basis of separating the face from the neck, advocates the use of porous polyethylene implants for mandibular augmentation.[50] He believes that patients with a high-mandibular plane-angle skeletal structure with poor definition of the mandibular border will potentially benefit from the procedure. Poor definition of the mandibular angle can also result from proximal segment rotation after a sagittal split osteotomy.

Implants of several different designs are available for mandibular angle augmentation.

Mandibular angle augmentation remains relatively uncommon, and it is usually performed by those surgeons trained in maxillofacial techniques. Implants always need to be placed in a submuscular position below the masseter and along the angle of the mandible. The lateral aspect of the mandible is approached intraorally. The masseter muscle is dissected off the lateral border of the mandible down to the inferior border. The pterygomasseteric sling is elevated off the inferior border, but it is not cut. The implant should conform to the contour of the border of the mandible. Because the mandibular border varies considerably from person to person and changes with age, some contouring of the available shapes is often required to achieve an appropriate fit. Because the masseter muscle overlies the lateral aspect of the implant, the implant should be fixed to the mandible to prevent the masseter from moving the implant. Caution must be exercised in the area of the mental nerve to avoid impinging on the nerve. This is especially true in elderly patients with atrophic mandibles where greater lengths of the nerve may be exposed. An absolute contraindication for the use of porous polyethylene is alveolar ridge augmentation. With any use in the mandible, the surgeon should keep in mind that the implant must be placed low enough on the mandible so that if dentures are to be worn, they do not press on mucosa that directly overlies an implant.

MALAR IMPLANTS

The surgical community has learned a great deal in recent years about the aesthetics and anatomy of the malar area. Much of our understanding of deep plane surgery and the importance of the soft tissue attachments to the facial skeleton has been gained from experience in reconstructive surgery. With the adoption of rigid fixation for the treatment of zygomatic fractures, extensive degloving is now performed to obtain adequate mobilization of the fracture fragments. Emphasis has been placed on the restoration of the facial buttresses and on obtaining the correct anterior/posterior facial relationships, rather than on the redraping of the soft-tissue envelope.[51] With the persistence of malar deficiencies after anatomic restoration of the skeletal structures, the role of soft tissue ptosis and the importance of soft tissue suspension became clear.[26] For this reason the use of an implant that allows for tissue ingrowth is particularly important in the malar region. Porous implants become attached to the facial skeleton, and the ingrowth of the overlying tissue suspends the soft tissue envelope of the face.

Analysis of the deficiencies in the malar region have been reviewed by a number of authors.[44] From an aes-

thetic surgeon's perspective, the malar region can be divided into the soft tissue portions that overlie the zygomatic arch, the area below the arch, and the area medial to the arch. The zygomatic arch can be divided into thirds.[44] The medial and middle thirds are those most amenable to augmentation. Augmentation of the posterior aspect of the zygomatic arch is rarely, if ever, indicated because of the unnatural appearance that would be produced and because of the danger of injuring the facial nerve.

The region immediately medial to the zygomatic arch, which is also referred to as the nasojugal groove, is separated from the arch by the infraorbital foramen. The soft tissue in this region is thin, and implants in this area should be precisely contoured and tapered. This area can be augmented with a small teardrop-shaped implant. The nasojugal region can also be augmented in conjunction with the zygomatic arch with a malar implant that includes a medial extension separated by a groove to allow for unobstructed passage of the infraorbital nerve.

The malar region inferior to the zygomatic arch has been referred to as the submalar triangle, and augmentation of this region with large shell-shaped silicone implants has been advocated by some authors.[44,52] Anatomically, the submalar area is not directly adherent to a bony structure, and other authors do not attempt direct augmentation with an implant. Soft tissue augmentation of the submalar region can also be achieved with soft tissue suspension techniques.

SURGICAL APPROACH

Malar implants are most often placed through the mouth, through a subciliary incision, or using a combined approach. When malar implants are used in conjunction with open or endoscopic facelifts, they can also be placed through the facelift or crow's foot incisions.[53] Whichever route is selected, the basic principles of creating the pocket remain the same. The area of the pocket is infiltrated with a solution containing epinephrine. The dissection of the pocket should be performed staying as close to the bone as possible. An adequate pocket needs to be created by gentle use of the sweeping action of an elevator. Traction on the infraorbital nerve must be avoided. A lighted retractor is helpful in visualizing the area.

The intraoral route is probably the most widely used. An incision is made in the buccal mucosa above the first molar. The soft tissue is incised down to the bone of the maxillary buttress at the apex of the gingival-buccal sulcus. The remainder of the dissection is carried out with a periosteal elevator. The insertion of the implant can be facilitated by placing traction sutures through the tail of the implant, which are brought out through the skin within the hairline of the temple.

With the subciliary approach, an ordinary blepharoplasty incision is made 3 mm below the lash line, and a skin muscle flap is developed down to the infraorbital rim. This approach provides excellent visualization of the inferior orbital rim and thus allows for accurate positioning of the implant (Fig. 20–5).

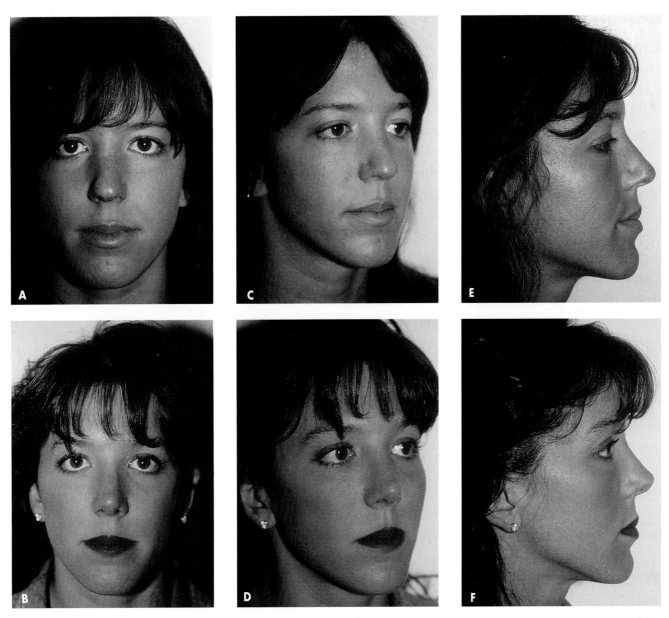

Figure 20–5. Preoperative **(A,C,E)** and 1-year postoperative **(B,D,F)** views of a patient after porous polyethylene malar implants and rhinoplasty.

PARANASAL IMPLANTS

The use of porous polyethylene implants in the paranasal region is an excellent solution to what is often a bilateral and asymmetric problem. This is particularly true in cleft patients and in non-Caucasian primary rhinoplasty patients. The ability to mold and carve the implants makes augmentation of the paranasal region easier than with autogenous tissue techniques. Preformed implants are available in right and left paranasal shapes. HA granules have also been used with success.[38]

CRANIAL APPLICATIONS

A variety of bony contour deformities can be found in the areas of the forehead or along the orbital rim.[54] Bony projections are easily corrected with a burr, being aware of the location of underlying sinuses. Bony depressions, as long as they are not in contact with open sinuses, are amenable to correction with a variety of alloplasts as onlay grafts.[55] When porous polyethylene is used, the onlays can be fixed in place with a suitable microscrew system, and final contouring can be performed in situ. For optimal results, it is necessary to taper the edges of the implant and to overlap the edges of the implant onto normal bone. A useful technique is to use an ultrathin sheet of material as an overlay to eliminate any minor irregularities or potentially visible implant edges. Specific shapes are available for both the temporal fossa and the orbital rim. HA, either in block or granular form, can also be useful for this purpose.

Custom implants are available for complex areas such as the supraorbital region of the forehead. These can either be prefabricated from a moulage or a piece of bone that has been removed, or they can be designed based on the basis of computed tomography (CT) data. CT data can be compiled to produce a three-dimensional model from which a custom implant can be manufactured.

POSTOPERATIVE COURSE

Most aesthetic facial surgery patients in whom alloplastic materials are used experience a relatively uneventful postoperative course. Fibrovascular ingrowth occurs in porous implants as early as 2 weeks, depending on the material. Nonporous implants invite formation of a pseudocapsule within 3 to 4 weeks. Once ingrowth or capsule formation occurs, the implants are stabilized and relatively resistant to infection. Despite this, the surgeon should remain aware of the possibility of extrusion or infection at all times. Persistent erythema in the skin overlying an implant is a harbinger of extrusion. Occasionally oral and possibly intravenous antibiotics can fend off an infection and salvage the implant. However, if a rapid response is not observed, rapid removal should be the next step.

SUMMARY

The chapter reviews the use of alloplastic implants in aesthetic facial surgery with an emphasis on malar and chin implants. The authors' highlight the use of several materials, including porous high-density polyethylene, Silastic, and expanded PTFE.

PEARLS

- Because of donor site morbidity, difficulty of use, and late changes of the implant, autogenous bone implants are used less frequently than alloplastic implants.
- Fixation of polyethylene implants is rarely necessary. If the potential exists for an implant to move before tissue ingrowth, the implant can be stabilized with sutures, K-wires, or screws.
- Patients who appear to need 15 mm or more projection in the chin should be considered for osteotomy of orthognatic treatments rather than implantation.
- Ethnic considerations play an important role in choosing the appropriate projection of the chin.
- Alveolar ridge augmentation is an absolute contraindication to the use of porous polyethylene.

REFERENCES

1. Farkas LG, Munro IR, Kolar JC. Relationships of profile segment inclinations in the faces of North American caucasians. In: Farkas LG, Munro IR, eds. *Anthropometric Facial Proportions in Medicine*. Springfield, Ill.: Charles C Thomas; 1987:57.

2. Bartlett SP, Wornom I, Whitaker LA. Evaluation of facial skeletal aesthetics and surgical planning. *Clin Plast Surg* 1991; 18(1):1–9.

3. Sheen JH, Sheen AP. *Aesthetic Rhinoplasty*. St. Louis: C.V. Mosby; 1987.

4. Gibson T, Davis WB. The distortion of autogenous cartilage grafts: Its cause and prevention. *Br J Plast Surg*. 1958; 10:257.

5. Young VL, Schuster RH, Harris LW. Intracerebral hematoma complicating split calvarial bone-graft harvesting. *Plast Reconstr Surg*. 1990; 86(4):763–765.

6. Frodel JL, Mereplette LJ, Quatela VC, Weinstein CS. Calvarial bone grafts. Techniques, considerations and controversies. *Arch Otolaryngol Head Neck Surg*. 1993; 119:17.

7. Adams JS. Facial augmentation with solid alloplastic implants: A rational approach to material selection. In: Glasgold AI, Silver FH, eds. *Applications of Biomaterials in Facial Plastic Surgery*. Boca Raton, FL: CRC Press; 1991:297–300.

8. Compton RA. Silicone manufacturing for long-term implants. *J Long-Term Effects Medical Implants* 1997; 7(1):29–54.

9. Ousterhout DK, Stelniki EJ. Plastic surgeon's plastic. *Clin Plast Surg*. 1996; 23:183–190.

10. Lewin SL, Miller TA. A review of epidemiologic studies analyzing the relationship between breast implants and connective tissue disorders. *Plast Reconstr Surg*. 1997; 100(5): 1309–1313.

11. Ahn ST, Monafo WW, Mustoe TA. Topical silicone gel: A new treatment for hypertrophic scars. *Surgery* 1989; 106(4): 781–787.

12. Robinson M, Shuken R. Bone resorption under plastic chin implants. *J Oral Surg*. 1969; 27:116–118.

13. Jobe RP, Iverson R, Vistnes L. Bone deformation beneath alloplastic implants. *Plast Reconstr Surg*. 1973; 51:169–175.

14. Lilla JA, Vistnes L, Jobe RP. The long term effects of hard alloplastic implants when put on bone. *Plast Reconstr Surg*. 1976; 59:14–18.

15. Wellisz T, Lawrence M, Jazayeri M, et al. The effect of alloplastic implant onlays on bone in the rabbit mandible. *Plast Reconstr Surg*. 1995; 96(4):957–963.

16. Wellisz T, Gade P, Zhou ZY, Golshani S. The persistence of orbital volume augmentation with the use of different implant materials. In Press.

17. Yaremchuk MJ, Rubin JP, Posnick JC. Implantable materials in facial aesthetic and reconstructive surgery: Biocompatibility and clinical applications. *J Craniofac Surg*. 1996; 7(6):473–484.

18. Dougherty W, Wellisz T. The fate of porous high density polyethylene implants placed adjacent to an open facial sinus. Canadian Society of Plastic Surgeons 45th Annual Meeting. Whistler, British Columbia, Canada, June 27, 1991.

19. Spector M, Harmon SL, Kreutner A. Characteristics of tissue growth into Proplast and porous polyethylene implants in bone. *J Biomed Mater Res*. 1979; 13:677–692.

20. Homsey CA. Bio-compatibility in selection of materials for implantation. *J Biomed Mater Res*. 1970; 4:341–356.

21. Rubin LR. Polyethylene as a bone and cartilage substitute: A 32 year retrospective. In: Rubin LR, ed. *Biomaterials in Plastic Surgery*. St. Louis: CV Mosby, 1983:477–493.

22. Bikhazi HB, Van Antwerp R. The use of Medpor in cosmetic and reconstructive surgery: experimental and clinical evidence. In: Stucker S, ed. *Plastic and Reconstructive Surgery of the Head and Neck*. St. Louis: C. V. Mosby, 1990:271–273.

23. Berghaus A, Mulch G, Handrock M. Porous polyethylene and Proplast: Their behavior in a bony implant bed. *Arch Otorhinolaryngol*. 1984; 240:115–123.

24. Wellisz T, Dougherty W. The role of alloplastic skeletal modification in the reconstruction of facial burns. *Ann Plast Surg*. 1993; 30(6):531–536.

25. Wellisz T. Reconstruction of the burned external ear using a Medpor porous polyethylene pivoting helix framework. *Plast Reconstr Surg*. 1993; 91(5):811–818.

26. Wellisz T. Clinical experience with the Medpor porous polyethylene implant. *Aesthet Plast Surg*. 1993; 17:339–344.

27. Romano JJ, Iliff NT, Manson PN. Use of Medpor porous polyethylene implants in 140 patients with facial fractures. *J Craniofac Surg*. 1993; 4(3):142–147.

28. Wellisz T, Kanel G, Anooshian RV. Characteristics of the tissue response to Medpor porous polyethylene implants in the human facial skeleton. *J Long-Term Effects Medical Implants*. 1993; 3(3):223–235.

29. Merritt K, Shafer JW, Brown SA. Implant site infection rates with porous and dense materials. *J Biomed Mater Res*. 1979; 13:101–108.

30. Sclafani AP, Romo T, Silver L. Clinical and histologic behavior of exposed porous high-density polyethylene implants. *Plast Reconstr Surg*. 1997; 99(1):41–50.

31. Sclafani AP, Thomas JR, Cox AJ, Cooper MH. Clinical and histologic response of subcutaneous expanded polytetrafluoroethylene (Gore-Tex) and porous high-density polyethylene (Medpor) implants to acute and early infection. *Arch Otolaryngol Head Neck Surg*. 1997; 123:328–336.

32. Eriksson C. Surface energies and the bone induction principle. *J Biomed Mater Res*. 1985; 19:833–849.

33. Gristina AG. Biomaterial-centered infection: microbial adhesion versus tissue integration. *Science* 1987; 237:1588–1595.

34. Williams JD, Romo T, Sclafani AP, Cho H. Porous high-density polyethylene implants in auricular reconstruction. *Arch Otolaryngol Head Neck Surg*. 1997; 123:578–583.

35. Choi JC, Sims CD, Casanova R, et al. Porous polyethylene implant for orbital floor reconstruction. *J Cranio-Maxillofacial Trauma*. 1995; 1(3):42–49.

36. Holmes RE, Hagler HK. Porous hydroxyapatite as a bone graft substitute in cranial reconstruction: a histometric study. *Plast Reconstr Surg*. 1988; 81:662–671.

37. Salyer KE, Hall CD. Porous hydroxyapatite as an onlay bone-graft substitute for maxillofacial surgery. *Plast Reconstr Surg.* 1989; 84:236.

38. Waite PD, Matukae VJ. Zygomatic augmentation with hydroxyapatite: A preliminary report. *J Oral Maxillofac Surg.* 1986; 44:349.

39. Rubin PJ, Yaremchuk MJ. Complications and toxicities of implantable biomaterials used in facial reconstructive and aesthetic surgery: A comprehensive review of the literature. *Plast Reconstr Surg.* 1997; 100(5):1309–1313.

40. Garner WL, Committee TPSEFD. Gore-Tex facial implants. *Plast Reconstr Surg.* 1997; 100(7):1899–1900.

41. Maas CS, Merwin GE, Wilson J, et al. Comparison of biomaterials for facial bone augmentation. *Arch Otolaryngol Head Neck Surg.* 1990; 116:551–556.

42. Sauer BW. Technical aspects of Porex Surgical Implants. In Janecka IP, Tiedemann K, eds. *Skull Base Surgery: Anatomy, Biology and Technology.* Philadelphia: Lippincott-Raven; 1997:367–375.

43. Eppley BL, Sadove AM, German RZ. Evaluation of HTR polymer as a craniomaxillofacial graft material. *Plast Reconstr Surg.* 1990; 86:1085–1092.

44. Terino EO. Alloplastic facial contouring: surgery of the fourth plane. *Aesth Plast Surg.* 1992; 16:195–212.

45. Flowers RS. Aesthetic surgery in the Oriental: Current trends. In: Marsh J, ed. *Current Therapy in Plastic and Reconstructive Surgery.* Philadelphia: BC Decker; 1988:483.

46. Flowers RS. Alloplastic augmentation of the anterior mandible. *Clin Plast Surg.* 1991; 18(1):107–138.

47. Ousterhout DK. Mandibular angle augmentation and reduction. *Clin Plast Surg.* 1991; 18(1):153–161.

48. Ousterhout DK. Aesthetic contouring of the craniofacial skeleton. Boston: Little, Brown; 1991.

49. Whitaker LA, Bartlett SP. Skeletal alterations as a basis for facial rejuvenation. *Clin Plast Surg.* 1991; 18(1): 197–203.

50. Epker BN. *Esthetic Maxillofacial Surgery.* Malvern, PA: Lea & Febiger Publishing; 1994.

51. Manson PN, Grivas A, Rosenbaum A, et al. Studies on enophthalmos: II. The measurement of orbital injuries and their treatment by quantitative computed tomography. *Plast Reconstr Surg.* 1985; 77:203–214.

52. Binder WE. Submalar augmentation. *Arch Otolaryngol.* 1989; 115:797.

53. Ramirez OM, Pozner JN. Subperiosteal minimally invasive laser endoscopic rhytidectomy: The SMILE facelift. *Aesthet Plast Surg.* 1996; 20:463–470.

54. Manson PN, Crawley WA, Hoopes JE. Frontal cranioplasty: Risk factors and choice of cranial vault reconstructive material. *Plast Reconstr Surg.* 1986; 77:1986; 77:888–900.

55. Wellisz T, Dougherty W, Gross J. Craniofacial applications for the Medpor porous polyethylene flexblock implant. *J Craniofac Surg.* 1992; 3(2):101–107.

Facial Resurfacing

The facial resurfacing section is the only section in this volume that we have separated into three parts with three contributors. Facial resurfacing, although an old and time-honored technique, has taken on a new form as a result of changes in technology and appreciation of the enhanced result that facial resurfacing can add to excisional and suspensory facial surgery techniques.

Dr. Farrior introduces the oldest and most time-honored technique of dermabrasion. Dermabrasion certainly was the most powerful method of facial resurfacing until the last half dozen years. It is experiential, or experience based, and for that reason it is frequently difficult to master a consistently aesthetically acceptable technique for many surgeons. However, in the hands of an expert such as Dr. Farrior, the technique yields results that are consistent, predictable, and highly desirable.

Dr. English reviewed meticulously what may be historically the most ancient of facial surgical techniques, the chemical peel. The chemical peel has been described as long ago as Egyptian times and in a sense may represent the first facial aesthetic treatment. The use and indications of the variety of chemical techniques have certainly been the foundation of the eventual evolution of laser techniques. Dr. English renders insightful information that clearly proves the continuing integral usefulness of chemical techniques used in conjunction with or as an alternative to modern laser resurfacing techniques.

Finally, Dr. Geronemus describes in detail what has certainly added a new tool in the armamentarium of the facial surgeon: laser resurfacing. Laser resurfacing itself is undergoing evolution even at the time of this printing, and the modalities of CO_2 and erbium: YAG and combined erbium: YAG/CO_2 technologies are discussed.

As with any advancement and introduction of newer techniques, no doubt exists that the successful surgeon will never forget and stop using older, time-honored techniques for the lure of newer technology. It is certainly the combination and synergy of all three modalities that enable the facial plastic surgeon to approach the perfect result.

Facial Resurfacing

Aesthetic Facial Plastic Surgery, edited by Thomas Romo, III, and Arthur L. Millman, Thieme Medical Publishers, Inc., New York, New York, Copyright © 2000.

CHAPTER 21

Dermabrasion
A Facial Plastic Surgeon' s Perspective

RICHARD T. FARRIOR*

Dermabrasion, or skin planing, has multiple uses in cervicofacial esthetic and reconstructive surgery. The aesthetic facial plastic surgeon is often not familiar with the variety of places that dermabrasion can be helpful or further improve results. Certainly the facial plastic surgeon should have this useful procedure in his or her armamentarium whether dealing with injury and scar revisions or changes in aging skin.

Dermabrasion is far from obsolete although it has had fluctuating degrees of popularity over the last twenty-five to thirty years, the span of the author's personal experience with the techniques. It is not the purpose of this chapter to compare the merits of laser, chemabrasion, and dermabrasion or particularly to champion one over the other. In general it might be said that the deeper the scar or the wrinkle the more dermabrasion is indicated. Each procedure requires some dermabrasion as indicated.

* Editors' Note: Much of this chapter is taken directly from Dr. Farrior's classic article "Dermabrasion in Facial Surgery" (Laryngoscope 1985; 98(5):534–545), which was used for a number of years by the American Board of Facial Plastic Surgery and American Board of Otolaryngology in their examinations. Rather than rewrite this material, we reproduce the article almost verbatim here. Dr. Farrior has updated the information where appropriate; these sections are called "An Update." All of Dr. Farrior's original references are included in the reference list and are recommended reading for a thorough and historical knowledge of dermabrasion. All art and text has been reproduced with permission of the publisher.

GENERAL CONSIDERATIONS

Dermabrasion, or one form or another of surgical planing, has been used in facial surgery since antiquity, probably since the traumatically abraded skin surface was first observed to heal smoothly and completely. The more recent and wide use of the dermabrasion techniques is credited to the early work of Iverson,[1,2] Kurtin,[3] Orentreich,[4] and other contributors from plastic surgery and dermatology.[5–7] Originally attention was drawn to dermabrasion by Kromayer,[5] with Iverson[2] repopularizing the procedure using motor driven abrasion cylinders. Dermabrasion is the treatment of choice for acne scars and other scars or irregularities of the skin surface. For the author it is the treatment of choice in a number of other conditions where chemoexfoliation or chemabrasion (chemical peel) is now widely used.

The precise mechanical control of the depth of dermabrasion, the ability to vary the depth of the dermabrasion according to the location of and degree of scarring, the early healing without concern for the penetration and absorption of chemical elements, especially phenol, and the predictability of healing have led the author to favor dermabrasion in most instances.

Healing occurs at the surface with a rapid proliferation of squamous epithelium, while in the depths a horizontal striation of collagenous patterns with which the described inter-island contraction leads to the smoothing out of the skin and perhaps some increased surface tightness.[8,9] Healing of the epithelium arises from the epithelial elements in the skin adnexae, which vary in location and number among individuals.[7] The deeper into the depths of the dermis one proceeds, the fewer of these skin elements there are found.

There is probably a greater collagen proliferation with chemical peel and some feel that this favors the smoothness of the skin.[8–10] However, in my observations over a quarter of a century with long-term follow-up, I have not noted a particular difference between the healing of the two techniques and feel that long lasting results may be obtained by both in regard to fine rhytids.[11] For acne scarring most authorities agree that dermabrasion is the treatment of choice.[9]

MATERIALS

For acne scarring per se we have preferred the disposable silicone cylinders on the motor driven unit originally described by Iverson[2] (Fig. 21–1A). Usually only the large and medium size cylinders are necessary although a smaller cylinder is available for use in the smaller crevices

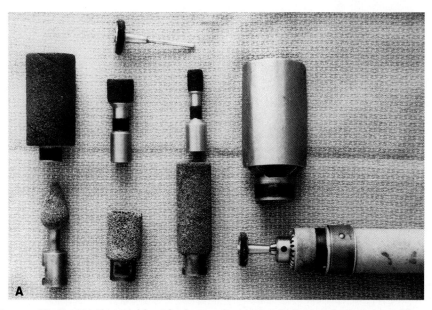
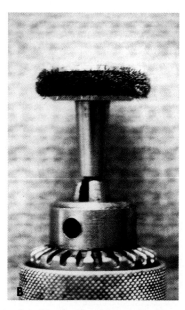

Figure 21–1. (A) Disposable cylinders and permanent abrasive cylinders used on the Stryker handpiece. Motor driven with cable attachment and accelerator-type foot control. **(B)** Fine wire brush, medium width. Used for fine rhytids or more precise deeper dermabrasion.

or where the angle for dermabrasion is difficult. The variable speed accelerator type foot pedal is preferred and recommended. For specific deep pitted scars, particularly deep rhytids or in association with scar revisions, the wire brush is used (Fig. 21–1B).

The list of materials given in Table 21–1 are those most commonly used by the author and are included to assist the surgeon. There are a number of excellent electrical or air-driven units in use and there are a variety of other abrasive cylinders. The cylinders can be of various shapes, in particular cone or tapered; the surgeon should select those with which he or she is most comfortable and proficient (Fig. 21–1). Proficiency can come only with practice and use in a variety of situations. Portable or battery driven units have been developed but some surgeons have found these to be of limited use, especially relative to adequate power or sufficient duration of power. They, perhaps, have some use in small areas for office surgery. Handpieces may range from the standard dental handpiece to the more elaborate. The author prefers the larger cylindrical handpiece which can be both firmly and lightly held and precisely controlled. The hand and knuckles are held on the back of the handpiece so that the revolving cylinder can be held as flat as possible against the skin surface.

An Update

The chief feature of the equipment that we use today is the ability to reverse the rotation of the cylinder or brush so

Table 21–1 Specific Equipment for Dermabrasion[*] **(See text and Fig. 21–2 also)**

Carbide cylinders	Small	1360–30
	Medium	1360–200
	Large	1360–100
Silicone cylinders	1″ × 2″	1360–10
	$\frac{1}{2}″ \times \frac{1}{2}″$	1360–20
	$\frac{1}{4}″ \times \frac{1}{4}″$	1360–30
Wire Brush	Regular	
Motor	115 volt motor power limit	
Cord	Flexible cable 1308	
Foot pedal switch	1307	
Iverson dermabrader handpiece	1360	
	Jacobs chuck & key	1355–4
	sleeve for 5/32″ chuck	1355–8
	Handpiece only	1360–5
	2″ × 1″ splash guard	1360–6
	Wire key	1360–7
Adaptic nonadhering dressing	3″ × 16″	2014
	Johnson & Johnson	
Adrenalin compresses	Adrenalin topical	1 : 1000–30 mL
	Normal saline	240 mL
	(1 : 8000 topical adrenalin)	

[*] Data for the 1300 series from the Stryker Corporation, Kalamazoo, Michigan.

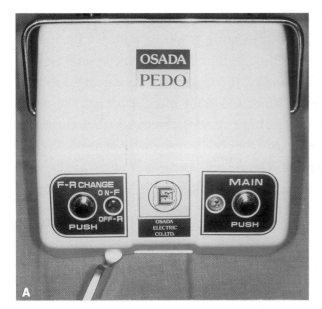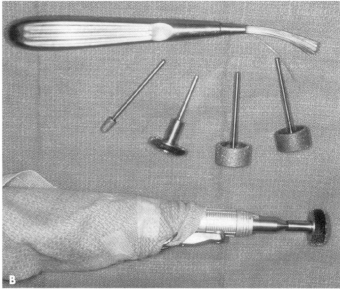

Figure 21-2. (A) Dermabrasion power source with reversible rotation. Note F (*forward*) and R (*reverse*). This is controlled by the surgeon by pushing the button with the foot. **(B)** Small handle that is sterile. The cord may be covered with a variety of available tubed drapes. The preferred wider dermabrasion brush is shown on the handle. Above is the wire brush for cleaning the dermabrasion brush.

that it is always rotating toward the anatomic margin, such as for the lip. When rotated away, the possibility always exist of grabbing into the particular margin, creating a tear or laceration. We have found the Osado (Pedo) dermabrader with its smaller, light handle most satisfactory (Fig. 21–2). Many of the pictures in the original article (see Figs. 21–1, 21–8, and 21–9) show the Stryker cable and handpiece with the Jacobs chuck, although the guard has been omitted in some photographs for demonstration.

The quality of the wire brushes also has improved, so that less spread of the bristles occurs, especially on the sides of the brush. Where possible, the wider the brush, the safer and more even the dermabrasion (Fig. 21–2B, *bottom*). More narrow brushes are, however, an advantage for varying the depth of the dermabrasion, such as into a narrow, deep rhytid or inverting scar. The wire brush is being used more frequently for segmental dermabrasion such as in the perioral and glabella areas (Fig. 21–3).

I still prefer the silicone cylinders of varying sizes for acne scarring and fine facial rhytids, especially when full-face dermabrasion is done (Fig. 21–9). Compared with the disposable cylinders, I have found the permanent

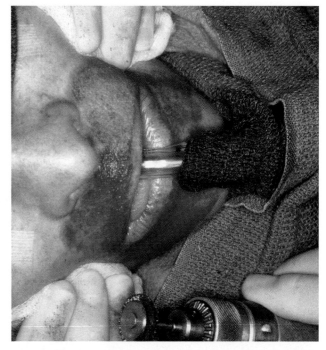

Figure 21-3. Segmental dermabrasion using the Stryker handle, cable, and motor with a guarded Jacobs chuck to hold the shaft. Note that the abrasion is carried over the vermilion roll onto the pink vermilion. Compare with Figures 21–6, 21–7, and 21–13. The white deeper dermis shown on the patient's left upper lip serves as a gauge as to the depth. The more delicate handle shown in Figure 21–2 is more frequently used today.

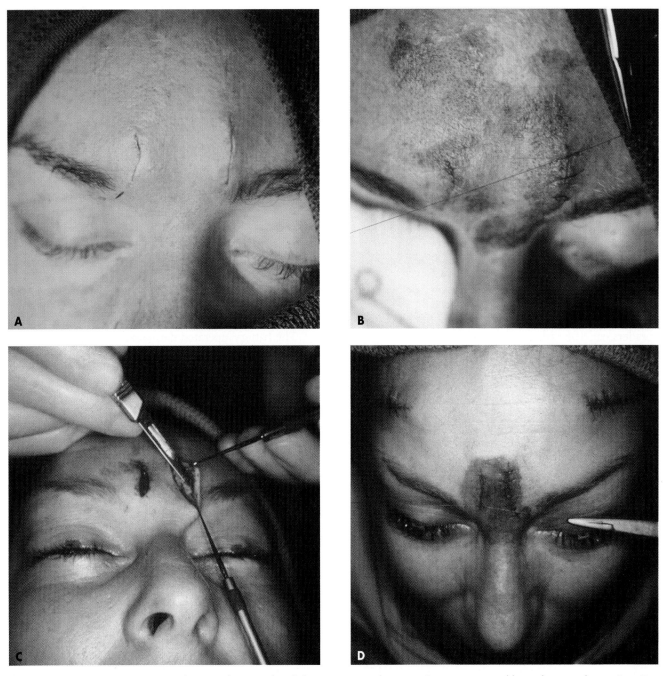

Figure 21–4. **(A)** Scar revision showing the completed deep interrupted sutures. Deep interrupted buried suture closure (see Figure 21–11). This step is followed by dermabrasion. **(B)** After dermabrasion over the incision and surrounding area, fine nylon skin sutures are placed. **(C)** and **(D)** For extreme glabellar rhytids with deep furrowing, this technique, for appropriate cases, is used in combination with dermabrasion. A beveled incision is made on either side of the furrow and each side elevated as for any plastic closure. The intervening skin is left in place and de-epithelialized, thus providing a dermal fat graft filler in place with its own blood supply. The corrugator muscles are then sectioned and partially resected. The skin is closed with interrupted buried subcuticular sutures over the "implant." Dermabrasion is carried out, and final closure is accomplished with interrupted nylon skin sutures.

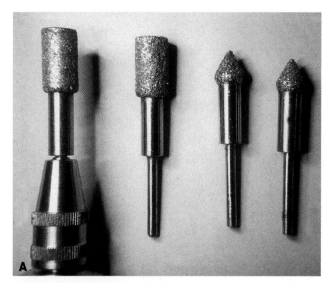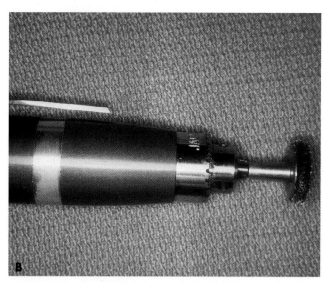

Figure 21–5. (A) Permanent dermabrasion cylinders versus the silicone "sandpaper" cylinders. **(B)** Battery-operated dermabrasion handle (see text). See Figure 21–1A and B.

abraders, such as carborundum and diamond, less satisfactory because they have a tendency to abrade or even "burn" the surface with more serum production. Their various shapes can be advantegeous in particular locations (Fig. 21–5A). Both the cylinders and the wire brushes can be effectively hand held and manually used without the motor in areas such as the eyelids and smaller scar revisions. This is accomplished by slight rotation while advancing the brush with side-to-side and axial movement.

The battery-operated dermabraders have proven satisfactory only for very small areas. The power to the rotating brush can vary, and the duration of power is limited (Fig. 21–5B).

In regard to the lips we are now going over the vermilion roll with a soft fine touch and getting better results at the skin mucosal junction as opposed to what is seen in Figure 21–6, where a more cautious approach was done at the time of that surgery (see also Figs. 21–3, 21–7, and 21–13).

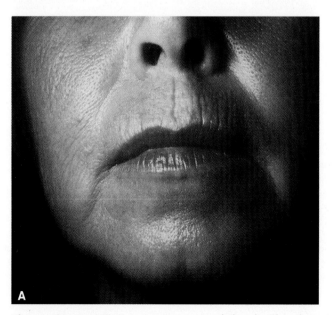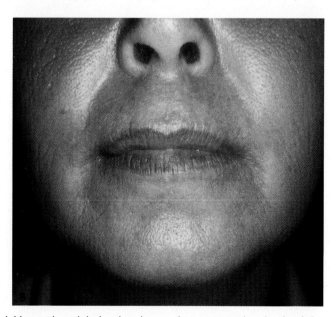

Figure 21–6. (A) Preoperative perioral rhytids. The photo is deliberately sidelighted to better demonstrate the depth of the rhytids. **(B)** Satisfactory result but note rhytids at vermilion roll. At the time this area was omitted but is now included in the technique. Compare to Figures 21–2, 21–8, and 21–13.

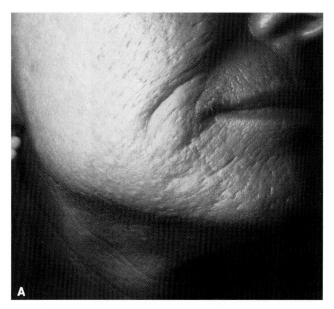 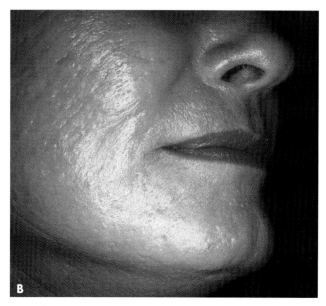

Figure 21-7. (A) Preoperative photo showing rhytids, acne scars, and weathering in an athletic woman. The sidelighting is deliberate. **(B)** Postoperative results with segmental dermabrasion combined with facelift. The patient did not want total facial resurfacing. See Figures 21–13C and D and 21–14.

PREOPERATIVE CONSULTATION

The patient presenting for dermabrasion requires considerable preoperative preparation in what to expect from the actual procedure and postoperative course. In addition to the degree of the activity of the acne and the nature of the patient's skin, the scars themselves must be precisely analyzed. Preferably the patient should be receiving no hormonal therapy. If birth control pills have been used, the patient should discontinue the pills for at least two full cycles in the hope that some of the related pigmentation problems can be prevented. The type of skin, particularly that with considerable sebaceous material, should be noted. The present degree of pigmentation and all degrees—from the thick, oily skin with deep punctate pits to the thin, fair skin—must be evaluated and these conditions pointed out to the patients.

In the preoperative evaluation and instructions the patient should be advised that the two most common complications of dermabrasion are hyper- or hypopigmentation and formation of milia (see complications below). Following the general information for any surgical procedure, the next main emphasis is placed on the need to remain out of the sun postoperatively. The patient is instructed, in as much detail as possible, what the immediate postoperative appearance will be; that they will want to "hide" for seven to ten days or, at least, might not want to make major social or business plans during this time.

SURGICAL TECHNIQUE

For a full face dermabrasion for generalized acne pitting, rhytids or generalized superficial keratosis,[12] hospitalization and general anesthesia are utilized (Fig. 21–8). For smaller areas or for areas of secondary dermabrasion, local anesthesia with infiltration is preferred to ethyl chloride spray.

Ethyl chloride is believed to prevent determining the exact depth of dermabrasion. Under general anesthesia the sanguineous and serosanguineous excretions help moisten the skin, preventing abrasive burning of the tissues which could occur if the freshly abraded area is too dry.

One learns to determine the depth of dermabrasion through the epidermis and into the outer layers of the

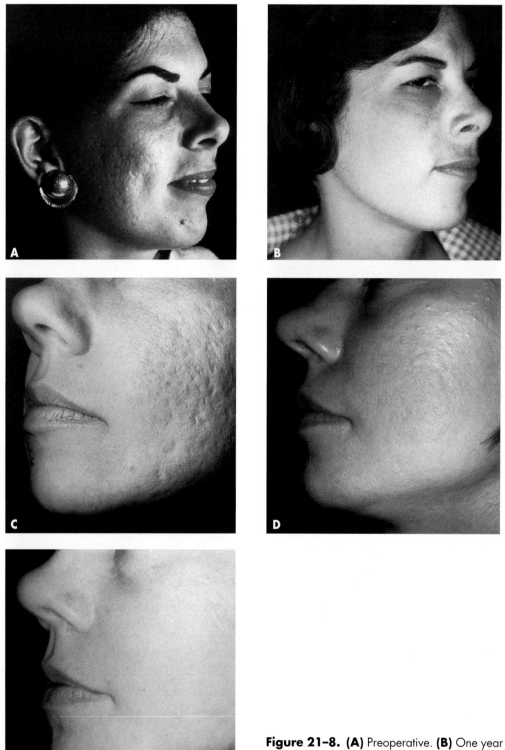

Figure 21–8. (A) Preoperative. **(B)** One year postoperative, slight hypopigmentation cheeks and hyperpigmentation of lips. **(C)** Second patient, preoperative. **(D)** Six months postoperative with a few persistent milia. **(E)** One year postoperative with final healing.

dermis both while the dermabrasion is in progress and after some hemostasis by the white appearance of the dermis and the actual texture of the skin with its variable thickness. Occasionally, for extremely deep pits, crosshatching or scoring of the bottom of the pit with the surgical blade or broken razor blade may be required. These deep pits, which may have originally extended through the thickness of the skin, can rarely be completely eliminated, but with the dermabrasion around their periphery, they usually flatten, and with contracture, the depth of the scar draws level, or nearly to the level, with the surrounding skin surface. Such deep scars lack the pilosebaceous adnexae of normal skin and therefore heal with an excessively smooth appearance.[7] The patient and the surgeon must be aware that extending the dermabrasion through these deep scars only produces additional scar.

Although lesser procedures can be done as outpatient or office procedures, full face dermabrasion is done under oral endotracheal anesthesia. Positioning of the endotracheal tube and the approach to the dermabrasion can be worked out systematically so that there is minimal movement of the tube. The preferable position in the various anatomic sites, taking into account the direction of rotation of the cylinder, can be used to best advantage. (Fig. 21–9).

With the patient in the supine position, the head is extended slightly and initially rotated to the patient's left with the endotracheal tube, which is not fixed, coming out of the far left side of the mouth and displaced slightly cephalically (Fig. 21–9A). The endotracheal tube has a flexible extension going towards the patient's chest which must be draped such that it is covered but able to be moved from side to side, allowing dermabrasion to be carried out with planing, such as on the left side of the lower lip and chin area. At all times the assistant applies countertraction with his fingers extending over the edge of a gauze sponge, both for a better grip and to prevent catching the sponge in the revolving cylinder (Fig. 21–10). In small areas the surgeon himself provides the countertraction, dermabrading between two fingers.

Dermabrasion commences on the left lower lip as far towards the left commissure or beyond as is mechani-

cally advantageous. On the other side of the endotracheal tube one of the assistant's hands is placed directly opposite the commissure and the other in the submandibular area to flatten the skin and provide countertraction. The surgeon uses his left hand to produce opposing traction. From the surgeon's eye, the dermabrasion cylinder, which revolves to the right (clockwise), is revolving towards the lip allowing dermabrasion to the very margins of the lip. If the opposite position was used there would be a tendency to bite into the loose lip which could create lacerations. This is of much more concern when utilizing the wire brush (Fig. 21–10).

Dermabrasion is then carried back towards the patient's right until the entire lower lip is dermabraded. This dermabrasion is carried beyond the shadow line of the chin and mandible. Dermabrasion is then commenced far laterally and posteriorly in the area of the mandible and the preauricular area. This is of some help regarding bleeding during dermabrasion carried out beyond the area which is now bleeding. The surgeon works from below upward or towards the center of the face. The adrenalin compress (1 : 8000 solution, topical) is placed over the previously dermabraded area. From this position, dermabrasion is carried up to the temple area, far forward into the nasolabial sulcus and on to the nose. One can go quite close to the thin eyelid skin but this is the shadow line and the area where the standard dermabrasion usually stops. With a slight change in the patient's position, the dermabrasion is carried out for the majority of the forehead, dermabrading right to and within the edge of the hair. The hair is brushed aside by the rotation of the burr (Fig. 21–9B). The eyebrows are not done at this time. From the head of the table the glabella area and the majority of the nose can be approached continuing to use the large cylinder.

The foot pedal, base of the dermabrasion motor and surgeon's position then shift to the left side. The endotracheal tube is brought out the right side of the mouth. From the left side attention is given to the eyebrow area and the upper lip (Fig. 21–9C). The medium size cylinder is used for the upper lip and for more precise

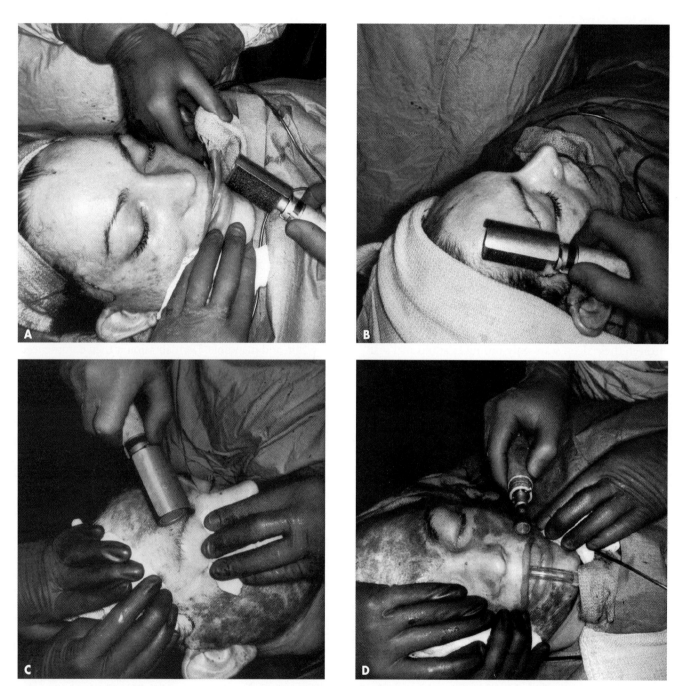

Figure 21–9. (A) Procedure started with endotracheal tube controlled on far side of lower lip dermabrading first parallel then perpendicular to lip margin. **(B)** Rotation of cylinder is clockwise from the operator. The forehead hairline is operated from the patient's right brushing the hair away. **(C)** Lower forehead dermabraded from the left side brushing the brow downward. **(D)** Medium cylinder for upper lip and where smaller cylinder is required for good positioning. This was a combined facelift and dermabrasion. See Figure 21–14.

dermabrasion around the nose (Fig. 21–9D). The large size cylinder can be used readily for most of the left side of the upper lip before reaching the nose. With the medium, or occasionally the small, dermabrasion cylinder one can go back over the now virtually hemostased area and look for deeper pits which may require addi-

tional dermabrasion. The wire brush is sometimes used to supplement in these areas. Occasionally it is necessary, as previously mentioned, to score or cross-hatch the depths of the wound or deep pits that might be the result of epidermal inclusion cysts beyond the simple acne scar. These more extensive scars may require surgical excision,

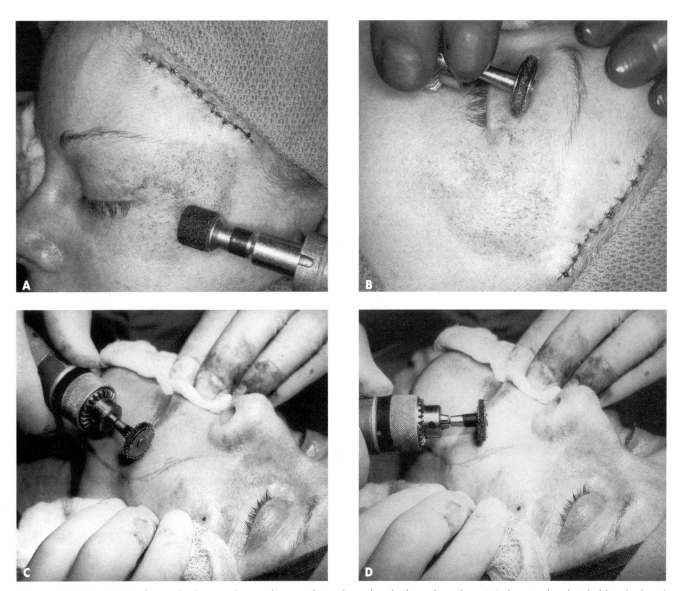

Figure 21–10. (A) Medium cylinder may be used motor driven lateral to the lateral canthus. **(B)** The wire brush is held in the hand and manual dermabrasion carried out for the eyelids. This may be carried to the lid margins. **(C)** Lip dernabrasion with the wire brush for fine rhytids. Wire brush first held parallel to the vermillion and extending slightly over the vermillion roll. **(D)** Second position, 45– to 60–degrees angulation to go to the lip margin and create mini 'Z' plasties. Note hand position for skin traction. Brush rotates toward the lip margin.

staying in favorable skin tension lines. As mentioned, in the management of scars when excision is necessary, the deep interrupted subcuticular suture may be placed first, additional dermabrasion carried out and then the skin sutures placed (Fig. 21–11).

Immediately following completion of dermabrasion, adrenalin sponges are placed over the entire operative field until the superficial bleeding is controlled. At the end of the procedure there is usually a mottled white appearance as the deeper layers of the dermis are apparent. In essence, the dermabrasion goes only into the superficial layers of the dermis but this can be modified relative to the thickness of the skin of the anatomic area and patient. At this time it is often advisable on particular patients with a large amount of sebaceous material, small sebaceous inclusion cysts or comedones to thoroughly go over the face and express as many of these small sites as possible. In some patients these can be quite numerous

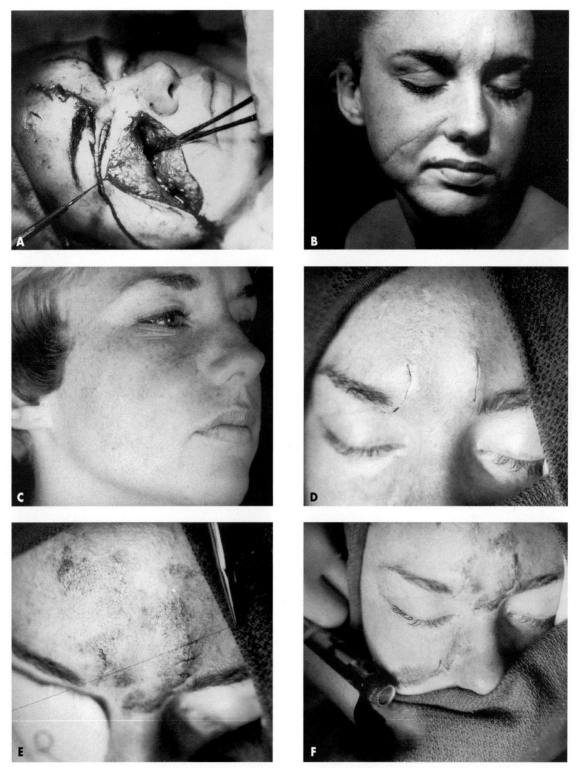

Figure 21–11. Dermabrasion in scar revision. (See also Fig. 21–4A and B.) **(A)** Original injury. **(B)** Less than ideal result after initial repair. **(C)** Final result after limited revision and dermabrasion. **(D)** Scar revision with meticulous closure using interrupted subcuticular sutures. **(E)** After deep closure dermabrasion is used and then the alternating spring loop and surgical twists surface nylon sutures applied. **(F)** Dermabrasion following 'Z' plasty on cheek.

but with this management and the aid of dermabrasion, tend to heal better than at any other time.

DRESSING

Following compression and hemostasis, Adaptic gauze is placed over the entire area with considerable overlap beyond the dermabraded sites to allow for some slippage or movement of the dressing. Flat gauze is placed immediately over this and then Kerlix fluff or Kerlix rolled gauze is applied in a wraparound type head dressing and held in place with light pressure using two and three inch Kling. The dressing is stabilized with adhesive tape. This mummy-type dressing stays in position until the following day when it is removed down to the Adaptic as described below. For small dermabraded areas, whether done under local or general anesthesia, modified pressure dressings to absorb the serum which comes through the larger mesh of the Adaptic is used. Adequate sedation and pain medication is given to the patient, who is kept in a semi-Fowler position and fed a liquid or a mechanical soft diet.

An Update

One advantage of the experience gained through all these years has been the introduction of various dressings that have been presented, such as N-Terface or Interface fine mesh Scarlet Red and Vigilon, and less porous dressings. However, despite these newer products, we have gone back to Adaptic covered with an absorbing gauze occlusive dressing with light pressure (Fig. 21–12A,B). The dressing is removed to the level of the Adaptic in 24 hr. At this point a dry technique as opposed to hydrating care is instituted. The Adaptic is left on 6 to 10 days or until it falls off. This dressing looks no worse than other dressings or than the natural crusting with weeping, which occurs with no dressing and the use of creams and ointments.

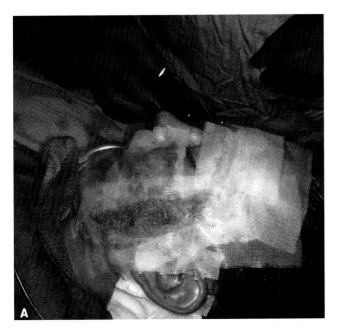 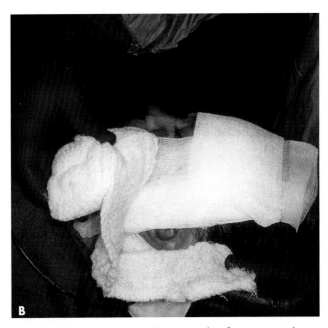

Figure 21–12. (A) Combined full-face dermabrasion and limited flap facelift, demonstrating the principle of a moist occlusive dressing for optimum epithelial healing. Adaptic gauze is placed over the wound after diluted adrenalin sponges have been applied for hemostasis. See Figure 21–13. **(B)** Flat gauze is placed over the Adaptic, creating a smooth dressing immediately over the wound. Kerlix gauze is then applied and held in position with light pressure by wraparound roll gauze (Kling). The dressing is secured by tape. The outer absorbent dressing is removed down to the Adaptic in 24 hr. After this dry treatment is instituted, using a drying lamp or hairdryer. This is opposed to the hydrating care given for the use of Interface. Some additional crusting occurs but comes off with the Adaptic at 5 to 8 days. During this time the patient looks no worse than with any other resurfacing technique and is free of crusting much earlier than with other types of postoperative care at the time the Adaptic is removed. See Figures 21–9 and 21–14

Postoperative patient instruction with this method is much simpler than for Interface for instance. All the crusting comes off with the Adaptic leaving the face looking better sooner than with other techniques (Fig. 21–12B). The mesh of the Adaptic seems to be the appropriate size for both epithelial healing and for the serum to seep through to the absorbing gauze during the first 24 hr.

SEGMENTAL DERMABRASION

When the areas of involvement are limited, dermabrasion is carried to natural skin lines or anatomic areas of limitation to camouflage the line of demarcation with the unabraded skin. The cheek, for instance, is surgically planed to the nasolabial area, the lower eyelid, and inferiorly and laterally to either the line of prominence of the cheek (rouge area) or to the hairline and mandible when there is greater involvement. Preferably the entire forehead is done going lateral to the point of the shortest distance between the hair and eyebrow, blending into the temple. In general, the nasolabial fold is a major demarcation line for completing the dermabrasion of the cheek and lips (Figs. 21–9 and 21–13).

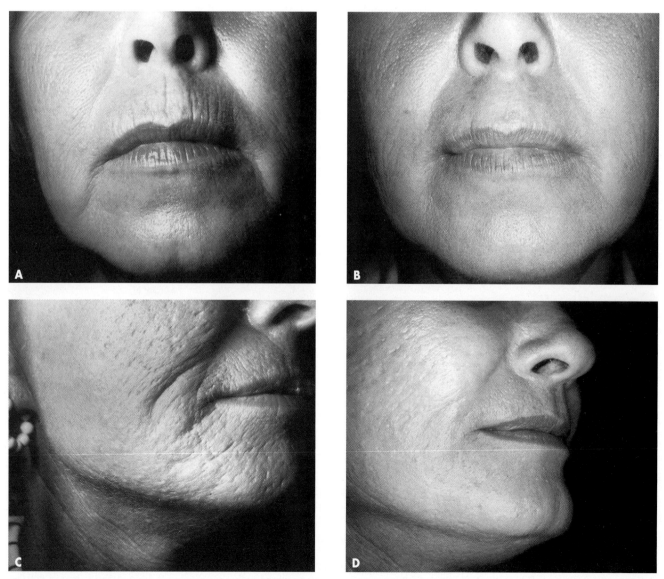

Figure 21–13. (A) Preoperative fine perioral rhytids, **(B)** Postoperative, 6 months, done before dermabrasion was carried over the vermillion roll as it is now executed. **(C)** Preoperative fine rhytids and pitting with sun exposure. **(D)** Postoperative limited facelift and dermabrasion of upper and lower lips and chin only. See Figures 21–6 and 21–7, color versions of these photographs.

Table 21–2 Indications for Dermabrasion in Facial Surgery

Acne scarring	Telangiectasia
Acne scarring with facelift	Tattoos
Fine rhytids	Scar revisions
Full face	
Perioral	Superficial lacerations
Periorbital	
Glabella	Overlay grafts
Rhinophyma	Hyperkeratosis
Scars lower third of nose	De-epithelization of flaps
Nasal supratip	Thinning of cartilage (otoplasty)

CONDITIONS FOR DERMABRASION

There are a number of conditions where dermabrasion is particularly useful for the facial plastic surgeon. These are not all simply cosmetic procedures but are medical conditions or anatomic considerations to which the surgeon should give special consideration (Table 21–2).

ACNE SCARRING (FIGS. 21–7, 21–8, AND 21–14)

It should be emphasized at the outset to the patient that dermabrasion is for the scars which are the result of the acne infections, not to treat the active lesions. Actually, in the older patient who may have only occasional active lesions, dermabrasion seems to help in reducing the number and appearance of these active infections. Generally one waits for the major period of acne infections to pass, which is usually the early twenties, if it is teenage acne with which we are concerned. Dermatologic consultation is strongly advocated, especially if the number of active lesions is great. The dermatologist is of great assistance in preparing the patient for surgery. If the patient is not already on antibiotics, broad spectrum antibiotics are given starting two to six weeks prior to

surgery to control any active lesions. Epidermabrasion, such as advocated by Orentreich,[4] is not encouraged in the immediate postoperative period. In the absence of a dermatology consult, we provide the patient with general instructions, particularly in regard to facial cleansing, perhaps using Therapads (Fuller), detergent soaps or Phisohex, and a course of antibiotic therapy.

Combined dermabrasion and face lift may be advisable in severe acne associated with loss of skin elasticity. This was done on the patient shown in Figure 21–9.

Full face dermabrasion is occasionally carried out as either a staged or a single procedure with what is usually a more limited facial rhytidoplasty. The use of the face lift for acne scarring should be emphasized. Often severe acne causes considerable loss of elasticity of the skin and the pitting cannot be improved significantly with dermabrasion alone. In these cases a limited face lift is done to increase the skin tension and to bring up the depth of the severe acne pits or surface depressions. For socioeconomic reasons, this is often done as a single stage procedure. I would prefer to do the face lift and follow this in three to six months with the dermabrasion. This combination can be used either for fine rhytids or acne scars.

An Update

We have done only a few dermabrasions combined with facelifts. These have been mostly with severe acne as in Figure 21–14, where premature loss of tissue elasticity is present, because of the acne. Both procedures complement each other in that the tightening of the skin seems to also pull the depth of the pits upward. This can be done for fine facial rhytids as well but in general is reserved for cases in which only a limited facial flap elevation is done because of the combination of the two different procedures.

FINE RHYTIDS

We prefer dermabrasion to chemical peel for fine rhytids whether done as described above for full face dermabrasion or doing segmental dermabrasion such as the more common sites of the upper lip or perioral

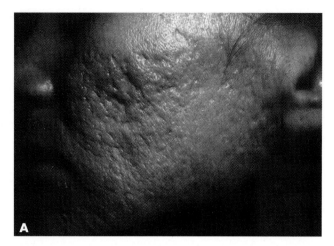 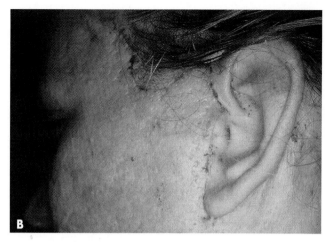

Figure 21–14. Combined dermabrasion and facelift. **(A)** Severe acne scarring with pitting and premature relaxation of skin. Side-lighting is done to demonstrate the preoperative condition and the depth of the pitting. **(B)** Patient 7 days postoperative from single-treatment with combined dermabrasion and facelift. The continuous subcuticular preauricular facelift suture is still in place. It is our opinion that the crusting and erythema subside quicker with this dressing than for other resurfacing techniques. See Figures 21–9 and 21–12.

rhytids (Figs. 21–10 and 21–13). For these rhytids or those of the glabella and lateral canthus the wire brush is preferred. We use the somewhat narrow, medium brush (Figs. 21–1B and 21–10). For large areas where there is a flatter surface, the wide brush is definitely better. For fine rhytids, where one may want to carry the dermabrasion to the bottom of the rhytid, the slightly narrower brush has proven best. Again, the technique should be described in some detail because an extremely efficient and somewhat dangerous machine is used. A slow speed is used with the foot pedal. The wire brush is carried horizontal to the lip margin at the vermillion first and then carried at approximately a 45-60 degree angle for the second pass with the brush rotating to brush the free margin of the lip away rather than biting into it (Fig. 21–10C,D). The positioning described above is required and is vital to this delicate procedure.

There has to be absolute quiet in the operating room and no unnecessary movements. Countertraction is vital and the traction hand position should not change as long as the motor is running (Fig. 21–9). Although previously we stopped short of the vermillion roll, now dermabrasion is quite often carried over this ridge and slightly into the mucosa or pink portion of the lip (Figs. 21–3, 21–4,

and 21–13). Two planings are done with the brush, one horizontal and the second at an angle. This obliterates any linear "scratch" marks and serves as micro 'Z' plasties at angles to the rhytids.

Utilizing the motor driven brush or cylinder, the lateral canthus can be dermabraded up to the thin eyelid skin and even here some dermabrasion can be carried out cautiously watching the direction of rotation of the brush. Quite often the brush is used manually in this area or over the entire eyelids near the ciliary margins (Fig. 21–10B). Manual dermabrasion of the eyelids can be quite precise. This was first learned from Dr. Oscar Becker who used a short stiff bristled nylon toothbrush to accomplish the same thing as can be done with the hand held wire brush. As proficiency is developed either the motor driven wire brush or medium cylinder can be used as long as all precautions are followed. Care must be taken not to get the epithelial debris in the eyes. Eyeglasses should be worn by the surgeon and assistants. Following this procedure the patient's eyes are thoroughly irrigated and antibiotic ointment (Polysporin) applied.

The glabella area creates particular problems. Dermabrasion is most helpful where there are deep permanent rhytids within the skin, but it does not help the ridging created by the action of the corrugator or pro-cerus muscles. In these instances the vertical rhytids from the corrugator or the horizontal rhytids from the pro-cerus are directly excised and closed with some eversion after sectioning the muscles themselves. After the skin is closed with the interrupted deep subcuticular suture, der-mabrasion is carried out. Following dermabrasion the final surface skin sutures are placed.

SCAR REVISIONS

Scar revisions have been described in previous publica-tions and when combined with dermabrasion are carried out essentially as described above for glabella wrinkles: The deep subcuticular closure is carried out first, then dermabrasion, then the application of skin sutures whether spring loop sutures, simple surgical twists or the continuous intradermal suture using 5-0 monofilament nylon (Fig. 21–11). W plasties, small Z plasties or other broken line camouflage techniques where surface tension varies and hills and valleys are created may require later dermabrasion.

SCARS ON LOWER ONE-THIRD OF NOSE

Whenever a scar is revised on the lower third of the nose in the thicker more sebaceous skin, the patient should be forewarned that six months later it is likely that a der-mabrasion will be advisable. This particular skin heals with some indentation rather than eversion and there is a tendency for deep sutures to be rejected or for skin sutures to bite in due to its friable, sebaceous nature. Describing the difference in this skin to patients and informing them of the likely need for secondary dermabrasion, whether the condition exists from lacerations, burns or for mar-gins of rotation flaps or grafts, is important.

LACERATIONS

Even for primary lacerations the above combination of suturing and dermabrasion can often be helpful, particu-larly if there are irregular surfaces. Thin sliced superficial epithelial cuts or the punctate cuts which can occur from shattered glass may definitely benefit from primary der-mabrasion. In the process of the dermabrasion small frag-ments of glass can often be detected.

TATTOOING

Whether tattooing from artistic tattoos or from injury with the impregnation of carbon matter or gunpowder, dermabrasion can be useful. Except in the most superfi-cial tattooing, dermabrasion alone is usually not ade-quate. Sometimes following the dermabrasion the pigment must be picked out using fine forceps and a broken pointed razor blade under magnification. Fol-lowing grafting or other techniques for the removal of tattoos, dermabrasion can also be helpful. Dermabrasion can reduce the area of visible tattoo the remainder of which must be excised.

An Update

For tattooing I have found nothing truly satisfactory. However, in the case of gunpowder tattooing, the der-mabrader does provide a diffuse smoothing of the sur-face and, with magnification, further wire brush dermabrasion can be carried out. Specific deeper tattooed material can be removed by use of the razor blade der-matome and picking out the material with the small otology Noyes forceps (Fig. 21–15D).

TELANGIECTASIA

Telangiectasia or small prominent vessels which can occur particularly around the nose or in the cheek area can often be helped with simple dermabrasion. We often combine this with microcoagulation of these vessels under magnification. Dermabrasion is carried only to the depth necessary to take off the surface of these vessels. Microcoagulation is done with the same fine needle used in epilation with a very low current.

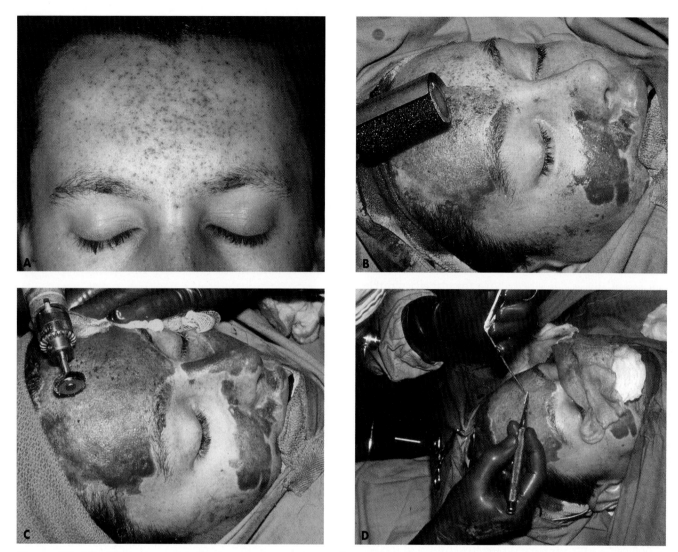

Figure 21–15. (A) Some gunpowder particles have penetrated quite deep into the dermis. **(B)** Generalized dermabrasion with the large silicone cylinder, Stryker/Iverson handle, and spray guard. The guard is held close to skin on the side and direction of the spray. **(C)** More specific and deeper dermabrasion is carried out for any more deeply impregnated foreign body. To demonstrate the Jacobs chuck the sleeve ordinarily covering it has been removed. **(D)** Finally, with magnification the deep particles are grasped with the fine Noyes otology forceps and excised with the razor blade knife.

ACTINIC KERATOSIS[12]

The use of dermabrasion for superficial keratoses or actinic keratosis must be approached with caution, making certain that no subtle skin malignancies exist. As long as patient selection is critical and there are not too many existing atrophic changes in the skin, especially of the older patient, this procedure, carried out usually quite superficially, can be most helpful in freshening the skin. With proper precautions regarding additional solar radiation, it also, I believe, serves some preventative purpose in the development of skin cancers.

NASAL SUPRATIP THICKENING

Following rhinoplasty or nasal injury for subtle supratip swelling and contouring, dermabrasion with the wire brush is often extremely helpful. This, of course, is done after all other primary or secondary rhinoplasty procedures are completed but should be in the rhinoplasty surgeon's armamentarium. Dermabrasion is delayed at least six months postoperatively. For this undesirable postoperative condition or for conditions where there may have been pustules leaving irregularities or pitting, dermabrasion can help.

ACNE ROSACEA (RHINOPHYMA)

In mild acne rosacea, dermabrasion may be all that is necessary. In more severe cases we utilize the hand dermatome, shaving off the more involved area, and then use the wire brush dermabrasion to blend at the edges of this shave (Fig. 21–16). Because of the sharpness of the wire brush this can even be used at the same procedure to smooth out surface irregularities where the dermatome had been used.[13]

OVERLAY GRAFTS

It has been advocated that over thick split thickness skin grafts the area may be dermabraded and covered with an overlay graft both for smoothness and to avoid further depression. I have not had personal experience with this but have used dermabrasion to create a de-epithelized surface of the skin over the carotid artery which is then covered with a pedicle flap of one type or another. This serves as an attached dermal graft. De-epithelization is

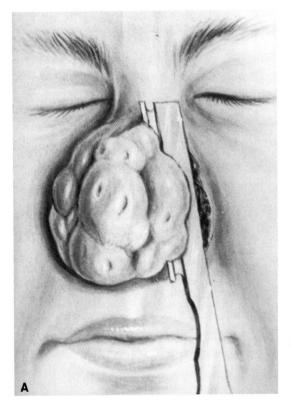

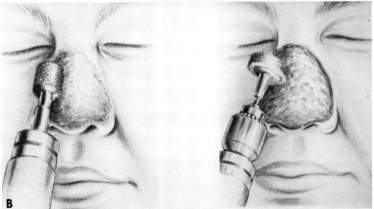

Figure 21-16. **(A)** Shave excision for bulk of rhinophyma with hand-held dermatome. **(B)** Use of the cylinder for blending with the skin about the margins of the shave and the wire brush, which may be used for blending and for smoothing irregularities over the previously dermabraded area. **(C)** Preoperative condition. **(D)** Postoperative.

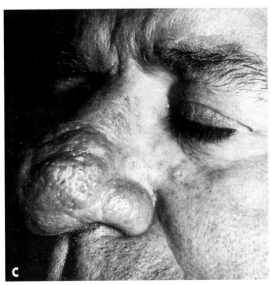

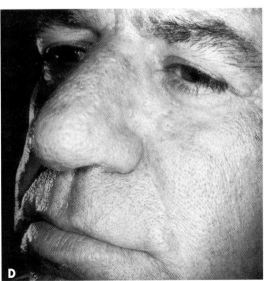

most commonly carried out by hand with a razor blade dermatome. The wire brush dermabrador may then be used to precisely deepen the area and further assure that no surface epithelium remains.

DE-EPITHELIZATION OF FLAPS

Dermabrasion, especially with the use of the more efficient wire brush, can be used to de-epithelize the end of regional pedicle flaps where there is a desire to imbricate the end of the flap around the margins of the defect to create a stepped closure. In the mid-portion of a flap or along the shaft the epithelization can be utilized to tunnel the graft and effect primary healing as when the pedicle is passed through the surface skin for inner lining.

OVERGRAFTING

Where it is desirable to remove the entire dermis, scars or previous grafts may be dermabraded to the desired level in the outer dermis and a thick split-thickness skin graft placed over this abraded area. In scar revisions or in the removal, for instance, of deep glabella wrinkles, the intervening skin may be dermabraded or de-epithelized and the margins, after incision, brought over this deep tissue in a straddling technique. This, in effect, serves as a deep dermal graft beneath the revised scar.

POSTOPERATIVE CARE

The dermabraded area must receive critical postoperative care and requires some patience, both on the part of the surgeon and the patient. The first axiom is to not rush the dressings or the debridement.

On the first postoperative day the larger absorbent and pressure dressing is removed down to the Adaptic. Immediately, moist Zephiran sponges are placed over this to absorb any serum seeping through. The Adaptic is then trimmed close to the actual edge of the dermabrasion and to release the lips and eyebrows. After compresses for

approximately ten minutes, one goes to the drying treatment which can be accomplished either with a drying lamp held eighteen inches from the face or a hair dryer set on low heat. Any continued serum secretions can be blotted by the patient. Drying is usually carried out for twenty to 30 minutes approximately every three to four hours. Usually two drying treatments are given before the patient actually leaves the hospital on the first postoperative day.

At home the drying technique is continued until it is complete, usually within the first twenty-four to forty-eight hours. The patient may be seen on the third to fifth postoperative days just for reassuranae and to assist if there should be any pockets of serum beneath the Adaptic. If this is the case, the Adaptic is incised, all excess material allowed to exude and drying is carried out. The re-epithelization and regeneration of the epidermis is quite rapid, usually occurring between the third and fifth days. One should not rush removal of the Adaptic; however, should it come off, the dry coagulum then serves as a dressing. We have found that healing is smoother and more rapid when the Adaptic is left on for seven to ten days. Usually it can then be peeled off, along with all of the accumulated crust, leaving the face cleaner than if one had to remove the crusts or frank scabs individually. In removing either the Adaptic or the crust, care should be taken not to create bleeding or to remove the re-epithelized, thin, healed tissue. If the crust or dressing adheres, one simply waits for two to three days more until it loosens up. Usually for the beard it is necessary to remove the Adaptic within one week as the beard begins to grow through.

Adaptic has proven very useful because of the inert impregnation material and because of the larger size of the mesh, which allows serum to come through into the absorbent dressing. This has been the most expeditious and least frightening technique for the patient and family. We tell patients preoperatively that they are going to want to "hide" for seven to ten days. This is the case whether a dressing is used or not used, or whether a chemical peel or dermabrasion is the method chosen.

For three days following the removal of the Adaptic or crust warm compresses using a soft washcloth and tap water are all that are used. No scrubbing or rubbing is done. If there are any raw areas or bleeding, Polysporin ointment is placed on these areas. The patient then shifts to washing with a mild soap, particularly if the skin is oily. The soap is rinsed off thoroughly and the face dried without rubbing. If there is continued crusting or the patient seems to have extremely dry skin, simple Burroughs Welcome Lanolin cream is applied. Make-up can usually be worn in ten to fourteen days. A make-up consultant is nice to have at this time to advise the patient but generally the patient must wear a lighter powder or base because the redness of the skin shows through. The erythema persists from a few days to three to four months, depending upon the patient. The skin is then smooth but red, almost as from a sunburn, for varying periods of time. Strong emphasis is placed on avoiding sun for a minimum of three months. During this time sunscreens are used progressing down from a sun protection factor number of 15 to no less than 10. The patient is encouraged to wear a hat and to go out primarily in the early and late parts of the day avoiding any direct or reflected sunlight. This is particularly important in Florida in that one must work to avoid the sun. Ideally, it is best to do dermabrasions in the fall, particularly for the more commonly operated on young group for whom outdoor activities are so important. Until the dressing is removed, broad spectrum antibiotics are used by mouth and topical antibiotic ointment is used only where there is a raw area after the dressings are off.

COMPLICATIONS

The patient is advised in the preoperative instructions that the two most common complications of dermabrasion are pigment changes and the formation of milia. Rounding off our own figures, approximately half of the patients can get either one of these two complications and some have both. These are relatively normal occurrences. Pigmentation is usually no more severe than that which may occur with taking birth control pills, other superficial abrasions or as in the chloasma of pregnancy.

Milia are generally a self-limited condition but can last for a number of weeks. As explained to the patient, these are simply plugged up normal skin glands which are caught in the re-epithelization. I rush the removal of milia for the patient's sake so they are totally healed in a shorter period of time. This treatment involves nicking the surface of the milia with either a #11 blade or a straight Keith needle and then removing the pearl-like concretion with the flat surface of the blade or needle.

If one does not go through the depth of the dermis (to the capillary layer) or too deeply within the dermis and if postoperative care, as described, has been carried out, additional complications are rare. Hyperplastic scars are always a concern but has occurred for me on only two occasions in a twenty-five year period. One occurred in areas where the new epithelium had been violated or removed with the Adaptic. These responded over a period of months to dilute Kenalog intralesional injections. The other was in a case where, it was later learned, the patient was a keloid former. Some of these scars had to be revised, particularly over the bony prominence of the mandible. Caution should be exerted over bony prominences and in regard to the careful removal of dressings.

Heavily pigmented people are not good candidates for dermabrasion. I would never perform full face dermabrasion in the black race for fear of keloid formation, even in a small area.

CONCLUSIONS

Dermabrasion, or skin planing, is a most useful tool in facial plastic and reconstructive surgery. Dermabrasion is the treatment of choice for acne scarring. The technique, using the powered handpiece, is appropriate for a variety of conditions and the author prefers its use over chemoexfoliation for fine rhytids.

The more frequent complications are milia formation and superficial pigmentation changes. Materials and methods are discussed in some detail to aid the surgeon. Technical precautions are emphasized.

Dermabrasion, as it is currently performed, with proper selection of cases and proper recognition of the limitations of the procedure is a valued and useful procedure.

AN UPDATE

Many surgeons and authors argue against dermabrasion because they claim the procedure takes more experience and requires technical expertise. However, these things are required in all properly perfomed facial plastic surgery techniques and most require some cutting or "cold steel" (knife) techniques. If one is advised to start with the laser because it is "easier," from where would the experience in dermabrasion come? If one looks at it objectively, the main argument for laser is that the surgeon has made a major investment in buying or leasing the equipment and it is, therefore, the best technique because he or she has to make it pay for itself. Dermabrasion can accomplish the same goals both in terms of cosmetic results and histologic changes in the dermis. In my observation, less edema, weeping, or long-term erythema has occurred with dermabrasion. I have noticed no difference in the pigmentation from the different techniques. Less hypopigmentation has been reported with the laser, but I have not been convinced or seen this well documented by an equal number of both procedures done by the same surgeon.

In nearly one-half century of experience I have never encountered any case of hepatitis, immune deficiency disease, or even conjunctivitis attributable to dermabrasion if the proper precautions are followed. The precautions are basic, including proper eye shields,

a spray-guarded dermabrasion wheel, maximum avoidance of peripheral spray, and thorough washing and irrigation for the surgeon, nurses, and assistants. In addition, the patient's eyes should be thoroughly irrigated with a buffered saline solution. Personally I have had no problem with infection by simply wearing larger glasses lenses. As with all surgery, we are concerned with body fluids, serum, blood, and in this situation, epithelium. An added safety feature of the laser might be that it does not, as with a knife or cylinder, carry the potential for infection. However, in our experience infection has not been a problem with dermabrasion. Each technique can have some superficial infection if an active staphylococcol infection is present in the skin or if material is allowed to accumulate beneath the dressing.

Microdermabrasion (particle beam) resurfacing with aluminum oxide crystals is an advance in skin care procedures which we wish to mention. It is placed somewhere between skin care and surgery in that it can be performed by a certified technician in several stages. An added feature is the combined suction which removes the epithelial debris. This was introduced in Italy in 1985 and reported in separate presentations by Dr. M. G. Rubin and Dr. S. A. Goldstein et al at the Annual Meeting of the AAFPRS in New Orleans in September 1999. The depth of the microdermabrasion can be controlled and an advantage could be that there is no need for anesthesia. Documentation, objective evaluation with long-term follow-up, and recording of the number and frequency of treatments needs to be done. Further objective evaluation is recommendend.

Despite the introduction of laser techniques, dermabrasion has withstood the test of time. *Laser* resurfacing, by the same token, should be endorsed as the technology becomes more and more sophisticated. Certainly LASER (light amplification by stimulated emissions of radiation) has come a long way since Charles Townes won the Nobel prize in physics for the pioneering its development particularly in medicine.

PEARLS

- Dermabrasion remains the treatment of choice in several procedures where chemoexfoliation or laser resurfacing is now widely used.
- If a patient presenting for dermabrasion is taking birth control pills, its is best to discontinue their use for at least two full cycles to prevent pigmentation problems that usually occur in patients taking hormonal therapy.
- Consultation with a dermatologist is recommended in cases of acne scarring, especially if the patient is still fairly young or has active lesions.
- Full-face dermabrasion is not recommended in patients with heavily pigmented skin.
- Meticulous observation and utilization of the direction of the cylinder or brush rotation is vital, especially in the vicinity of anatomic borders such as the lips, nostrils, eyelids, or eyebrows.

REFERENCES

1. Iverson PC. Surgical removal of traumatic tattoos. *Plast Reconstr Surg.* 1947; 2:427.
2. Iverson PC. Further developments in the treatment of skin lesions by surgical abrasion. *Plast Reconstr Surg.* 1953; 12:27.
3. Kurtin A. Corrective surgical planing of skin, new technique for tratment of acne scars & other skin defects. *Arch Dermat Syph.* 153; 68:368.
4. Orentreich N. Dermabrasion. *J.A.M.W.A.* 1969; April: 331–336; and Personal communication.
5. Kromayer E. Totationinstrumente: Ein neues technisches Verafahren in der dermatologischen Kleinchirurgie. *Chir Dermat Ztschr Berlin.* 1905; 12:26.
6. McEvitt WG. Treatment of acne pits by abrasion with sandpaper. *J.A.M.A.* 1950; 142:647.
7. Campbell R. Surgical and chemical planing of the skin. In: Converse B, ed. *Reconstructive Plastic Surgery.* Vol. I. Philadelphia: W. B. Saunders Co.; 1964:187–207.
8. Behin F, Feuerstein S, Marovitz W. Comparative histological study of mini pig skin after chemical peel and dermabrasion. *Arch Otolaryngol.* 1977; 103:271–277.
9. Baker TJ. Chemical face peeling and dermabrasion. *Surg Clin North Am.* 1971; 51:387–400.
10. Rees T, Wood-Smith D. Chemabrasion and Dermabrasion. *Cosmetic Facial Surgery.* Philadelphia: W. B. Saunders Co; 1973: 213–220.
11. Farrior RT. Facial irregularities. *Current Therapy in Otolaryngology–Head and Neck Surgery, 1982–1983.* Gares: B.C. Decker; Inc., 1982:146–151.
12. Pickerell K, Matton G, Huger W, Pound E. Dermabrasion of extensive keratotic lesions of the forehead and scalp. *Plast Reconstr Surg.* 1962; 30:32.
13. Farrior RT. Corrective and reconstructive surgery of the external nose. In: Naumann HH. *Head & Neck Surgery.* Vol. 1. Stuttgart, Germany: Georg Thieme; 1980:173–277.

SUGGESTED READINGS

Baker TJ, Stuzin JM, Baker TM. Facial skin resurfacing. In: Baker, (ed.) St. Louis: Quality Medical Publishing Inc.; 1998.

Baker TM. Dermabrasion as a complement to aesthetic surgery. *Clin Plastic Surg.* 1998; 25:81–88.

Branbam GH, Thomas RJ. Rejuvenation of the skin surface: Chemical peel and dermabrasion. *Facial Past Surg.* 1996; 12: 125–133.

Campbell JP, Terhune MH, Shorts ST, Jones RQ. An ultrastructural comparison of mechanical dermabrasion and carbon dioxide laser resurfacing in the minipig model. *Arch Otolaryngol Head & Neck Surg.* 1998; 124:758–760.

Converse JM, Robb-Smith AHT. The healing of surface cutaneous wounds: Its analogy with the healing of superficial burns. *Ann Surgery* 1944; 120:873–885.

Epstein E. Present status of dermabrasion. *JAMA.* 1968; 206: 607–610.

Farrior RT. Corrective and reconstructive surgery of the external nose. In: Naumann HH, (ed.) *Head and Neck Surgery.* Vol. 1. Stuttgart, Germany: Georg Thieme; 1980:173–277.

Farrior RT. Dermabrasion in facial plastic surgery. *Laryngoscope.* 1985; 95:534–546.

Farrior RT. Facial Irregularities. *Current Therapy in Otolaryngology–Head and Neck Surgery, 1982–1983.* B.C. Decker, Inc.: 1982:146–151.

Frodel JL. Wound healing. In: Papel, (ed.) *Facial Plastic and Reconstructive Surgery, 1992.* Mosby–Year Book, Inc.; St. Louis: 1992: 14–21.

Hrurza GJ. Laser skin resurfacing. *Arch Dermatol.* 1966; 132: 451–455.

Keller GS. Cutaneous laser surgery. *Facial Plast Surg.* 1989; 6:137–192.

Mechlin DC, Foote JE. Dermabrasion. *Ear, Nose, & Throat J.* 1981; 102:79–83.

Orentreich N, Orentreich DS. Dermabrasion as a complement to dermatology. *Clin Plast Surg.* 1998; 25:63–80.

Parsons RW. The management of traumatic tattoos. *Clin Plast Surg.* 1975; 2:517–522.

Rubach BW, Schoenrock LD. Histological and clinical evaluation of facial resurfacing using a carbon dioxide laser with the computer pattern generator. *Arch Otolaryngol Head Neck Surg.* 123:929–934.

Stegman SJ. A study of dermabrasion and chemical peels in an animal model. *J Dermatol Surg Oncol.* 1980; 6:490–496.

Facial Resurfacing

Aesthetic Facial Plastic Surgery, edited by Thomas Romo, III, and Arthur L. Millman, Thieme Medical Publishers, Inc., New York, New York, Copyright © 2000.

CHAPTER 22

Chemical Peel

A Facial Plastic Surgeon's Perspective

JIM L. ENGLISH

In antiquity, our ancestors understood the ravages of the sun and its effect on the aging process. The Egyptian Pharaohs and their court could be easily distinguished by their lack of sun exposure and delicate skin. Sun damage was a cultural stigma that belonged to the working class, which today, ironically, is just the opposite. They used oils and alabaster and bathed in sour milk (lactic acid) to maintain their skin and social status. The Holy Scriptures also bore witness to the daily use of emollients and perfumes to soften and cleanse the skin among the wives of the Jewish and Babylonian kings. With time's progression, other cultures developed their own sine qua non remedies for the enhancement of their aged skin envelopes. For instance, Middle Eastern men and women used urine mixed with an abrasive compound and fire to exfoliate the outer layers of their skin. During the 1700s Madame Pompadour of France bathed in red wine (tartaric acid) to create a more supple look and feel to her countenance.

It has only been in the last 120 years or so that a more scientific approach was used to identify and measure the results of applying things to the skin's surface for its improvement. In 1882, German dermatologist P.G. Unna worked with and described different types of peeling agents such as trichloroacetic acid (TCA), phenol, and resorcinol.[1] Phenol was later used for war wounds during World War I, and that experience translated into techniques brought to the United States and practiced by "lay peelers" near Los Angeles and Southern Florida during the 30s and 40s. Others went on to work with these dermatologic methods over the next decade, culminating in the work of Brown and coworkers on the effectiveness of various phenol preparations.[2] In addition, Litton published his work on a nonsaponified phenol formula during the late 50s and early 60s.[3] Various results and complications followed that placed the practice of skin peels in a state of disrepute until Baker and Gordon presented their results with before and after photographs at a national conference in 1972.[4] This brought a resurgence of interest in facial peeling for the improvement of wrinkling, and their particular saponated

peel formula has in some form or fashion become the mainstay of treatment for deep rhytids ever since.

TCA, resorcinol, and other chemical agents have had similar histories within the annals of skin resurfacing. They have been used with increasing frequency for the improvement of these and other skin problems, especially with the advent of national seminars that tout their results and teach their techniques.[5] In addition, the use of such products as Retin-A and the alpha hydroxy acids (glycolic and lactic) have received national attention over the past decade and a half. This widespread exposure has positioned chemical peels as a part of our armamentarium into the twenty-first century for the improvement of the skin's appearance.

EFFECTS OF AGING

Prerequisites to performing skin peels are a thorough knowledge of the anatomy of the epidermis and dermis, the depth of injury required to achieve the desired results (Fig. 22–1), and the series of events that follow the injury produced by the application of the "peel

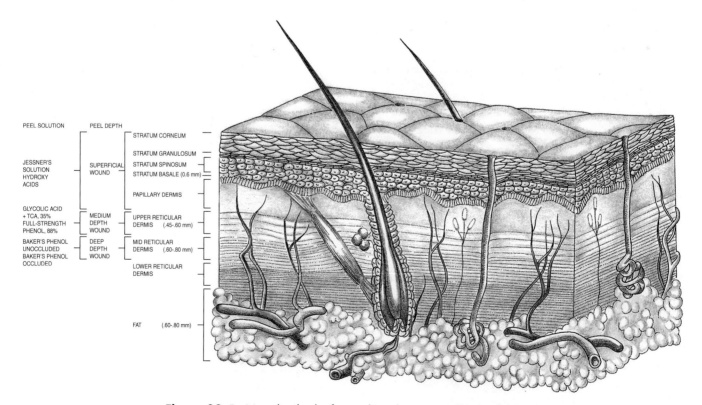

Figure 22-1. Note the depth of wounds and corresponding peel agents.

solution." In normal skin, the dermis can be 20 to 30 times thicker than the epidermis, and it is in this foundational layer that architectural changes are sought to obtain the desired enhancement for the overlying wrinkled epidermis. Simple changes in the epidermis alone do very little for wrinkled skin because dermal factors are largely responsible for this condition. As we age and our skin becomes photodamaged, the papillary dermis becomes thinner because of dermal collagen and elastin degeneration. The overlying epidermis will eventually come to rest either on the lower papillary or upper reticular dermis. This loss of upper dermal thickness requires the more *inelastic* epidermal layers to shrink, and its inability to do so helps produce wrinkling. (Simply stated, this physiologic process constitutes the main reason for the deeper chemical peels, i.e., to insult the remaining dermal components in a controlled fashion expecting a response of dermal regrowth with enhanced vertical thickness and a realignment of the collagen bundles parallel to the skin's surface, all of which help tighten the overlying skin.) This process of upper dermal degeneration is noted histologically by a decrease in dermal collagen production, an increase in collagen breakdown by collagenases, an increase in solar elastosis, a state of disarray within the melanocytic system producing variations in skin color, and a diminution of papillary dermal blood flow. Decrease in the number and length of the rete pegs at the dermal epidermal junction also create a more loose and mobile skin envelope. Coupled with the fact that as we age our facial skeleton gets smaller and the layer of subcutaneous fat may atrophy, it is a wonder that we are not all "prune faced."

CHOICE OF SKIN PEEL

This histologic information helps the surgeon or peeler in choosing the appropriate wounding agent to carry them to the depth necessary to achieve the desired response. For instance, if superficial exfoliation is indicated, the alpha hydroxy acid peels with glycolic acid will suffice because only the epidermal layers need be involved. This particular acid tends to restore keratinocyte adhesion to normal by creating their detachment at the junction of the stratum granulosum and enhancing the process of desquamation. If depigmentation or a more homogenous pigmentary color of the face is desired, peels such as a 35% TCA with or without epidermal vesiculation can produce wounds down to and below the basement membrane of the epidermis, where alteration of the melanocytic system can occur. Of note, pigmentation can be epidermal, dermal, or both. In any of these the wound should not extend to the deepest levels of pigmentation so as to avoid unnecessary morbidity. For this particular problem, more frequent and more superficial skin peels are indicated to achieve improvement and avoid a significant loss of pigmentation. If wrinkle improvement of thin skin is desired where a flatter dermal-epidermal interface exists, such as the eyelids, a medium-depth peel is warranted and can be produced either by a 35% TCA in conjunction with glycolic acid or a straight 88% phenol (carboxylic acid) solution because the depth of injury required for this response is the mid papillary to upper reticular dermis (Fig. 22–2). (The latter is my preference and will be discussed later in this chapter. To place a deep peel solution on the lower lids within the confines of the orbit will lengthen the healing time and in some instances produce ectropion as a result of vertical contracture of the lower lid.) If, however, deeper rhytids exist as on the forehead or other areas of the face with thicker skin, a deep surgical peel such as a Baker-Gordon peel with or without occlusion is recommended because the level of response required is the midreticular dermis. Dermal wounds into and below the lower reticular dermis respond with scar formation, and this complication can be prevented by limiting the depth of injury above this level. Given today's range of peeling agents, it has become fashionable to diagnose and treat each cosmetic unit of the face with whatever modality is warranted. Such an approach will limit morbidity and unwanted complications but may produce differing lines of demarcation if the peel solution is not carefully applied and blended.

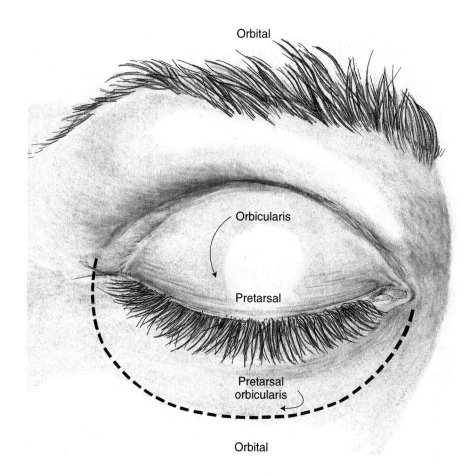

Orbital

Orbicularis

Pretarsal

Pretarsal
orbicularis

Orbital

Figure 22–2. Anatomy of the eyelid with thinner skin in the pretarsal regions and thickening with outward migration.

THE HEALING PROCESS

Regardless of the depth of injury produced down to the midreticular dermis, the response of the individual to this controlled wounding is fairly predictable. The surgeon or peeler must understand this process completely so as to provide postoperative reassurance when needed and early intervention before a complication occurs if that is also needed. Patients need to understand that certain types of peels are very inconvenient and stressful procedures to undergo, but that they produce a type of result when nothing else can (Fig. 22–3). It is incumbent on the originator of the wound to walk the patient through this process as skillfully as possible. Much misinformation about chemical peels exists among the lay community, and one of the biggest challenges for the surgeon or peeler is in correcting these myths on the basis of a large body of existing knowledge and their own clinical expe-

rience. Wrinkling is within the substance of the skin, and the treatment modality needs to address that particular area. Surgery, per se, is not for wrinkling and so the treatment of rhytids lies within the domain of the chemical peel, laser resurfacing, or dermabrasion.

Chemical peels are partial-thickness injuries that heal rapidly by secondary intention provided that certain parameters are met. Because the first phase is coagulant and inflammatory, nothing else should be done to increase or for that matter to decrease this response after the initial insult. Although this phase is mandatory for proper healing, additional trauma such as chemical, mechanical, radiant, or infection should be avoided because an exacerbation at this time could be detrimental to the final result. In the past many who performed the deep Baker-Gordon peels attempted to prolong this initial phase by the occlusion of the wound with tape. It was thought that the tape trapped moisture in the wound bed

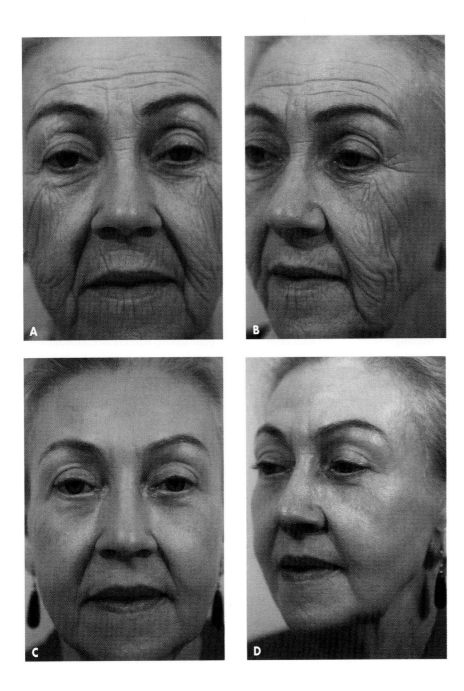

Figure 22-3. Preoperative frontal (**A**) and side (**B**) views. Note the "sleep lines" on each cheek. Five months postoperative frontal (**C**) and side (**D**) views from a full-face Baker-Gordon peel. Note slight thickening of each lower eyelid. This patient had a mild ectropion of each lower lid for approximately 3 months. It resolved with intralesional steroid injections and massages.

and increased the absorption and penetration of the phenol through maceration. With this particular formula of phenol, its high 88% concentration had a keratocoagulant effect on the skin, but when diluted with any type of moisture such as tears or tissue fluid, it became keratolytic and went deeper. Recent data suggest that taping may not have this particular effect after all.

The body's response to these partial-thickness wounds is immediate, with the formation of the platelet fibrin clot and activation of the kinin and complement inflammatory pathways that produce chemotactic mediators at the wound site such as leukotrienes, kallikreins, growth factors, and fibrin lysis products. These factors increase local blood vessel permeability and attract neutrophils, monocytes, and lymphocytes.[6] This chemoattraction is necessary for stability, protection, and the initiation of wound healing.

Neutrophils are the first line of defense to a breach in the integumentary system and are present for at least 3 to 7 days. Careful attention with good wound management is necessary during this critical phase of wound healing to prevent infection from monilial, herpetic, or opportunistic bacterial organisms, thus avoiding deeper wounds, delayed healing, and possible scar formation. Monocytes arrive 3 to 10 days after the initial wound and differentiate into macrophages. These are the most important cells in the resolution of inflammation and are largely responsible for initiating the proliferative phase of dermal wound healing by directing the development of granulation tissue. This type of tissue is a collection of cellular components such as fibroblasts, cellular by-products such as fibronectin and collagen, and ground substances, which include glycoaminoglycans (GAGs), sulfonated and nonsulfonated. The lymphocyte is found in the wound bed after the first week and continues the processes begun by the macrophages. Early intervention during this phase by the patient or physician can interfere with the natural healing process by slowing down the buildup of granulation tissue. Corticosteroids, which are a great treatment alternative later on, would adversely affect the accumulation of these "building blocks" and should not be used unless specifically indicated.

The next phase is re-epithelization of the defect, and this occurs initially by migration of the epithelium from the involved adnexal structures (Fig. 22–4 and 22–5) within the first 24 to 72 hours of a peel initiated by fibrin and platelet products. The density of the pilosebaceous units per square centimeter is important to the rapidity of re-epithelization, and this lack of density explains the differences in healing between the face and the neck because the neck has less units per area. Although this process is measured in hours, the next step that requires proliferation of epithelial cells at the periphery of the defect and continued growth from the adnexal remnants is measured in days. Keratinocytes migrate on a scaffold of dermal matrix consisting of fibronectin, which is cross linked to collagen, fibrin, and elastin. Fibronectin allows adhesion to these dermal structures and surrounding cells. After migration and coverage are obtained, cell proliferation at the wound edge shifts centrally, providing the needed depth to the epidermis (Fig. 22–6). This process continues for 60 to 90 days after a deep chemical peel. Early re-epithelization of the wound bed, although monocellular in initial thickness, is paramount to the pre-

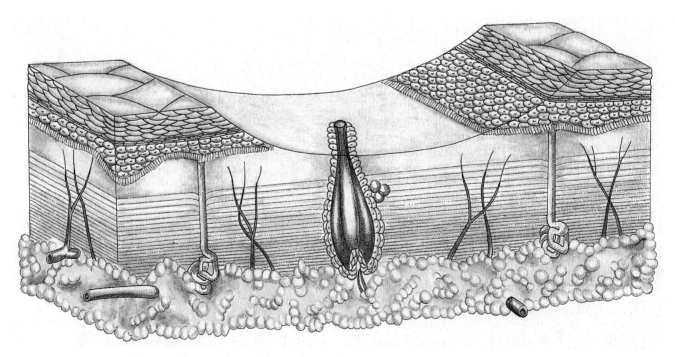

Figure 22–4. Suface of the epidermis-dermis immediately after a chemical peel.

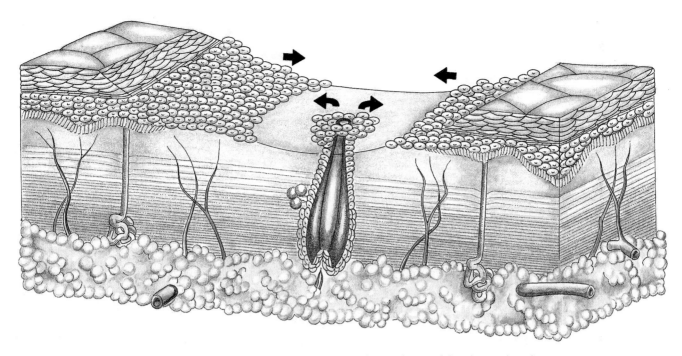

Figure 22–5. Keratinocyte migration within 72 hours of the chemical peel.

vention of complications. The longer a wound is left uncovered with epithelium, the greater the chances for healing abnormalities. Maibach and Rovee provided good insight into this early process of healing during their studies in the late 60s and early 70s.[7] They found that a moist wound with a high water content healed much faster than a dry wound. (This is not to be confused with the reasons for taping a deep surgical wound obtained by a peel agent such as Baker-Gordon. This technique is used solely for the purpose of driving the wounding agent

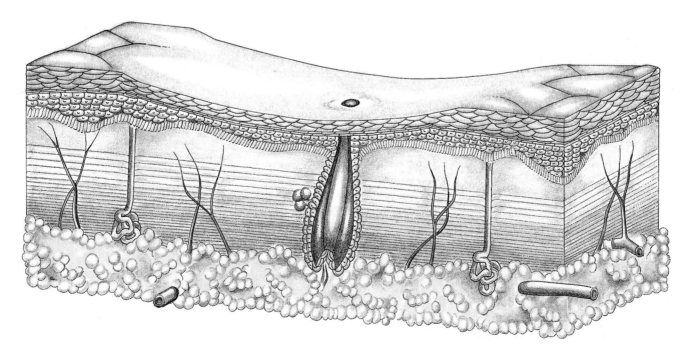

Figure 22–6. Epithelialization is complete. Dermal and epidermal height regeneration will be ongoing for 2 to 3 months.

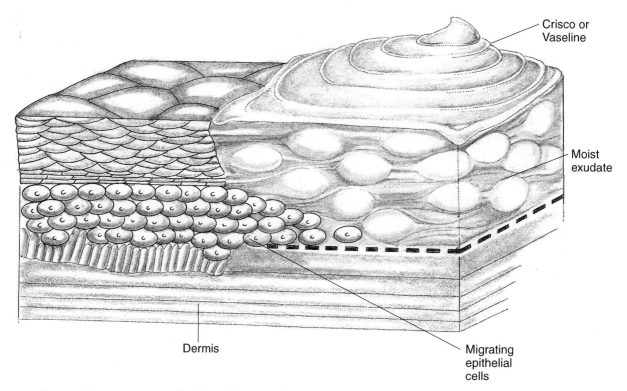

Crisco or Vaseline

Moist exudate

Dermis

Migrating epithelial cells

Figure 22–7. Moist wound with overlying emollient and a more superficial layer of bridging keratinocytes.

deeper through maceration. For this reason, I do not place an emollient on any deep surgical peels for 4 to 6 hours to prevent dilution of residual phenol and possibly a deeper wound.)

Because the leading edge of epithelium must seek a sustaining layer of hydration to bridge the defect, it need not travel as deeply when an emollient or a bio-occlusive dressing is kept on the wound bed in such a way as to trap moisture. This allows the advancing epithelium to bridge the defect more efficiently and more superficially (Fig. 22–7). A desiccated wound makes it necessary for the advancing epithelial cells to descend further down into the dermis and subsequently delays healing and runs the possibility of compromising the final results (Fig. 22–8). Placing a desiccant such as thymol powder on a deep peel is physiologically incorrect and should be avoided. Also, a dry wound is a rich breeding ground for facultative microaerobes that will interfere with the advancing edge of keratinocytes in their attempt to cross this denuded expanse of epidermis

and dermis. Good wound management dictates frequent washings and application of a suitable emollient or the use of a bio-occlusive dressing in an effort to trap dermal moisture. This in turn enhances the substance within the dermis previously alluded to as GAGs. This material absorbs water up to 1000 times its own volume and is critical to the health of the wound. Without this hygroscopic material, the wound would desiccate and the healing process would be delayed and possibly compromised.

Because the acute phases of inflammation are ongoing for the first 2 weeks, the dermal matrix cannot begin to replicate until this inflammatory smolder has decreased. The first signs of replication are noted by the increased presence of granulation material that continues to proliferate until the wound has epithelialized. One of the tissue's components as previously mentioned is fibroblasts, and their activity produces collagen, elastin, and other needed materials. A differentiated fibroblast, the myofibroblast, produces wound bed contracture. Studies have

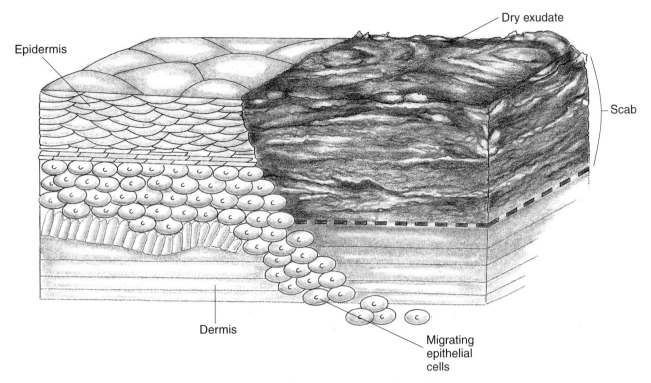

Epidermis

Dry exudate

Scab

Dermis

Migrating
epithelial
cells

Figure 22–8. Dry wound with scabbing and a deeper layer of bridging keratinocytes.

suggested that these steps can be improved with the preoperative use of tretinoin[8,9] and the postoperative use of a zinc-containing compound such as bacitracin.[10] Topical retinoids increase fibroblast and epidermal migration, possibly by decreasing the desmosomal and tonofilament attachments. They also increase mitosis in regenerating epidermal cells. Systemic retinoids on the other hand increase collagen synthesis, decrease collagenase production, and increase fibronectin production. This alteration in collagen degradation may be the factor in the accumulation of excessive collagen and hypertrophic scarring.[11] Head and neck studies have also suggested that vitamins with additional zinc may have added benefit in this early postoperative healing phase as well. During this stage of granulation tissue buildup, close attention must be paid to excessive fibroblastic activity, especially in an area where regrowth of epidermis has been slow. These areas can produce prolonged erythema and potential scarring if not closely monitored and appropriately dealt with. Once the wound bed is covered with epidermis, the formation

of granulation tissue essentially stops, and the regrowth of dermal components begins. This regrowth of vertical dermal height and its remodeling is ongoing for 2 to 3 months and needs to be monitored and encouraged because this buildup of dermal thickness, its alteration, and reorientation of existing structures are the main histologic reason for the chemical peel when the improvement of wrinkles is desired. Good nutrition, lack of stress, and the absence of sun exposure combined with good common sense can make this phase most fruitful and create the desired outcome with an enhanced dermal foundation for the overlying epidermis.

Angiogenesis is extremely important during this phase and is noted within the first 72 hours of wounding with endothelial buds that travel along the dermal matrix, providing oxygen to the area of healing. Smoking at this time is very harmful to this neoproliferative process because it not only impedes vascular bud generation but also robs the hemoglobin of its transported cargo, oxygen. A sensitization of the raw area to smoke also will create symptoms of increased burning and stinging if allowed to come in contact with the areas peeled before complete epithelization has occurred.

A later concern for patient and physician is that of prolonged erythema or hyperpigmentation. Although erythema may represent a sentinel finding of trouble, it need not always be such an indicator. Regardless, however, it can be a concern to the patient, and they need to be reassured that this is a normal healing process and should subside when the healing is completed. An exception would be that of telangiectasias. This vascular abnormality is more noticeable with the thinner layers of regenerating dermis and epidermis, and the patient needs to be encouraged that they should obtain a prepeel appearance. However, their number maybe increased at the conclusion of a medium to deep peel when healing is completed. This is an issue that must be addressed with the patient preoperatively; however, the advent of newer lasers have made this sequela less problematic. Hyperpigmentation, on the other hand, is not a favored response to the peel process and can persist if not prevented with good patient selection and adequate preoperative preparation with complete sun avoidance. If developed, the problem is managed with retinoic acid and hydroquinone with or without steroids. The process of lightening with these agents is slow, but the enzymatic disruption of tyrosine to melanin is certain if the patient is consistent in their use.[11]

Collagen remodeling is the last healing phase to start and finish. This process usually manifests itself 60 to 90 days after surgery, depending on the depth of the wound; the deeper the wound the longer it is before remodeling begins and the longer it takes to complete the process. Corticosteroids to help decrease swelling during these phases delays all aspects of wound healing and should be used sparingly unless an overproduction of fibroblastic material or of pigmentation occurs. Also, it stands to reason that immunosuppressive agents are to be avoided during and after a peel for at least 3 to 6 months.

PHENOL
PATIENT SELECTION

Patient selection is extremely important to the successful outcome of a facial peel. The normal prepeel evaluation should include a thorough head and neck examination, especially noting the amount of photodamage, sebaceous activity, and the presence or lack of pilosebaceous units. The Fitzpatrick classification of sun-reactive skin types and Glogau classification of photoaging are two of the best tools used today for categorizing patients for two purposes: first, to help in choosing the best peel formula and technique, and second, to help in predicting the postoperative response. The Fitzpatrick classification gives a subjective but reliable measure of the skin's responsiveness to sun exposure; when considering the patient's eye color and the choice of wounding agent, the postoperative course is fairly predictable (Table 22–1). Types I through III skin types are ideal candidates for all the favored chemical peel solutions. Type IV skin begins that gray area when the surgeon or peeler must anticipate and attempt to avoid pigmentary changes such as postinflammatory hyperpigmentation, noticeable lines of demarcation, and hypopigmentation. These concerns are paramount in skin types V and VI, and these patients should undergo test spots before a medium or deep facial peel, although the test spot's response is not a guarantee of the face's response.

The Glogau classification describes the structure of the rhytids with and without expression and the

Table 22–1 The Fitzpatrick Classification

Skin Type/Color	Reaction of First Summer Exposure
I—White	Always burn, never tan
II—White	Usually burn, tan with difficulty
III—White	Sometimes mild burn, tan average
IV—Moderate brown	Rarely burn, tan with ease
V—Dark brown	Very rarely burn, tan very easily
VI—Black	No burn, tan very easily

patient's attempt to overcome their appearance (i.e., through the use of makeup) (Table 22–2). Although each group is individual, overlap exists, and the surgeon or peeler should use common sense in assigning a patient to a particular class. As previously mentioned, it may also be necessary to assign each of the cosmetic units a particular classification to tailor each to the appropriate wounding agent.

Another important aspect of performing chemical peels is assessment of lifestyle and emotional stability. The superficial to medium depth peels provide little-to-moderate disruption to either, whereas the deeper peels are indicated only when the patient and physician can come to a mutual understanding concerning the amount of morbidity and encroachment on the patient's day-to-day routine. Additional information obtained before medium and deep peels should include a prior history of isotretinoin (Accutane), previous surgery, radiation or peels, a history of smoking, future plans for sun exposure, the use of hormones, a history of herpes simplex, and the patient's cardiac and renal status.

Whether isotretinoin is a culprit remains to be seen, however, because it is in the literature as a potential contraindication, planning a medium-to-deep peel within a 6-to 18-month time frame after its use needs to be dis-cussed with the patient, including its possible ramifications, the need for test spots, or a delay of the procedure.[12] Previous peels and facial plastic surgery are usually good indicators of history and compliance. Neither are contraindications if sufficient time has elapsed. A history of radiation should alert the surgeon or peeler that normal skin anatomy may not exist. The number of pilosebaceous units should confirm that suspicion if less than normal and lead to a more superficial attempt to improve the skin's surface if the decision to proceed with a chemical peel is acceptable to both parties. Smoking is detrimental to the immediate and the long-term healing process in the form of oxygen depletion and the formation of free radicals within the healing skin that will damage existing and regenerating dermal components such as collagen. Sun exposure can also produce these free radical scavengers and stimulate the less covered melanocytes to produce melanin and cause subsequent postinflammatory hyperpigmentation. A good sunscreen both before and as soon after a peel is always indicated. Hormones may also exacerbate the stimulation of the exposed melanocytic system and should be discontinued at least 2 weeks before and 2 to 6 weeks after a peel. This request to forego hormone therapy for 4 to 8 weeks or longer seems to be one of the biggest hardships for the

Table 22–2 Glogau's Classification

Group I (Mild)	Group II (Moderate)	Group III (Advanced)	Group IV (Severe)
No keratoses	Early actinic keratoses—slight yellow skin discoloration	Actinic keratoses—obvious yellow skin discoloration with telangiectasis	Actinic keratoses and skin cancers have occurred
Little wrinkling	Early wrinkling—parallel smile lines	Wrinkling present at rest	Wrinkling—much cutis laxa of actinic, gravitational, and dynamic origin
No scarring	Mild scarring	Moderate acne scarring	Severe acne scarring
Little or no makeup	Little makeup	Wears makeup always	Wears makeup that does not cover, but cakes on

patient and their family to endure. If depression or anxiety is a postoperative complaint, the decision to restart the hormones versus their potential harm should be weighed and acted on accordingly. Any history of herpetic infections of the face should necessitate the addition of an antiviral agent to be given with their postoperative medications. If a blister is present or the suspicion of one is evident the day of the procedure, it is prudent to cancel and reschedule. Routine laboratory studies should include a complete blood count, an electrolyte panel, liver enzymes, and a creatinine level to assess kidney function. An electrocardiogram and medical clearance is always indicated if prior history of renal and/or cardiac problems exists.

PREOPERATIVE PREPARATION

Preparation of the skin before a peel is necessary to prevent or to reduce the chances of postoperative complications in all skin types, especially in Fitzpatrick IV through VI types or Glogau groups III and IV. Once scheduled, the patient needs to be taking retinoic acid for 2 to 6 weeks before surgery to enhance wound healing and decrease the possibility of postinflammatory hyperpigmentation. If the skin type suggests, twice daily additions of a hydroquinone 2 to 4% are indicated. Higher concentrations initially can produce skin irritation. If either or both are not tolerated, then decrease their frequency of use. These preoperative difficulties may lead to choosing a lighter peel if the skin's inability to tolerate these products is significant. It is also a good idea to have the patient on a proper suncreen before the peel to determine compliance and to protect the skin before wounding. These proactive precautions are helpful to ensure good wounding at the time of the procedure, lack of postoperative sequelae, and adaptation of the patient's schedule and skin to ensure its good health and maintenance.

TECHNIQUE

With the introduction of the transconjunctival blepharoplasty, the need for lower eyelid skin tightening at the time of surgery has led me to modify my existing technique for this cosmetic unit. In the past, when a "pinch technique" was not indicated and skin tightening was still required, the peel of choice was the Baker-Gordon peel with minimal skin preparation because peeling in this area with the thin dermal-epidermal interface would produce a deeper wound than necessary, resulting in delayed healing and on occasion a mild ectropion. Also, the length of time for healing was in weeks or months if the depth of peel matched that of the rest of the face where thicker skin predominated (Fig. 22–3C, D). Because the standard formula for the Baker-Gordon peel solution included distilled water, septisol soap, croton oil, and 88% phenol, simply removing all adulterants and using only the straight phenol prevented many of these previous concerns. Instead of weeks or months in healing, the time was cut to days. The concentration of the phenol was such that when applied to the thinner skin of the lower eyelid, frosting was immediate, and the process of keratocoagulation limited its penetration. When I first performed this procedure, the initial concern was the speed and the amount of frosting for fear of too much skin destruction. However, experience proved that the straight 88% phenol was so concentrated that its destructive properties were self limited and created the desired wound without going too deep. The result was that of a medium-depth wound, and healing was usually complete in 7 to 10 days if the wound was kept moist and clean. In retrospect, the results may not be quite as good as a Baker-Gordon peel in this particular area, but the significant decrease in morbidity outweighed the small loss in improvement. Also, if necessary, this type of medium depth peel can be repeated within 4 to 6 months if additional skin tightening is needed and no contraindications exist. It is best to repeel with a medium-depth peel than contend with the sequelae left from peeling with a deep peel in an area that may not tolerate it without increased morbidity and increased healing time. The other good thing about this type of wound is that no appreciable change occurs in skin color or texture in the Fitzpatrick type I to IV. Skin tests are performed on types V to VI.

As far as the technique is concerned, after the transconjunctival blepharoplasty, any blood or residual moisture on the lower eyelids is removed and the dry skin is degreased lightly with acetone, taking precautions not to get the liquid or fumes in the patient's eyes. Because the surgical plane is beneath the orbicularis oculi muscle, peeling the lids concomitantly is not a concern. An 88% phenol solution to be used is poured from the stock bottle into a glass container on the back table and a cotton-tipped applicator is dipped into the phenol and the excess solution is wrung out by rimming the applicator on the lip of the glass. The first stroke is at the orbital rim, where the junction of lid and cheek skin exists and the skin is thicker. This first pass dispenses the most peel solution and subsequent strokes cephalically will contain less solution as the strokes are carried from lateral to medial and within 2 to 3 mm of the free lash margin. At all times, a dry cotton-tipped applicator is kept ready to absorb any tearing that might dilute the peel solution and create a keratolytic effect especially in the lateral fornix of the eyelid. Tearing can be minimized by anesthetizing the conjunctiva with an appropriate topical anesthetic. Before the other lower lid is peeled, the lowest stroke of peel is feathered onto the upper cheek and over the zygomatic region to prevent any lines of demarcation even though this medium-depth peel is not usually known for producing any significant variation in pigment.

POSTOPERATIVE COURSE

After both lids are peeled, the patient should stay on the table for at least another 15 minutes to watch for tearing and to monitor them for cardiac dysrhythmias, although the amount of phenolic uptake is negligible for such a small area peeled. When released from the recovery room, the patient is instructed to apply an emollient on the skin surface in approximately 4 hours. The facial rinsings are not required until the next morning when they are instructed to allow a gentle stream of clean water to lightly rinse the area for 3 to 5 minutes followed by drying with unscented facial tissues. The emollient is then applied, and the process is repeated four to six times daily. Patients are seen in follow-up the day after surgery and either at day 6 or 7. If delayed healing is suspected after 10 to 14 days, Duoderm, a hydrocolloid dressing that is occlusive and oxygen impermeable, should be applied to the raw areas for 48 to 72 hours. In most instances, this will complete the re-epithelization.

COMPLICATIONS AND SEQUELAE

Although hypopigmentation is not an issue, postinflammatory hyperpigmentation is a concern and may be prevented with good preoperative management and proper patient selection. If there is any redness or pinkness turns light brown after 2 or 3 weeks, a 2% hydroquinone should be applied twice daily with close follow-up visits. Most of the hyperpigmentation that develops is gone after this type of treatment in 2 to 4 weeks. If not, increase the percentage of hydroquinone and consider the concomitant use of retinoic acid or a nonfluorinated steroid. The patient should be reassured that the final result is forthcoming in approximately 3 months and that the patient needs to minimize sun exposure for that period and avoid squinting, which can induce mechanical disruption and encourage increased fibroblastic activity. Again, if agreed on by both parties, repeeling for additional improvement can be done in 4 to 6 months if no contraindications exist.

BAKER-GORDON DEEP PEEL

The "Cadillac" of chemical resurfacing is the Baker-Gordon peel. The formula is 3 mL of 88% phenol (carboxyclic acid), 3 gtts, of croton oil, 2 mL of distilled water, and 8 gtts of Septisol soap. Although this formula has been modified over the years, most surgeons or peelers find this particular concentration fairly predictable in results and satisfaction.

The technique is operator dependent and requires the aforementioned body of knowledge, some type of previous training with a skilled surgeon or peeler, and the experience that comes with a graduated and conservative approach to peeling one's own patients. To take the position of simply applying the solution to the skin and expecting the same results every time is foolhardy and unrewarding for both patient and physician in the postoperative stages of healing. Although the actual application is matter of fact, the preparation before and the care after its application is paramount to consistent results and requires the most experience.

PATIENT SELECTION

Before a deep peel with a Baker-Gordon solution, a thorough evaluation should include a prior history of isotretinoin; previous surgery, radiation, or peels; a history of smoking; the use of hormones; a history of fever blisters; and the cardiac and renal status with appropriate medical clearance. All candidates should be adequately photographed and thoroughly educated in the follow-up care.

PREOPERATIVE PREPARATION

Two to 6 weeks before peeling, the patient is placed on a formula of Retin A that had been handed down to me by Jack Anderson during a conference in 1986.[11] That formula contains 0.05% Retin A and Shepherd's lotion, which is an emollient that offsets the skin's reactivity to the retinoic acid. This is applied to the skin at night and rinsed off in the morning. If indicated, the patient is also placed on a skin bleacher such as 2 or 4% hydroquinone in the morning to be followed by an application of a sunscreen that protects against both ultraviolet A and ultraviolet B radiation. If patients are not compliant with these preoperative requests, it is a safe assumption that they will be noncompliant with the postoperative instructions.

TECHNIQUE

On the day of the peel, the patient needs to have been NPO from the night before, have showered well, and on arrival, will need to perform the first of that day's skin preparation. This includes the patient washing his or her own face with a degreasing solution such as Septisol soap.[12] This removes the oils and dirt along with any type of makeup that may still remain on the facial skin. An oral preoperative medication is then given an hour before their transfer into the operating room, where an IV is started and cardiac monitoring is begun. With appropriate IV push sedation and regional nerve blocks, the surgeon or peeler begins to prepare the patient's face to his or her satisfaction. This includes aggressive corneocyte epiabrasion with a 2 × 2 gauze soaked in acetone and wrung out. Some use alcohol first to be followed by acetone, but acetone alone is sufficient. A fan to blow away the fumes from the acetone is necessary to prevent inhalation and eye irritation.

The peel solution does have a shelf life; however, the low cost of the ingredients should be reason enough to have the formula constituted fresh each morning before a peel of any sufficient size on the patient's face. When the skin has been adequately prepared by degreasing with the acetone (i.e., when the surgeon or peeler can feel and hear a light scraping with the 2 × 2 gauze without inducing purpura), the peel solution can be applied. Most advocate the use of a cotton-tipped applicator. However, broad strokes with these can place a lot of solution at the beginning of the stroke and little at its end. For that reason, small "blocks" of facial skin are peeled within a cosmetic unit at a time (Anderson J, personal communication, 1986), waiting 15 to 20 minutes per cosmetic unit to allow uptake of the phenol and its sequestration by the bladder to prevent cardiac dysrhythmias. Where deep rhytids exist as around the mouth, I break the cotton stick applicator at an angle, dip the wooden end into the solution, and apply it directly into the depth of the rhytid with light pressure. Visible signs of retained solution may be present within the depth of the rhytid, but if no pooling exists, one should not be alarmed. With constant monitoring, the areas of the face are sequentially peeled. If full-face peeling is performed, the entire process should take about 2 hours. By then, approximately 1000 to 1500 mL of IV fluids should have been infused and processed by the body if not medically contraindicated. The patient is allowed to stay on the table for an additional length of time while monitoring is ongoing. After an additional 15 to 30 minutes, if the patient can tolerate transfer, he or she is taken to recovery. In keeping with the need not to dilute the remaining phenol on the face, no emollient is placed on the face for at least 4 to 6 hours. The patient is allowed to fully recover and sent home. Follow-up consists of a phone call that night and an office visit the next morning for further instructions and reassurance.

POSTOPERATIVE COURSE

The daily care consists of showers with body temperature water for 5 to 10 minutes every 4 to 6 hours. Drying is accomplished either by room air or unscented facial tissue. After these two steps, petroleum or nonbuttered flavored shortening is applied to the peeled areas. Eucerin will not stick to a raw wound early on and, if used, needs to be reserved until after epithelization. The head should be elevated at 30 to 40 degrees during sleep to retard swelling, and eating consists of soft foods with care not to get any on the face.

Medication consists of a cephalosporin four times daily with a Medrol dose pack and a nonsteroidal anti-inflammatory (NSAID) such as generic ibuprofen, 800 mg, every 8 to 12 hours as needed for discomfort. A narcotic can also be dispensed for any discomfort not controlled by the NSAIDs. Follow-up visits include the day after, postpeel day 4 and 7, and then weekly for at least a month for reassurance and troubleshooting. The visits become biweekly or as indicated for an additional 2 months and then monthly, depending on the patient and their needs. The final result may be as long as 6 to 9 months in coming, and the patient is observed for at least that length of time to ensure that all is well (Fig. 22–9).

COMPLICATIONS AND SEQUELAE

The most common mistake or postoperative problem is uneven uptake of the peel solution and subsequent skip areas of varying degrees of texture and color. The use of preoperative retinoic acid and hydroquinone coupled with good preoperative degreasing will limit this problem but will not totally eliminate it. If the areas of skip are noticeable after 9 to 12 months, a light feathering across the borders of these areas will help camouflage the situation. Although this problem is potentially distressful for patient and physician, nothing is more troublesome than scar formation that is obvious to the naked eye. This happens when the depth of injury proceeds below the lower layer of reticular dermis either from the initial insult or by subsequent trauma from the patient such as scratching or some type of infectious process from the lack of good wound care. As mentioned previously, frequent visits and topical or intralesional steroids can minimize or eliminate this condition if dealt with in an appropriate time frame.

The other sequela that is more common that all others and can only be predicted but not totally eliminated is that of skin lightening. Most of the time in the Fitzpatrick type I through IV, the degree of lightening is one-half shade. This is more pronounced in darker skinned individuals and proper patient selection will keep this problem to an acceptable level.

CONCLUSION

Time and space have prevented a complete exegesis of the known peel techniques that are in existence today. If further information is required, Brody[14] has an excellent compendium concerning most of the peels that are presently performed. Also, specific articles exist for other types of peels not covered in this chapter such as Monheit's articles on the combined use of TCA and Jessner's solution.[16,17]

Chemical peels can produce some of the best results and some of the worst long-term complications for patient and surgeon or peeler. However, with proper attention to detail, patient selection, good skin preparation, and common sense from proper training and clinical experience, the risks and complications are few and far between and should not be a significant factor for either party with good education and appropriate follow-up.

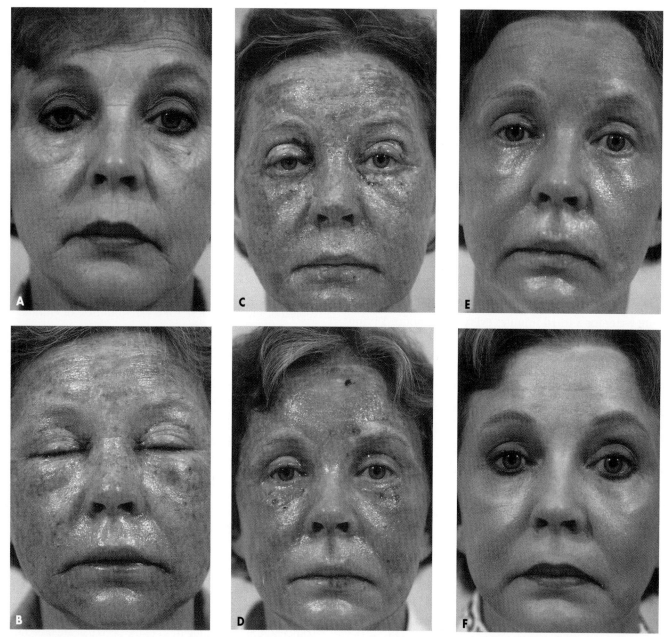

Figure 22–9. (A) Preoperative full-face Baker-Gordon chemical peel. This patient had had previous surgery but continued to have facial rhytids. **(B)** Postpeel day 1. Swelling normally peaks in 48 to 72 hours. **(C)** Postpeel day 5. The patient has allowed crusting to form on each of the upper and lower lids. This is secondary to the use of full-strength Baker-Gordon solution. These and other incidences led the author to alter the depth of peel in these areas to that of a medium depth. **(D)** Postpeel day 14. Note the lower eyelids are delayed in their healing. **(E)** Postpeel day 21. Duoderm application to the lower lids resulted in faster reepithelization. **(F)** Postpeel day 28. Note the persistant erythema that will subside over the next 3 to 6 months.

PEARLS

- If depigmentation or a more homogenous pigmentary color of the face is desired, peels such as a 35% TCA with or without epidermal vesiculation can produce wounds down to and below the basement membrane, where alteration of the melanocytic system can occur.
- Wrinkling is within the substance of the skin, especially the dermis, and the treatment modality must address that particular area. Surgery, per se, is not for wrinkling and so the treatment of rhytids lies within the domain of the chemical peel, laser resurfacing, or dermabrasion.
- My patients wear $\frac{1}{2}$-inch brown paper tape on their scar revisions for several months postoperatively. This provides good wound apposition and traps moisture, providing a better milieu for the healing process.

REFERENCES

1. Letessier SM. Chemical peel with resorcin. In: Roenigk RK, Roenigk HH, eds. Dermatologic Surgery. New York: Marcel Dekker; 1989.
2. Brown AM, Kaplan LM, Brown ME. Phenol induced histological skin changes: hazards, techniques, and uses. Br J Plast Surg. 1960; 13:158.
3. Litton C. Chemical face lifting. Plast Reconstr Surg. 1962; 29:371.
4. Baker TJ, Gordon HL. The ablation of rhytids by chemical means: A preliminary report. J Fla Med Assoc. 1961; 48:541.
5. Rubin MG. Manual of Chemical Peels, Superficial and Medium Depth, Philadelphia: J.B. Lippincott Co.; 1995.
6. Sams WM Jr., Lynch PJ. Principles and Practices of Dermatology. New York: Churchill Livingstone Inc.; 1990.
7. Maibach HF, Rovee DT. Epidermal Wound Healing. St Louis: Mosby; 1972.
8. Hevia O, Nemeth AJ, Taylor JR. Tretinoin accelerates healing after trichloroacetic acid chemical peel. Arch Dermatol. 1991; 127:678–682.
9. Hung VC, Lee JY, Zitelli JA, et al. Topical tretinoin and epithelial wound healing. Arch Dermatol. 1989; 125:65–69.
10. Geronemus RG, Mertz PM, Eaglstein WH. Wound healing: the effects of topical antimicrobial agents. Arch Dermatol. 1979; 115:1311.
11. Goodman LS, Gilman AG. The Pharmacological Basis of Therapeutics. New York: MacMillan; 1980:973.
12. Alt TH. Avoiding complications in dermabrasion and chemical peel. Skin Allergy News. 1990; 21:2.
13. McCollough EG, Lanston PR. Dermabrasion and Chemical Peel, a Guide for Facial Plastic Surgery. New York: Thieme Medical; 1988: 53–112.
14. Brody HJ. Chemical Peeling and Resurfacing, 2nd ed. St. Louis: Mosby; 1997.
15. Monheit GD. Combination medium-depth peeling, the Jessner's and TCA peel. Facial Plast Surg. 1996; 12:00–00.
16. Monheit GD. Advances in chemical peeling. Facial Plast Surg Clin North Am. 1994; 2:00–00.

Facial Resurfacing

Aesthetic Facial Plastic Surgery, edited by Thomas Romo, III, and Arthur L. Millman, Thieme Medical Publishers, Inc., New York, New York, Copyright © 2000.

CHAPTER 23

CO₂ Laser

A Dermatologist's Perspective

LEONARD J. BERNSTEIN AND ROY G. GERONEMUS

Over the years, the desire to return to one's youthful appearance has stimulated the development of rejuvenating products and procedures. In the past several decades, various topical agents have emerged to remove rhytides, fine wrinkles, and blemishes. The early chemical peeling agents, including trichloracetic acid, resorcin, salicylic acid, and phenol, are used to create a superficial wound of the epidermis and dermis. Subsequent collagen neogenesis and remodeling within the wound creates a tightening of the skin and a smoother texture. Newer agents include the alpha-hydroxy acids, which produce a very superficial peel and aid in removal of only very fine rhytides. The overwhelming response of the public to facial rejuvenation has lead to the production of topical agents that can be used at home on a regular basis to help reduce the signs of aging. Retinoic acid (tretinoin), a vitamin A analog that has been shown to stimulate new collagen growth within the dermis and lighten superficial skin dyschromias, was one of the first topical agents proven to have a long-term effect on rhytides. The alpha-hydroxy acids, such as glycolic, lactic, and ascorbic acids, have recently been introduced in low-concentration topical agents to help reduce the effects of chronic actinic damage.

Surgical rhytidectomy and blepharoplasties are among the common surgical approaches to improve the effects of elastolytic changes resulting from aging and sun damage. Chemical peeling and dermabrasion are popular methods of removing rhytides by chemical or physical manipulation of the surface of the skin. Recently, advances in laser technology have allowed lasers to become the latest modality in the field of facial rejuvenation.

PRINCIPLES OF CO_2 LASER THERAPY

The CO_2 laser was first developed in 1964 by Patel.[1] However, only in the past two decades has the usefulness of this laser in medicine been appreciated. The CO_2 laser is a laser system consisting of helium, nitrogen, and CO_2 gases as the gain media within a sealed tube that is stimulated either by high-voltage currents or by radio frequency discharge to produce an energy output at a wavelength of 10,600 nm.[2] The optical penetration depth has been calculated to be 20 to 30 μm.[3] The main chromophore for CO_2 energy is water. Because 70% of the

content of living tissue, and particularly skin, is water, the CO_2 laser has become a useful tool in both dermatology and surgery.[4,5]

The early CO_2 lasers were continuous wave (CW) lasers that produced a continuous steady low-level power output over time. The operator controlled the duration of the exposure time by the use of shutters. Subsequently, CW CO_2 lasers were modified with a revolving shutter that emitted continuous wave power output in a "chopped" manner. Despite the ability to control the duration of laser emission with either manual, electronically controlled, or "chopped" shutters, the power output remained low and uniform throughout the laser emission.[6,7] (Fig. 23–1).

The two most important characteristics of CO_2 laser interaction with tissue are the power density, or irradiance, of the laser emission and the rate of energy delivered to the tissue. The power density determines the volume of tissue vaporization, and the rate of energy delivery determines the thermal effects to the surrounding tissue. A high-power density delivered to tissue at a slow rate will vaporize a large volume of tissue with a large area of surrounding thermal damage. Conversely, a low-power density delivered at a rapid rate will vaporize

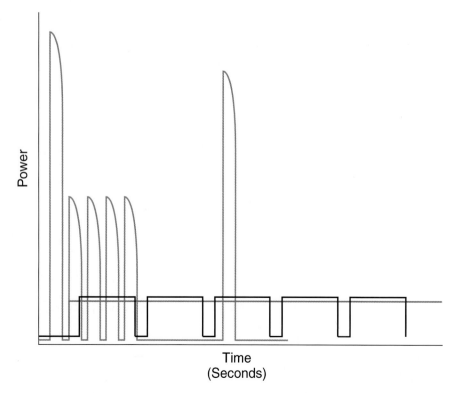

Figure 23–1. Power output versus time of laser emission for three types of laser systems: Low-power "chopped" CW CO_2 emission; "superpulsed" train of high-power CO_2 emission; high-power, short-pulsed CO_2 emission.

a small volume of tissue with little thermal damage. Ideally, a CO₂ laser would provide both a high-power density and a rapid rate of delivery. The power density of a CW CO₂ laser with a steady low-level power output is manipulated by varying the spot size of the laser beam. In a focused mode the spot size is at a minimum, and power density is at a maximum. As the beam is defocused, the spot size increases and the power density decreases. The fluence, or power density–time relationship, needed to vaporize tissue has been determined to be 5 J/cm^2. [8,9]

In a focused mode the CW CO₂ laser has a high-power density and vaporizes a large volume of tissue. As the target tissue is vaporized by the rapid change in tissue temperature with laser emission, the heat generated diffuses to the surrounding tissue over time. Although this transfer of energy is not adequate for tissue vaporization, it creates several zones of thermal damage.[9–12] (Fig. 23–2). The depth of thermal injury is directly proportional to the exposure time of the laser

energy. Immediately adjacent to the impact crater is a rim of thermal necrosis caused by tissue temperature changes between 60 and 100° C, leading to protein coagulation and denaturation with subsequent cell death. This area represents irreversible thermal damage. Beyond this layer is a zone of reversible thermal damage dependent on the duration of thermal exposure. To prevent unwanted thermal injury to the surrounding tissue and to control the depth of ablation, the laser emission must be rapidly moved across the desired tissue plane. This latter point becomes the limiting factor in performing fine, accurate cutting of tissue or to control superficial ablation with the CW CO₂ laser.

By adhering to the principle of selective photothermolysis, described by Parrish and Anderson in 1983, laser systems have been developed that minimize this collateral tissue damage.[13,14] This principle states that by confining the duration of a pulse of energy at a wavelength specific for a given target, or chromophore, to a time

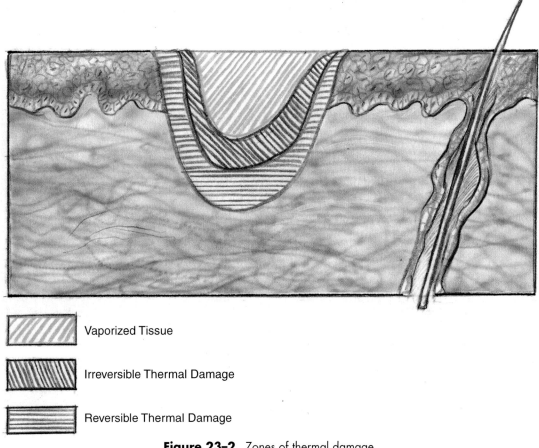

▨ Vaporized Tissue

▨ Irreversible Thermal Damage

▤ Reversible Thermal Damage

Figure 23–2. Zones of thermal damage.

period shorter than the thermal relaxation time of that target, the time period in which diffusion of 50% of the thermal energy produced will occur, selective destruction of the target can be accomplished. The thermal relaxation time for tissue heated by the CO_2 laser is less than 1 ms.[15]

This principle stimulated the next generation of CO_2 laser, the pulsed CO_2 lasers. The "superpulsed" CO_2 laser is able to generate peak powers 2 to 10 times higher than conventional CW CO_2 lasers, with pulse durations ranging from 0.1 to 0.9 ms[15-18] (Fig. 23–1). However, this system does not deliver the energy required to generate a power density adequate to vaporize tissue in a practical fashion with a single pulse. "Superpulsed" lasers use a train of such pulses in a quasicontinuous manner that increases the time of thermal tissue interaction. A high-energy, short-pulsed CO_2 laser was subsequently developed that creates a single pulse of CO_2 laser emission with a very high peak power and a short exposure time, between 600 and 950 ms.[19-23]

Another approach in the development of CO_2 lasers for tissue ablation was the development of a computer-driven opticomechanical scanner for CW CO_2 lasers. This device precisely guides a focused beam of CW CO_2 energy in a spiral pattern over tissue with a tissue "dwell" time of less than 1 ms (Fig. 23–3). Because of the small spot size, 0.2 mm, the power density generated by the lower power CW CO_2 laser is high enough for tissue vaporization, and the computer-driven rapid movement of the laser emission around the preset pattern

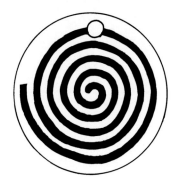

Figure 23–3. Spiral pattern of laser emission of a CW CO_2 laser with a computer-driven opticomechanical scanner.

allows for precision ablation with minimal collateral thermal damage.[24,25]

The histologic changes induced by CO_2 laser include vaporization of the target tissue with a variable thickness of surrounding thermal necrosis.[26-34] Using redundant skin that was to be excised along with skin used for skin grafts during facial reconstructive procedures, Kauvar et al, studied the histologic effects of the various CO_2 lasers that have been used for skin resurfacing procedures.[35] The four laser systems evaluated were a CW CO_2 laser (Surgicenter 40; Sharplan Lasers Inc., Allendale, NJ) (10 W and 0.2 s exposure time), a high-energy, short-pulsed CO_2 laser (Ultrapulse 5000C, Coherent Laser Corp., Palo Alto, CA) (3-mm spot size, 450 mJ, 4W), a CW CO_2 laser with computer-controlled opticomechanical scanner (Surgicenter 40 with SilkTouch scanner, Sharplan Lasers Inc., Allendale, NJ) (6-mm spot size, 18 W, 0.2 s exposure time), and a "superpulsed" CO_2 laser (Surgipulse XJ150, Sharplan Lasers Inc., Allendale, NJ) (3-mm spot size, 10W). With both the CW CO_2 laser with scanner and the "superpulsed" lasers, the epidermis was ablated completely by one pass of laser emission with a depth of ablation measuring 30 to 50 μm. The high-energy, short-pulsed CO_2 laser ablated the epidermis with foci of intact epithelium along the dermoepidermal junction. The depth of ablation with this laser was measured at 20 to 30 μm. The depths of thermal necrosis varied from 50 to 150 μm proportional to the number of laser passes over the target tissue. The CW CO_2 laser produced depths of thermal necrosis measuring 500 μm with a single exposure time.

CO_2 LASER RESURFACING

As techniques for facial rejuvenation have expanded and improved over the past several years, the interest and expectations of the prospective patient for such procedures have also been elevated. The process of safely and effectively treating a patient with a laser for facial rejuvenation consists of several steps that are all essential to the best outcome. These steps can be divided into four categories, including proper operator laser training, preoperative patient evaluation and preparation, operative techniques, and postoperative wound care.

OPERATOR LASER TRAINING

Although laser technology has advanced in the past several years, allowing the creation of laser systems that seem "user-friendly," the importance of training in the proper selection and use of particular lasers cannot be underestimated. In fact, the emergence of a great number of new lasers that consist of variable laser media, pulse widths and durations, energy outputs, and delivery mechanisms has made the need for proper laser training more important.

Traditional laser training over the past several years has been through preceptorships with experienced laser surgeons. These programs could consist of a formal "fellowship" training program over a course of 1 to 2 years with extensive theoretical and practical training or a less formal environment of periodic practical experience with a local laser surgeon. With the recent popularity of laser therapy in dermatology and plastic surgery, weekend courses on laser theory and demonstration of laser application have been developed. Although these later courses are useful to help understand the basics in laser use, alone they do not provide the foundation for the clinical use of lasers. The need for clinical training under the supervision of an experienced laser surgeon is essential. This type of training will lead to an understanding of laser physics and laser-tissue interactions and will provide the laser surgeon with the ability to adapt the use of the laser to best suit the particular need in a given situation.

PREOPERATIVE PATIENT EVALUATION

One of the most important elements of a facial rejuvenation procedure is the preoperative evaluation. Preoperative considerations for laser therapy are the following.

- Assessment of patient's concern
- Physical examination
- Pertinent medical history
- Determination of treatment options
- Discussion of patient's expectations
- Discussion of procedure, risks, and benefits

This evaluation should include an assessment of a patient's concerns and desires for laser surgery, an examination of the physical nature of the problem, a review of pertinent medical history, a determination of the appropriateness of a given procedure, an assessment of a patient's expectations of outcome from a laser procedure, and a discussion of the elements of performing the procedure, including the risks and benefits.

The first step in the evaluation for facial resurfacing is to determine what is the nature of the patient's concern regarding his or her skin. It is often helpful to have a patient point out the fine lines, or rhytides, and other tissue changes with a mirror and bright lighting. It is not uncommon for patients to notice other areas of concern when looking at their face with better lighting than they may have at home. Rhytides in the periorbital and perioral areas are a common focus for facial resurfacing patients because these areas are not greatly affected by other surgical modalities, such as facelifting procedures and blepharoplasties. Elastolytic changes of the skin caused by sun damage, creating a yellow, pebblelike texture to the skin, most notably on the lateral cheeks, also are affected little by facelifting procedures. Muscular creases or folds of the face that are present with muscle contraction or at rest do not benefit greatly over the long-term from CO_2 laser resurfacing procedures. These muscular folds, such as the melolabial fold and glabellar crease, may be tightened by collagen contraction with the CO_2 laser; however, the creases and folds subsequently return.

While discussing with the patient his or her concerns, a thorough examination of the facial skin should be performed. Important considerations in this evaluation include skin color, texture, laxity, actinic damage, pigmentation irregularities, and the presence or absence of scarring. This examination should be conducted with the patient in a sitting position after having all cosmetic products removed from the skin. To properly evaluate the presence of mild ectropion changes from previous surgical procedures, one should evaluate the lower eyelid retraction from the globe of the eye while the patient is sitting upright, eyes looking superiorly, and with the mouth open wide.

Along with a general evaluation of a patient's past and present medical condition, particular attention should be focused on previous facial surgery, radiation therapy, the use of isotretinoin, and a history of scar formation. Previous facial surgery, in particular lower eyelid blepharoplasties, will have induced a degree of dermal fibrosis, which greatly affects the laxity of the skin in the periorbital area. Because the CO_2 laser causes both immediate and delayed contraction of the skin, the presence of previous fibrosis may lead to excessive contraction with time. This contraction is most notable at the free borders of the skin, such as the eyelid, which could lead to ectropion formation. In addition, a history of previous dermabrasion or chemical peel, especially a phenol peel, is significant with regard to pigmentary changes of the skin. These techniques can often lead to a degree of irreversible hypopigmentation, which may be accentuated by further resurfacing procedures.

Previous radiation treatment to the skin will have a significant effect on the healing ability of a patient after a resurfacing procedure. Radiation therapy and certain connective tissue disorders, such as scleroderma, alter the viability of adnexal structures within the skin. During the wound healing process, re-epithelialization is initiated from healthy epithelium within these adnexal structures, in particular the pilosebaceous unit. One could expect delayed and incomplete healing of injured skin with diminished adnexal structures. These patients should not undergo facial resurfacing procedures.

Although, the cause is not well known, keloids generally form on the central chest, back, shoulders, and face of a person after trauma or inflammation. Patients who are prone to keloids developing after trauma are discouraged from undergoing laser resurfacing procedures. In addition, atypical hypertrophic scarring has been reported for patients undergoing chemical peels, dermabrasion, and laser procedures while receiving isotretinoin therapy and for as long as 9 months after its discontinuation.[36-38] Isotretinoin is an oral synthetic vitamin A analog used in the treatment of severe acne. One of the observed actions of isotretinoin is an alteration in the pilosebaceous unit. We recommend waiting a period of 18 months after the discontinuation of isotretinoin therapy before an elective cosmetic surgical procedure.

As with any cosmetic surgical procedure, a clear understanding of a patient's expectation of outcome from a laser resurfacing is very important to achieve a patient's satisfaction in the procedure. Because every patient is different, it is important to stress to the patient that the outcome will vary from person to person. Showing several series of photographs of other patients, both before and after laser resurfacing, will help illustrate the variation in response to a given procedure. With recent technologic advancement in digital imaging and photography, a photograph of a patient can be taken during the preoperative evaluation and displayed on a computer monitor. This image can then be modified to simulate an expected outcome. However, the variability in the extent of improvement must be stressed to the patient, and no guarantees of outcome on the basis of preoperative digital photography are given.

PREOPERATIVE PATIENT PREPARATION

In an effort to improve the results of CO_2 laser resurfacing and decrease the potential for complications, several topical and oral medications are used before the laser

Table 23–1 Medications Used Preoperatively for CO₂ Laser Resurfacing

Topical		
Retinoic acid, 0.025%, cream	Nightly	2–6 wk before treatment
Hydroquinone, 4%, cream/solution	Twice daily	2–6 wk before treatment
Oral		
Dicloxacilin, 250 mg,	Every 6 h	1 d before and 7 d after
or clarithromycin, 500 mg	Every 12 h	laser treatment
Acyclovir, 400 mg	3 × d	1 d before and 7 d after
		laser treatment

procedure[39-42] (Table 23–1). To minimize the potential for postinflammatory hyperpigmentation, most notably seen in darker skin phototypes, topical hydroquinone creams are applied to the treatment areas from 2 to 6 weeks before laser resurfacing. Hydroquinone inhibits the protein tyrosinase and decreases the formation and increases the destruction of melanosomes within the melanocytes.[43] Because postinflammatory hyperpigmentation is a result of melanocyte stimulation and melanosome production after injury to the skin, the use of hydroquinone can minimize the potential for postoperative hyperpigmentation.

Retinoic acid cream is also applied to the treatment areas nightly for 2 to 6 weeks before laser resurfacing. Mandy studied the time of re-epithelialization after dermabrasion with and without the use of preoperative retinoic acid.[44] In 113 patients studied, 88 were treated preopereratively with retinoic acid, 0.05%, cream. All 88 patients were re-epithelialized by day 7 postoperatively, with 68% re-epithelialized by day 5 postoperatively. In the control group of 25 patients not treated with retinoic acid, none were re-epithelialized by day 7 postoperatively, but all were re-epithelialized by day 11 postoperatively. In addition, less postinflammatory hyperpigmentation and milia were observed in the pretreated group of patients.

To minimize infection, oral preparations, including both antiviral and antibiotic agents, are initiated 24 hours

before laser resurfacing.[39,42] A broad-spectrum penicillin derivative with adequate coverage for both streptococcal and staphylococcal organisms is recommended. In addition, acyclovir is started the day before the laser procedure. Acyclovir is used empirically in all patients regardless of a previous history of herpes infection because some individuals may have had a subclinical infection in the past. Also, because of the de-epithelialized state of the skin after CO₂ laser resurfacing, significant risk for a widespread primary infection as a result of casual contact with another individual with an active clinical or subclinical herpes infection is present. These oral agents are continued for a period of 9 days postoperatively.

Immediately before the start of the CO₂ laser resurfacing, the skin in the treatment area is cleansed with a mild soap and water to remove any residual creams or cosmetics. If alcohol is to be used in this capacity, it must be allowed to dry completely before CO₂ laser resurfacing to avoid the potential for a fire.

OPERATIVE TECHNIQUE
Anesthesia

Anesthesia should be obtained before laser resurfacing to overcome the pain associated with the thermal effect of the laser on the skin. Various agents have been used to accomplish anesthesia, including topical, local, regional, and general anesthetics. Topical agents, such as eutectic mixture lidocaine anesthesia (EMLA), (Astra Pharmaceutical Production, Sodertalje, Sweden), require application under occlusion to the treatment areas for a period of 1 to 11/2 hours before the procedure. The anesthetic effect of the topical agents is often incomplete; it begins to wane after removal from the skin surface and dissipates almost completely within 20 to 30 minutes. These topical agents may be useful for laser resurfacing of small areas or as an adjunct before local and regional anesthesia with injectable agents.

Small areas of the skin can be anesthetized completely with injectable agents either locally or by regional nerve blocks. Regional nerve blocks of the supraorbital, infraorbital, and mental nerves provide a large area of anesthesia to the central face while using a minimum volume of anesthetic agent. The use of a combination of fast-acting, short-duration agents with slow-acting, long-duration agents can provide adequate anesthesia in a short time with long-lasting patient comfort. Although effective for pain control, the use of local anesthetic agents will increase the degree of edema in the immediate postoperative period.

Sedative anesthesia is a preferred method for anesthesia for full-face CO_2 laser resurfacing used by itself or in conjunction with local and regional anesthetic techniques. The anesthesia is accomplished by the administration of a variety of sedative analgesics, including meperidine, midazolam, and diazepam. Careful cardiac and oxygen perfusion monitoring should be done when sedation anesthesia is used. Our preferred anesthetic regimen includes the combination of fentanyl, a narcotic analgesic, and propofol, a sedative hypnotic agent, administered by an anesthesiologist with proper monitoring devices.

The use of general anesthesia for CO_2 laser resurfacing is a less common but effective practice to achieve complete anesthesia. However, special care must be taken with regard to the prevention of fires in the operating room. The use of open oxygen delivery systems, such as nasal cannulas and face masks, is incompatible with CO_2 lasers. When general anesthesia is being used for a laser procedure, a closed endotracheal system, such as a laryngeal mask airway or an endotracheal tube, must be used with a further recommendation of covering the airway device with water-soaked gauze.[45]

Laser Procedure

After anesthesia has been achieved, the area surrounding the treatment area is carefully draped with water-soaked towels to prevent accidental fires. A water-based lubricant (Surgilube, E. Fougera & Co., Melville, NY) is applied to the hair-bearing regions surrounding and within the treatment area, notably the eyebrows, eyelashes, and surrounding hairline, to prevent unintentional burning of the hair. The patient's eyes are protected by internal stainless steel eye shields when resurfacing involves the periorbital region or by water-soaked gauze when the periorbital region is not involved. Plastic laser eye protection should not be used on the patient because of its ability to burn or melt if accidentally contacted by the CO_2 laser emission.

The method of CO_2 laser resurfacing is based on many variables, including type of laser used, size and location of treatment area, previous surgical procedures, and degree of rhytid formation. As noted previously, it is essential to understand the effects of an individual laser and how it relates to these variables before beginning laser resurfacing.

The two most common lasers used today for facial laser resurfacing are the high-energy, short-pulsed CO_2 laser and the CW CO_2 laser with scanning device. Prototypes of these lasers are the Ultrapulse 5000C (Coherent Laser Corp., Palo Alto, CA) and the Surgicenter 40 with SilkTouch handpiece (Sharplan Lasers Inc., Allendale, NJ), respectively. The Utrapulse 5000C laser with a 3-mm handpiece can produce a collimated beam of energy with a peak power output of 500 mJ and a pulse duration of approximately 0.9 ms. A subsequent modification of the laser's delivery system with a scanning device allows for a series of rapid collimated laser pulses 2.5 mm in diameter to be generated in various patterns

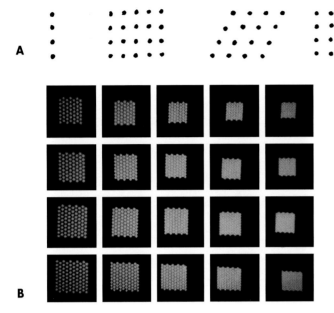

Figure 23–4. (A) Pattern selections available on scanning device for high-energy, short-pulsed CO_2 laser. **(B)** Various sized laser patterns versus density of overlap: The higher the degree of density, or pulse overlap, the smaller the treated pattern on tissue with the greater depth of thermal injury.

and sizes (Fig. 23–4). In addition, the scanning device allows for overlap of adjacent pulses ranging from −10 to 60%. The higher the degree of overlap of these pulses when resurfacing, the greater will be the depth of ablation.

The Surgicenter 40 CW CO_2 laser with SilkTouch scanner allows a CW CO_2 emission to be delivered to the target tissue in a controlled manner with a high-power density and a tissue dwell time of approximately 1 ms. Various spot sizes can be generated ranging from 2 to 16 mm. Adjustment of the power output will directly affect the depth of tissue ablation. Conversely, adjustment of the laser spot size will inversely affect the depth of ablation at a given power.

Carbon dioxide laser resurfacing of a region of the face should include the entire surface of that particular cosmetic unit (Fig. 23–5). The treatment of partial cosmetic units can lead to visible inconsistencies of the skin with regard to postoperative erythema, relative hypopigmentation (the removal of actinically induced bronzing and lentigines), and texture. Similarly, patients who have a significant degree of actinic damage, such as a diffuse bronze pigmentation or extensive lentigines, or who are of a darker skin phototype (Fitzpatrick types IV to VI) are best served by undergoing a full-face CO_2 laser resurfacing.[46] Partial-face laser resurfacing in this patient population leads to incon-

sistent pigmentation across treated and untreated regions over both the short and long term after the laser procedure.

When laser resurfacing the periorbital region, the treated areas should include the infraorbital area (Fig. 23–6) extending from and including the infraorbital crease inferiorly, the inner canthus medially, the lateral canthus inclusive of lateral extending rhytides ("crow's feet") laterally, and the eyelid margin superiorly; and the supraorbital area extending from the eyelid margin inferiorly, the medial canthus medially, the lateral canthus laterally, and the eyebrow superiorly. Similarly, treatment of the perioral area (Fig. 23–7) would include the entire upper and lower lips with lateral borders defined by the melolabial folds and inferiorly to the base of the chin. Laser resurfacing of the entire face (Fig. 23–8) should extend from the edge of the hairline superiorly and laterally to just below the mandibular ridge. Often the lower portion of the ear lobe is treated as well.

The entire target area should be uniformly treated with individual nonoverlapping pulses of the CO_2 laser in a confluent manner. Although the depth of ablation will vary from one laser system to another, using more common CO_2 lasers, the first pass of laser pulses will ablate the epidermis to the epidermal-dermal junction. Additional passes of the the laser pulses will produce

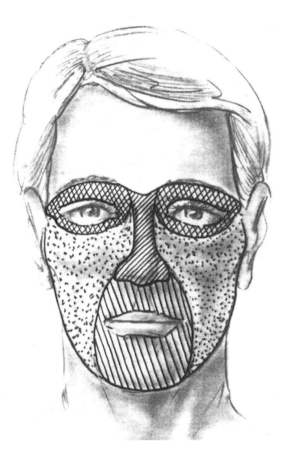

Figure 23–5. Cosmetic units of the face for CO_2 laser resurfacing.

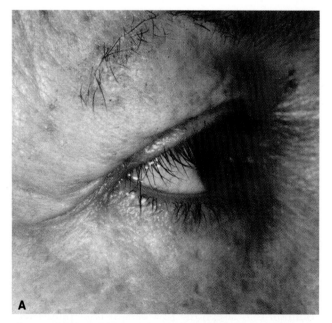

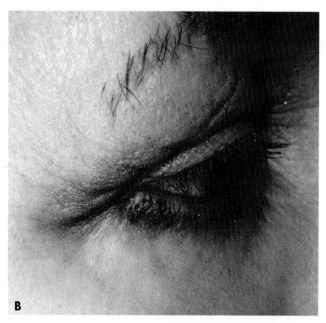

Figure 23–6. **(A)** Preoperative and **(B)** three month postoperative right eye for CO_2 laser resurfacing of the infraorbital area with extension to the limits of lateral canthal rhytides ("crow's feet").

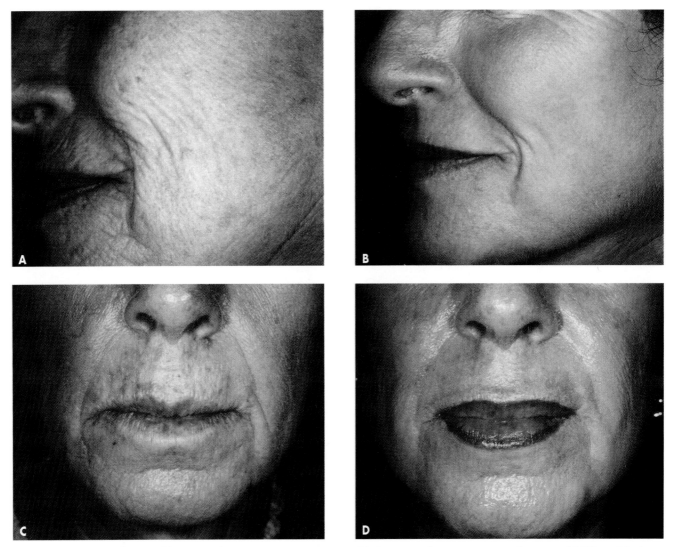

Figure 23–7. Resurfacing of the perioral area. **(A)** Preoperative and **(B)** two month postoperative side views of full face CO$_2$ laser resurfacing with significant reduction of perioral rhytides. **(C)** Preoperative and **(D)** two month postoperative front views of CO$_2$ laser resurfacing of the perioral unit.

deeper levels of ablation with wider bands of thermal necrosis. The number of laser passes to a given treatment area will vary with the desired clinical outcome. Fine rhytides within the periorbital and cheek regions are adequately treated with one to two passes of CO$_2$ laser pulses, whereas coarse rhytides of the perioral region often require two to three passes of CO$_2$ laser pulses.

Two regions of the face that deserve particular caution while resurfacing with the CO$_2$ laser include the infraorbital area and the lower half of the mandibular ridge

(Fig. 23–9). The thickness of the periorbital skin is considerably less than the skin of the cheek. To avoid hypertrophic scarring and ectropion formation, either the number of laser passes over this region or the energy output of the laser should be decreased. Similarly, the skin of the lower mandibular region is more sensitive to the development of hypertrophic scar formation. When treating this region of the face, it is recommend that only one pass of the CO$_2$ laser at standard energy output be used with or without a second pass of the CO$_2$ laser at a lower energy.

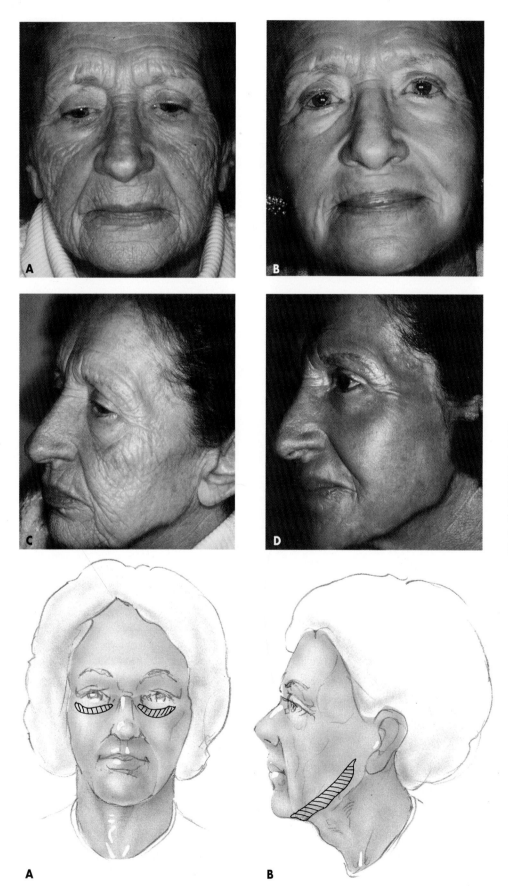

Figure 23–8. CO$_2$ laser resurfacing of the entire face with significant reduction of both fine and coarse rhytides. **(A)** Preoperative and **(B)** one month postoperative front views. **(C)** Preoperative and **(D)** one month postoperative side views.

Figure 23–9. Areas of the face at higher risk for scar formation. Caution should be used when resurfacing the **(A)** infraorbital and **(B)** lower mandibular ridge.

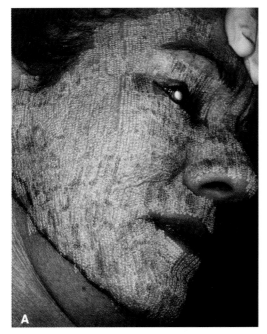
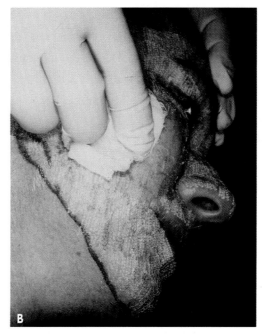

Figure 23–10. (A) The surface of the skin becomes white and grainy with dehydrated proteinaceous debris following a pass of CO₂ laser resurfacing. **(B)** This debris is removed by gentle wiping of the surface with a water-soaked gauze.

The skin in the treated areas immediately becomes white and grainy after CO₂ laser treatment (Fig. 23–10A). This layer of dehydrated proteinaceous debris must be removed between laser passes to allow the laser emission from subsequent passes to reach its target chromophore, intercellular and intracellular water (Fig. 23–10B). This task is accomplished by the gentle wiping of this debris from the treated areas with water-soaked gauze. Before performing an additional pass of the laser over this region, the skin surface must be dried of residual moisture. Surface water will absorb the laser emission and greatly attenuate the effect of the laser on the targeted tissue.

The first pass of the CO₂ laser vaporizes either the entire epidermis or a large fraction of this layer with little observed contraction of the skin (Fig. 23–11). Subsequent passes of the laser reach the papillary and

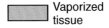 Vaporized tissue

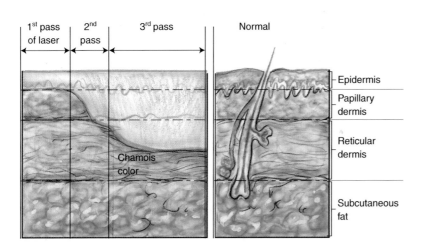

Figure 23–11. Tissue vaporized by the first, second, and third passes of the CO₂ laser.

superficial reticular dermis with immediate and notable contraction of the skin. As the depth of injury reaches the reticular dermis, a chamois color is evident. Caution must be taken at this depth of injury because the risk for hypertrophic scar formation becomes significant.

POSTOPERATIVE CARE

Immediately after the laser resurfacing procedure, the skin is gently debrided of residual proteinaceous debris using cold water compresses. A thick layer of a bland emollient ointment is applied to the entire region. The patient is instructed to soak the treatment area with cold water compresses five times daily followed by the application of the bland emollient ointment throughout the first 5 days postoperatively. This routine is then modified to three times daily until re-epithelialization is complete. Generally, re-epithelialization is complete within 10 to 14 days. The use of cold water compresses reduces the amount of swelling and diminishes the sensation of heat after the laser procedure. In addition, throughout the re-epithelialization phase, the treatment area is steamed for 5 to 10 minutes daily to help remove serous crusting on the surface of the skin.

An alternative to this "open-wound" care plan just described is the use of occlusive dressings applied to the skin immediately after debridement of the proteinaceous debris. This "closed-wound" method allows for less patient work at home. However, the risk for infection with this method is greater than with the "open-wound" method.[40,47] To help avoid infection, the dressings must be changed daily and the skin gently debrided with cool water compresses.

The time to complete re-epithelialization varies from person to person, but on average, it is complete within 7 to 14 days. Two important side effects can develop during this period, pruritus and hypersensitivity reactions. Pruritus in the treatment area is common during the second week of re-epithelialization. Oral antihistamines and low-potency topical corticosteroid ointment, applied to the affected areas twice daily, are used to relieve the pruritus. In addition, it is sometimes recommended that patients sleep with white cotton gloves at night to diminish the possibility of nocturnal excoriation caused by the pruritus. Hypersensitivity to topical agents is another side effect often seen during this healing period. To avoid hypersensitivity reactions, only bland topical ointments are used on the skin. Although topical antibiotic agents may reduce the risk of infection, the incidence of hypersensitivity reactions increases with the use of these agents.[48]

SIDE EFFECTS AND COMPLICATIONS

As with any surgical procedure, the possibility of side effects and complications exists. These side effects and complications can be divided into short-term and long-term effects[38,49] (Table 23–2). Furthermore, some of these side effects are an expected outcome as a result of the procedure.

The short-term side effects of CO_2 laser resurfacing include erythema, pain, discomfort, edema, pruritus,

Table 23–2 The Short-term and Long-term Side Effects and Complications of CO_2 Laser Resurfacing

Side Effect	Duration (average)
Short term	
Erythema	1–8 mo (3 mo)
Discomfort/pain	1–3 d (2 d)
Edema	3–10 d (6 d)
Pruritus	1–7 d (5 d)
Milia/acneiform papules	1–4 wk (3 wk)
Hypersensitivity	5–7 d (6 d)
Infection	Variable
Long term	
Pigmentary change	
Hypopigmentation	Variable—often permanent
Hyperpigmentation	2–10 wk (4 wk)
Scarring	Variable—often permanent

milia, acneiform eruptions, and hypersensitivity reactions. Erythema is an expected outcome in 100% of CO_2 laser resurfacing patients. The degree of erythema and its duration is directly proportional to the depth of laser ablation and adjacent thermal injury. With most CO_2 lasers having pulse or laser dwell times of 1 ms, the erythema often persists from 1 to 8 months, with an average of $3\frac{1}{2}$ months. Although CO_2 lasers with very short pulse widths, ~ 60 ms, create less thermal damage and have less persistent erythema. The erythema gradually decreases from a sunburned, red appearance initially to a faint pink glow over time. After re-epithelialization is complete, patients can camouflage the erythema with a green-tinted cosmetic foundation.

Immediately after the CO_2 laser procedure, patients describe a sensation of heat lasting 2 to 3 days. This discomfort is often controlled by the use of cold water compresses. Interestingly, the use of some occlusive dressings postoperatively can diminish the incidence of his symptom. Pain, as defined by the need for oral analgesics, is a rare symptom after the laser procedure, only reported by 2.8% of patients.

Edema is an expected consequence of CO_2 laser resurfacing usually subsiding within 2 weeks of the procedure. The use of injectable local anesthesia preoperatively will increase the degree of swelling. Cold water compresses and ice packs will decrease the edema. Oral corticosteroids can also be used to diminish the edema; however, the risk of postoperative infection may be slightly higher when using this agent.

Pruritus is a symptom in greater than 90% of patients after CO_2 laser resurfacing. The pruritus usually begins during the second week of re-epithelialization and can persist from 1 to 3 weeks. Rarely the pruritus can be severe, leading to both conscious and subconscious excoriation of the skin. The use of oral antihistamines and topical corticosteroids can relieve these symptoms. The use of cotton gloves at night helps prevent nocturnal subconscious excoriation.

Milia and acneiform eruptions are present in more than 80% of patients after CO_2 laser resurfacing. These lesions become apparent between the third and sixth week and gradually dissipate over subsequent weeks. These lesions are a result of thick oily emollients used during the immediate postoperative period and the re-epithelialization process of denuded skin. The use of retinoic acid before and after laser resurfacing may help diminish the severity of these outbreaks. Milia can be removed by careful extraction with little risk of scarring.

Hypersensitivity reactions occur in less than 5% of patients after CO_2 laser resurfacing. This type of reaction can be due to either an allergic reaction to a product applied to the skin or an inherent hypersensitivity reaction after trauma. To minimize allergic reactions, only bland ointments are used immediately postoperatively. During the first several weeks after re-epithelialization, while the skin is more likely to be sensitive, hypoallergenic moisturizers and cosmetics are used. Posttraumatic hypersensitivity, or eczema, has been described after trauma to the skin that is significant enough to cause tissue damage with an inflammatory or regenerative response. This hypersensitivity usually begins within weeks of injury and persists for a variable time.

An uncommon short-term complication after CO_2 laser resurfacing is wound infection. Wound infections can be due to bacterial, viral, or candidal organisms. Streptococcal and staphylococcal organisms are the most common agents of bacterial infection with gram-negative organisms being less common. Rarely, a localized bacterial skin infection can become systemic and possibly progress to sepsis and shock. Close monitoring of the infection and aggressive therapy is essential to help prevent this later scenario. The use of prophylactic antibiotics before and after a CO_2 laser resurfacing procedure decreases the incidence of bacterial infections. In addition, "open wound" care allows for close monitoring of the skin and the subsequent early detection and treatment of infection.

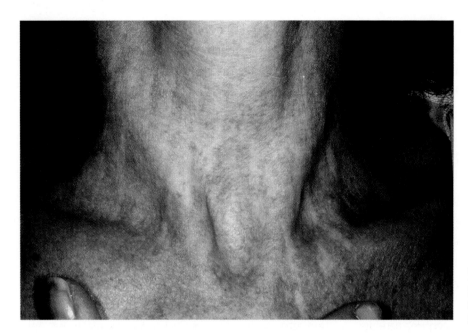

Figure 23–12. Permanent pigmentary and textural changes of the skin on the neck following CO_2 laser resurfacing.

Viral infections, namely herpes simplex, can occur in patients with and without a history of a previous infection. During the re-epithelialization period while the skin is denuded, it is susceptible to widespread herpetic infection. This can occur from either a reactivation of a dormant labial herpes infection or from contact with an individual with either a clinical or a subclinical infection. A severe herpes viral infection of the skin can lead to ulceration and subsequent atrophic scarring. Therapy for such an infection is urgent. Local wound care in conjunction with high doses of oral or intravenous acyclovir is essential. The use of prophylactic antiviral agents in all patients helps to decrease the incidence of these infections.

Candidal infection of the skin is rare after CO_2 laser resurfacing. This type of infection, however, may become more likely because of the use of prophylactic antibiotics. Candidal infections can be scaly and resemble an eczematous reaction or be erosive in nature. Treatment with topical and oral antifungal agents provides quick resolution of this type of infection. As with any infection, maintaining a high level of alertness to infection and obtaining proper samples for culture is essential for the quick detection of infection and identification of the organism.

Long-term complications of CO_2 laser resurfacing include pigmentary changes of the skin and scarring

(Fig. 23–12). Pigmentary changes of the skin include both hyperpigmentation and hypopigmentation. Postinflammatory hyperpigmentation has been reported in between 3 and 36% of patients treated with CO_2 laser resurfacing.[39,42,50] Hyperpigmentation becomes evident between 1 and 3 months after the laser procedure. It is more common among darker skin phototypes (Fitzpatrick types III to VI) after inflammatory injury to the skin. The hyperpigmentation is generally temporary, persisting from weeks to months and is diminished by the use of topical hydroquinones. Protection from ultraviolet A exposure during the first 2 to 3 months after laser resurfacing is important in all skin phototypes to reduce the risk of postinflammatory hyperpigmentation.

Hypopigmentation has been seen in approximately 16% of patients after CO_2 laser resurfacing.[39] This hypopigmentation is often delayed in onset until after the complete resolution of the postoperative erythema. Although the cause is unclear, this pigmentary change is thought to be a relative hypopigmentation of the treated skin compared with the bronzed and actinically damaged untreated skin. Patients who have experienced this hypopigmentation are generally older patients with moderate-to-severe actinic damage. The significance of this pigmentary change is grossly apparent when partial-face resurfacing is performed. As stated previously, patients of darker phototypes and those with actinically bronzed skin should only undergo full-face CO_2 laser resurfacing to avoid obvious pigmentary transitions from treated to untreated areas.

Last, scar formation is a rare but significant complication of CO_2 laser resurfacing. As one would expect with any surgical modality that injures the skin, a risk of scarring exists, which can be either hypertrophic or atrophic. The risk of scarring will increase with the depth of laser ablation. Specific areas of the face that are prone to hypertrophic scarring include the periorbital region and the mandibular rim. Hypertrophic scars are best treated with a combination of intralesional injections of corticosteroid, application of silicone gel, and pulsed dye laser. Proper laser training, careful patient selection, and attentiveness to wound care will minimize the risk of scarring from CO_2 laser resurfacing.

OTHER USES OF CO₂ LASER

Beyond its use in facial skin laser resurfacing, the CO_2 laser has proven to be useful for the treatment of many skin lesions.[51-65] The CO_2 laser can be used in either the conventional CW, scanned CW, or in a pulsed mode when treating skin lesions. However, the degree of thermal necrosis and subsequent time to heal will be affected by the mode selected.

Benign neoplasms of the skin can be categorized as either epidermal or dermal in origin (Table 23–3). In the

Table 23–3 Epidermal and Dermal Lesions Treated with the CO₂ Laser

Epidermal	Dermal
Epidemal nevi	Syringoma
Seborrheic keratosis	Adenoma sebaceum
Verruca vulgaris	Xanthalasma palpebrum
Lentigines	Myxoid cyst
Actinic keratosis/cheilitis	Lupus pernio
Bowen's disease	Tattoo
Familial benign chronic pemphigus	Rhinophyma

treatment of epidermal neoplasms, it is essential to limit the depth of thermal injury to minimize the risk of scarring. The high-energy, short-pulsed and the scanned CW CO_2 lasers produce depths of ablation ranging from 30 to 50 μm with each pass with depths of thermal necrosis proportionate to the number of laser passes. The method of treatment will depend on whether the epidermal neoplasm is exophytic, flat, or endophytic. Exophytic lesions are treated with repetitive passes of the laser and the removal of proteinaceous debris until the lesion is flush with the surrounding skin. Flat lesions can generally be eradicated with one to two passes of the laser. An endophytic lesion, such as an actinic keratosis, may have significant extension along adnexal structures and should be treated similar to a dermal neoplasm. Wound care consists of gentle cool water compress soaks followed by a topical antibiotic ointment application.

The complete removal of benign dermal neoplasms is difficult without creating a scar or visible pigmentary and textural change (Fig. 23–13). Often the partial removal of the exophytic portion of the neoplasm is the desired effect. For example, syringomas in the periorbital area of the face are skin-colored papules that consist of a neoplastic growth of eccrine sweat ducts. Because this lesion is a dermal adnexal tumor with variable depth, the complete removal of a syringoma may require injury to the deeper portion of the reticular dermis, resulting in scar formation. However, by vaporizing the exophytic portion of the neoplasm, a fine layer of dermal fibrosis will develop over the remaining neoplasm and prohibit the regrowth of the visible exophytic portion of this neoplasm. It is better to be conservative in the number of CO_2 laser passes used in the treatment of a dermal neoplasm, and perhaps retreat the neoplasm a second time, rather than to excessively treat a lesion and create an irreversible scar.

The CO_2 laser has been particularly useful and is the treatment of choice for rhinophyma and actinic cheilitis.[66-68] (Fig. 23–14). Rhinophyma results from a hyperplasia of the soft tissue and sebaceous tissue of the nose. The cause is unclear. The hyperplastic tissue can be

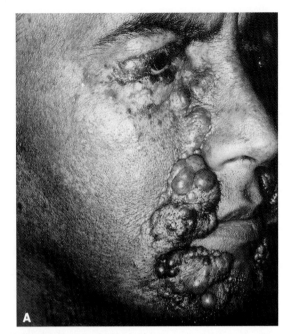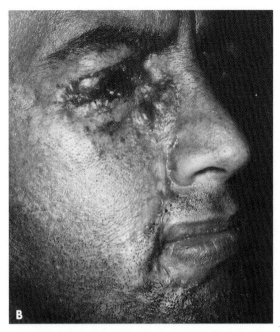

Figure 23-13. Removal of benign dermal neoplasms may create scarring and pigmentary change. **(A)** Preoperative side view of a patient with xanthoma disseminata with ocular, perinasal, and perioral involvment. **(B)** Postoperative side view following CO_2 laser resurfacing of the perinasal and perioral area with significant improvement with limited scarring.

removed by repetitive pulses using the pulsed or scanned CO_2 lasers. Alternately, most of the hyperplastic tissue can be debulked using the CW mode of the CO_2 laser with fine contouring of the nose with the resurfacing modes.

Actinic cheilitis is a premalignant change in the epithelium of the vermillion of the lip caused by exces-

sive solar radiation. Because of the paucity of adnexal structures within the mucosa of the lip, this neoplasm is often superficial. The high-energy, short-pulsed, or CW-scanned CO_2 lasers are the lasers of choice in the treatment of actinic cheilitis, requiring only one to two passes of laser pulses to eradicate this process. The use of

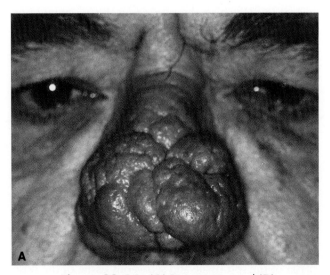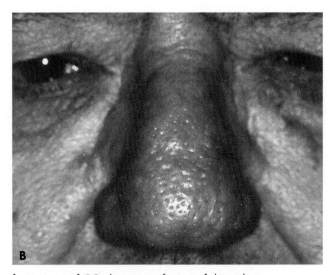

Figure 23-14. (A) Preoperative and **(B)** postoperative front views of CO_2 laser resurfacing of rhinophyma.

the traditional CW CO$_2$ laser is also highly effective for this condition; however, the depth of thermal injury leads to a longer healing time and a higher risk of scar formation.

Techniques for the revision of surgical and traumatic scars have included dermabrasion and scalpel surgery. The resurfacing CO$_2$ laser systems have proven to be useful in flattening elevated scars and improving the contour of depressed scars.[69] Multiple passes of the laser over the complete surface of the scar and the adjacent tissue with a concentration of laser pulses on the elevated edges of a scar are required.

Improvement of acne and varicella scars has also been demonstrated with the CO$_2$ laser.[50] Generally, broad-based, shallow scars improve more dramatically than pitted, narrow, and deep acne scars. Laser resurfacing of entire cosmetic units or the entire face is recommended in the treatment of acne scars. Because the degree of clinical improvement of acne scars after laser resurfacing is highly variable and related to the overall composition of the scarring, a clear understanding of this variability must be understood by the patient and match his or her expectations.

Last, CO$_2$ lasers have proven to be useful in hair transplantation procedures.[70–74] Variably sized recipient site holes can be created with little or no bleeding and with little thermal injury to the surrounding dermis. Results with CO$_2$ laser–assisted hair transplantation have been as successful as traditional methods.

NEWER LASERS FOR THE TREATMENT OF RHYTIDES

ERBIUM:YAG LASER

The erbium:YAG laser emits radiation at a wavelength of 2940 nm matching the peak of the absorption spectrum for water. Because of the 10-fold higher degree of absorption by water of the erbium:YAG energy, the optical penetration depth is 1 μm compared with 30 μm for the CO$_2$ laser.[75–77] The erbium:YAG laser produces a maximum pulse energy of 2 J with a 200 ms "macropulse" train of 1 ms pulses at a frequency of 10 Hz. The high degree of absorption by water of erbium:YAG irradiation leads to a very rapid rise in tissue temperature, creating an explosive ablation of the tissue with very little thermal necrosis.

Compared with one pass of the high-energy, short-pulsed CO$_2$ laser, the erbium:YAG laser requires three passes to reach the dermoepidermal junction. The thermal necrosis ranges from 10 to 30 μm.

Because of the small degree of thermal injury with the erbium:YAG laser, the time to re-epithelialization and the duration of the postoperative erythema is greatly reduced. However, because the thermal effects of this laser are well confined to the target chromophore, little thermal coagulation of vessels occurs, resulting in bleeding from capillaries in the papillary dermis.[78–81] In addition, the number of passes of the erbium:YAG laser required to achieve a similar depth as the CO$_2$ laser is three times greater. This latter fact requires longer procedures and therefore slightly higher risks for anesthetic complications.

Despite these potential drawbacks, the erbium:YAG laser has become useful for the eradication of fine rhytides on the face. We often use the erbium:YAG laser in combination with traditional CO$_2$ laser resurfacing to reduce the time of healing. When used in this manner, the skin that has been treated with the CO$_2$ laser is also treated with one pass of the erbium:YAG laser. Although the histologic aspects of the wound healing after such a treatment is still being explained, the improved healing time may be related to the removal of CO$_2$ laser–induced thermal necrosis.

NONABLATIVE LASER TREATMENT OF RHYTIDES

In an effort to remove facial rhytides without producing injury to the epidermis, a new laser has been produced with a solid-state neodymium:yttrium-aluminum-garnet

(Nd-YAG) laser with an emission at 1320 nm on the electromagnetic spectrum.[82] This laser is used in combination with a dynamic cooling device that produces a burst of a cryogen spray 10 to 20 ms before laser emission. The laser produces three pulses of 300 ms duration at 100-Hz pulse repetition frequency and pulse radiant exposures extending to 15 J/cm^2. This laser is designed to create sufficient thermal injury to the papillary dermis to activate collagen synthesis and fibroblast production of extracellular material without creating any epidermal damage (Fig. 23–15).

Preliminary results of ongoing studies with this laser show mild-to-moderate improvement of periorbital rhytides with little or no side effects. The immediate post-treatment area is slightly edematous and erythematous for 1 to 2 days. Purpura and epidermal damage is not seen. Long-term benefits and extent of improvement are not known at this time.

PEARLS

- The two most important characteristics of CO_2 laser interaction with tissue are the power density (or irradiance) of the laser emission and the rate of energy delivered to the tissue.
- Patients who have undergone radiation therapy or who have certain connective tissue diseases should not undergo facial resurfacing procedures.
- The method of CO_2 laser resurfacing is based on many variables, including the type of laser used, the size and location of the treatment area, previous surgical procedures, and degree of rhytid formation.
- If during CO_2 laser resurfacing the depth of injury extends to the reticular dermis, the surgeon should remain cautious because the risk for hypertrophic scar formation is significant.

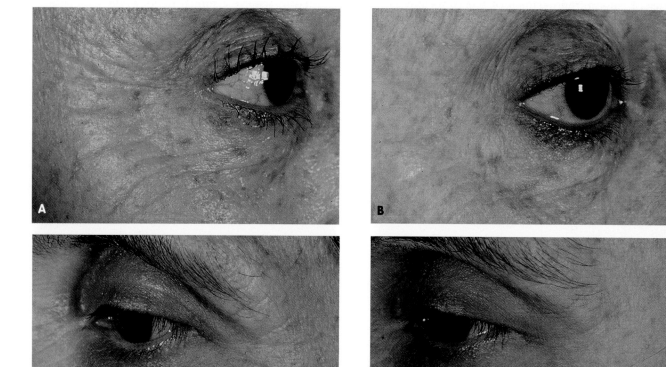

Figure 23–15. Treatment of lateral canthal rhytides with a Nd: YAG laser (1320 nm) with dynamic cooling (CoolTouch™). **(A)** Preoperative and **(B)** postoperative right eye. **(C)** Preoperative and **(D)** postoperative left eye.

REFERENCES

1. Patel CKN, McFarlane RA, Faust WL. Selective excitation through vibrational energy transfer and optical maser action in N_2-CO_2. *Phys Rev.* 1964; 13:617–619.

2. Wheeland RG. History of lasers in dermatology. *Clinic Dermatol.* 1995; 13:3–10.

3. Anderson RR, Parrish JA. The optics of human skin. *J Invest Dermatol.* 1981; 77(1):13–19.

4. Spicer MS, Goldberg DJ. Lasers in dermatology. *J Am Acad Dermatol.* 1996; 34:1–25.

5. Alster TS, Lewis AB. Dermatologic laser surgery: A review. *Dermatol Surg.* 1996; 22:797–805.

6. Ratz JL. Laser physics. *Clinics Dermatol.* 1995; 13:11–20.

7. Lanzafame RJ, Naim JO, Rogers DW, Hinshaw JR. Comparison of continuous wave, chop-wave, and super pulse laser wounds. *Lasers Surg Med.* 1988; 8:119–124.

8. Walsh JT, Deutsch TF. Pulsed CO_2 laser tissue ablation: Measurement of the ablation rate. *Lasers Surg Med.* 1988; 8:264–275.

9. Ross EV, Domankevitz Y, Skrobal M, Anderson RR. Effects of CO_2 laser pulse duration in ablation and residual thermal damage: Implications for skin resurfacing. *Lasers Surg Med.* 1996; 19:123–129 properties *IEEE Trans Bio Eng.* 1989; 36(12):1195–1201.

10. Reid R. Physical and surgical principles governing carbon dioxide laser surgery on the skin. *Dermatol Clin.* 1991; 9(2):00–00.

11. Ben-Baruch G, Fidler JP, Wessler T, Bendick P, Schellhas HF. Comparison of wound healing between chopped mode-superpulse CO_2 laser and steel knife incision. *Lasers Surg Med.* 1988; 8:596–599.

12. Green HA, Domankevitz Y, Nishioka NS. Pulsed carbon dioxide laser ablation of burned skin: In vitro and in vivo analysis. *Lasers Surg Med.* 1990; 10:476–484.

13. Parrish JA, Anderson RR, Harrist T, Paul B, Murphy GF. Selective thermal effects with pulsed irradiation from lasers: From organ to organelle. *J Invest Dermatol.* 1983; 80(6):75–80.

14. Anderson RR, Parrish JA. Selective photothermolysis: Precise microsurgery by selective absorption of pulsed radiation. *Science.* 1983; 220:524–527.

15. Walsh JT, Flotte TJ, Anderson RR, Deutsch TF. Pulsed CO_2 laser tissue ablation: Effect of tissue type and pulse duration on thermal damage. *Lasers Surg Med.* 1988; 8:108–118.

16. Walsh JT, Deutsch TF. Pulsed CO_2 laser ablation of tissue: Effect of mechanical properties. *IEEE Trans Bio Eng.* 1989; 36:1195–1201.

17. Hobbs ER, Bailin PL, Wheeland RG, Ratz JL. Superpulsed lasers: Minimizing thermal damage with short duration, high irradiance pulses. *J Dermatol Surg Oncol.* 1987; 13(9):955–964.

18. Venugopalan V, Nishioka NS, Mikic BB. The effect of CO_2 laser pulse repetition rate on tissue ablation rate and thermal damage. *IEEE Trans Bio Eng.* 1991; 38(9):1049–1052.

19. Fitzpatrick RE, Goldman MP, Satur NM, Tope WD. Pulsed carbon dioxide laser resurfacing of photoaged facial skin. *Arch Dermatol.* 1996; 132:395–402.

20. Lowe NJ, Lask G, Griffin ME, Maxwell A, Lowe P, Quilada F. Skin resurfacing with the ultrapulse carbon dioxide laser: Observations on 100 patients. *Dermatol Surg.* 1996; 21:1025–1029.

21. David LM, Sarne AJ, Ungar WP. Rapid laser scanning for facial resurfacing. *Dermatol Surg.* 1995; 21:1031–1033.

22. Hruza G, Dover JS. Laser skin resurfacing. *Arch Dermatol.* 1996; 132:451–455.

23. Yang CC, Chai CY. Animal study of skin resurfacing using the ultrapulse carbon dioxide laser. *Ann Plast Surg.* 1995; 35:154–158.

24. Lask G, Keller G, Lowe NJ, Gormley D. Laser skin resurfacing with the SilkTouch flashscanner for facial rhytides. *Dermatol Surg.* 1995; 21:1021–1024.

25. Waldorf HA, Kauvar ANB, Geronemus RG. Skin resurfacing of fine to deep rhytides using a char-free carbon dioxide laser in 47 patients. *Dermatol Surg.* 1995; 21:940–946.

26. Fitzpatrick RE, Tope WD, Goldman MP, Satur NM. Pulsed carbon dioxide laser, trichloroacetic acid, Baker-Gordon phenol, and dermabrasion: A comparative clinical and histologic study of cutaneous resurfacing in a porcine model. *Arch Dermatol.* 1996; 132:469–471.

27. Kamat BR, Carney JM, Arndt KA, Stern RS, Rosen S. Cutaneous tissue repair following CO_2 laser irradiation. *J Invest Dermatol.* 1986; 87:268–271.

28. Gardner ES, Reinisch L, Stricklin GP, Ellis DL. In vitro changes in non-facial human skin following CO_2 laser resurfacing: A comparison study. *Lasers Surg Med.* 1996; 19:379–387.

29. Alster TS, Kauver ANB, Geronemus RG. Histology of high-energy pulsed CO_2 laser resurfacing. *Semin Cutanes Med and Surg.* 1996; 15:1–6.

30. Haina DH, Landthaler M, Braun-Falco O, Waidelich W. Comparison of the maximum coagulation depth in human skin for different types of medical lasers. *Lasers Surg Med.* 1987; 7:355–362.

31. Trelles MA, David LM, Rigau J. Penetration depth of ultrapulse carbon dioxide laser in human skin. *Dermatol Surg.* 1996; 22:863–865.

32. Cotton J, Hood AF, Gonin R, Beeson WH, Hanke W. Histologic evaluation of preauricular and postauricular human skin after high-energy, short pulse carbon dioxide laser. *Arch Dermatol.* 1996; 132:425–428.

33. Fitzpatrick RE, Ruiz-Esparza J, Goldman MP. The depth of thermal necrosis using the CO_2 laser: A comparison of the superpulsed mode and conventional mode. *J Dermatol Surg Oncol.* 1991; 17:340–344.

34. Kauvar ANB, Bernstein LJ, Grossman MC, Geronemus RG. Tissue effects of computerized scanners for char-free CO_2 lasers. *Lasers Surg Med.* 1996; 16(suppl 8):34.

35. Kauvar AN, Geronemus RG, Waldorf HA. Char free tissue ablation: A comparative histopathological analysis of new carbon dioxide laser systems. *Lasers Surg Med.* 1995; 16(suppl 7):50.

36. Zachariea H. Delayed wound healing and Keloid formation following argon laser treatment or dermabrasion during isotretinoin treatment. *Br J Dermatol.* 1988; 118:703–706.

37. Rubenstein R, Roenigk HH, Stegman S, Hanke CW. Atypical keloids after dermabrasion of patients taking isotretinoin. J Am Acad Dermatol. 1986; 15:280–285.

38. Bernstein L, Geronemus RG. Keloid formation with the 585 nm pulsed dye laser during isotretinoin treatment. Arch Dermatol. 1997; 133:112–113.

39. Bernstein LJ, Kauvar ANB, Grossman MC, Geronemus RG. The short and long term effects of carbon dioxide laser resurfacing. Dermatol Surg. 1997; 23:519–525.

40. Haedersdal M, Poulsen T, Wulf HC. Laser induced wounds and scarring modified by antiinflammatory drugs: A murine model. Lasers Surg Med. 1993; 13:55–61.

41. Goldman MP. Pre- and Postoperative care of the laser resurfacing patient. Int J Aesth Restorative Surg. 1997; 5:46–49.

42. Lowe NJ, Lask G, Griffin ME. Laser skin resurfacing: Pre- and posttreatemnt guidelines. Dermatol Surg. 1995; 21:1017–1019.

43. Swinyard EA, Pathak MA. Surface acting drugs: demelanizing agents—hydroquinones. In: Goodman AG, Goodman LS, Rall TW, Murad F, eds. Goodman and Gillman: The Pharmacological Basis of Therapeutics. 7th ed. New York: MacMillan Publishing Co.; 1985:954–955.

44. Mandy SH. Tretinoin in the preoperative and postoperative management of dermabrasion. J Am Acad Dermatol. 1986; 15:878–879.

45. Waldorf H, Kauvar AN, Geronemus RG, Leffell D. Remote fire with the pulsed dye laser: Risks and prevention. J Am Acad Dermatol. 1996; 34:503–505.

46. Ho C, Nguyen Q, Lowe NJ, Griffin ME, Lask G. Laser resurfacing in pigmented skin. Dermatol Surg. 1995; 21:1035–1037.

47. Sriprachya-Anunt S, Fitzpatrick RE, Goldman MP, Smith SR. Infections complicating pulsed carbon dioxide laser resurfacing for photoaged facial skin. Dermatol Surg. 1997; 23:527–536.

48. Fisher AA. Lasers and allergic contact dermatitis to topical antibiotics, with particular reference to Bacitracin. Cutis. 252–254.

49. Kilmer SL. Laser resurfacing complications: How to treat them and how to avoid them. Int J Aesth Restorative Surg. 1997; 5:41–45.

50. Alster T, West T. Resurfacing of atrophic scars with a high-energy, pulsed carbon dioxide laser. Dermatol Surg. 1996; 22:151–155.

51. Don PC, Carney PS, Lynch WS, Zaim MT, Hassan MO. Carbon dioxide laserbrasion: A new approach to management of familial benign chronic pemphigus (Hailey-Hailey disease). J Dermatol Surg Oncol. 1987; 13:1187–1194.

52. Lanigan SW, Sheehan-Dare RA, Cotterill JA. The treatment of decorative tattoos with the carbon dioxide laser. Br J Dermatol. 1989; 120:819–825.

53. Magid M, Garden JM. Pearly penile papules: Treatment with the carbon dioxide laser. J Dermatol Surg Oncol. 1989; 15:552–554.

54. Ruiz-Esparza J, Goldman MP, Fitzpatrick RE. Tattoo removal with minimal scarring: The chemo-laser technique. J Dermatol Surg Oncol. 1988; 14:1372–1376.

55. Baldwin HE, Geronemus RG. The treatment of Zoon's balanitis with the carbon dioxide laser. J Dermatol Surg Oncol. 1989; 15:491–494.

56. Fitzpatrick RE, Goldman MP, Ruiz-Esparza J. Clinical advantages of the CO_2 laser superpulsed mode: Treatment of verruca vulgaris, seborrheic keratoses, lentigines and actinic cheilitis. J Dermatol Surg Oncol. 1994; 20:449–456.

57. Landthaler M, Haina D, Brunner R, Waidelich W, Braun-Falco O. Laser therapy of Bowenoid papulosis and Bowen's disease. J Dermatol Surg Oncol. 1986; 12:1253–1257.

58. Stack Jr BC, Hall PJ, Goodman AL, Perez IR. CO_2 laser excision of lupus pernio of the face. Am J Otolaryngol. 1996; 17:260–263.

59. Sunde D, Apfelberg DB, Sergott T. Traumatic tattoo removal: Comparison of four treatment methods in an animal model with correlation to clinical experience. Lasers Surg Med. 1990; 10:158–164.

60. Geronemus RG. Laser surgery of the nail unit. J Dermatol Surg Oncol. 1992; 18:735–743.

61. Boixeda P, Sanchez-Miralles E, Azana RM, Arrazola JM, Moreno R, Ledo A. CO_2, argon, and pulsed dye laser treatment of angiofibromas. J Dermatol Surg Oncol. 1994; 20:808–812.

62. Wheeland RG, Bailin PL, Kantor GR. Treatment of adenoma sebaceum with carbon dioxide laser vaporization. J Dermatol Surg Oncol. 1985; 11:861–864.

63. Apfelberg DB, Maser MR, Lash H, White DN. Treatment of xanthalasma palpebrum with the carbon dioxide laser. J Dermatol Surg Oncol. 1987; 13:149–151.

64. Apfelberg DB, Maser MR, Lash H. Superpulse CO_2 laser treatment of facial syringomata. Lasers Surg Med. 1987; 7:533–537.

65. Ratz JL, Bailin PL, Wheeland RG. Carbon dioxide laser treatment of epidermal nevi. J Dermatol Surg Oncol. 1986; 12:567–570.

66. Robinson JK. Actinic cheilitis: A prospective study comparing four treatment methods. Arch Otolaryngol Head Neck Surg. 1989; 115:848–852.

67. Whitaker DC. Microscopically proven cure of actinic cheilitis by CO_2 laser. Lasers Surg Med. 1987; 7:520–523.

68. Wheeland RG, Bailin PL, Ratz JL. Combined carbon dioxide laser excision and vaporization in the treatment of rhinophyma. J Dermatol Surg Oncol. 1987; 13:172–177.

69. Bernstein LJ, Kauvar ANB, Grossman MC, Geronemus RG. Scar resurfacing with high-energy, short pulsed and flash-scanning carbon dioxide lasers. Dermatol Surg. 1998, in press.

70. Ho C, Nguyen Q, Lask G, Lowe N. Mini-slit graft hair transplantation using the ultrapulse carbon dioxide laser handpiece. Dermatol Surg. 1995; 21:1056–1059.

71. Ungar WP, David LM. Laser hair transplantation. J Dermatol Surg Oncol. 1994; 20:515–521.

72. Ungar WP. Laser hair transplantation II. Dermatol Surg. 1995; 21:759–765.

73. Ungar WP. Laser hair transplantation III. *Dermatol Surg.* 1995; 21:1047–1055.

74. Fitzpatrick RE. Laser hair transplantation: Tissue effects of laser parameters. *Dermatol Surg.* 1995; 21:1042–1046.

75. Kaufmann R, Hibst R. Pulsed erbium:YAG laser ablation in cutaneous surgery. *Lasers Surg Med.* 1996; 19:324–330.

76. Hohenleutner U, Hohenleutner S, Baumler W, Landthaler M. Fast and effective ablation with an Er:YAG laser: Determination of ablation rates and thermal damage zones. *Lasers Surg Med.* 1997; 20:242–247.

77. Walsh JT, Deutsch TF. Er:YAG laser ablation of tissue: Measurement of ablation rates. *Lasers Surg Med.* 1989; 9:327–337.

78. Kaufmann R, Hartmann A, Hibst R. Cutting and skin-ablative properties of pulsed mid-infrared laser surgery. *J Dermatol Surg Oncol.* 1994; 20:112–118.

79. Kaufmann R, Hibst R. Pulsed 2.94um erbium-YAG laser skin ablation: Experimental results and first clinical application. *Clin Exp Dermatol.* 1990; 15:389–393.

80. Walsh JT, Cummings JP. Effect of the dynamic optical properties of water on midinfrared laser ablation. *Lasers Surg Med.* 1994; 15:295–305.

81. Ziering CL. Cutaneous laser resurfacing with the erbium YAG laser and the char-free carbon dioxide laser: A clinical comparison of 100 patients. *Int J Aesth Restorative Surg.* 1997; 5:29–37.

82. Lask G, Lee PK, Seyfzadeh M, et al. Nonablative laser treatment of facial rhytides.

Otoplasty

Two authors who have extensive experience with this aesthetic surgical technique have contributed this section on otoplasty. Dr. Farrior, a facial plastic surgeon, has been writing about otoplasty since 1959. Dr. Ordon, a plastic surgeon, has contributed extensively to the literature.

Both authors review the embryology and anatomy of the preoperative otoplasty patient. Dr. Farrior stresses a progressive or advanced technique as the degree of auricular anomaly progresses. He has provided detailed and elaborate illustrations that demonstrate his surgical techniques. Great care and review of these illustrations are required to glean understanding of his specific techniques. The effort of reviewing the illustrations will be worth the time in that a superior otoplasty result will ultimately be produced.

Dr. Ordon emphasizes careful diagnosis and patient selection and notes specific aesthetic goals be established to produce a superior result. Dr. Ordon uses a composite technique, which is a compilation of current techniques in the literature that he describes in detail. Both authors emphasize the use of the simplest procedure to obtain the maximal effect, and both stress cartilage-sparing techniques and only excise cartilage in the rarest of cases.

The plethora of information provided in these chapters is such that the reader will find them a key to excellence in otoplasty.

Otoplasty

Aesthetic Facial Plastic Surgery, edited by Thomas Romo, III, and Arthur L. Millman, Thieme Medical Publishers, Inc., New York, New York, Copyright © 2000.

CHAPTER 24

A Facial Plastic Surgeon's Perspective

RICHARD T. FARRIOR

The correction of the protruding ear is a relatively simple surgical technique that produces satisfying results and uniformly gratified patients.

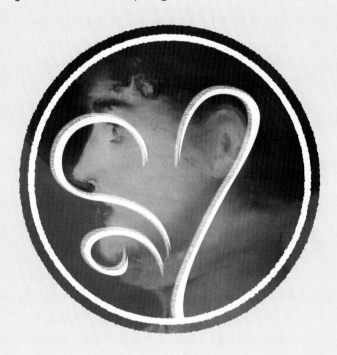

EMBRYOLOGY

The embryology of the auricle for an external structure is actually quite complex considering that it usually creates an auricle that has near uniform structural characteristics. This phenomenon is emphasized by the fact that the follicles or hillocks arise on either side of the mandibular (first branchial) and hyoid (second branchial) arches and are usually seven or eight in number with epithelial valleys between each one. Nearly 85% of the external ear forms from the hyoid arch and only two of the hillocks are from the caudal border of the first branchial or mandibular arch (Fig. 24–1). In the embryo the primordia of the auricle is discernible during the sixth week.

ANATOMY

The anatomy of the auricle is complex, but in reality we are addressing simply the contour of the cartilage, which requires sculpturing and artistic judgment but no interference with the complex anatomy.[1] The contour is detailed in Figure 24–2.

Without further review of the anatomy, embryology, or historical review of the types of otoplasties that are performed, suffice it to say that the most common pathologic anatomy of the protruding ear is incomplete development or contouring of the antihelix. The angle between the outer rim of the concha and the antihelix is inadequate. In the normal ear the angle across the antihelix, scaphoid fossa, and helical rim is approximately 90 degrees with the conchal rim (Fig. 24–3). To reconstruct the antihelix, incisions in the auricular cartilage are not only acceptable but sometimes essential. When incisions, partial or through the thickness of the cartilage, and excision of cartilage are used, the incisions must be precisely placed. The surgeon must know the anatomy of the external ear and the subtleties of the contour in the lateral and oblique view (Figs. 24–2 and 3; see also Fig. 24–11).

Valid objections exist to making incisions in the cartilage, but these usually are related to improper placement and poor execution. With due precision it is frequently helpful both to have weakened and broken the spring of the resilient cartilage. Certainly for the surgeon trained in the principles of aesthetics, not to mention microsurgical techniques, the correct positioning of the incisions should create no problems in this simple and gratifying procedure.

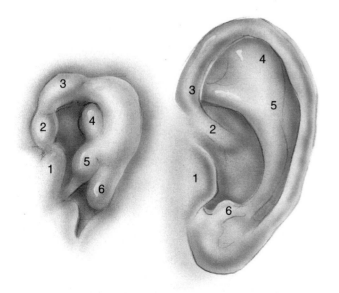

Figure 24–1. Embryology. Development of the ear from the first branchial (mandibular) arch and the second branchial (hyoid) arch. See text.

SURGICAL PRINCIPLES

Since 1956, the year I developed an original technique to overcome some of the shortcomings of procedures done at that time, modifications to the technique have been made regularly and newer techniques developed when appropriate.[2] A progressing or advancing technique has been used for many years, which is considered in patient evaluation and for surgical planning. The minimal procedure required for correcting a particular defect, taking into consideration the abnormal anatomy involved, is the one described below. It may extend from a simple suture creation of the antihelix to an extension of my technique. In most cases I consider the antihelix in my approach to the defect. For example, a favorable combination for the young ear with pliable cartilage is the

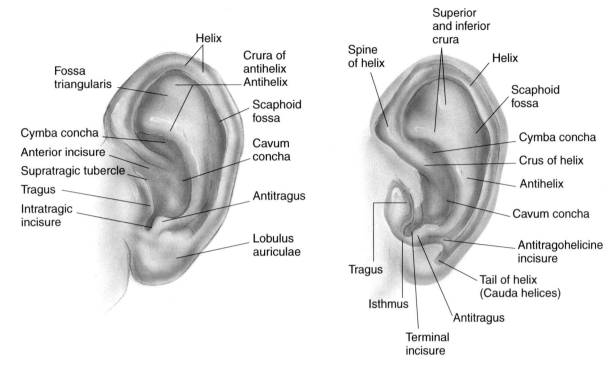

Figure 24–2. Anatomy. Contours of the auricle as seen on the lateral view. Lateral and oblique photography are recommended for critical evaluation of surgical results. Emphasis is placed on the "level of the junction of the crura" (anterior and inferior) with the anti-helix proper (about the concha). There is blending of the crura without angulations across the inferior crus at the junction, the gradual convexity of the superior crus, and the acute convexity of the antihelix proper inferior to the junction of the crura; the distinct scaphoid fossa, which becomes more shallow as it extends superiorly, blends with the superior crus. The superior crus also blends gradually with the fossa triangularis anteriorly. The cavum conchae is cupped to varying degrees. The cauda helices may be thick and resilient, contributing to the protrusion of the lower portion of the ear and lobule. The inferior crus is sharply angled and may create a stiff post or pillar effect that influences protrusion. In reconstruction the new antihelix should not be so prominent as to hide the helical rim.

simple suture technique combined with both conchal and fossa triangularis setback procedures.[3–5]

Beyond this approach some form of partial or through-and-through incision procedure is advocated. This progressing technique is addressed in some detail in the references 6 to 11 (see also Fig. 24–7).

CHOICE OF PROCEDURE

Any otoplasty technique should be kept in perspective and the technique selected only after careful analysis of the abnormal anatomy of the individual ear. When assessing the ear, the surgeon must consider the degree of prominence, the resilience or stiffness of the auricular cartilage, and the existing or nonexisting contour of the cartilage, including the prominence of the antihelix and depth of the conchal cavity. Procedures that have

been developed through the years often can be combined or incorporated into the time-tested technique that is described below. The technique considers all anatomic components and has produced uniformly satisfactory results over a 40-year span. The originally described technique continues to be modified, refined, and improved, and so it remains a contemporary operation.

Particular attention must be given to the *degree* of development and contour of the antihelix, the depth and cupping of the conchal cavity, and, to a lesser degree, the development of the scaphoid fossa. The stiffness or pillar effect of the inferior crus and its angulation from the side of the head may be contributing to the prominence.

In essence, the operation combines weakening the cartilage spring, reducing the cupped concha, and reinforcing the new contour with permanent sutures in the cartilage (suture technique). Both partial and complete

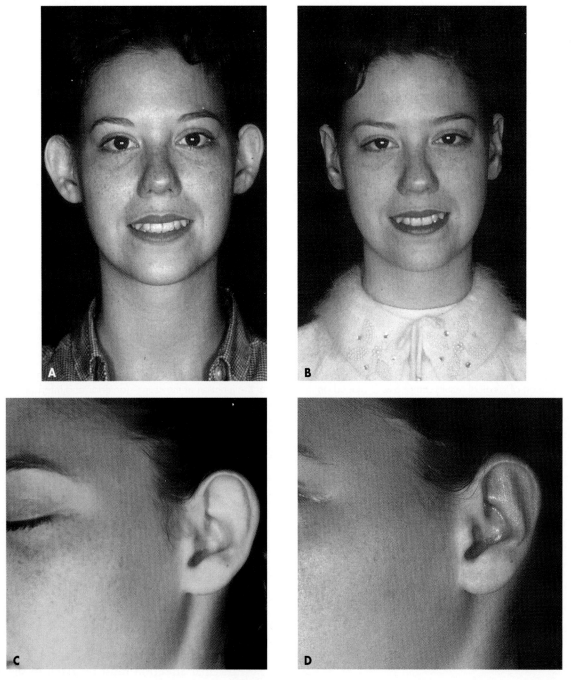

Figure 24–3. (A, C) Preoperative photographs and **(B, D)** Postoperative results in a patient who underwent the original technique. For the suturing in this technique horizontal mattress sutures were used from the scaphoid to the concha not picking up the rim of the new antihelix, which then overrode the two fossa margins. This is satisfactory for the less resilient cartilage. More control is obtained by the vertical mattress suture, picking up all four cartilage margins as described in the text and seen in Figures 24–4, 24–7, and 24–8. See also Figure 24–11.

incisions are made through the cartilage. Important to the success of the operation is the surgeon's anatomic and artistic judgment of the *degree* to which each of the three above-mentioned elements is addressed for the particular ear. These elements determine how the procedure is to be

modified, simplified, or extended; thus a progressing method is used and a rigid single technique is not used. By learning in detail the contributing factors for a particular ear the surgeon is prepared to manage the differences that occur from ear to ear. The basic procedure may be combined with reduction otoplasty, the cupped (constricted) ear, conchal setback, or the simple suture technique. The continuous longitudinal wedges may be substituted by beveled incomplete incisions that allow the partially folded cartilage to override, thus weakening the spring of the cartilage and with sutures maintaining the new contour.

It is important that the antihelix and, therefore, the conchal rim and crura be precisely outlined. The Mersilene (braided Dacron sutures) creates and maintains contour and favorable reduction of the antihelix toward the reduced concha (Fig. 24–4, p. 432).

Most techniques are directed at correcting the basic anomaly, which is underdevelopment or inadequate angulation or curvature of the antihelix. Other techniques attempt to camouflage the anomaly, as with setback procedures that do not address the antihelix. In most protruding ears the objective should be to reconstruct the antihelix with proper contour and width.

A number of techniques provide satisfactory results for correcting the protrusion. The technique chosen should be determined by the anatomic variables for the particular ear, and results should be evaluated over several years using critical criteria to assess the contour of the ear as seen from the side and obliquely (Fig. 24–3; see also Fig. 24–11). The degree of satisfaction varies with different patients and surgeons. Therefore, the surgeon should examine the ear critically and select a technique, that is appropriate, taking care to pay attention to details in preoperative analysis, technical precision at surgery, and proper evaluation after surgery.

PATIENT SELECTION AND TIMING OF SURGERY

For the common protruding ear, patient selection is not a major problem. The prominence of the ear is apparent, certainly to the parents and often even to the young patient. The older the child gets, and perhaps as the child becomes the subject of some jests, even from family and friends, the more he becomes conscious of his ears. It is preferable that the child desires the operation as much as the parents. Ideally, the surgery should be performed at about age 5 years, before the child enters "regular school" and after major growth of the auricle has occurred.

Although the *adult* and his or her family may have adjusted to the prominence, most adult patients who present to the surgeon do not like their ears. Awareness of the prominence usually is compounded if the person is in a business that requires interaction with clients. When these older patients seek surgery, the motivation and goals are usually realistic.

The psychiatric aspect of this simple deformity can be severe. Some patients have a very poor self-image, whereas others insist on having a particular hairstyle. Rather than *adjusting* to the deformity, the anomaly can be simply corrected and permanently shed.

Of course, photography, preoperative analysis, and documentation are essential and should be used for instructing patients and for familiarizing them with the goals of the surgery.

INTRAOPERATIVE TECHNIQUE
AURICULAR CONTOUR

The surgeon should strive to create a normal auricular contour, constructing a new antihelix to provide a gradual convexity for the superior crus, which blends gradually with the shallowing superior scaphoid fossa posteriorly and the fossa triangularis anteriorly (Figs. 24–2 and 3; see also Fig. 24–11). Inferiorly, at the level of the antihelix proper, the convexity is more acute, creating a deep scaphoid fossa between the new antihelix and the helix. There should be a blend of the superior and inferior crus at the level of the junction of the crura and the antihelix proper; no incision lines or angulations should extend across this junction, for example, from the anterior border of the superior crus to the conchal rim at the anterior border of the antihelix. Most protruding ears have a deep concha that must be reduced. Occasionally a pillar effect is present from the inferior crus that protrudes with

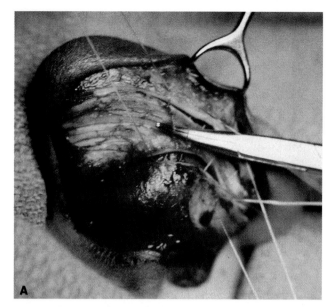
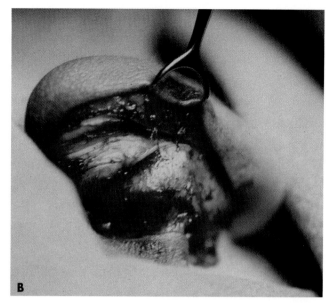

Figure 24–4. Left ear, posterior surface. **(A)** Demonstrating the position of the vertical mattress sutures starting inferiorly. All sutures are placed first then tying is done from inferior to superior, observing the contour on the anterior surface as each suture is secured. With the vertical mattress suture less tendency exists for flattening of the antihelix proper. **(B)** Braided Dacron (Mersilene) sutures have been tied. By having no incision through the cartilage about the superior crus and no sutures above the level of the junction of the crura, the desired gradual convexity of the superior crus blending with the fossa triangularis anterior and the shallowing scaphoid fossa superiorly is obtained. The tunneling, or dead space, has not created a problem.

resistance straight out from the head. When this post exists, it must be broken (see Fig. 24–9). A normal auriculomastoid sulcus should be maintained.

General techniques for otoplasty include (1) suture only, (2) weakening the cartilage spring, (3) breaking the cartilage spring, (4) conchal reduction, (5) conchal setback, and (6) combinations of any of the above.

The cartilage spring may be weakened by (1) wire brush dermabrasion, (2) longitudinal beveled partial incision (Fig. 24–5A; see also Fig. 24–7), (3) longitudinal parallel wedge excisions (Fig. 24–5B; see also Fig. 24–7), (4) cartilage shave, (5) fish scale incision (shingle overriding technique), or (6) scoring of the anterior surface. The last technique may leave irregularities that can be seen through the thin skin on the anterior surface of the auricle. This technique, with incisions in the antihelix on the anterior surface, has not been favored by me, especially for the heavier adult cartilage (Figs. 24–5B and 24–6). Our goal is to weaken

the spring from the posterior surface of the cartilage without these incisions on the anterior surface.

When incisions are made through the cartilage, to break the elastic cartilage spring one must know the detailed anatomy of the external ear, the incision must be precisely placed, and the maneuvers precisely performed.

The author advocates a progressing or advancing surgical technique designed to approach the anatomic deficiency of the individual ear (Fig. 24–7). The surgery is individualized with no more being done than is necessary for the particular correction. In young children, who have more pliable cartilage, fair development of the helix-antihelix relationship and not too deep a concha, a simple suture technique (Fig. 24–7), or a combination of the simple suture technique and conchal setback (concha-mastoid sutures) are the best options. The author also uses setback sutures for the fossa triangularis, as well as the concha. The suture technique is not satisfactory if

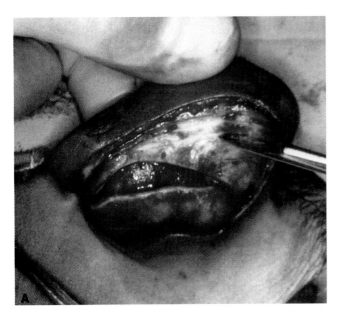
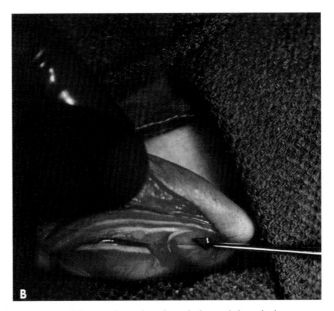

Figure 24–5. Left ear, posterior surface. **(A)** Weakening the cartilage spring of the newly outlined antihelix with beveled incisions extending only part way through the cartilage. The anterior perichondrium is preserved. **(B)** Heavier adult cartilage, as in the patient in Figure 24–6. Incisions through the cartilage paralleling the scaphoid fossa to the level of the junction of the crura and about the reduced concha. The cartilage is weakened by removing longitudinal cartilage wedges, being accomplished here with the Farrior cartilage knife. Again, the wedges extend only partially through the cartilage. There are no incisions through the cartilage for the superior crus. The wedges preserve the normal resilience of the intervening cartilage and are closed when the sutures are secured. This is accomplished on the posterior surface with no weakening incisions on the anterior surface of the cartilage with the thin anterior auricular skin.

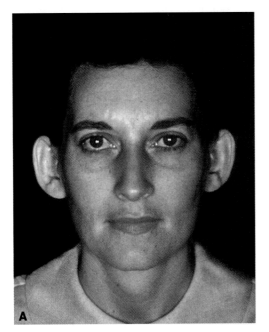
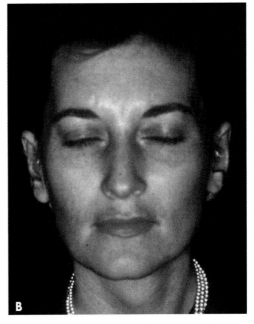

Figure 24–6. Adult patient with thicker cartilage and more resistance to contouring as in Figure 24–5-B. The simple suture technique will not get a satisfactory result in such a case. **(A)** Preoperative. **(B)** Postoperative.

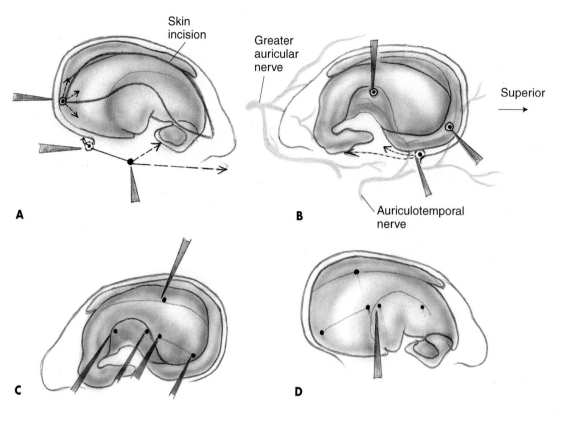

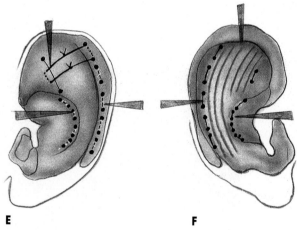

Figure 24–7. Artist rendition of the details of surgery (including modifications and extensions). In E to O, the ear is shown upright to assist in anatomic interpretation. On the operating table, the ear would be horizontal as in A to D. **(A)** Injection sites from the *posterior* aspect of the ear. Injection is made midway in the auriculomastoid sulcus (*right pointer*) and carried immediately to block the main nerve supply from the great auricular nerve. The ear canal is ballooned out from posterior, and injection is extended superiorly to make a wheal from which the injection, along the anterior border of the auricle, is made when the ear is turned over (*middle pointer*). Infiltration from this single injection site is then carried onto the posterior surface of the ear as much as possible. The left pointer indicates the injection at the superior extent of the incision. The skin incision is an elliptical dumbbell, slightly wider at either end and usually, at its widest point, is no more than 1.0 cm. **(B)** Injection sites as seen from the anterior surface. The left pointer indicates the posterior injection extending to the ear canal. *Right pointer,* The injection at the superior extent of the antihelix. *Center pointer,* The wheal made at the top of the ear for extension along the anterior border to block the auriculotemporal nerve. **(C)** Anterior view, The pointers indicate the anatomic landmarks for inserting the Keith or straight cutting needles, marking the anterior border of the antihelix and the rim of the concha. There is a jump across the inferior crus. The outer pointer (*above*) is an optional needle to outline the width of the antihelix and the level of the junction of the crura as seen on the posterior surface **(D)**. The cartilage is scored slightly with the knife. The needles serve as a guide outlining the proposed new antihelix. The procedure, through outlining the new antihelix, is the same whatever technique is to be used. **(E)** (*Posterior surface*), The simple suture technique using horizontal mattress sutures that fan out from a central hub and most often include a suture about the superior crus. This is the posterior view as seen from behind. Top pointer indicates horizontal suture in cartilage at anterior border of the new antihelix at fossa triangularis and passed across the superior crus to the outer margin of the antihelix. The other pointers mark the conchal rim to scaphoid fossa sutures. **(F)** Anterior view, showing the placement for anatomic orientation of the mattress sutures, in this case combining any one of several techniques for weakening the spring. *Top pointer,* I usually use longitudinal beveled incisions, which, with contouring, can overlap, or longitudinal cartilage wedge resections from the posterior surface. *(Continued on p. 435.)*

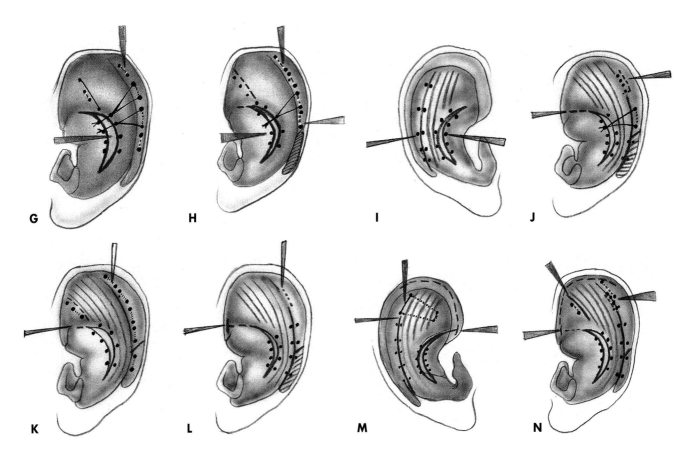

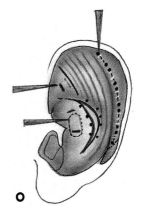

Figure 24–7. *(Continued from p. 434.)* **(G)** The addition of conchal reduction *(left pointer)*. This uses the combined horizontal-vertical mattress sutures with horizontal mattress sutures being placed on the outer aspect of the antihelix *(top pointer)* and vertical mattress sutures to pick up the anterior border of the antihelix and the reduced concha *(indicated by dots)*. This effectively brings the new antihelix down to the conchal margin. **(H)** The horizontal-vertical *(left pointer)* mattress suture with conchal reduction has been extended to include removal or thinning of the cauda helices *(right pointer)* and extension or deepening of the incisions along the anterior border of the superior crus and further into the inferior crus. *Top pointer*, Horizontal mattress suture, outer aspect of superior crus. **(I)** This is my technique as seen from the anterior surface. The technique incorporates weakening of the cartilage spring, usually with removal of longitudinal continuous parallel wedges as depicted with the blue lines, vertical mattress sutures indicated by the pointers and as dots, conchal reduction, and further breaking of the cartilage spring by an incision along the scaphoid fossa from inferiorly to the level of the junction of the crura. **(J)** My technique, viewed posteriorly, is extended by further extending the incision through the cartilage along the scaphoid fossa *(right pointer)* and into the inferior crus *(left pointer)*. **(K)** Further extension is made by incorporating a horizontal mattress suture around the superior crus *(top pointer)* and (deepening the incision at the anterior border of the superior crus *[dotted line]*). The lower pointer shows extension into the inferior crus. The cauda helices is removed or thinned without removal, allowing the placement of horizontal mattress sutures. This particular technique uses the combined horizontal-vertical mattress suture *(dots on either side of the conchal reduction)*. **(L)** Further extension superiorly along the scaphoid fossa and outer rim of the superior crus with sectioning of the cartilage to break the spring for the pillar effect. **(M)** Extension of the technique as seen on the anterior surface with the work being done on the posterior surface. The pillar effect of the inferior crus is broken *(right pointer)* and incision through the cartilage is carried over the entire superior extent of the ear. The outer antihelix incision is extended superiorly *(left pointer)*, and a horizontal mattress suture is used around the superior crus *(top pointer)*. **(N)** Further extension as seen from the posterior aspect of the ear, including a deeper incision along the anterior border of the superior crus *(top left pointer)*. *Left pointer*, Breaking at anterior extent of inferior crus. *Right pointer*, Breaking spring of outer rim of antihelix to higher level *(dots)*. **(O)** Conchal setback sutures may be combined with breaking or weakening of the cartilage spring. The setback sutures are placed in the fossa triangularis, the cimba conchae, and the cavum conchae *(left pointers)*. About the superior crus a horizontal mattress suture *(top pointer)* is combined with further weakening of the anterior border.

the concha is too deep or if in reducing the concha with placement of the sutures only the antihelix is made abnormally wide. The *conchal setback* disturbs too much soft tissue over the mastoid away from the ear, alters the opening of the ear canal, and may reduce too much the auriculomastoid sulcus.

At the other extreme of the spectrum is the adult whose cartilage is more firm and who therefore may require fracture of the cartilage spring, reduction of the concha, removal of the cauda helicis, or even extension of the technique around the superior aspect of the ear (Figs. 24–5B, and 24–6; see also Fig. 24–9). In a systematically progressive approach the following steps should be considered: (1) skin incision and excision, (2) outlining the new antihelix with small Keith needles only, (3) conchal setback, (4) simple suture, horizontal mattress, (5) simple suture with weakening of spring, (6) simple suture with reduction of concha (combined horizontal-vertical mattress sutures), (7) simple suture and combined conchal setback, and (8) Farrior technique with vertical mattress sutures combining weakening the spring, breaking the spring, conchal reduction, suture technique, and modifications for cupped or constricted ear.

When the cartilage spring is weakened, either longitudinal wedges are excised that parallel the curvature of the new antihelix or partial beveled incisions are made to allow the cartilage to fold backward by overriding (Fig. 24–5A). The latter incisions are also longitudinal, following the axis of the antihelix (Fig. 24–7E, I). This method of weakening the spring might be the first progression from the simple suture technique (Fig. 24–7F). The next step would entail incisions and the removal of a crescent of cartilage from the conchal rim (along the anterior border of the antihelix) both to break the cartilage spring and to reduce the deeply cupped concha (Fig. 24–7G).

From this point the original technique—weakening the cartilage spring, breaking the cartilage spring, reduc-

ing the concha, and using sutures to stabilize and ensure proper contour and angulation—may be indicated (Figs. 24–4, 24–5B, 24–6 to 24–8).

In general, further extension of the technique addresses the resistant upper fourth to third of the auricle. Incisions made through or deeper into the cartilage may be extended higher on the anterior and posterior borders of the superior crus, into the inferior crus, or over the entire dome of the ear hidden beneath the helix (Fig. 24–7H, M-N and Fig. 24–9). Horizontal mattress sutures on either side of the superior crus, which are not ordinarily used in the standard technique, may be required (Fig. 24–7 K-N and O).

Longitudinal beveled cuts are an increasingly frequent expedient (Fig. 24–5A). These partial incisions retain the resilience of the cartilage but allow contouring. The incisions extend continuously over the full length of the antihelix on the same principle as the fish scale or overlapping shingle technique. Therefore less irregularity occurs with this incision than with the other less precise methods. As with the longitudinal beveled wedges, the outer two incisions extend the full length of the antihelix (Fig. 24–7 F-O). The remainder jump the area of the junction of the inferior crus and the antihelix proper and provide contouring of the superior crus, where no incisions are made through the thickness of the cartilage, effecting the desired gradual convexity of the superior crus, which blends smoothly with the fossa triangularis and the shallowing scaphoid fossa posteriorly. Ordinarily, no sutures are placed on either side of the newly formed superior crus (Figs. 24–4 and 24–7I, J, and L).

When the wedges are removed after the same contour, several purposes are served: the spring is weakened, resilience and thickness of the cartilage are maintained, the intervening space allows molding but is closed when the sutures are applied, and a convexity is created on the anterior surface. The normal contour is followed and visible incisions on the anterior surface of the cartilage are

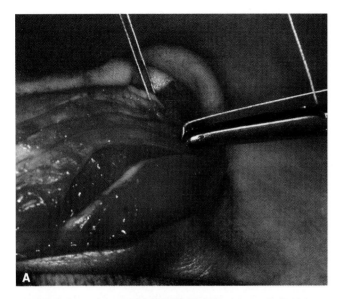

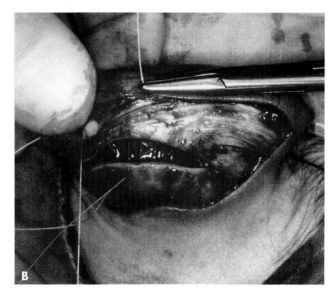

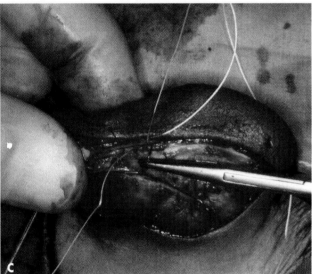

Figure 24–8. Details of suture placement. The suture is 4-0 braided Dacron on a full half-curved cutting needle. **(A)** The reduced and thinned remaining cauda helices is used for the first (*inferior*) suture passing to the outer margin of the antihelix then to the anterior border of the antihelix and then to the conchal rim. The tip of the needle is just seen passing through the reduced conchal cartilage margin. **(B)** and **(C)**. Opposite ear (left) picking up the scaphoid margin and walking the suture to the outer margin of the new antihelix. These demonstrate the partial incisions and the incisions through the cartilage so as to accentuate the scaphoid fossa and effectively reduce the antihelix to the now less-cupped concha.

avoided, leaving the anterior perichondrium intact (Figs. 24–3, 24–6; see also Fig. 24–11).

The precisely placed incisions around the concha and paralleling the scaphoid fossa are hidden by the overriding new antihelix and follow a normal shadow line. Where the crescent of cartilage is removed from the conchal rim, immediately anterior to the newly formed antihelix, the redundant skin further masks the incisions through the cartilage (see Fig. 24–11).

The cauda helicis may be removed or thinned as indicated for the lower portion of the ear or as the cauda helicis influences the lobule. If left thick, it disturbs the contour of the inferior extent of the new antihelix. Often partial excision is carried out with thinning so that a portion of the cauda helicis remains for placement of the inferior outer vertical mattress suture. For the soft tissue portion of the lobule additional excision of skin may be required.

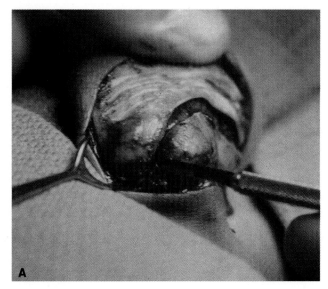 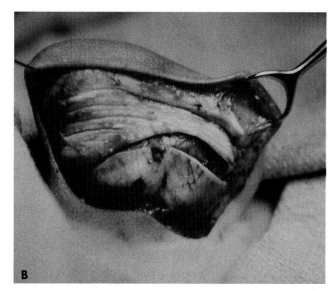

Figure 24–9. Extending the technique. **(A)** The incision is extended the full length of the inferior crus, and the spring at the anterior extent of the crus is broken to correct the pillar effect the inferior crus may have. The incision is then carried over the superior dome of the ear for the resistant upper third. This incision parallels the helix. **(B)** The above incisions have been accomplished. Note the cartilage spring has been broken to the level of the junction of the crura, the pillar effect of the inferior crus has been negated, the cartilage of the new antihelix has been weakened, and the cauda has been shortened. A thick cauda such as this will also be thinned but allowed to remain to receive the first vertical mattress suture. The deeply cupped concha has been reduced. In the resistant upper third of the ear it may be necessary to place a horizontal mattress suture about the superior crus.

For correction of the more complicated constricted or cupped ear and reduction for the large shell ear of macrotia the technique described for reconstruction of the antihelix and reduction of the cupped concha can be incorporated.

Summary of Surgical Technique

Our technique for positioning, anesthesia, excision of the skin off the posterior surface of the auricle, and outlining the new antihelix is the same in each procedure (Fig. 24–7A, B, C and D).

1. A minimal amount of skin is excised on the posterior aspect of the auricle immediately posterior to the antihelix. The auriculomastoid angle is preserved (Fig. 24–7A).
2. Small straight Keith cutting needles are inserted from the anterior surface for the identification of landmarks and outlining the incisions. No dye is used (Fig. 24–7C and D).
3. The cauda helicis is usually removed or reduced and thinned (Fig. 24–7J, K, and L; Fig. 24–8A, B; and Fig. 24–10A, B).
4. A strip of cartilage of variable width is removed around the conchal rim below the anterior aspect of the antihelix proper (Fig. 24–5, 24–8B).
5. Incisions through the full thickness of the cartilage are made only around the conchal rim, sometimes extending slightly into the inferior crus and along the posterior border of the antihelix proper along the scaphoid fossa to the level of the junction of the crura. This superiorly widening cartilage will eventually override the underlying cartilage from the concha and scaphoid fossa to form the prominent new antihelix proper (Figs. 24–4B, 24–7I, 24–8C, and 24–11).

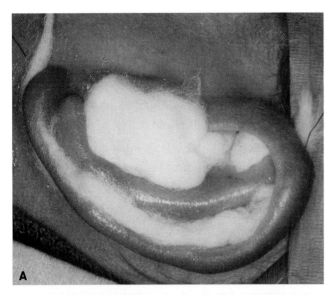

Figure 24–10. Dressing. **(A)** The ear is carefully contoured with cotton moistened with sterile mineral oil, supporting the reconstructed auricle. Another strip of moistened cotton is placed over the posterior incision, which is directly posterior to the new antihelix. **(B)** Kerlix gauze is wrapped around the ear, staying perpendicular to the side of the head. This creates a doughnut round the ear and a fluff over the ear. On the first ear done this final dressing can be held in position for immediate pressure by the head drape. It is unnecessary to compare the ears at the end of surgery because appropriate measurements were made on the first ear to be applied to the second ear. **(C)** A splinting wraparound head dressing is secured with lightly placed adhesive. Two-inch fine gauze mesh with selvedged edges or Kling dressing may be used. This dressing is a secure splint for the reconstructed ear, not a simple mastoid dressing.

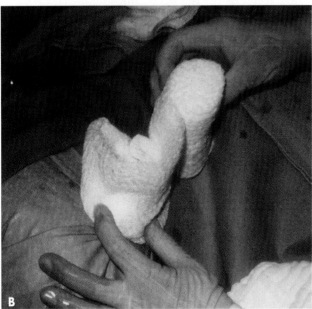

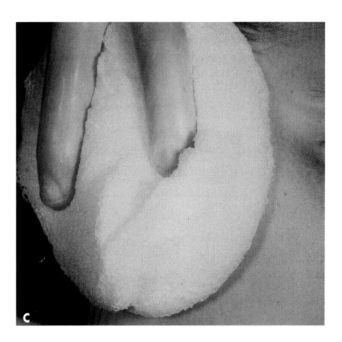

6. No through-and-through incisions of the cartilage are made in the area of the superior crus, and no continuous incision extends from the conchal rim across the junction of the crura to the anterior border of the superior crus. A break is made here to effect a more natural contour and blending of the two crura. Parallel longitudinal cartilage wedges or beveled partial incisions are removed along the entire antihelix (Figs. 24–4 and 24–7F and I-O).

7. In the area of the through-and-through incision, vertical mattress sutures incorporating the margins of both the outer cartilage and the overriding cartilage may be used. This suture incorporates the margin of the scapha, both margins of the new antihelix, and the conchal rim (Figs. 24–4A and B, 24–7I and J, and 24–8). For the cartilage, 4-0 braided Dacron (Mersilene) on atraumatic half-curved needles is used (Fig. 24–8). When the superior cartilage suture is placed, the distance of the

helix from the mastoid is measured (usually approximately 1.5 cm). This measurement is carried to the second ear so no need exists for visual comparison of the two ears, and the first ear can be dressed with pressure as soon as it is completed.

8. The skin is closed with a continuous subcuticular suture of 5-0 monofilament nylon on an atraumatic cutting edge needle. Buried interrupted subcuticular sutures are used at the widest portion of the skin excision.

9. The contour is molded with cotton moistened with mineral oil, and a soft pressure dressing is applied (Fig. 24–10A, B and C).

SIMPLE SUTURING TECHNIQUE

The simple suturing technique has become popular again because of the satisfactory results that it can achieve, particularly in young children with delicate cartilage, provided the normal anatomy is critically analyzed in regard to placement of the sutures. In the simple protruding ear in the young patient without too much cartilage resistance and not too deep a conchal cavity, the simple suturing technique will work.

The simple suturing technique is a procedure with which every surgeon should be familiar. More consistent results can be expected in young children with delicate auricular cartilage. The surgical technique is simple and may be incorporated after some of the steps of the method of otoplasty already described. The outline of the anterior and posterior extent of the new antihelix for the placement of the sutures should be made critically; the surgeon should accurately draw the new antihelix on the posterior surface of the ear before placing the sutures. (see steps 1 and 2 above; Fig. 24–7C, D, E, and F).

Despite its simplicity and excellent results, the *simple suturing* technique does not take into account all factors contributing to the particular deformity. Among these, one would have to consider the pillar effect of the inferior crus that may be encountered. Success depends on the degree of the existing convexity of the antihelix, the degree of the existing concavity of the scaphoid fossa, and the development of the antihelix. The simple suturing technique produces a backward tilting and flattening posterior to the antihelix, which may occur in a flat ear in which no scaphoid fossa and a minimal helical rim exists. The suturing technique does nothing to create the scaphoid fossa. The antihelix may end up being relatively prominent compared with the helix, an undesirable postoperative appearance.

In addition, nothing in the simple suturing technique accounts for the deep cupped conchal cavity in which it is essential to remove some cartilage to reduce the size of the cup. To reduce the concha by placing the suture further into the depth of the cavity creates an antihelix that is too wide. It is interesting that since the revival of the simple suturing technique, many surgeons are now adding modifications and performing more complicated procedures. This is happening in some cases because of improper analysis of the contributing abnormalities.

POSTOPERATIVE CARE

At the end of surgery, the ears are carefully molded with contoured cotton moistened with mineral oil (Fig. 24–10A) and a wraparound head dressing (splint) is applied (Fig. 24–10B and C). An intraoperative bolus of appropriate antibiotics is given and postoperative oral antibiotics are prescribed until the dressing is changed on the fourth postoperative day.

The dressing is changed on the fourth postoperative day, although it may be removed earlier if indicated. The anterior contoured cotton is left in place; the posterior cotton over the incision is removed. Surgical twists are removed and antibiotic ointment is applied over the skin incision. A lighter wraparound splint is applied.

On the seventh postoperative day, the dressing is removed and the incision is cleaned. Polysporin ointment is applied. The patient is instructed to wear a stocking cap at night.

The patient returns 2 weeks postoperatively for removal of continuous subcuticular suture. At four weeks postoperatively, the patient is instructed to discontinue use of the stocking cap. Postoperative visits are scheduled for 6 weeks, 3 months, 6 months, and 1 year after surgery. When possible, longer follow-up is suggested. Postoperative photographs should be obtained at 6 months, 1 year, and long term (Fig. 24–11).

COMPLICATIONS AND SEQUELAE

Over four decades there have been no major complications after this technique, including thorough hemostasis, dressings, and postoperative management. Minor complications have been limited. No hematomas or infections, including chondritis, have occurred. One patient bled significantly into the dressing but not subcutaneously. The source of bleeding was from the skin edge where one margin slightly overlapped the other. In two different patients, a total of three of the permanent sutures required simple removal with no untoward results when they presented through the skin. Fewer than five patients showed hardly appreciable angulation of one of the partial incisions on the anterior surface; the incisions had been carried too deep. This was corrected by limited posterior exposure and diffusion of the angulation by further weakening the spring on either side of the visible angulation. One patient required opening the superior third of the incision for placement of a horizontal mattress suture near the superior crus. This had been inadequately corrected by omitting this suture above the level of the junction of the crura as is usually and preferably done to create more normal contour.

CONCLUSION

The imperativeness of thorough knowledge of the anatomy of the normal external ear and the need to tailor the surgical approach to the abnormal anatomy of each ear cannot be overemphasized. The procedure selected is based on the existing contour and degree of angulation, cupping, or depth of the concha, the development of the antihelix; and the inherent resilience or spring of the auricular cartilage.

The techniques that require incisions in the cartilage were presented in a progressing sequence. For some auricles, incisions through the cartilage are thought to be necessary and, if precisely placed, present no problems. For most ears my original method incorporating updated techniques provides a sound standard approach for the trainee because it considers all the contributing factors for the protrusion, requires knowledge of the anatomy, and, when properly performed, overcomes any shortcomings in analysis of the deformity or artistic judgment of the surgeon. If only one of the large number of operations devised for this simple problem could be used, my basic technique would stand the surgeon in good stead. The procedure described in Figure 24–7 E to O incorporates the basic principles of properly outlining the antihelix, breaking the cartilage spring, weakening the cartilage spring, reducing the deep concha, and maintaining the desired contour with permanent sutures in the cartilage. As first described, the technique has been modified mainly by placing vertical mattress sutures through the cartilage around the antihelix rather than *horizontal* mattress sutures placed only from the scaphoid fossa to the concha and by the more frequent use of partial beveled incisions into the cartilage rather than the removal of the longitudinal wedges.

As the surgeon becomes more skilled in analysis of the abnormalities of the ear and more critical of the postoperative result, he or she may then modify the selection of procedures, using techniques that are more easily

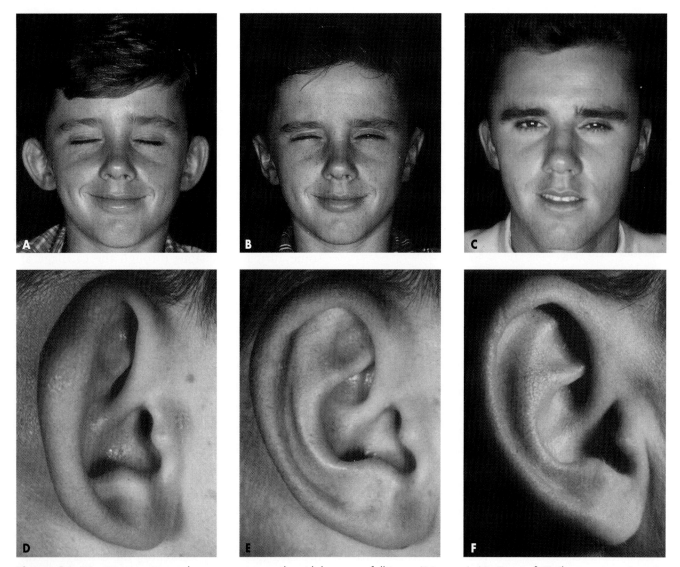

Figure 24–11. Preoperative and postoperative results with long-term follow-up (12 years). **(A, B, and C)** The postoperative pictures in the anterior view demonstrate the normal projection from the head without obliterating the auriculomastoid sulcus. **(D)** In the lateral view the cupping of the concha and loss of angulation of the antihelix with the conchal rim is demonstrated in the preoperative picture. **(E and F)** The two postoperative pictures show proper contouring with blending of the crura into the antihelix proper without incisions across the inferior crus and the definition of the scaphoid fossa and the associated acute convexity of the antihelix proper. There is a gradual convexity of the superior crus blending into the fossa triangularis anterior and the shallowing scaphoid fossa posterior. Compare with Figure 24–2 of the normal anatomy. In neither of the postoperative pictures are incisions visible on the anterior surface, even with the 12-year follow-up **(F)**.

executed or even more advanced than the basic technique for the resistant auricle.

The technique presented herein is not an exhaustive review. The subject is covered in detail in previous publications. The technique described here and advocated over four decades, with modifications, is most commonly used, especially in the teaching setting. It requires the trainee to learn the details of anatomy and to develop

skills for precise placement of the incisions and sutures. The technique takes into account virtually all anatomic variables and pitfalls and will aesthetically correct quite satisfactorily most protruding ears. There will be fewer disappointments if the resident physician or the occasional operator follows the full technique. Although this method has the disadvantage of being slightly more complicated than some techniques, this is offset by the advantage of more consistent results. In addition, the technique is valuable because it teaches the contributing factors and may be modified for particular abnormalities. If the surgeon pays attention to the details and follows the refinements described, a better otoplasty will be done no matter which technique is chosen.

PEARLS

- A thorough knowledge of the anatomy of the ear prepares the surgeon to properly manage otoplasty, no matter which technique is used.
- When selecting a procedure, the surgeon must consider the degree of prominence, the resilience or stiffness of the auricular cartilage, and the existing (or nonexisting) contour of the cartilage, and depth of the concha.
- A simple suture technique or a combination of the simple suture technique and conchal setback are the best options for correction deformities in some young children. The adult usually will require a more complex combination of techniques. See text.
- To obtain the best results, a progressing technique that is designed to approach the anatomic deficiency of a particular patient's ear is advocated.

REFERENCES*

1. Weerda H. Embryology and structural anatomy of the external ear. *Facial Plastic Surgery.* 1985; winter:85–91.
2. Farrior RT. A method of otoplasty. *Arch Otolaryngol.* 1959; 69:400–408.
3. Farrior RT. Otoplasty. Surgery for protruding ears. In: English. *Otolaryngology,* rev. ed. Philadelphia; Harper & Row; 1984.
4. Farrior RT. Surgery for protruding ears (otoplasty). In: Gates G, ed. *Current Therapy in Otolaryngology-Head and Neck Surgery 1984-1985.* Toronto: BC Decker; 1985.
5. Farrior RT. Modified cartilage incisions in otoplasty. *Facial Plastic Surgery.* 1985; winter:109–118.
6. Farrior RT. Contemporary otoplasty. Seventh International Symposium. Facial plastic surgery (panel). Orlando, Florida, 1998.
7. Farrior RT. Modified cartilage incisions for otoplasty. *Symp Otorhinol.* 1986; 21:177–187.
8. Furnas DW. Correction of prominent ears by concha-mastoid sutures. *Plast Reconstr Surg.* 1968; 42:189–193.
9. Mustarde JC. The correction of prominent ears using simple mattress sutures. *Br J Plast Surg.* 1963; 16:170–176.
10. Romo Thomas III. Protruding ears (otoplasty). In: Gates G. *Current Therapy in Otolaryngology–Head and Neck Surgery 1998.* 6th ed. St. Louis: Mosby; 1998.
11. Stambaugh K. Outstanding ears (otoplasty). In: Gates G. *Current Therapy in Otolaryngology–Head and Neck Surgery 1994.* 5th ed. St. Louis: Mosby; 1994.

*Two particular volumes of *Facial Plastic Surgery* are recommended to the reader in their entirety. These are *Facial Plastic Surgery,* Thieme-Stratton, Volume 2, No. 2 Winter, 1985, and *Facial Plastic Surgery,* Thieme Medical Publishers, Inc., NY, Stuttgart, Vol. 10, No. 3, July, 1993.

Otoplasty

CHAPTER 25

A Plastic Surgeon's Perspective

ANDREW PAUL ORDON

Aesthetic Facial Plastic Surgery, edited by Thomas Romo, III, and Arthur L. Millman, Thieme Medical Publishers, Inc., New York, New York, Copyright © 2000.

Otoplasty is aesthetic surgery performed to reshape or form the external ear. The term *otoplasty* most commonly refers to surgery designed to correct the overly prominent pinna or auricle. It also refers to surgery to correct associated deformities, including the constricted ear (lop ear or cup ear), cryptotia (invaginated ear), shell ear, and Stahl's ear. It is a common misconception that the correction of prominent ears is easy. Otoplasty is a complex procedure, requiring careful analysis of the deformity and careful selection of the appropriate treatment plan, and perfect results remain elusive. However, our history of performing several hundreds of these operations suggests that experience, technical knowledge, and ability are all required to obtain consistent and predictably good results.

Congenital prominence of the ear is caused by multiple factors. It may be due to failure of the antihelix to fold correctly, overgrowth of the concha, malposition of the concha with a concha-scapha angle greater than 90 degrees, a prominent tail of the helix, a prominent auricular lobule, and/or varied helical rim deformities, including invagination (cryptotia), shelling, cupping, and lopping (constricted ear deformities). The correction of congenital prominence of the ears has remained a constant topic in plastic surgical literature, with many chapters and articles dedicated to techniques and technical refinements. Unfortunately, most of these techniques have focused solely on correction of the antihelical roll. More recently, aesthetic surgeons have begun to diagnose and treat the concomitant problems of the concha, lobule, and tail of the helix. Surgeons now realize that a variety of operative techniques are needed to address the specific deformities, hence the title "composite otoplasty." The perspective of this plastic surgeon/otolaryngologist dictates a sequential approach to otoplastic surgery similar to the one we follow during rhinoplastic surgery.

EMBRYOLOGY

A clear understanding of the embryologic formation of the auricle is essential in understanding the pathogenesis and the anatomic aberrations that contribute to the prominent ear. The external ear develops from the first branchial cleft and portions of the juxtaposed first mandibular and second hyoid arches (see Fig. 25–1). The auricle forms from six hillocks (of HIS) clustered about the first branchial cleft, which appear in the 5-week embryo. These include three hillocks on the posterior border of the first arch and three hillocks on the anterior border of the second arch. Research shows a specific relationship between these hillocks and spe-

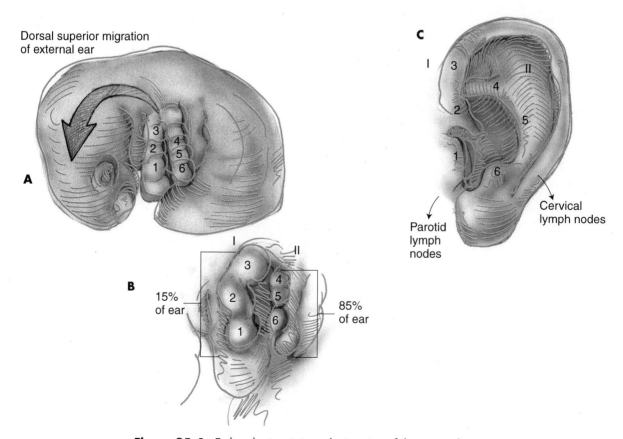

Figure 25–1. Embryologic origin and migration of the external ear.

cific pinnal structures. The three hillocks from the mandibular arch contribute to the tragus, crus of the helix, and conchal floor. Contributions from the hyoid branchial arch constitute most (approximately 85%) of the adult auricle, specifically all the remaining anatomic areas not derived from the mandibular arch. The first and sixth hillock maintain a fairly constant position, marking the sites of development of the tragus and antitragus, respectively. The fourth and fifth hillocks expand and rotate across the dorsal end of the cleft, giving rise to the anterior and superior helix and the adjacent portion of the body of the auricle. Suppression studies show that the auricular portion of the mandibular arch contributes only to the formation of the tragus and anterior crus helix. The auricle and external auditory meatus originally lie ventrally on the head but later migrate in a dorsal and superior direction. With further migration, the primary auditory meatus and tympano cavity reach the level of auricular migration, and amal-

gamation of the external, middle, and inner ear occurs. Because of the greater contribution of the second branchial arch hillocks, anomalies related to the antihelix, concha, antitragus, and lobule are the ones that most often need to be addressed and surgically corrected during otoplasty.

ANATOMY

The diagnostician must understand the normal external anatomic landmarks of the auricle to assess the abnormal and to correct the pathologic condition. Allison[1] gives us an excellent review of the anatomy of the external ear (see Fig. 25–2). The framework of the auricle comprises three tiers forming four planes of delicately convoluted cartilage: the conchal complex (floor and wall), the antihelix-antitragus complex, and the helix-lobule complex (see Fig. 25–3). The auricle consists of a single piece of yellow fibrous cartilage that gives a complicated relief

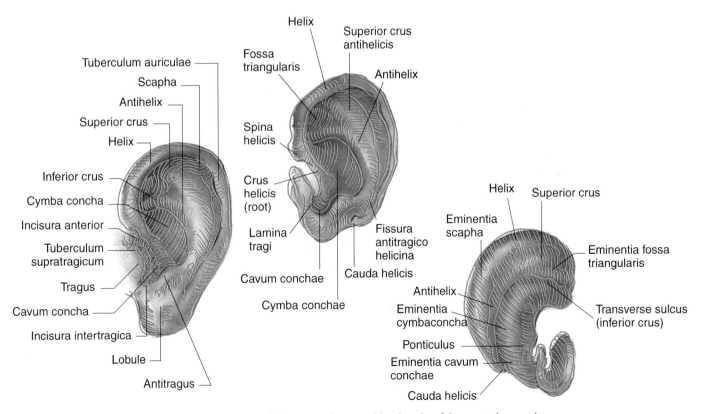

Figure 25-2. Anatomy of the external ear and landmarks of the auricular cartilage.

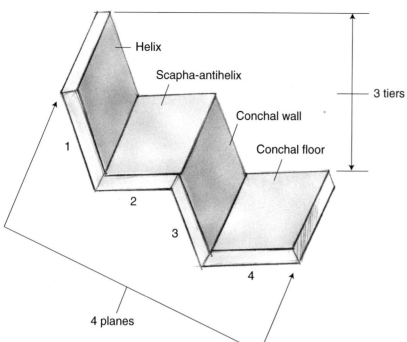

Figure 25–3. Four-plane, three-tier concept of auricular design. (1) Conchal floor; (2) posterior conchal walls; (3) scapha-anthelix complex; and (4) helix.

on the anterior, or concave, side and a smoother configuration on the posterior, or convex, side. Anteriorly the covering skin is thin and firmly adhered, whereas posteriorly it is freely moveable. The Darwinian tubercle, which is prominent in some people, lies in the descending part of the helix and corresponds to the true ear tip of long-eared mammals. The ear lobule alone contains subcutaneous tissue.

Although the external ear is a convoluted three-dimensional form; no sharp edges or peaks are present in its contour and relief. The helical rim arises anteriorly and inferiorly from the crus, extending in a horizontal direction from the external auditory meatus. The helix then continues superiorly and curves inferiorly to merge with the cauda helicis and join the lobule. The antihelix rises superiorly as the anterosuperior and anteroinferior crura that merge to form the antihelix body. This separates the helix posteriorly from the concha rim and concha proper. The scapha is a low, shallow fossa lying between the antihelical crura. Enclosed between the two crura is the fossa triangulares. The concha cavity com-

prises the cavum, the bowl, and cymba conchi superiorly and meets the antihelix. The conchal rim is bounded anteriorly by the tragus and the external auditory meatus. It is bounded posteriorly and inferiorly by the antitragus, which is separated from the tragus by the intratragal notch. The lobule presents varying degrees of development and attachment to the adjacent scalp and cheek.

Blood to the auricle is supplied by the superficial temporal and posterior auricular arteries. Sensation is supplied by anterior and posterior branches of the greater auricular nerve, reinforced by the auricular temporal and lesser occipital nerves. A small portion of the posterior wall of the external auditory meatus is supplied by the auricular branch of the vagus nerve (Arnold's nerve).

HISTORY

Four concepts of otoplastic surgical repair form the basis from which current techniques have been developed.

Diffenbach in 1845[2] advocated a simple excision of skin from the postauricular cephalic sulcus to decrease the prominent ear. Subsequently, Morestin[3] noted the necessity of breaking the spring of the cartilage to obtain a more permanent correction. This was accomplished by excising a crescent of conchal cartilage near the auricular cephalic sulcus, in addition to excising a skin strip. Luckett in 1910[4] recognized the failure of the antihelical fold and the superior crus. His technique involved making vertical curved incisions through virtually the whole length of the ear cartilage, following the line of the proposed antihelical fold and retaining the antihelix in its new folded position with Lembert sutures. Luckett's[4] concept formed the basis for subsequent developments in otoplastic surgery.

The next step in the evolution of otoplastic techniques was to devise methods to overcome the sharpness of the antihelical fold, which characterized the Luckett approach. Barsky[5] was the first to suggest incising the borders of the proposed fold of the new antihelix and superior crus to permit proper tubing of this structure, but he still retained the Luckett incision along the rest of the fold. Converse in 1961[6] and later Tanzer in 1962[7] further refined methods of rolling the antihelix and superior crus into a smooth three-dimensional structure by using an abrader to thin the cartilage when necessary and of tubing the auricular cartilage with multiple mattress sutures. Most recently, Elliott in 1984[8] has advocated varying the operative technique by using all the above-mentioned concepts, while simultaneously addressing specific ancillary deformities such as those found at the tail of the antihelix and the lobule and excessive proportions of the auricle itself. Composite sequential otoplasty, therefore, emphasizes the use of multiple techniques tailored to the specific complex of deformities. This represents the latest generation in the evolution of otoplastic surgery.

Until the late 1960s most surgeon/authors focused their attention on producing a more natural antihelix and ignored the concha in their efforts to do so. Thinning or through-and-through incisions to define the antihelix were combined with subcutaneous or buried sutures to secure the new position. Most important were contributions made by Mustarde in 1963[9] who proposed a reversible suture technique without incisions, and Stenstrom in 1963[10] who broke the cartilage spring by scratching the anterior surface. These two techniques were later combined, virtually eliminating the incidence of recurrence. Eventually, Mustarde's technique was refined to create a more gently curved antihelix and superior crus by using a greater number of smaller mattress sutures. Stenstrom's observation that cartilage springs toward the intact surface led to prompt acceptance of anterior scoring of the cartilage, but suture fixation of the cartilage fold was clearly preferable to the skin excision Stenstrom had proposed.

Little was written about the concha in otoplastic literature through the 1970s. In 1972, Elliot and Hoehn[11] wrote about conchal reduction and their experiences with more than 100 cases performed by means of an anterior approach. This facilitated redraping of the anterior conchal skin coverage. In 1973, a posterior approach to conchal reduction was proposed by Courtiss et al.[12] Repositioning of the concha was addressed by Owens and Delgado[13] in a 1965 publication describing their experience with a conchal-mastoid suture technique. Furnas's 1968 article[14] popularized this technique and Elliot suggested the development of a conchal pocket as a modification.

Prominence of the lobule as a topic is routinely included in recent otoplastic literature, although surgeons are still confused about which technique will successfully eliminate the deformity. The value of skin excision as a viable technique has been overstated. Fixation techniques were advocated by Spira et al[15] and Furnas.[14] Spira's technique involved suturing the lobule skin to the scalp periosteum; Furnas recommended fixation of the fibrofatty lobule tissue to the sternocleidomastoid muscle. Webster[16] recommended repositioning the tail of the helix to control the lobule, and this valuable contribution was subsequently published in 1969 and cited by Beernick et al[17] in a report 10 years later that documents 131 corrections using this technique.

ETIOLOGY AND PATHOGENESIS

A prominent ear may form as a result of any aberration of the normal migration and fusion of the six hillocks derived from the first and second branchial arches. Because 85% of the external ear develops embryonically from the second branchial arch, the structures derived from this area represent the most common pathologic abnormalities. In order of occurrence, these are the following.

1. Absence of proper antihelical folding
2. Conchal excess contributing to an excessive cephalo-conchal angle of greater than 90 degrees
3. Prominence in the tail of the helix, resulting in an excessive scapha-conchal angle of greater than 90 degrees
4. A prominent ear lobule, whether it be ptotic, excessive soft tissue, or simply overly abundant
5. Helical rim deformities derived embrionically from the first branchial arch, including the invaginated ear, shell ear, cup ear, and lop ear

It is not uncommon for prominent ears to manifest significant asymmetry between the two sides. Any of the preceding anatomic sites may contribute to this asymmetry.

PATIENT SELECTION

Successful aesthetic surgery begins with astute patient selection. As aesthetic surgeons, our first objective must always be to identify the well-motivated, realistic patient and at the same time to eschew the unfavorable patient. The undesirable patient has unrealistic expectations, emotional instability, and other signs of underlying psychopathologic conditions. Any patient with an excessive preoccupation with relatively minor defects raises a red flag to the discerning surgeon.

The strongest indication for successful surgical treatment of prominent ears is well-motivated patient desire. Family and friends who are aware of the deformity may influence the patient to have corrective surgery. How-ever, it is important for a patient of any age to express personal interest in the treatment and to undergo the procedure for himself or herself. The very young patient may first become aware of an unusual prominence of his or her ears as a result of uninhibited ridicule by peers. Many children have become emotionally disturbed by being reminded again and again of this deformity, and the primary reason for operating on prominent ears is to avoid or correct these adverse psychologic consequences. The ideal time to correct prominent ears is during the year or two before the child starts school. Preschoolers often do not notice this deformity in their schoolmates, so the psychologic trauma is minimized. The motivation of adults seeking otoplastic surgery, particularly young men, is more difficult to assess. The surgeon must be particularly critical of his or her preoperative assessment and must pay attention to proper patient selection in this group. Patient dissatisfaction, despite a good result, can be averted by spending appropriate time on preoperative counseling, discussing unrealistic expectations, and being sensitive to underlying emotional problems.

When considering otoplastic surgery for a patient of any age, it is critical to listen to the patient and to document exactly what bothers the patient. Most people have asymmetric ears. Many patients desire correction of only the more prominent ear when in fact both ears could be improved. The surgeon and patient must understand and agree on those areas that will be helped and those that will not be altered. The overly prominent auricle represents a congenital anomaly, and it behooves the operating surgeon to obtain a proper patient and family history to determine whether other congenital anomalies and deformities merit medical attention.

DIAGNOSTICS

Performing a careful preoperative physical examination, taking precise preoperative measurements, and having a clear knowledge of average auricular dimensions all help

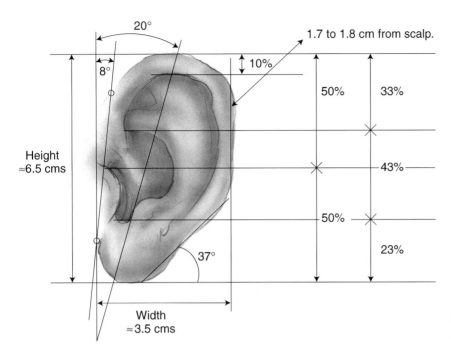

Figure 25–4. Diagnostics. Normal auricular measurements.

the surgeon to correctly identify the cause of ear prominence, which is crucial to selecting a proper treatment plan (see Fig. 25–4).

Architecturally, the auricle can be conceptualized as consisting of four planes: the conchal floor, the conchal wall, the scapha-antihelix complex, and the helix, all joined in a series of right angles (see Fig. 25–3). The defect in any specific patient should be analyzed in terms of these planes, and deformities then corrected.

An average auricle is 6.5 cm long and 3.5 cm wide, an approximate length width ratio of 2 : 1. The helical rim ideally should measure 1.7 cm to 1.8 cm from the mastoid area, and it is the aim of the surgeon to create a helical rim that maintains a 2-cm excursion from the mastoid area. The normal pinna lines up at a 30-degree tilt between the upper orbit and nasal spine and is parallel to the nasal bridge. The normal external ear has a scapho-conchal angle of 90 degrees and a cephalo-conchal angle of 90 degrees. A scapho-conchal angle that exceeds 90 degrees indicates failure of antihelical folding, a common cause of ear prominence. This deformity is evident from all views. An abnormally large and deep or malpositioned concha is another cause of ear prominence. Although hypertrophy is not readily detected on the lateral view,

malposition of the concha can be seen because the ear tilts forward and obscures some or all of the scapha. These guidelines, explained preoperatively to the patient, help determine which anatomic sites need to be altered.

During the preoperative consultation, I recommend standing behind the patient in front of a mirror and manually curling back the pinna with a cotton-tipped applicator to simulate the postoperative displacement of the corrected auricle. In this way the surgeon is able to point to those areas (antihelix, concha, helix, lobule) that need alteration, to create a properly positioned ear.

Computer imaging, which I have used in my practice for more than 12 years, has limited application in otoplasty. The usual frontal projection on the computer screen will give the patient some idea of how facial appearance would be improved by appropriate setback of the pinna. However, I find it more useful to use a plaster model of an external ear to demonstrate to the patient what is lacking in his or her anatomic configuration. Pointing to the areas requiring correction and allowing the patient to participate in his or her own preoperative surgical plan, prevents postoperative problems and confusion.

In terms of surgical timing it is accepted that the external ear is 85% grown by the age of 5 and fully grown by age 8. Therefore corrective otoplasty can be considered for preschoolers to avoid the psychologic problems associated with prominent ears. Adolescents and young adults have various reasons for deciding on otoplastic surgery. Whether their reasons be related to hair styling, personal grooming, or occupational necessity, they usually come in for a consultation when they are most motivated and prepared emotionally and financially to undergo the surgery.

AESTHETIC GOALS

The primary goal of any aesthetic surgical procedure is patient satisfaction. However, it is important for the surgeon to predetermine the aesthetic goals of the procedure and present them simply to the patient. The surgeon's goal is to refine, recontour, or reposition the ear with resolute effort to duplicate a normal ear. In attempting to realize this goal, the surgeon should strive for a result that will be undetected by the most discerning and critical eye. The following five otoplastic tenets will help the surgeon achieve his or her aesthetic goals.

1. *Correct any upper pole protrusion.* The lateral plane of the reconstructed ear should be singular from the upper pole, and when measured at the midpoint of the concha, should lie 1.8 cm from the skin of the mastoid prominence. A significant protrusion in the upper and lower poles, known as telephone ear deformity, or the reverse, a protrusion of the middle third of the outer ear, is totally unacceptable.
2. *Ensure that the helical rim beyond the antihelix is frontally visible.* An ear with a hidden helix has an abnormal appearance.
3. *Ensure that helix and antihelix are smooth and regular, without sharp or abrupt edges.* Most prominent ears require a correction to the antihelix. Preserving or reconstructing the curvature, width, and smooth roll, including the superior crus, is essential. Deformities involving the helix, such as transverse bar (helix root extends across conchal floor), Darwin's tubercle (outer border of upper pole is wide and prominent), or an abnormal prominence of the tail of the helix should be corrected to eliminate complications or unwanted results such as sharp ridges, irregular contours, vertical post, or a malpositioned roll—all of which can be created by the injudicious surgeon.
4. *Ensure that the postauricular sulcus is normal.* This component is important to the ear's aesthetic appearance, particularly from the posterior view. Relocation and fixation of the tail of the helix controls lower-third deformities. Excess skin may need to be removed to make the postauricular sulcus appear normal.
5. *Avoid a plastered-down look.* Both overcorrection and undercorrection of the prominent ear can result in an unnatural, plastered-down look, which the patient at first may believe is desirable.

By carefully analyzing the deformity and determining the existing pathologic abnormality, the surgeon can tailor his or her surgical procedure to achieve a desired goal. I recommend following a sequential process with five discrete steps (as is done for rhinoplastic surgery) when evaluating the prominent ear for otoplasty.[18]

1. Examine skin envelope and determine the necessary excision.
2. Determine what other soft tissue adjustments may be needed.
3. Incise and excise prominent cartilage.
4. Correct the lobule if necessary.
5. Correct any miscellaneous auricular deformities.

SURGICAL PRINCIPLES

The main principle of otoplastic surgery is to select a simple procedure that will yield the maximum aesthetic result with low risk of recurrence and the lowest possible risk to the patient. As with all surgical procedures, a sterile environment and careful hemostasis are essential. The otoplastic surgeon must develop a clear strategy and technique for handling each tissue type as well.

CARTILAGE

The character and consistency of cartilage varies from patient to patient. Some patients have soft, malleable cartilage that is forgiving, whereas some have cartilage that is stiff and heavy. Regardless of the type, ear cartilage may need to be thinned, excised, relocated, or have its spring released. Any combination of these procedures may cause sharp edges and distortions, and a miscalculation may not be reversible. Beveling and approximation of edges may mitigate these unwanted effects. Other than excision, incisions through the cartilage should be avoided if possible.

SKIN

A limited need for skin excision occurs in otoplasty. It is usually limited to the removal of excess in the posterior sulcus. The occasional lobule reduction can be performed without skin excision if the tail of the helix is preserved and used for this purpose.

SUTURES

When using nonabsorbable sutures, a chance of localized infection exists; however, these sutures retain their strength and cause less tissue reaction than absorbable ones. Because they are available in clear or white material, nonabsorbable sutures are less noticeable than dark sutures beneath the skin cover. In the absence of tension, absorbable sutures can be used for posterior skin closure. If plain catgut is used, removal of these sutures is not necessary. Chromic catgut and polyglass sutures, however, are not absorbed as quickly and may result in unwanted suture tracks. Likewise, nonabsorbable sutures should be removed within a week to avoid these epithelial tracks.

SPLINTING

A soft compression dressing is needed to position the reconstructed ear and to protect it while it heals. The dressing provides comfort for the patient and decreases edema and ecchymosis. The dressing will not prevent a hematoma, however, so careful hemostasis is essential. Persistent pain is a harbinger of possible complications and requires prompt attention.

SURGICAL TECHNIQUE

My preferences and perspectives regarding surgical techniques have evolved from 20 years of personal experience as both a plastic surgeon and otolaryngologist with a keen interest in otoplasty. My techniques are a composite of the those described in surgical literature, along with my own methods.

PREPARATION

The patient's hair is washed the evening before and again immediately before surgery. By this time surgical consent forms, laboratory data, and other administrative paper work have been completed. General anesthesia is administered to young children; older children and adults are premedicated with a local anesthetic and intravenous sedation and are treated as outpatients.

DRAPING

The entire head is cleansed and left exposed in the operative field. Plastic drapes may be used to isolate the ears, but drapes often shift during the operation and have little advantage. Meticulous sectioning of the hair with rubberbands can provide the surgeon with a hairless field, without the necessity of shaving the patient's head.

ANESTHESIA

Anesthesia is provided by injecting a solution of 2% lidocaine with 1:50,000 epinephrine beneath the skin of the anterior and posterior surfaces of the ear, as well as into the posterior sulcus. The local anesthesia facilitates hemostasis and aids dissection. Young patients under general anesthesia should be locally injected in the same way for the same reasons.

MARKING

The auricle is examined, palpated, and the deformities analyzed in a sequential fashion. Analysis is facilitated by applying pressure to the scapha region, folding the ear back manually to form the desired antihelix and demonstrating the scaphal depression and posterior border of the superior crus of the antihelix. Conchal excess and skin excess are noted (see Fig. 25–5).

With the ear folded back and expected tubing visualized, a marking pen is used to delineate the centerline of the antihelix, posterior border of the antihelix, and anterior border of the superior crus of the antihelix. The conchal rim is marked on the anterolateral aspect of the auricle, extending superiorly into the cymba conchae and inferiorly to the external auditory meatus. The amount of excess, based on the desired amount of inset, is also marked. The tail of the helix is palpated and its position noted on the anterior skin surface. Incisions for lobular or pinna reduction are marked as the appropriate pie-shaped wedges.

The ear is then folded forward to mark the posterior skin for excision. The ellipse of skin to be excised extends from pole to pole and is centered on the new antihelical roll. Its width corresponds to the amount of inset desired. If indicated by prominent poles, skin excisions may be extended and ended as M-plasties to help prevent telephone ear deformity.

APPROACH

Usually it is best to correct the more prominent ear first, so it may guide correction of the second ear. Proceeding in a sequential fashion allows the surgeon to limit the correction to those components of the ear that contribute to the specific deformity. The flexibility of this sequential technique, with immediate evaluation and reversibility, makes it particularly efficacious (see Figs. 25–6 and 25–7).

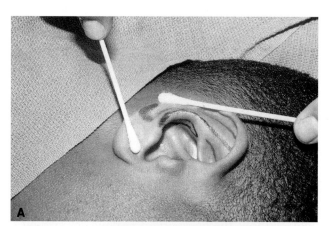

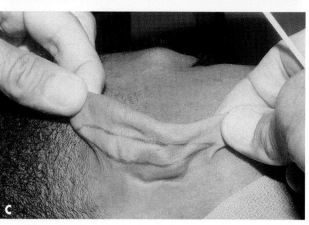

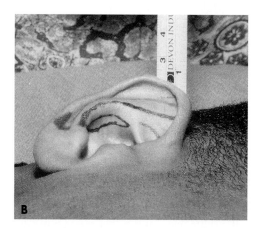

Figure 25–5. Preoperative markings. **(A)** Ear is folded back by gentle pressure on the helical rim and lobule. **(B)** Conchal excess, proposed antihelical roll, and tail of helix are marked according to the desired amount of inset. **(C)** An ellipse of postauricular skin to be excised is marked according to the degree of setback to be achieved and centered on the proposed antihelical roll extending from upper pole to the inferior limit of the concha and tail of the helix.

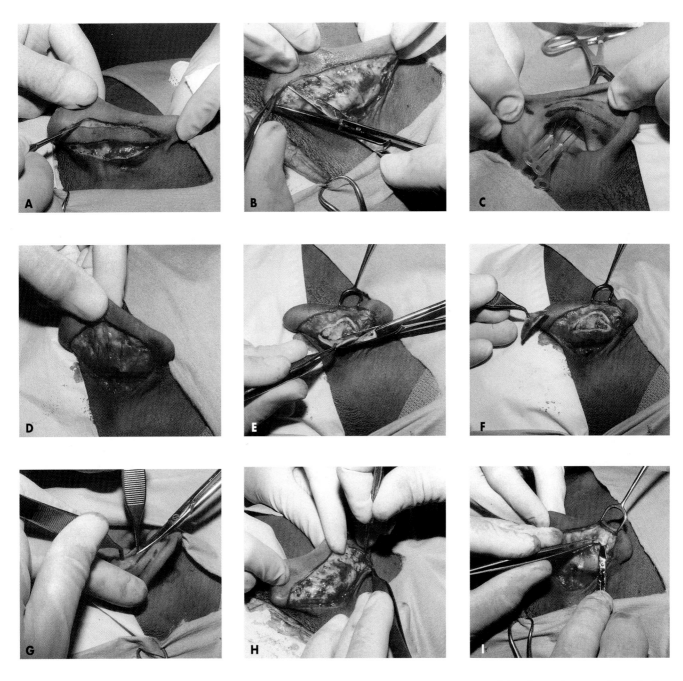

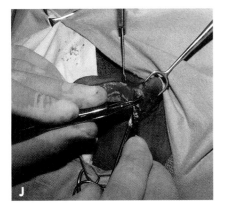

Figure 25–6. Operative sequence. **(A)** Excision of the ellipse of previously marked postauricular skin and subcutaneous tissue. **(B)** Perichondrium is exposed. Further undermining of the posterior skin and subcutaneous tissue exposes the perichondrium of the helical rim and tail, as well as the entire posterior aspect of the concha down to its junction with the mastoid process. **(C)** Superior aspect of conchal excess to be excised is marked by needles. **(D)** Posterior view, needles determine site for conchal incision. **(E)** Conchal cartilage is dissected and exposed. **(F)** A lunar-shaped segment of conchal excess is excised on the basis of preoperative markings. A pocket is prepared to reposition and set back the concha. **(G)** Skin lying on the anterolateral aspect is undermined 3 to 4 mm. Excess skin that does not redrape may be excised and closed with 6-0 nylon suture. **(H)** Tail of the helix is exposed on its posterior surface. **(I)** Tail of helix is only dissected out if it is excessively firm and severely angulated in an anterior vector. **(J)** A suture may be placed to draw the tail of the helix onto the posterior surface of the concha until the lobule is in the desired position.

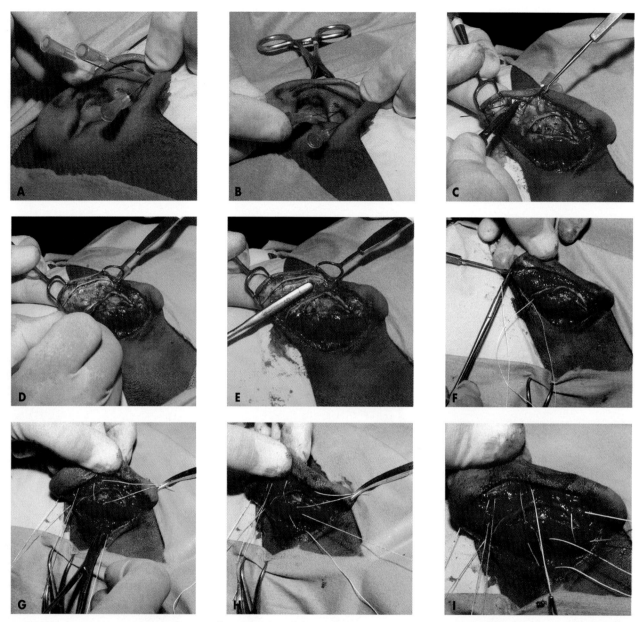

Figure 25–7. Operative sequence. **(A)** Needles placed to delineate posterior border of antihelix. **(B)** Needles placed to delineate superior crus of antihelix. **(C, D)** Incisions are made through the cartilage of the proposed antihelical roll. **(E)** Thinning of antihelical roll by means of a sharp No. 5 rasp. **(F)** Tubing of antihelix is achieved with 4-0 Mersilene mattress sutures starting superiorly. **(G)** Further placement of antihelical roll mattress sutures. **(H)** Placement of "conchal-mastoid inset" mattress suture. **(I)** Row of "5" mattress sutures placed (including tail of helix). Radial placement produces curved roll. *(Continued on p. 457.)*

SKIN EXCISION

Begin exposure of the antihelix and concha posteriorly, with excision of the ellipse of previously marked postauricular skin and subcutaneous tissue. The center line of this ellipse is determined by introducing needles from the anterolateral aspect of the auricle through the center

line of the body of the antihelix and the superior crus. The excision extends from the upper pole of the ear to the inferior limit of the concha and tail of the helix. The width of the skin excision must be estimated to match the anticipated amount of inset.

Removing the ellipse of skin exposes the perichondrium. Further undermining of posterior skin and sub-

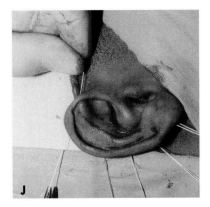

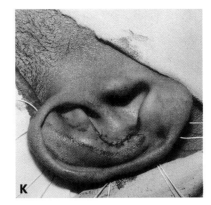

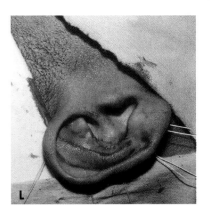

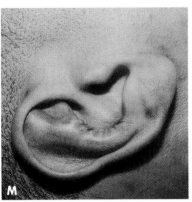

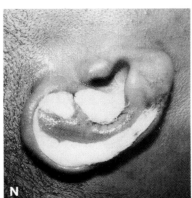

Figure 25–7. *(Continued from p. 456.)* **(J)** Sutures are tied superior to inferior for antihelix, superior crus, and lobule control. **(K,L)** All sutures tied in place. Each suture tightened only enough to achieve the desired effect at that level. **(M)** Appearance after skin closure. Note the closure of conchal skin excision. **(N)** Cotton impregnated with mineral oil used to bolster and protect new antatomy before mastoid dressing.

cutaneous tissue exposes the perichondrium of the helical rim and tail, as well as the entire posterior aspect of the concha down to its junction with the mastoid prominence. This facilitates complete control of the auricular structure and also permits predraping with skin closure.

CONCHAL REDUCTION AND REPOSITIONING

Conchal reduction begins with auricular setback. A conchal rim incision is made corresponding to the preoperative markings. An ellipse of conchal cartilage is removed from the appropriate portion of the concha rim, medial to the previous conchal rim incision. The precise location and extent of the ellipse depends on the correction that is planned. Both surfaces of the cartilage are undermined, which allows the ear to be recessed into the desired position. Skin lying on the anterolateral aspect is undermined for a distance of 3 to 4 mm from the edges of the new conchal rim. Excess skin that does not redrape may be excised and closed with a running 6-0 nylon suture. The

length of the incision must be planned to avoid distortion as the defect is closed by edge-to-edge approximation of cartilage with two clear 5-0 nylon sutures.

To reposition the concha, a definite pocket must be prepared by excising the posterior auricular muscle and the fatty tissue overlying the mastoid fascia. The concha may be fixed to the mastoid fascia with two tacking sutures, although the surgeon must take care not to distort the external auditory meatus.

ANTIHELIX, SUPERIOR CRUS, AND LOBULE

These structures are considered a unit and should be addressed together. Begin by lifting the skin to expose the bare surface of the scapha and superior crus all the way down to the tail of the antihelix. The surgeon may then pass 28-gauge needles from the lateral aspect of the auricle to delineate the previously marked posterior border of the antihelix and superior crus and the superior and anterior borders of the superior crus and conchal rim. Incisions are made corresponding to these points through the cartilage to, but not including, the perichondrium over the lateral auricular cartilage. These are relaxing incisions, and they must not be joined to allow formation of a smooth and gradual antihelical roll. When antihelical cartilage is particularly thick and not readily malleable, it may be necessary to gently thin the ear to facilitate proper tubing. Thinning may be done by means of sharp No. 7 or No. 5 Parkes rasps or with a wire brush and dermabrader.

Tubing of the antihelix roll and tail may now be achieved and maintained with a row of four or five sutures of 4-0 Mersilene or 4-0 clear nylon or Gor-tex suture. The sutures are laced posteriorly in a radial fashion from superior to inferior and are not tied until all sutures have been placed. Mattress sutures are placed securely into the cartilage, adjacent to but not through the relaxation incisions. Each suture is tested when placed, then left to be tied in order from superior to inferior. We have found the superiormost mattress suture to be the most important, but it is also the most difficult to place. Therefore we start there and proceed inferiorly, taking care to adjust the tightness of each suture just enough to produce the desired effect at that level. If anything, it is better to overcorrect in anticipation of some loosening of the sutures. Any distortion will be readily apparent and may be immediately corrected by replacing the offending suture or by adding supplementary sutures.

The tail of the helix is exposed on its posterior surface and only dissected out if it is excessively firm and severely angulated in an anterior vector. A single suture may be placed to draw the tail of the helix onto the posterior surface of the concha until the lobule is in the desired position. The effect is immediate and this permanent suture may be repositioned as necessary until the desired anatomic correction is seen. Usually this technique is sufficient to control the lobule. Occasionally, a relaxation incision (forming a swinging door) is made through the tail of the antihelix at the point of maximum

deflection, being careful not to form a sharp break. Likewise, a small posterior skin excision or reduction of the lobule may be necessary, but it is best deferred until final skin adjustments and closure.

COMBINED DEFORMITIES

Naturally the preceding procedures may be recombined to suit the diagnosis and the surgical plan. In some cases it will be better to correct the antihelix before reducing and repositioning the concha. In any case, the surgeon must take care if making the anterior incision through the conchal cartilage to avoid interfering with any folding sutures. As a general rule, I prefer to address conchal excess and then proceed in a superior-to-inferior fashion, addressing helical rim, antihelix, tail of helix, and any lobular abnormalities to be corrected.

MISCELLANEOUS DEFORMITIES

Once prominence has been corrected, the surgeon may evaluate and treat any remaining deformities, such as an overly broad scapha or a prominent Darwin's tubercle. It is very important for the aesthetic surgeon to pause before completing these procedures and to assure himself or herself that he or she has constructed the most pleasing ear. It is much better to make an additional correction during the initial surgery and not to compel the patient to return for additional correction at some later time.

Macrotia, or truly large ears, are most effectively reduced with full-thickness wedge excisions placed appropriately (lobule superior or middle third). Large ear lobes are also reduced with full-thickness wedge excisions. It is paramount to approximate the rim border exactly and with eversion to prevent notching; Z-plasties may be needed to prevent notching. The surgeon should exercise those principles available for ablative surgery to remove auricular malignancy.

The *lop ear deformity* refers to the lidlike turning down of the helix with a compression or narrowing of the scapha and fossa triangularis. It usually occurs at the level of Darwin's tubercle. More simply stated, the upper posterior portion of the ear hangs downward. Failure of normal unfurling of the superior helix over the antihelix during the third to fourth month of gestation most probably causes the deformity. The lop ear may or may not also be prominent with indistinct antihelix and conchal excess.

Because the basic pathologic abnormality is a shortening of the helix, correction involves lengthening. The helical crus and ascending part of the helix are cut free so that the ear can be unfurled. Undermining and release of cartilage with incisions further relaxes the shortened helix. The anterior helix is then raised to a more superior location by a V to Y advancement and closure.

The *cup ear* is essentially a protruding ear. An overdeveloped, deep, and cup-shaped concha, a deficient superior part of the helical margin and antihelical crura, and small vertical height are typical features of this deformity. Whether unfolded or fully developed, the body of the antihelix is often wider and it tends to exaggerate the cupping deformity. The helical margin or fold, in some cases, drapes forward and over the scapha in a hoodlike fashion.

Cryptotia (invaginated ear) is a deformity in which the upper portion of the ear is more or less embedded beneath the scalp. This "invagination" is, in fact, an abnormal adherence of the ear to the temporal skin and is associated with cartilage malformation in the scaphal/antihelix complex. The cause is suspected to be a result of abnormalities of the intrinsic transverse and intrinsic oblique ear muscles. In terms of natural history the condition is rare in Caucasians but significantly more common in Asians (1 : 4 ratio). Like microtia, the right ear is affected more often than the left, and the deformity is bilateral in about 40% of cases.

Early splinting is fairly successful. Surgical correction requires direct division of the abnormal muscles with addition of skin to the deficient retroauricular sulcus. Additional skin is usually obtained by expanding the tissue and advancing and rotating a flap of expanded,

postauricular and scalp tissue. Cartilage reconstruction may also be indicated and necessitates modification of an existing helical rim or cartilage addition. Mutimer and Mulliken in 1988[19] and Hirose in 1985[20] share their experiences in treating this condition.

Stahl's ear (satyr ear, "Spock" ear) is another helical rim deformity. This condition was first reported in the nineteenth century by Schwalbe.[21] Patients manifest a pointed contour and incomplete curling at some point along the horizontal portion of the helix, as well as an abnormal posterior crus, flat helix, and malformed scaphoid fossa. In neonates, when ear cartilage is soft and pliable, Stahl's ear can be corrected with proper ear splinting. Older children and adults require operative correction. Nakajima et al in 1989[22] and Nakayama and Soeda in 1986[23] have advocated combining Z-plasty, cartilage reversal, and a periosteal tethering maneuver to recreate normal external ear configuration.

Shell ear is best described as a prominent ear with little or no concomitant curling of the helix and an absence of the antihelix and crura. In the resulting configuration the concha and scapha merge directly into each other.

My suggested approach to this problem is composite otoplasty to correct the prominent features of this ear. Once this has been achieved, increasing curling of the helix can be addressed. This can be done by excising appropriate wedge-shaped pieces based at the rim of the auricle. The defect is then sutured, shortening the external rim of the ear to create the required curvature of the helix. Care must be taken not to distort correction of the prominent ear. Posterior skin excision fine tunes the repair.

As an alternative, the Stenstrom technique of posteriorly scratching the helical roll will result in the desired anterior curling of the helix. This is achieved by undermining a 1-cm wide zone of cartilage from below and has the advantage of not directly exposing and violating the margin of the helix. Again, careful attention must be paid to trace the curl of the newly created antihelix and crura and to score the cartilage in a graduated fashion to achieve the desired contour.

CLOSURE

Close posterior wounds in a single layer using a continuous 5-0 plain prolene suture. Supplement the main suture with interrupted sutures as required to maintain eversion of the edges. Close anterior incisions with nonabsorbable 6-0 nylon everting sutures. Cover the incisions with medicated gauze. Once the wound is closed, a cotton patch impregnated with mineral oil is trimmed to accommodate the concha and placed behind the ear. The anterior recess of the ear is also packed with mineral oil–saturated cotton. A strip of tape extending from the neck to the forehead holds the dressing in place. A mastoid-type compression dressing made of a soft gauze roll and an elastic bandage may also be wrapped around the head and over the ear. Patients usually find this dressing quite comfortable. It also protects the ear from injury and may help reduce swelling and bruising.

POSTOPERATIVE CARE

All patients receive routine postoperative instructions. These include limited activity, back elevation, and medication for pain management. After an antihelix reconstruction or a conchal repositioning, the patient is advised to wear the compression dressing for 1 week. After less invasive procedures (conchal reduction for example), the dressing may be removed in 3 or 4 days. A protective ski or sports headband is then recommended for sleeping and should be worn for at least a month to avoid any traction on the ears. Cleanliness is important, and the outer ear may be gently cleansed with a cotton-tipped applicator and mild soap. Bacitracin ointment is beneficial on all incisions, and any areas where skin was penetrated and the underlying cartilage should be protected.

Soft tissue swelling dissipates over several weeks and the new auricular contour is visible in a matter of months. Final results may take 6 months to a year after surgery (see Fig. 25–8).

RESULTS AND COMPLICATIONS

Elliott,[24] Mustarde,[25] Webster and Smith,[26] Tan,[27] and Heftner[28] have all examined, from their own perspectives, unsatisfactory results of otoplasty for patients of either the Mustarde or Stenstrom technique.

Elliott separated unsatisfactory results of otoplasty into two separate groups. The first group, *complications*, includes pain, bleeding, pruritus, infection, chondritis, and necrosis early on. The second group of *undesirable sequelae* experience dissatisfaction, unsightly scars, suture problems, and dysesthesias later on.

Residual or recurrent deformity is the most common unsatisfactory result of otoplasty. These deformities may be any or a combination of the following: incomplete correction, overcorrection, recurrence of prominence, telephone and reverse telephone deformity, sharp ridges along the antihelical fold, a vertical post (lack of normal curvature of the superior crus), irregular contours, a too small or malpositioned antihelical roll, an excessively large scapha, and a narrow ear.

Examining the results of 264 ears in a 10-year survey, Mustarde[25] cited several potential problems with the otoplastic procedure that bears his name. Kinks in the antihelix, sutures cutting out, sinus tract formations, recurrence of prominence, and horizontal projection of the antitragus and lobule were conditions listed. In a subsequent article, Mustarde noted that of 600 ears he surgically corrected over a 20-year period, only six patients had sinus tracts develop, and none rejected the silk sutures. He continued to note that of the 600 ears, only 10 ears required additional surgery for recurring prominence.

Mustarde's technique (posterior suturing) has not been totally embraced by some of his colleagues. With this technique, Spira and Hardy encountered a relatively high number of minor complications and partial recurrence of deformities. Tan, comparing Mustarde's technique with the anterior scoring technique, discovered that the white stitches, particular to the Mustarde proce-

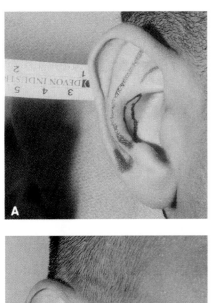

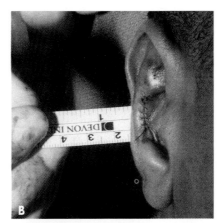

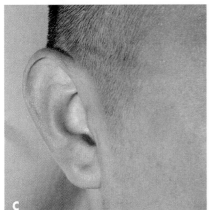

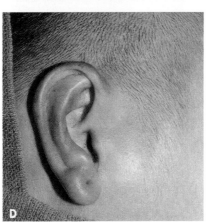

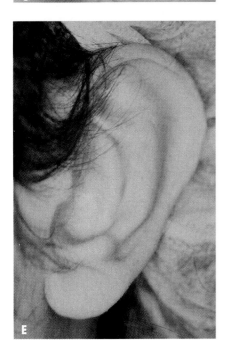

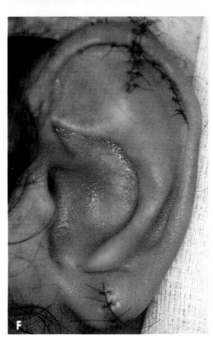

Figure 25–8. Postoperative results.
(A) Intraoperative preoperative view with proposed changes.
(B) Intraoperative postoperative view, degree of inset based on preoperative goals. Strive for 1.8 to 2.0 cm excursion of helix from mastoid. **(C,D)** Intraoperative preoperative and postoperative views. Note gentle roll and no sharp edges of antihelix. Lobule controlled with tail of helix suture.
(E–H) Intraoperative preoperative and postoperative views, showing correction of shell ear deformity and macrotia. Curling of helix achieved with helical wedge-shaped and shortening of the external rim.
(Continued on pp. 462 and 463.)

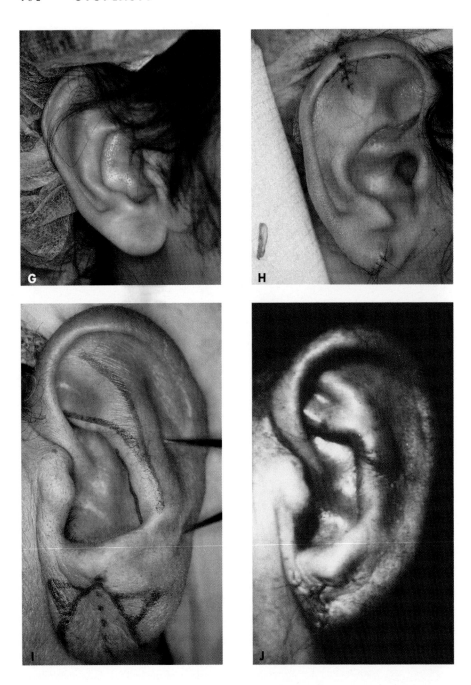

Figure 25–8. (I) Preoperative and postoperative views showing correction of macrotia and composite otoplasty with wedge excision of lobule.
(Continued on pp. 461 and 463.)

dure, caused sinus tracts and wound infections, and a significant number of patients required reoperation.

Hefner, surveying cases in which Stenstrom otoplasties had been performed, found that of 167 patients, 40% were very satisfied, 49% were satisfied, and 4% were fairly satisfied.

The techniques discussed here produce aesthetically pleasing results and satisfied patients in most cases. The composite approach allows the surgeon to correct most deformities and to achieve a natural-looking ear. Overcorrection and undercorrection do occasionally occur, primarily as a result of inexperience on the surgeon's part. Fibrous fixation generally holds the correction (which is what makes these techniques permanent), and this phenomenon is the reason secondary procedures often are more difficult than the primary procedure.

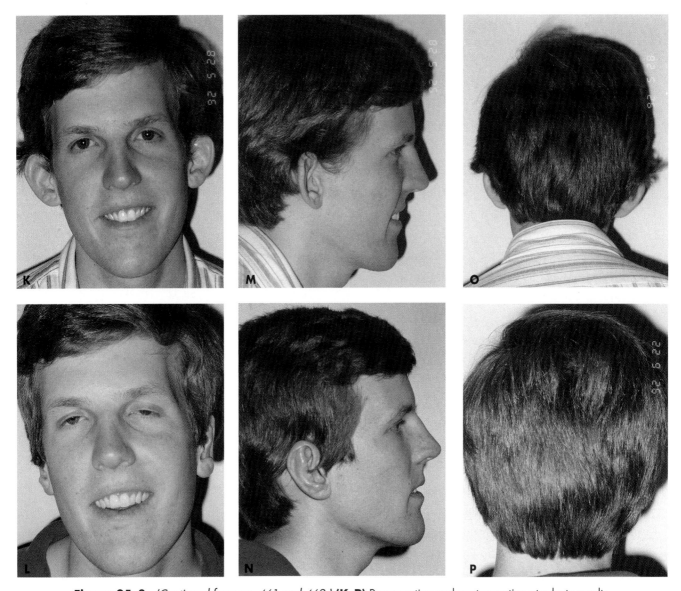

Figure 25-8. *(Continued from pp. 461 and 462.)* **(K-P)** Preoperative and postoperative otoplasty results.

Postoperative trauma is the most common cause of the deformity recurring. However, the surgeon must discover the precise cause of the failure if a second operation is to succeed. Similarly, successful correction of surgical error depends on careful analysis of the condition. Undercorrections usually can be improved by secondary surgery, but overcorrections generally require release of the fibrous fixation and replacement of the missing tissues with uncertain results.

CONCLUSION

Otoplasty is a complex procedure, requiring careful analysis of the deformity and careful selection of the appropriate treatment plan, and perfect results remain elusive. Although difficult, experience, technical knowledge, and ability are all that are required to obtain consistent and predictably good results. Composite otoplasty, the latest approach to defects of the ear, emphasizes multiple techniques tailored to the specific deformities.

Success with this technique is high if the surgeon pays careful attention to patient selection and detail.

PEARLS

- Preoperative analysis of the deformity is essential to good surgical planning.
- Use a "sequential approach," dealing with each of the anatomic components of the malformation one at a time. Steadfastly maintain adherance to the preoperative assessments.
- Use percutaneous 25 guage by $1\frac{1}{2}$-inch needles to assist in cartilagenous incision placement when creating the antihelix, thus avoiding "sharp edges" that look unnatural.
- Do not forget the tail of the helix. An otherwise acceptable result may resemble "telephone ear deformity" if the tail of the helix goes unaddressed. This is an intraoperative decision that should be considered on every patient.
- Dress the patient with an ENT style dressing. Compression alone is not enough. Each delicate curvature of the new ear must be gently packed with mineral oil soaked cotton, sparing the canal. The sulcus must also be filled with cotton before external compression is applied. This helps insure against collection and actually diminishes pain.

REFERENCES

1. Allison GR. Clin Plast Surg. 1978; 5:000–000.
2. Diffenbach JF. Die operative Chirurgia. Leipzig: Brockhaus; 1845.
3. Morestin H. De la reposition et du plissement cosmetiques du pavillon de l'oreille. Rev Orthopedie. 1903; 14:289.
4. Luckett WH. A new operation for prominent ears based on the anatomical deformity. Surg Gynecol Obstet. 1910; 10:635.
5. Barsky AJ. Plastic Surgery. Philadelphia: W. B. Saunders Co.; 1938.
6. Converse JM. Technical details... Lop ear deformity. Plast Reconstr Surg. 1963; 31:118.
7. Tanzer RC. The correction of the prominent ear. Plast Reconstr Surg. 1962; 30:236.
8. Elliott RA. Otoplasty. In: Regnault P, ed. Aesthetic Plastic Surgery. Boston: Little Brown; 1984.
9. Mustarde JC. The correction of prominent ears using simple mattress sutures. Br J Plast Surg. 1963; 16:170.
10. Stenstrom SJ. A "natural" technique for correction of congenitally prominent ears. Plast Reconstr Surg. 1963; 32:509.
11. Elliott RA, and Hoehn JG. Otoplasty. Int Micr J Aesthet Plast Surg. 1972A.
12. Courtiss EH, Webster RC, White MF. Otoplasty: Direct surgical approach. In: Masters FW, Lewis JR Jr., eds. Symposium on Aesthetic Surgery of the Nose, Ears, and Chin. St. Louis: Mosby; 1973.
13. Owens N, Delgado DD. The management of outstanding ears. South Med J. 1965; 58:32.
14. Furnas DW. Correction of prominent ears by concha mastoid sutures. Plast Reconstr Surg. 1968; 42:189.
15. Spira M, et al. Correction of the principal deformities causing prominent ears. Plast Reconstr Surg 1969; 44:150.
16. Webster GV. The tail of the helix as a key to otoplasty. Plast Reconstr Surg. 1969; 44:455.
17. Beernick JH, Blocksma R, Moore WD. The role of the helical tail in cosmetic otoplasty. Plast Reconstr Surg. 1979; 64:115.
18. Ordon AP. Correction of the overprojected nasal tip. Am J Cosmet Surg. 1994; 11:3.
19. Mutimer KL, Mulliken JB. Correction of cryptotia using tissue expansion. Plast Reconstr Surg. 1988; 81:601.
20. Hirose T. Cryptotia: Our classification and treatment. Br J Plast Surg. 1985; 38:352.
21. Schwalbe G. Das Darwinsche Spitzohr beim menschlichen Embryo. Anat Anz. 1887; 4:176.
22. Nakajima T, Yoshimura Y, Kami T. Surgical and conservative repair of Stahl's ear. Aesthet Plast Surg. 1984; 8:101.
23. Nakayama Y, Soeda S. Surgical treatment of Stahl's ear using the periosteal string. Plast Reconstr Surg. 1986; 77:222.
24. Elliott RA. Complications in the treatment of prominent ears. Clin Plast Surg. 1978; 5:479.
25. Mustarde JC. The treatment of prominent ears by buried mattress sutures—A ten years' survey. Plast Reconstr Surg. 1967; 39:382.
26. Webster RC, Smith RC. Otoplasty for prominent ears. In: Goldwyn RM, ed. Long-term Results in Plastic and Reconstructive Surgery. Boston: Little Brown; 1980.
27. Tan KH. Long term survey of prominent ear surgery: A comparison of two methods. Br J Plast Surg. 1986; 39:270.
28. Heftner J. Followup study on 167 Stenstrom otoplasties. Clin Plast Surg. 1978; 5:470.

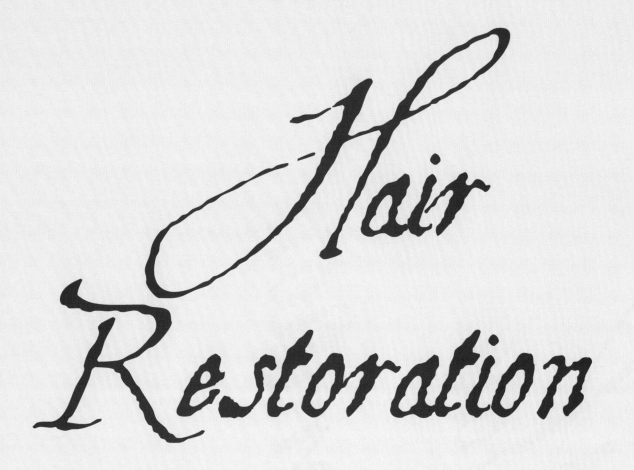

Hair Restoration

The chapter on hair restoration features two major innovators in the field. The chapter by Drs. Fleming and Mayer, both facial plastic surgeons, stresses the operative assessment, including present and future evaluations of alopecia. A historical review encompasses the development of basic hair restoration techniques. A detailed review of the alternative techniques for hair restoration includes punch grafting, alopecia reduction techniques, the Fleming-Mayer flap, inferior-based temporoparietal fascia flap, superiorly based preauricular and postauricular flap, and tissue expansion is presented. Drs. Fleming and Mayer are internationally known for their techniques and flap use in hair restoration, and an elegant review of patient selection and specific treatment modalities is presented. The chapter is thoroughly illustrated.

Alternately, the chapter by Drs. Orentreich and Orentreich, both dermatologists, reviews the history of punch grafting, which is their preferred modality for hair restoration. Patient evaluation and workup are stressed. A thorough review of the procedure planning and extensive review of the surgical procedure of punch grafting, including graft size and placement techniques, are accurately presented and illustrated.

These chapters completely cover the multiple modalities of current hair restoration techniques with a bias toward each of their particular preferred approaches.

Hair Restoration

Aesthetic Facial Plastic Surgery, edited by Thomas Romo, III, and Arthur L. Millman, Thieme Medical Publishers, Inc., New York, New York, Copyright © 2000.

CHAPTER 26

A Facial Plastic Surgeon's Perspective

RICHARD W. FLEMING AND TOBY G. MAYER

We have made every attempt in this chapter to present an honest, well-documented assessment of our experience with aesthetic hair replacement surgery. We present an overview of preoperative evaluation, surgical planning, operative technique, and postoperative care for each approach because we use all hair replacement techniques. The brief history of each procedure emphasizes the significant change in hair replacement surgery over the past 25 years. We refer the reader to the suggested reading list for a thorough discussion of the various approaches and alternate techniques.

CLASSIFICATION OF MALE PATTERN BALDNESS

The most important consideration before any surgical hair replacement procedure is an accurate assessment of the amount of existing baldness and the potential extent of progressive alopecia. Therefore a classification system is necessary to determine whether the patient is a candidate for hair replacement surgery and to compare the various procedures so the surgeon can make appropriate recommendations and establish reasonable expectations.

In 1951, Hamilton[1] published the first useful classification of male pattern baldness. In 1973 this was modified by Norwood,[2] who classified baldness into seven categories plus a variant type. Although such classification is useful for scientific purposes, we have simplified the classification of baldness in the following manner (Fig. 26–1).

Class I—Frontal baldness only, with or without an anterior tuft.

Class II—Frontal and midscalp baldness with no thinning of the crown
Class III—Frontal to occipital (vertex) baldness
Class IV—Crown baldness only.

The purpose of this classification is to define the ultimate pattern of baldness. Most balding men have or will have a Class III pattern. If any question exists regarding the final extent of alopecia, it is best to wait until the pattern is more clearly established.

PUNCH GRAFTING

Although Okuda[3] first described hair transplantation in 1939, credit for the popularity and evolution of hair transplantation belongs to Orentreich.[4] He realized the applications of this technique and described his experience in his classic paper "Autografts in Alopecia and Other Selected Dermatologic Conditions" in 1959.

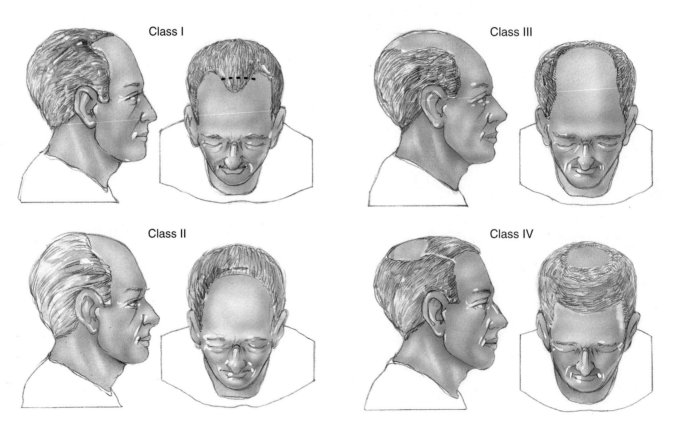

Figure 26–1. Classification of male pattern baldness, which represents a simplified method of evaluating most common types of male pattern baldness.

Because millions of men experience male pattern alopecia, which society deems undesirable and unattractive, Orentreich's operation to transplant hair-bearing autografts quickly became the most common cosmetic procedure in men. This has not changed in nearly 50 years.

Initially, the goal of transplantation was the elimination of as much alopecia as possible. Physicians advocated maximum density transplanting with 4- or 5-mm grafts, ideally containing 15 to 20 hairs. The major disadvantage of this technique was the "row of corn" or "doll's hair" appearance. Over the past 10 years "minigrafting" and "micrografting" have become state-of-the-art techniques in hair transplantation. Although the micrografts (containing one or two hairs) and the minigrafts (with three to five hairs) sacrifice the greater density achieved with the original plugs, a more natural result can be achieved. However, more grafts are necessary to transplant an equal amount of hair.

PATIENT EVALUATION AND SELECTION

At the time of initial evaluation the basic question of "supply and demand" is critical. The ultimate relative size of the bald and donor areas must be thoroughly assessed and discussed with the patient so that reasonable expectations are clearly established.

In patients with class I baldness that will *never* extend beyond the frontal scalp, maximum density transplantation can be achieved. A very large number of grafts can be concentrated in a relatively small area of alopecia. However, in these patients with limited baldness we prefer to use flaps because the results can be achieved immediately. The patient can return to work within a week with hair of normal, uniform density. The equivalent of 5000 to 10,000 minigrafts and micrografts can be transferred in one surgery. Most younger men want maximum density as quickly as possible.

In patients with class II or class III baldness a thin but natural appearance can be achieved using only minigrafts and micrografts. Older men are more likely to accept this appearance. In men with extensive class III alopecia,

diffuse placement of micrografts will provide thin, "see-through" hair. Another alternative is the establishment of a limited frontal forelock as described by Marritt and Dzubow.[5,6] In all patients we must strive to achieve a careful balance between density and natural appearance. Acknowledging that most men who experience male pattern baldness will progress in class II or III alopecia, a thin undetectable appearance is a reasonable, honest goal.

ASSESSMENT OF DONOR SITE

Dark hair covers better than light hair, but tufting is more apparent because of the contrast with the underlying skin. Therefore micrografts or smaller minigrafts should be used in dark-haired patients to minimize tufting.

Hair texture including hair caliber and curl will affect the ultimate result. Curly or wavy hair gives the illusion of more body and greater density, when in fact this may not be the case. Of course, transplanting this type of hair is advantageous when the density is adequate. Although large-caliber hair gives the appearance of thicker hair, smaller grafts should be used because tufting is more obvious. The patient should also be aware that hair texture may change after punch grafting; transplanted hair may be more coarse and curly.

Although the results of punch grafting are improved with curly hair, the results of punch grafting in African-Americans and Caucasians with kinky hair frequently is not as satisfactory. In our practice we always recommend transposition flaps over punch grafts in these patients because they usually have poor density. It is also more difficult to harvest grafts from kinky hair without injuring the underlying follicles. Other surgeons who have had similar experiences during transplantation of kinky hair often refer these patients to our office for flap surgery.

ASSESSMENT OF RECIPIENT SITE

Each patient, regardless of age, must be evaluated in light of the ultimate pattern and extent of alopecia. With maximum density transplantation using standard, minigrafts or micrografts, the surgeon attempts to eliminate all the bald skin. However, this should be avoided in a young patient with limited alopecia. Unfavorable results occur when most of the available grafts are used to achieve the best possible density in a young patient when he has the potential for additional hair loss in the future. A very conservative approach is best with a man in his 20s or 30s. This can be accomplished using minigrafts and micrografts, leaving spaces between each smaller graft. In these patients grafting as a frontal forelock may be done initially. With extensive progression of the alopecia, this may become an isolated frontal forelock. If this does not occur, the donor area can be re-evaluated, and grafting can be done more densely in the frontal scalp. If donor scalp is adequate, grafting may proceed more posteriorly.

Punch grafting should be avoided in recipient areas with minimal thinning. The surgical insult of placing grafts in parts of the scalp with moderate-to-thin hair may actually accelerate the genetically determined progression of hair loss. These lost hairs usually start to regrow about 3 months later. However, they return as finer hairs with less density, and the net gain of the transplant procedure may be insignificant. A patient should be aware that the surgeon may have to transplant thinning portions of the scalp as if they were bald rather place a few grafts simply to increase the existing density.

HARVESTING TECHNIQUE

Debate is ongoing concerning the advantages and disadvantages of punch harvesting versus strip harvesting. Minigrafts can be harvested by bisecting or quadrisecting 4- or 5-mm round grafts. It is much more difficult to harvest micrografts from circular punches than from strips of donor hair. Regardless of graft size, we believe that strip harvesting is more efficient because less injury occurs to the donor hairs and therefore yield is increased. In addition, less residual scarring occurs in the donor area. All size grafts can be harvested from strips 1 to 4 mm wide.

GRAFT PLACEMENT

Micrografts are placed in small slits created with a sickle-type knife. With larger minigrafts, we prefer to place the grafts in small holes created by the removal of bald skin with 1- to 2-mm punches. In this way the amount of bald skin is decreased.

Some surgeons place these minigrafts in slits created with a No. 15 blade. Compression of these grafts always occurs because no bald skin is removed. A tufted appearance with abnormal density may occur, especially in patients with coarse, dark hair.

POSTOPERATIVE COURSE

Analgesics are necessary the evening of the surgery; pain is common in the donor area. Methylprednisolone is given over 6 days postoperatively. This will minimize the edema and ecchymosis of the forehead and eyes when hair replacement has been done in the frontal scalp. By controlling the amount of swelling, the surgeon also minimizes postoperative pain.

The dressing is removed 48 hours after surgery. The patient is instructed to wash the hair daily, obviously being gentle in the recipient area so the grafts are not dislodged. With smaller grafts scabbing and crusting are kept to a minimum. The patient is advised to avoid strenuous activities for 1 week after surgery. Sutures in the donor wound are removed in 1 week.

COMPLICATIONS

Serious complications are relatively few, and when they occur, are most often a result of poor planning or poor technique. A hairline that has been placed too low or hairlines that are blunted and rounded at the frontotemporal junction can be very difficult to correct. Scalp reductions, coronal incisions with a forehead lift, or excision with repositioning the grafts will improve the appearance of the hairline, but the ideal result is rarely achieved. Random orientation of the grafts will make styling almost impossible. These transplants can be cut again and repositioned. These are complications that should be avoided. Poor hair growth or lack of growth may result from inadequate circulation in the recipient area, but most often is the result of placing too many grafts in one procedure. Although mega sessions of 1000 to 3000 grafts are done, it is still uncertain how many can be done without compromising yield. Parameters such as the size of the graft used and the size of the recipient area are still being evaluated. Poor hair growth may also result if the grafts are not kept moist or the fat is aggressively trimmed from the deep surface of the transplants.

Bleeding can be troublesome, but gentle pressure will usually provide hemostasis. The occasional site of persistent bleeding can be controlled with a suture or the use of oxidized cellulose gauze.

Although a few cases of infection after hair transplantation have been reported, the excellent blood supply of the scalp makes this an unusual complication. Prescribing prophylactic antibiotics is not necessary.

A decrease in scalp sensation and even numbness always occurs after transplantation. In most cases relatively normal sensation gradually returns over several months.

ALOPECIA REDUCTION

In 1976 Blanchard and Blanchard[7] published their experience with alopecia reduction surgery, which was a technique similar to that described by Hunt[8] in 1926. They excised bald paramedian scalp up to 3-cm wide and 7- to 10-cm long. They waited 4 to 6 weeks between reductions and performed as many as six procedures in some patients. In 1978 Sparkhul[9] and Stough and Webster[10] presented their experience with scalp reductions with midline longitudinal excisions. Since then, Unger and Unger[11] in 1978, Bosley et al[12] in 1979, and Fleming and Mayer[13] in 1980 have presented their modifications and refinements of the Blanchard technique. Alt[14] presented and published his paramedian method of scalp reduction

in 1980. In 1984 Marzola[15] described his method of extensive scalp reductions, including ligation of the occipital arteries with stretching of the temporal-parietal-occipital scalp superiorly and anteriorly. He performed this procedure with paramedian incisions on each side at different sessions to maintain blood supply to the posterior scalp. In 1984, Bradshaw[16] extended the Marzola incision around the entire superior margin of the fringe, elevating and advancing the entire temporal-parietal-occipital scalp bilaterally at the same sitting. In 1988, Unger[17,18] described a very high incidence of necrosis with this technique. In 1986, Brandy[19,20] described the bilateral occipitoparietal flap and subsequently the bitemporal and the modified bitemporal flap. Although Brandy[21,22] significantly decreased the size of necrosis at the nuchal ridge with horizontal "incision ligation" of the occipital arteries before scalp lifting, he virtually eliminated this complication by performing "vertical incision" ligation of both occipital arteries 4 to 8 weeks before the actual extensive scalp-lifting procedure. At present Brandy will perform the extensive reduction in only 10% of his patients when he wants to achieve anterior movement of the frontotemporal scalp (Brandy, personal communication, July 1997). Marzola[23] continues the extensive scalp-lifting procedure with an "M-shaped" incision at the superior margin of the fringe with identification and preservation of the occipital arteries. However, he no longer attempts to eliminate the midscalp baldness, which causes a midline scar with divergent hair growth. He now reduces the bald area and treats the residual alopecia with grafts.

In 1993, Frechet[24] described his extender. The device consists of two thick elastic bands placed under the scalp and attached to the fringe on each side with metal clips. By raising the fringe hair before reductions, more bald skin could be removed and the wound could be closed with minimal tension.

With the development and refinement of minigrafts and micrografts, most surgeons who have used reductions before punch grafting have changed their philosophy about this technique. Some no longer do reductions; very few attempt to eliminate the midscalp and crown alopecia.

PATIENT SELECTION
Alopecia Reduction With Hair Transplantation

Scalp reductions and the use of the large 4 mm grafts were appropriate when the surgeon's goal was maximum bald skin removal. After reductions, the grafts could be concentrated in a smaller bald area, decreasing the "doll's hair" appearance. However, because most men with alopecia ultimately have more extensive baldness, maximum density without the unnatural pluggy look is not possible.

With minigrafts and micrografts, the tufted appearance is lessened. Therefore placement of smaller grafts with a more uniform, thin, natural appearance is a more reasonable goal. However, density must be sacrificed when using the technique.

With the advent of minigrafts and micrografts, the disadvantages of scalp reduction surgery have become more apparent as follows.

1. *Unnatural hair direction as the baldness progresses.* Hair direction at the superior margin of the temporal and the parietal fringe changes from anterior (the natural direction of hair on top of the head) to vertical (the hair is directed toward the ears). Because the vertically oriented fringe is elevated superiorly with reduction surgery, this hair will grow in opposite directions on top of the scalp. Also, the angle between the hair shaft and the skin on the side of the head is much more acute than it is on top of the head. Therefore, after reduction, the hair will lie much flatter in the midscalp.

2. *Scars.* Even with ideal maturation of the reduction scar, it may be visible. If not hidden with transplants in the scar line, the patient must carefully style his hair at all times to hide the scalp scar. With adequate grafting to hide the scar, the density may be greater over the scar than the surrounding scalp, where thin-

ner or see-through hair is present. The surgeon may be forced to use grafts in the posterior scar instead of concentrating them in the frontal or forelock region.

3. *Stretch back.* With stretching of the bald scalp, maximum tension as a result of the scalp reduction is placed in the tissue adjacent to the incision line. The amount of stretching of the bald scalp after reduction has generally been found to be in the magnitude of 10 to 20%, and it has been reported as high as 30 to 40%.[25] Therefore it is difficult to justify the extent of improvement with alopecia reduction when the surgeon's goal is a thinner, more uniform appearance, not maximum bald skin removal.

We use alopecia reduction with or without expansion before transplantation only in men with limited baldness when the ultimate extent of baldness is present or clearly defined. The best results are achieved in patients with anteriorly directed hair at the superior margin of the fringe. For these patients divergent hair growth will not be present after alopecia reduction.

Alopecia Reductions Before Fleming/Mayer Flaps

Although we rarely use alopecia reductions before hair transplantation, we frequently use this technique before development and rotation of a Fleming/Mayer flap. The reduction scar will be eliminated with flap rotation. We obviously decrease the size of the bald area to be removed with a flap, but, more importantly, we expand the donor area. A smaller percentage of the donor scalp is removed with the flap so we can achieve more uniform distribution of the scalp hair after completion of hair replacement surgery. In addition, we are able to design a longer flap when necessary and stay away from the thin hair at the superior border of the donor scalp.

The reductions before Fleming/Mayer flaps are not advised in patients with tight scalps. A certain amount of elasticity will be lost during the alopecia reduction, which may make it difficult to close the donor defect at the time of flap rotation. In these patients, we use tissue expansion before flap development and rotation.

Alopecia Reductions
After Fleming/Mayer Flaps

After Fleming/Mayer flaps have been moved into place, the remaining bald skin can be excised, stretching the flaps by more than 50% in some cases. The typical 4.0-cm wide flap may be stretched from 6 to 7.5 cm in width. In patients with only frontal baldness, reductions may be done behind the hairline flap if necessary or when baldness progresses. Also crown scalp reductions are performed behind the second flap to reduce the bald area in the vertex.

CONTRAINDICATION TO ALOPECIA REDUCTION
Patients With Tight Scalps

Alopecia reduction is most useful in patients with good scalp elasticity. Conversely patients with very tight scalps are not good candidates for this procedure because the amount of gain does not justify the time and expense involved. Fortunately, this is a very small percentage of people.

Patients Older Than 50 With Only Frontal Loss

Older patients with no evidence of midscalp and crown thinning will not benefit from a midline reduction, which does nothing for frontal alopecia.

Young Patients With Only Frontal Loss

If any evidence of thinning within the midscalp or crown exists, a midline alopecia reduction would be considered before flap surgery. However, the surgical intervention with the midline reduction may accelerate the genetically programmed progression of alopecia. These reductions should not be performed if it is possible that the future progression of loss will not be cosmetically significant. Alopecia reduction may be performed at a later date if necessary.

TECHNIQUE

The procedure is normally done with local anesthesia, but if a patient is extremely apprehensive, intravenous sedation may be used. Before flaps and punch transplantation surgery, we use the inverted Y incision. The central line of the incision extends through the frontal and midscalp region. The lateral limbs of the Y are placed at the anterior margin of the crown.

With a No. 10 blade, the scalp incision is made parallel to the hair follicles, if present, and through the underlying galea. The skin is elevated and the dissection carried in the avascular plane between the galea and the periosteum.

After the dissection is completed, the appropriate amount of bald skin is excised. In most cases, one can accurately gauge the amount of tissue to be excised with the reduction on the basis of the preoperative mobility of the scalp. Sometimes more or less scalp is removed than one would expect. Therefore skin should not be removed before completion of the undermining to avoid creating a defect that is too large to comfortably close. We have never found galeatomies (incisions in the galea) to be effective in significantly increasing the amount of tissue removed at each session.

The galea is approximated in a sequential fashion by placement of multiple 0 polydioxanone (PDS) inverted interrupted sutures along the course of the incision. The epidermal margins of the wound are closed with staples.

POSTOPERATIVE COURSE

Oxycodone is used postoperatively for pain. Methylprednisolone is prescribed for 6 days after surgery to minimize the edema, bruising, and pain. A direct relationship exists between the tension placed on the wound closure and the severity of postoperative pain, which usually lasts 4 to 6 hours.

The fluff and kling dressing is removed the day after surgery. Patients are instructed to wash their hair daily. A subjective feeling of scalp tightness will last for approximately 2 weeks. The staples are removed 12 to 14 days after surgery. The scalp will continue to loosen for 3 to 4 months.

COMPLICATIONS

Of all the cosmetic procedures we do, scalp reduction surgery has the smallest incidence of complications. Only one patient, 3 days after surgery, had a hematoma develop. This was drained through the wound without any problem. One staphylococcus infection in a hospital employee, has been encountered. It was confined to a small portion of the incision site, which was drained and treated without sequelae. On rare occasions, a wound will spread several millimeters during scar maturation. Scar revision has been done on two separate patients who had reductions done in conjunction with hair transplantation. These reductions did not have an excess amount of tension on the wound closure nor did the patients have a history of keloid or hypertrophic scar formation. A good scar is usually obtainable with proper wound closure. The tension should be taken up at the galea level with maximum eversion of skin edges.

FLEMING MAYER-FLAP (MODIFIED AFTER JURI)

When Juri[26] published his experience with more than 400 temporoparietaloccipital flaps in 1975, we were immediately interested because of our dissatisfaction with the punch graft technique. We believed that his results were superior to those of the punch graft method that we used at that time. Our initial work was based on Juri's flap. Although many modifications have been made, the following basic elements of his design and technique are still used in our flap.

1. The flap is based on the posterior branch of the superficial temporal artery.
2. Two delays are always performed.
3. The flap is long enough to traverse the entire bald area whenever possible.
4. The flaps are designed so that a flap can be taken from each side.

The Fleming-Mayer flap has been modified in the following ways.

1. Flap width varies from 3.75 to 4.5 cm.
2. The superior margin of the flap is cut in an irregular design to create a more natural hairline.

3. The-hairline is designed with frontotemporal recessions to avoid a rounded or apelike appearance.
4. Midline scalp reductions are performed before flap rotation except in patients with baldness limited to the frontal scalp and patients with extremely tight scalps.
5. Tissue expansion of the donor scalp is frequently used before flap development and rotation. Flap width is 5 to 7 cm after tissue expansion.
6. A donor graft of bald skip removed from the recipient site is frequently used to help close the donor area to avoid raising the postauricular hairline and assist in the closure of the donor defect in a tight scalp.
7. With second flaps the anterior margin of the recipient site is delayed at the same time as the first delay.
8. A browlift (forehead rhytidectomy) is frequently performed before the Fleming-Mayer flap procedure.

FLAP DESIGN

The posterior branch of the superficial temporal artery is identified with the Doppler flowmeter. The inferior edge of the flap starts at a point approximately 3.0 cm above the anterior attachment to the helix. The superior edge of the flap begins 4.0 cm anterior and superior to this point at an angle of 30 to 45 degree to the horizontal, so the flap is centered over the superficial temporal artery (Fig. 26–2A,B). The proposed lines of the incision extend posteriorly and superiorly through the temporoparietal region and then curve inferiorly into the occipital scalp. The width of the flap is constant throughout its length. We must anticipate the total extent of alopecia when designing the flap so that the superior edge of the flap that will establish the new hairline is not taken from an area of the scalp where further hair loss will occur.

The distal two thirds of the flap will form the new hairline. Therefore the design of this part of the flap should correspond to the shape of the proposed hairline. The superior margin of the distal two thirds of the flap is cut in an irregular fashion to mimic the naturally occurring irregular hairline.

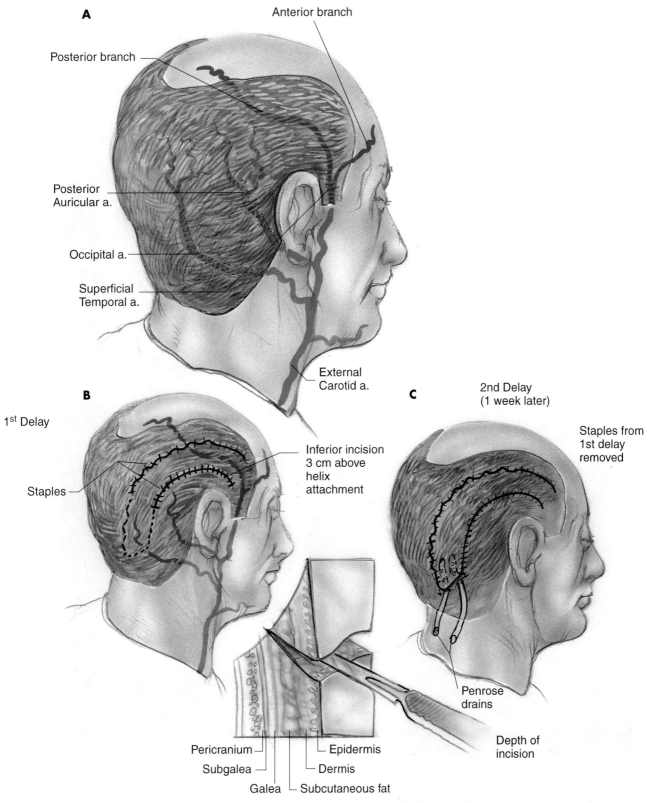

Figure 26–2. (A) Arterial blood supply of scalp, showing course of superficial temporal artery, posterior auricular artery, and occipital artery. **(B)** First delay of Fleming-Mayer flap. Parallel incisions made along three fourths of flap. Incision is closed. The superior border of flap is cut in an irregular fashion to mimic the naturally occurring hairline. The posterior branch of the superficial temporal artery is centered in the base of the flap. **(C)** One week later, second delay of Fleming-Mayer flap. Distal 25% of flap is incised and tail is elevated from deep tissue. Occipital artery is severed. Incision is closed with staples. *(Continued on pp. 476 to 478.)*

TECHNIQUE

The first two delays are performed with local anesthesia. Intravenous sedation is occasionally used for the apprehensive patient. In the first delay procedure incisions are made parallel to the hair follicles of the flap along three fourths of its length (Fig. 26–2B). The incision is closed with staples. The dressing is removed the next morning, the scalp shampooed, and the patient can resume normal activities. One week later, the second delay procedure is performed. Incisions are made at the margin of the distal flap, which is elevated from the underlying tissues to sever the vessels that penetrate the deep layers of the scalp posterior and inferior to the galeal attachment at the level of the nuchal ridge. Penrose drains are placed under the tail of the flap, and the incision is closed with staples

(Fig. 26–2C). The Penrose drains and bandages are removed in the office the next morning. These delays enhance the circulation through the base of the flap, which is frequently 25 to 29 cm long.

One week later (2 weeks after the first procedure) the flap is rotated into place in the office outpatient surgery center with the patient under general inhalation anesthesia.

The flap is elevated in the subgaleal plane and kept moist at all times with saline solution. The inferior margin of the donor defect is raised in the subgaleal plane until the lower limit of the hair-bearing scalp is reached. The dissection is then continued subcutaneously as in a facelift operation. The postauricular skin is elevated to the helical rim, and the dissection is carried as far inferiorly as necessary to close the donor defect in a tension-free manner (Fig. 26–2D). The frontal hairline incision is then made,

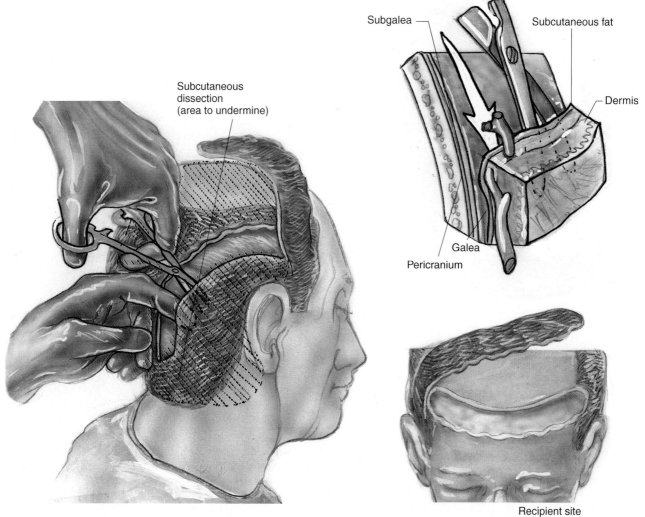

Figure 26–2. *(Continued from p. 475.)* **(D)** Transposition of flap 1 week later. Extent of undermining for donor closure is outlined. *(Continued on pp. 477 and 478.)*

bevelling the cut in an inferior direction to correspond to the angle of the cut on the superior border of the flap. The frontal, parietal, and occipital scalp posterior to this incision is elevated deep to the galea so that it can be rotated posteriorly and inferiorly to help in closure of the donor wound.

The donor wound is closed with 0 PDS sutures at the galeal level. The skin edges are then approximated using staples (Fig. 26–2E). The donor defect should be closed in a tension-free manner. Frequently we will use a full-thickness skin graft harvested from the recipient scalp to avoid undue tension on the donor closure, which would caused telogen or necrosis. The graft also minimizes elevation of the postauricular hairline. The graft acts as a physiologic dressing that can be removed after wound maturation with return of the scalp laxity (Fig. 26–2F).

Two millimeters of the anterior border of the flap is de-epithelialized, and the flap is sutured to the forehead with a 5-0 polypropylene suture (Fig. 26–3). Hair will grow from follicles buried beneath the hairline skin closure, establishing a new hairline and camouflaging the scar (Fig. 26–4). The appropriate amount of frontal scalp skin is removed, and the remaining incisions are closed without tension with staples (Fig. 26–2F).

POSTOPERATIVE COURSE

A dressing is in place for 4 to 5 days after surgery. The hairline sutures are removed 6 to 7 days postoperatively, and the staples are removed approximately 1 week later.

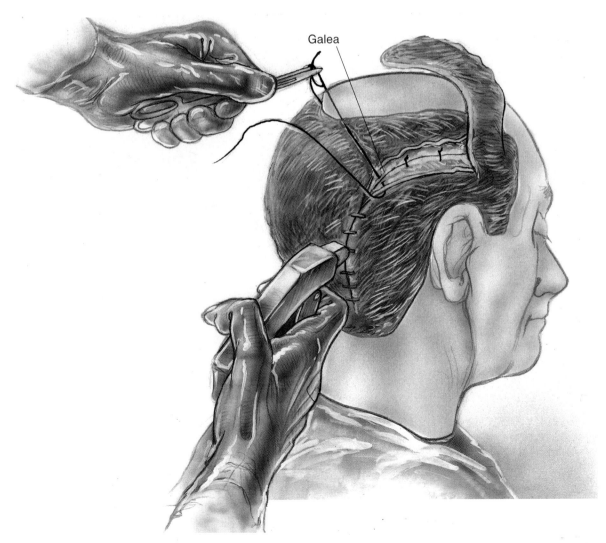

Figure 26–2. *(Continued from pp. 475 and 476.)* **(E)** Galea is approximated in tension-free manner before skin edges are approximated with staples. *(Continued on p. 478.)*

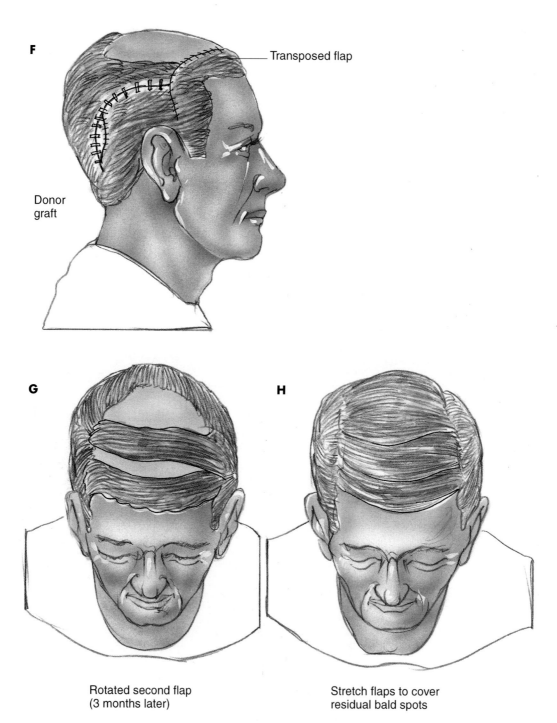

F

Transposed flap

Donor graft

G

Rotated second flap
(3 months later)

H

Stretch flaps to cover
residual bald spots

Figure 26–2. *(Continued from pp. 475 to 477.)* **(F)** Flap is sutured across hairline. Excess bald skin is removed in recipient site. A full-thickness skin graft is frequently used to avoid tension on donor closure and minimize elevation of postauricular hairline. **(G)** Second flap can be rotated 3 mo later or when baldness progresses to midscalp and vertex. **(H)** Residual bald skin between flaps and posterior to second flap can be excised by stretching flaps so all bald skin can be removed in most patients.

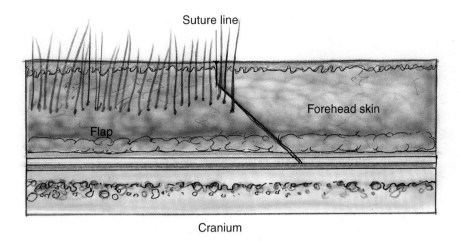

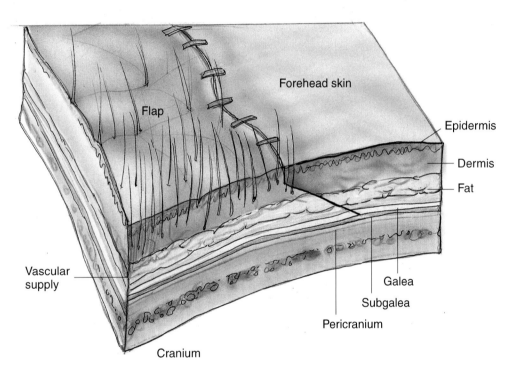

Figure 26–3. Hairline closure. Cross section through junction of flap and forehead skin. Anterior border of flap is de-epithelialzed. Growth of hair from follicles buried beneath epidermal closure establishes new hairline and camouflages scar.

If the patient is from out of town, the staples may be removed in their home town.

Eyelid and forehead edema frequently occurs after procedures performed in the frontal scalp. This problem has been virtually eliminated with the use of methyl-

prednisolone, 24 mg, on the day of surgery. The dosage is gradually tapered over the next 5 days. There may be tenderness of the ear on the donor side that persists for a few days because of sensitivity of the cartilage after surgical manipulation. Some swelling and ecchymosis of the

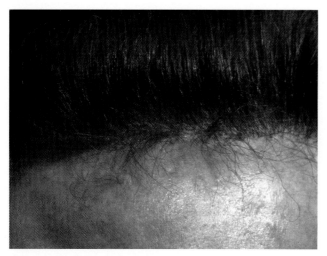

Figure 26–4. Hairline more than 1 year postoperatively. Hair growth through undetectable scar with normal uniform density of irregular flap hairline.

lateral neck in the area of undermining will occur. Stiffness of the neck will last for several weeks. Patients may return to work 1 week after surgery. There will be erythema of the hairline incision for 6 to 8 weeks as hair grows through and in front of this line.

Although serious complications are possible with any flap procedure, they are rare. Minor complications can and do occur but are easily treated. Complications with the Fleming-Mayer flap are classified into two groups: those occurring in patients with normal scalp circulation and those occurring in patients with compromised or impaired scalp circulation.

Patients With Normal Circulation

Flap necrosis is the most severe complication that can occur with this surgery. Even when we have seen flaps done by other surgeons with little experience, loss of even a small portion of the end of the flap is rarely present. This has occurred three times our experience with more than 3000 Fleming-Mayer flaps. In one patient this was a result of trauma after the second delay; in the second patient, it was due to heavy cigarette smoking; in the third patient the cause was never determined. In all these patients, the loss of the distal portion of the flap was 3.0 cm or less.

This can be reconstructed with a small flap from the opposite side to complete the hairline or serial excision of the alopecia, depending on the extent of loss.

If the donor area is closed under excessive tension, necrosis of the surrounding donor scalp may occur, usually inferior to the donor defect. This is a rare complication. If any question exists about undue tension, a small skin graft harvested from the recipient scalp can be used to assist in the donor closure. This can be excised after return of scalp laxity.

We have never seen permanent hair loss without associated skin necrosis in the flap or donor scalp. Temporary hair loss (telogen effluvium) almost always occurs with hair transplantation but is rarely seen in flap surgery. Hair within the portion of the tail of the flap or the donor scalp may undergo temporary shock. Hair growth resumes in 2 to 3 months.

Hematoma formation is unusual but, if present, will occur within several hours of surgery. Therefore all patients are carefully evaluated before discharge from the recovery room. In all cases this complication occurred in the donor area and was immediately evacuated. No long-term problem occurred after this complication.

Infection, always involving staphylococcus organisms, also has been very rare because of excellent scalp circulation. When the infection occurs after the second delay, the wound is drained, the patient placed on antibiotics, and the transposition delayed. All cases were successfully treated without permanent sequelae.

Patients With Impaired Scalp Circulation

The complications previously described may also occur in patients with compromised scalp circulation. Patients who have had previous hair transplantation with scarring in the donor scalp, nylon fiber implantation with infection, or forehead lifts with interruption of the superficial temporal artery carry a greater risk because of their impaired circulation.

In patients who have had hair transplantation we try to avoid taking the flap from scalp that has been scarred by transplant harvesting. If this is not possible, we frequently use tissue expansion before development and rotation of the Flaming-Mayer flap.

Patients who have had nylon fiber implantation have greater risk because of impaired circulation or chronic infection.

Two of our patients had the superficial temporal artery ligated as part of a previous forehead rhytidectomy performed elsewhere. In both of these patients the flap looked normal before rotation. However, both had necrosis of the distal 3 cm of their flaps develop. Even with two delays, we believe significant risk of distal flap necrosis exists. Therefore we no longer do the Fleming-Mayer flap in patients in whom the posterior branch of the superficial temporal artery is not intact.

ADDITIONAL PROCEDURES

A dog-ear will occur at the junction of the new flap hairline and the existing temporal hairline because of flap stiffness and the creation of the temporal "gulf." This gulf establishes the normal fronto-temporal recession. Six weeks after rotation of the flap, the dog-ear is divided at the junction of the frontal and temporal hairlines. The divided ends are rotated posteriorly and superiorly, taking advantage of the excess hair-bearing skin within the flap.

When necessary, a second flap may be rotated from the opposite side months after the initial flap rotation (Fig. 26–2G). Depending on scalp laxity, approximately 3 cm of bald skin is left between the two flaps, which is later removed with scalp reductions and stretching of the anterior flap. Total excision of bald skin in the crown and vertex can be accomplished with scalp reductions and further stretching of the posterior flap (Fig. 26–2H). We have not attempted a third (retroauricular or occipital) flap described by Juri.

In patients with thick coarse hair or abruptness of the hairline, further refinement of the irregular trichophytic hairline can be achieved with the use of micrografts placed at the new hairline to soften the appearance (Fig. 26–5). This is done in approximately 10% of patients, although most patients are satisfied without their use.

During every consultation for hair replacement surgery, the eyelid-eyebrow complex should always be evaluated. If the patient would benefit from a browlift and forehead rhytidectomy, this should be done before hair replacement surgery. The scar in the frontal scalp

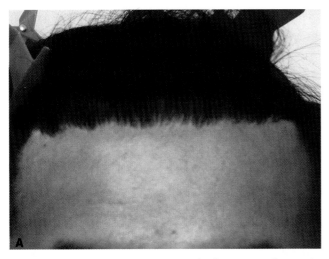
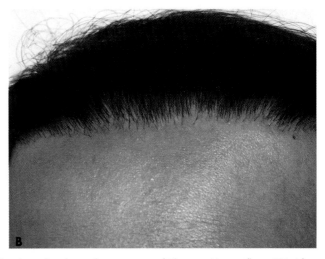

Figure 26–5. (A) Asian patient with abruptness of irregular trichophytic hairline after rotation of Fleming-Mayer flap. **(B)** After single session of micrografts to soften hairline. Patient has natural hairline with normal uniform density of frontal scalp.

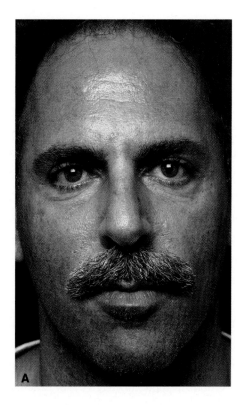 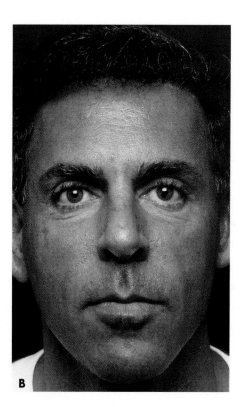

Figure 26–6. Patient with brow ptosis and frontal baldness. Patient had frontal rhytidectomy through frontal scalp incision followed by Fleming-Mayer flap 6 weeks later. **(A)** Preoperative. **(B)** After forehead rhytidectomy and Fleming-Mayer flap.

resulting from forehead rhytidectomy is temporary and will be eliminated with flap rotation 6 to 8 weeks later (Fig. 26–6).

OTHER SCALP FLAPS

With few exceptions, we believe the Fleming-Mayer techniwue is the best flap procedure for surgical hair replacement for most men. Limited indications exist for other transposition flaps.

INFERIORLY BASED TEMPOROPARIETAL FLAPS

Passot,[27] Elliot,[28] and Heimburger[29] described their application of this short flap. We presented our modifications in 1979. Temporoparietal flaps are narrower, shorter, inferiorly based flaps that are nondelayed and based on the posterior branch of the superficial temporal artery. They do not extend across the entire forehead. A second flap must be rotated from the contralateral side to complete the hairline.

Design

The flap, 2.5- to 3.0-cm wide, follows a gentle curve superiorly and posteriorly over the ear and then into the

parietal or anterior occipital scalp, depending on the length required. The first flap is cut long enough to extend beyond the midpoint of the new hairline, so risk of hair loss in the tail of the shorter second flap from the contralateral side is less. Furthermore, it is better to err on the side of making flaps longer than to be caught with flaps that are too short and therefore fail to join.

The tail of the first flap is designed to dovetail with the flap of the opposite side at an angle of 45 to 60 degrees. This angle will prevent the scar from being seen at the junction of the two flaps (Fig. 26–7).

Our design of the inferiorly based temporoparietal flap differs in several important respects from those described by other authors. Some have designed the flap without regard to the artery, and therefore its vascular supply is at risk. All scalp flaps should be axial whenever possible. This ensures maximum survival of the sensitive hair follicles and does not compromise flap design or make the procedure more difficult. Although narrowing of the base of the flap and delaying it have been described, we rarely delay these flaps. Narrowing of the base of the flap will decrease dog-ear formation at the point of flap rotation but may cause flap ischemia, neces-

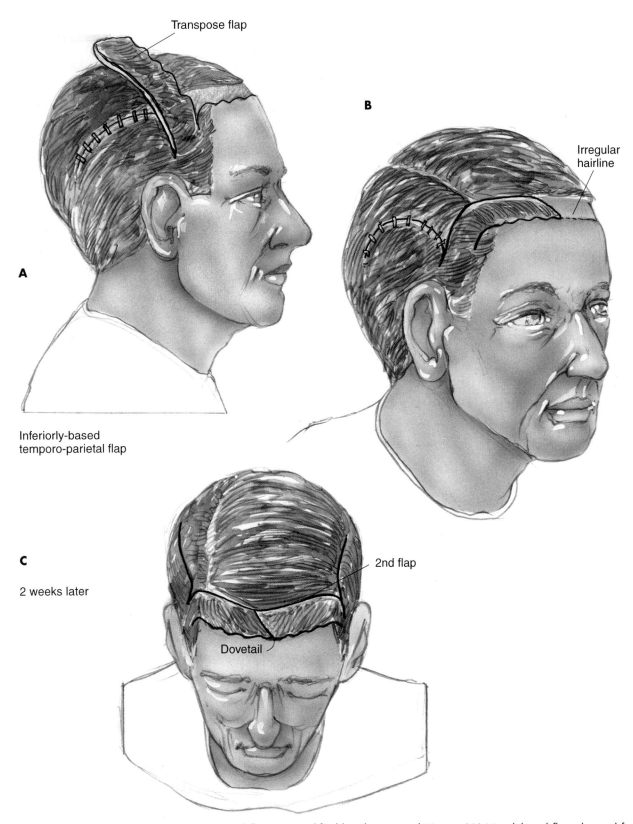

Figure 26–7. Inferiorly based temporo/parietal flaps as modified by Fleming and Mayer. **(A)** Nondelayed flap elevated from donor scalp. Only one flap performed at a time. Flap being transposed and donor area closed. **(B)** Well-defined frontotemporal recession with irregular hairline. Flap does not extend across entire forehead. Location of future second flap scratched so proper symmetry can be achieved. **(C)** Two weeks later, second flap from opposite side is used to complete hairline. Junction of flaps dovetailed to prevent visible scar.

sitating the delay procedure. The pedicle is the source of blood supply and decreasing its width may be risky.

The flaps are transposed 2 weeks apart. Although this has never occurred, if distal necrosis of the first flap did occur, the second flap may be delayed and extended to complete the hairline.

Disadvantages

The significant disadvantage of temporoparietal flaps is the fact that two temporoparietal flaps will give only one fourth as much coverage as two Fleming-Mayer flaps. Both sides of the donor scalp are used to establish a hairline. The baldness posterior to the flaps can be treated only with scalp reductions and punch grafts. In patients in whom baldness is more advanced or will be more advanced than frontal baldness, total or near total hair replacement cannot be achieved with temporoparietal flaps. This is possible with two Fleming-Mayer flaps followed by scalp reductions.

In our practice the short flaps are used primarily with individuals who wear hairpieces and are not candidates for hair replacement surgery. The short flaps produce the same natural hairline as the Fleming-Mayer flap, enabling individuals to improve the appearance achieved with hairpieces.

Surgical Technique

The surgical technique, including flap elevation (without delays), lateral scalp and neck dissection for donor closure, preparation of the recipient site, and flap placement, is identical to that previously described for the Fleming-Mayer flap.

The postoperative course, including dressings, suture removal, and morbidity, is also identical.

Complications

Infection, hematoma, and temporary or permanent hair loss are possible but rare complications. Necrosis and the resultant permanent hair loss, whether within the flap or donor area, would be the most serious complication. In our experience with short flap procedures only one instance of distal hair loss (1.5 cm in second short flap that had been traumatized postoperatively) occurred. When necrosis occurs in the distal portion of the second flap, it is more difficult to correct than in the Fleming-Mayer flap because hair loss occurs in the central portion of the hairline. The problem may be corrected by excising the area of alopecia and advancing the flaps medially to obtain complete closure. The area can also be punch grafted, although the cosmetic result is less desirable. Careful handling of the flap to avoid pressure on the flap or twisting of its base should ensure that the incidence of this complication is quite low.

Additional procedures

A second flap will be done 2 weeks later. A dog-ear will occur at the point of rotation at the junction of the frontal and temporal hairlines. With these smaller flaps, the dog-ear may spontaneously resolve. If necessary, the dog-ear revision can be performed approximately 6 weeks after flap rotation. Two or 3 months after the flaps have been rotated, they can be stretched with scalp reductions to increase their width by approximately 25%.

SUPERIORLY BASED PREAURICULAR AND POSTAURICULAR FLAPS

Nataf et al[30] described superiorly based preauricular and postauricular flaps. As originally described, the postauricular flap gives little advantage over the inferiorly based flaps previously described because the improvement in hair direction is minimal. Although the superiorly based preauricular flap has excellent hair direction after rotation, it is useful only for partial hairline restoration because the flap rarely reaches the midline. Using Marzola's technique[15] of extensive scalp reductions with anterior and superior enhancement of the temporal hairline, the surgeon can lengthen the donor area for the flap and at the same time shorten the intertemporal (hairline) distance. When used in this manner, the preauricular flap can reach the midline and beyond if scalp laxity permits adequate reduction before flap rotation.

Because we believe the indications for superiorly based flaps, whether preauricular or postauricular, are quite limited, we refer the reader to Nataf's and Marzola's descriptions of their techniques.

Disadvantages

These flaps have only one advantage over the other inferiorly based flaps: the hair grows in the anterior direction. This would be desirable if it were not for the following important disadvantages.

1. The Fleming-Mayer flap and most other inferiorly based flaps are axial flaps. The superiorly based temporoparietal flaps are random flaps and, therefore, more susceptible to necrosis. Marzola no longer performs the post-auricular flap in conjunction with his extensive lateral reductions because of compromised circulation within this longer flap. After his extensive lateral scalp reductions, Marzola now uses the preauricular flap or inferiorly based temporal parietal flaps if greater length is necessary (Marzola, personal communication, July 1997).
2. The hair in the distal end of these flaps, when taken from the preauricular hair just above the sideburn, is often of poor quality and low density.
3. If distal necrosis occurs, it results in alopecia in the center of the hairline that is more difficult to correct.
4. The temporal hairline is pulled posteriorly to close the donor defect and will appear more receded.
5. The donor defect can be difficult to close because it is vertically oriented. The donor closure of the Fleming-Mayer flap and the inferiorly based temporoparietal flaps are horizontal.
6. The most important drawback of the superiorly based flaps is the same as that with short inferiorly based temporal parietal flaps. Only 2.5 to 3 cm of alopecia in the frontal scalp is eliminated. The remaining alopecia posteriorly must be treated with scalp reductions or hair transplantation. We do not believe the final results compare with two Fleming-Mayer flaps (Fig. 26–8).

Indications for Superiorly Based Flaps as Modified by Fleming and Mayer

Despite the disadvantages of the superiorly based flaps, they are occasionally apropos in cases that meet the following requirements.

1. The patient must have only mild, fully established, frontal baldness and not be a candidate for the Fleming-Mayer flaps.
2. The temporal hairline must be very high, superiorly and anteriorly placed.
3. Good hair quality in the temporal scalp, including the preauricular area.
4. No punch graft or scalp reduction scars should be in the bald scalp superior and posterior to the flap base, which would compromise flap circulation.

With our modification of the superiorly based flaps, we use a rectangular tissue expander placed in the temporal scalp before flap development and rotation in all cases.

If hair direction obtained with the inferiorly based flaps were a serious problem, the superiorly based flaps would have much more advantage. However, in practice, a change in hair direction rarely presents more than a minor styling problem to the patient.

TISSUE EXPANSION

Tissue expansion is the single greatest advance in scalp reconstruction in our lifetime. Selected applications also exist in aesthetic scalp surgery. Argenta,[31] Radovan,[32] Manders at al,[33] and Anderson[34] made significant contributions to tissue expansion before bald scalp removal in scalp reconstruction and the treatment of male pattern baldness. Along with Kabaker et al,[35] and Anderson, we presented our experience with expansion at the Sixth International Symposium on Hair Replacement Surgery in 1988.

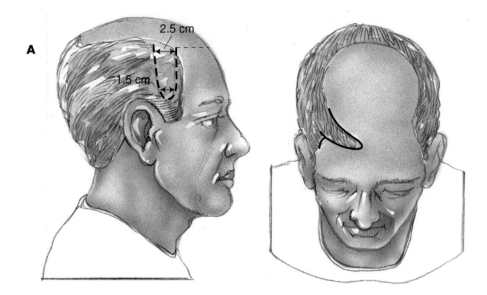

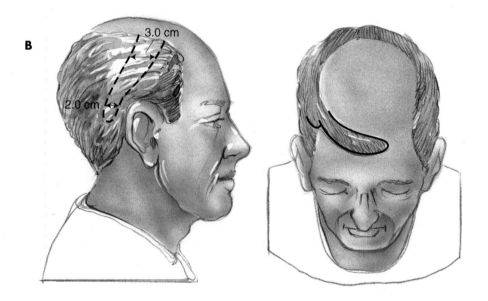

Figure 26–8. (A) Preauricular flaps. Closure of donor area may be difficult. Flap is quite narrow and usually will not reach the midline except when used in conjunction with extensive lateral scalp reductions before flap rotation. **(B)** Postauricular flap rarely crosses entire hairline. Circulation compromised because flap is superiorly based.

Although manufactured by different companies, we use the expanders from PMT Corporation (Chanhassen, MN). They are available in any size or shape. We have developed three expanders for use in the treatment of male pattern baldness. The type we use most commonly is the Fleming-Mayer type A expander. This "banana-shaped" expander, used in conjunction with the Fleming-Mayer flap, is placed under the hair-bearing scalp, where the flap will be harvested. The type B expander is a shorter version of the type A and is used in conjunction with short inferiorly based temporoparietal flaps. The type C expander is a rectangular expander used with the superiorly based temporal flaps. Types A, B, and C expanders are regular stock items at PMT. All are designed with a smooth surface and remote port.

Technique

Expander placement is done with the patient under local anesthesia. After 10 days, the staples are removed, and the expansion begins with injections of normal saline twice a week for 10 to 12 weeks. For convenience, most patients will have friends or family members inject the expander whether they live in our community or distant locations. For example, with the type A expander, in which we inject a total of 350 mL, 15 to 20 mL is injected each time. With the smaller expanders, less saline is injected each time, but the time necessary to achieve full expansion is typically the same.

Application of Tissue Expansion

Tissue expansion with alopecia reduction

We rarely do reductions before punch graft transplantation because we do not use maximum transplanting procedures in patients with Class II or Class III alopecia. We will use tissue expansion as an adjunctive procedure with scalp reductions in patients with the following characteristics.

1. Patients with tight scalps. Most patients with loose scalps would prefer to undergo two or three scalp reduction procedures rather than tissue expansion.
2. Patients with a fully established pattern of alopecia, where the size of the involved area will not increase with age.
3. Patients in whom the superior fringe hair in the midscalp is directed anteriorly and not inferiorly. This permits the surgeon to eliminate the baldness without resultant midscalp divergent hair growth.
4. Patients in whom hair transplantation rather than flaps will be used to treat the frontal hair loss and reestablish the hairline.

Expanders are placed bilaterally to increase the size of the hair-bearing scalp. After expansion, the fringe on each side is advanced superiorly to meet in the midline.

Tissue Expansion with the Fleming-Mayer Flap

The type A expander is used to stretch the donor scalp before flap design and rotation. We use tissue expansion in combination with this flap in the following cases.

1. In a patient with an extremely tight scalp.
2. In a marginal candidate with narrow fringe and dense hair.
3. In a patient requiring a great deal of length to cover a large intertemporal (hairline) distance.
4. In a patient who wishes no change in the configuration of the postauricular hairline, which will be raised slightly when closing the donor defect without tissue expansion.
5. In a patient in whom the size of the donor scalp will be increased to avoid taking the flap from scalp scarred as a result of trauma or previous HTP harvesting.

After the expansion is completed, the Fleming-Mayer flap is twice delayed because we do without expansion. The balloon is removed at the time of flap rotation.

Tissue expansion with superiorly based temporal flaps

The type C rectangular expander is placed under the temporal scalp. After expansion, a 3-cm flap is then outlined and incisions are made around the entire margin of the flap. One week later the flap is transposed. As previously stated, the superiorly based flaps are rarely used.

Morbidity

The most significant disadvantage of tissue expansion is the cosmetic deformity, which is most obvious the last 2 to 3 weeks of expansion, when the size of the expander becomes quite large. We have had professionals such as physicians lawyers, and entertainers work right up to the time of transposition with long hair and careful hair styling. As long as the expander is not overinflated at each injection, discomfort is minimal.

Complications

Postoperative complications such as hematoma and infection are rare. Port leaks have occurred as a result of poor injection technique, but this can be avoided with careful education.

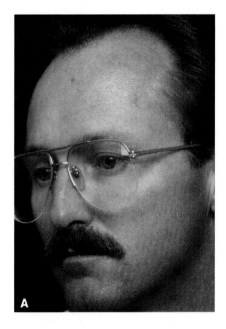
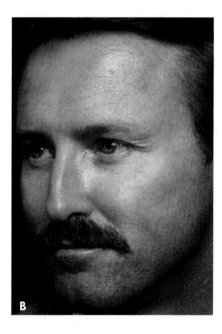

Figure 26–9. (A) Patient with frontal loss. **(B)** After Fleming-Mayer flap rotation. Uniform density allows freedom of styling. Hair direction within flap does not compromises styling.

CHOOSING A PROCEDURE

In our practice most men select the transposition flaps after all alternative techniques are presented. We have a bias toward these flaps because the results are immediate. The temporary hair loss that accompanies punch grafting usually does not occur with flaps. The hair texture and density within the flap are identical to the donor scalp. No additional hair replacement is ever needed in the area of the flap. Uniform density means the hair can be combed in any style, even straight back. It looks natural,

regardless of where the hair is parted, even if it is wind-blown or wet (Fig. 26–9).

FRONTAL BALDNESS ONLY (CLASS I)

In patients with an established pattern of alopecia limited to the frontal scalp, the Fleming-Mayer flap can be done with immediate, total elimination of the baldness (Fig. 26–10). If one flap does not eliminate all the patient's frontal baldness, scalp reduction(s) can be done behind the flap (Fig. 26–11). As previously

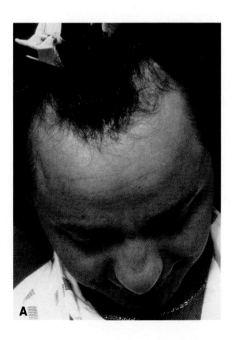
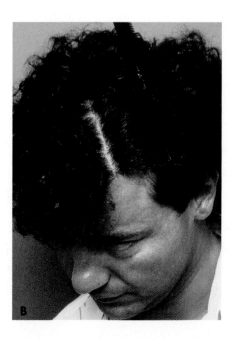

Figure 26–10. (A) Bilateral fronto-temporal loss. **(B)** Single Fleming-Mayer flap has totally eliminated baldness.

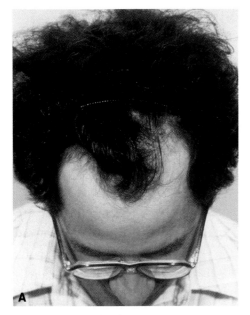
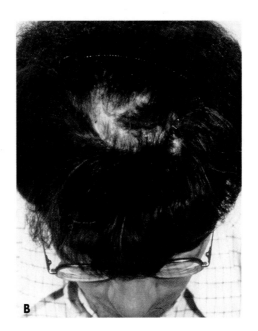
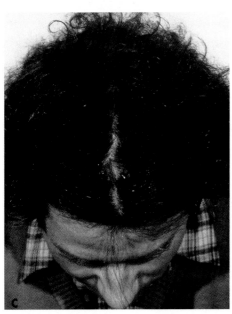

Figure 26-11. (A) Thirty-year-old patient with frontal baldness and thinning of frontal tuft. **(B)** After one Fleming-Mayer flap, residual baldness persists posterior to flap. **(C)** After scalp reduction behind frontal flap. Flap blends well with remaining hair in midscalp and crown. A second flap is available for future use if alopecia progresses.

described, these patients can have maximum density transplantation, but they will sacrifice density and take from 1 to 2 years to achieve a completed result. Two short flaps will also eliminate the baldness in these patients, but two short flaps are more work than a single Fleming-Mayer flap.

CROWN BALDNESS ONLY (CLASS IV)

The same considerations that apply to class I patients apply to class IV patients. This area can be treated with punch graft transplantation over a 2-year period. The same area can be treated with a single flap, with or with-

out subsequent scalp reductions. The improved density, texture, and hair direction achieved with the flap make this procedure advantageous for most patients with crown baldness.

FRONTAL AND MIDSCALP BALDNESS (CLASS II)

Class II baldness is the least common of the four balding patterns described. Two Fleming-Mayer flaps can be done on these patients with or without scalp reductions after flap transposition with total elimination of the bald skin with maximum density.

FRONTAL TO OCCIPITAL BALDNESS (CLASS III)

Most patients have or will have class III male pattern baldness. In general, patients with this degree of loss are least satisfied with punch grafts. As previously stated, a compromise must be made with graft placement because of the large bald area. For class III patients who select grafting, the most natural result can be achieved with (1) the diffuse placement of minigrafts or small micrografts resulting in thin "see-through" hair or (2) the creation of a frontal forelock. Two Fleming-Mayer flaps combined with scalp reductions between the flaps and behind the second flap will eliminate the baldness in most patients (Fig. 26–12). If we do not eliminate all the alopecia, residual baldness is limited to the vertex and crown, a natural pattern of alopecia in some virgin scalps.

CONCLUSION

In this chapter we discussed all methods of hair replacement surgery. No single best procedure exists because the application of these techniques should be individualized. Before consultation, the patient is given general information consisting of a printed brochure and video tape. Patient satisfaction, the ultimate goal, can be achieved only after a careful, honest discussion with the patient during consultation. A preference for one procedure over another is based on the results that can be achieved with that procedure for a given patient. The patient should clearly understand the advantages and disadvantages of each technique so he can make an educated, well-informed decision, choosing the approach that best fulfills his expectations.

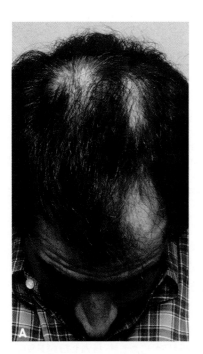
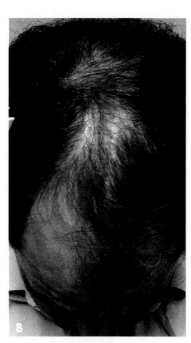
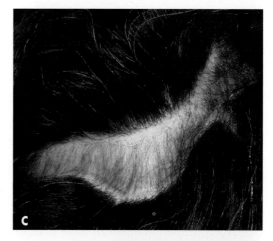
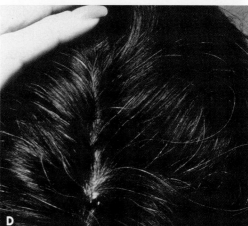

Figure 26–12. (A) Patient with class III baldness. **(B)** After midline scalp reduction. **(C)** After two Fleming-Mayer flaps. **(D)** After reductions between flaps and posterior to second flap with total elimination of alopecia.

PEARLS

- Baldness is *progressive*. All decisions regarding treatment should be based on the *ultimate* extent of alopecia.
- If a patient wants thick uniform density with more immediate results, transposition flaps are the alternative of choice.
- Tissue expansion with advancement or transposition flaps is beneficial in patients with tight scalps, in marginal candidates with a narrow fringe, and patients with compromised circulation of the donor scalp.
- Although micrografts and minigrafts sacrifice the greater density achieved with the traditional 4- or 5-mm plugs, a more natural result can be achieved.
- Regardless of graft size, strip harvesting is more efficient than punch harvesting in hair transplant surgery.

REFERENCES

1. Hamilton JB. Patterned loss of hair in men: Types and incidences. Ann NY Acad Sci. 1951; 53:708.
2. Norwood OT. Hair transplant surgery. Springfield, Ill: Charles C Thomas; 1973.
3. Okuda S. The study of clinical experiments of hair transplantation, Jpn J Dermatol Urol. Oct 1939; German abstract, klinishe und experimentelle untersuchunhen uber die transplantation von lebenden haaren, Jpn J Dermatol Urol. 1939; 46(6):135.
4. Orentreich N. Autographs in alopecia and other selected dermatological conditions. Ann NY Acad Sci. 1959; 83:463.
5. Marritt E, Dzubow LM. The isolated frontal forelock. J Dermatol Surg. 1995; 21:523–538.
6. Marritt E, Dzubow LM. A redefinition of male pattern baldness and its treatment implications. J Dermatol Surg. 1995; 21:123–135.
7. Blanchard G, Blanchard B. La reduction tonsurale (detonsuration): Concept nouveau dans le traitement chirurgical de la calvitie. Rev Chir Esthet. 1976; 4:5.
8. Hunt HL. Plastic Surgery of the Head, Face, and Neck. New York: Lea & Febiger; 1926.
9. Sparkhul K. Scalp reduction: Serial excision of the scalp with advancement. International Hair Transplant Symposium, Lucerne, Switzerland, Feb. 4, 1978.
10. Stough DB, Webster RC. Esthetics and refinements in hair transplantation. International Hair Transplant Symposium, Lucerne, Switzerland, February 4, 1978.
11. Unger MG, Unger WP. Management of alopecia of the scalp by a combination of excisions and transplantations. J Dermatol Surg Oncol. 1978; 4:670.
12. Bosley LL, Hope CR, Montroy RE. Male pattern reduction (MPR) for surgical reduction of male pattern baldnes. Curr Ther Res. 1979; 25:281.
13. Fleming RW, Mayer TG. Short vs. long flaps in the treatment of male pattern baldness. Arch Otolaryngol. 1981; 107:403.
14. Alt TH. Scalp reduction as an adjunct to hair transplantation: Review of relevant literature and presentation of an improved technique. J Dermatol Surg Oncol. 1980; 6:1011.
15. Marzola M. An alternative hair replacement method. In: Norwood OT, Shiell RC, eds: Hair Transplant Surgery, ed. 2. Springfield, Ill: Charles C. Thomas; 1984.
16. Bradshaw W. Quarter-grafts: A technique for minigrafts. In: Unger W, Nordstrom RE, eds. Hair Transplantation, 2nd ed. New York: Marcel Dekker, Inc; 1988:333–351.
17. Unger MG. Postoperative necrosis following bilateral lateral scalp reduction. J Dermatol Surg Oncol. 1988; 14:541–544.
18. Unger MG. Counterpoint: The risks of the bilateral lateral scalp reduction. J Dermatol Surg Oncol. 1988; 14:353–354.
19. Brandy DA. The bilateral occipitoparietal flap. J Dermatol Surg Oncol 1986; 10:1062–1066.
20. Brandy DA. The Brandy bitemporal flap. Am J Cosm Surg. 1986; 3:11–15.
21. Brandy DA. The modified bitemporal flap for the treatment of bitemporal recessions. Aesthet Plast Surg. 1989; 13:203–207.
22. Brandy DA. Effectiveness of occipital artery ligations as a priming procedure for extensive scalp-lifting. J Dermatol Surg Oncol. 1991; 17:946–949.
23. Marzola M. A new alopecia reduction design: No visible scars, no slots, no Frechet flaps. Am J Cosm Surg. 1997; 14:166.
24. Frechet P. Scalp extension. J Dermatol Surg Oncol. 1993; 19:616–622.
25. Nordstrom REA. Stretch-back in scalp reductions for male pattern baldness. Plast Reconstr Surg. 1984; 73:422.
26. Juri J. Use of parieto-occipital flaps in the surgical treatment of baldness. Plast Reconstr Surg. 1975; 55(4):456.
27. Passot R. Chirurgie Esthetique Pure: Technique et Resultats. Paris: G Dion; 1931.
28. Elliot RA. Lateral scalp flaps for instant results in male pattern baldness. Plast Reconstr Surg. 1977; 60:699.
29. Heimburger RA. Single stage rotation of arterialized scalp flaps for male pattern baldness. Plast Reconst Surg. 1977; 60:789.
30. Nataf J, Elbaz JS, Pollet J. Etude critique des transplantations de cuir chevalu et proposition d'une optique. Ann Chir Plast. 1976; 21(3):199.
31. Argenta LC. The principles of scalp expansion. American Society of Plastic and Reconstructive Surgeons Surgery Forum, Kansas City, Mo, 1985.
32. Radovan C. Tissue expansion in soft tissue reconstruction. Plast Reconstr Surg. 1984; 74:482.
33. Manders EK, et al. Skin expansion to eliminate large scalp defects. Ann Plast Surg. 1984; 12:305.
34. Anderson RD. Expansion-assisted treatment of male pattern baldness. Clin Plast Surg. 1987; 14(3):477.
35. Kabaker S, et at. Tissue expansion in the treatment of alopecia. Arch Otolaryngol. 1986; 112:720.

Hair Restoration

Aesthetic Facial Plastic Surgery, edited by Thomas Romo, III, and Arthur L. Millman, Thieme Medical Publishers, Inc., New York, New York, Copyright © 2000.

A Dermatologist's Perspective

DAVID S. ORENTREICH AND NORMAN ORENTREICH

In 1939, in a report virtually unrecognized in the English-speaking world, Okuda, a Japanese dermatologist, described the use of small full-thickness autografts of hair-bearing skin for the correction of alopecia of the scalp, eyebrow, and mustache areas.[1,2] This method was almost identical to that of Orentreich, reported in 1959.[3] Okuda constructed special metal trephines (circular punches) with diameters of 2 to 4 mm and used these to bore out grafts from hair-bearing areas of the scalp. A similar instrument was used to prepare recipient sites in the area of alopecia into which the grafts were placed. Okuda noted that better cosmetic results were achieved if slightly smaller trephines were used for the recipient holes. A total of 200 patients, most of whom had cicatricial alopecia, was successfully treated with this technique. Okuda did not, however, specifically note its use in patients with male pattern baldness.

Unfortunately, because of World War II, Okuda's work was not recognized outside Japan until many years later. This was generally true for other relevant publications and for the proceedings of various Japanese dermatologic and plastic surgery societies, which were written entirely in Japanese. Thus knowledge and trial of these techniques outside Japan were long delayed.[4] It was not until 1970 that Friederich mentioned Okuda's significant contribution and designated the free punch graft method as the Okuda-Orentreich technique.[5]

More than 40 years have elapsed since the first controlled experiments with autografts in 1954 that led to the 1959 publication of "Autografts in Alopecias and Other Selected Dermatological Conditions."[3] Hair-bearing scalp punch grafts transplanted into areas of male pattern baldness (androgenetic[6] or androchronogenetic alopecia[7]) still continue to grow hair more than four decades later. In the interim, hundreds of lectures, symposia, workshops, papers, books,[8] and other media on this and related techniques of hair replacement surgery have been held or published. Some 200 physicians have observed the basic transplant technique at our medical facility, and today hair transplantation is one of the most commonly performed office-based plastic surgery procedures in the United States.

THE PRINCIPLE OF HAIR TRANSPLANTATION

The success of hair-bearing autografts (hair transplants) for the correction of androgenetic alopecia (AGA) and certain other alopecias depends on the principle of donor and recipient dominance, terms introduced by Orentreich in 1959.[3] Donor- dominant grafts retain the characteristics of the donor site after transplantation to a new site, whereas recipient-dominant grafts take on the characteristics of the tissue at the recipient site. These concepts of dominance were developed out of studies investigating the localization of various dermatoses, including several types of alopecia. The research use of such autografts, with appropriate multiple controls, helped to further understanding of certain physiologic and pathologic cutaneous phenomena.

With his 1959 publication of "Autografts in Alopecias and Other Selected Dermatological Conditions,"

Orentreich realized that AGA could be treated surgically. The 1959 article illustrated the aesthetic placement of grafts in the frontal scalp in a pattern that reconstructed the anterior hairline, with allowance for an appropriate degree of temporal recession and frontal peaking. The hairline continued to recede, and the grafts aesthetically placed in front of the pre-existing hairline continued to show stable hair growth, increasingly anterior to the receding hairline.

The results of the 1954 experiment with autografts for the treatment of AGA corroborated that "the capacity for development of baldness appears to be controlled by factors resident in localized areas of the scalp,"[9] that is, the pathogenesis of AGA is inherent in each individual hair follicle. The phenomena explained the occasional clinical observation of singular, normally growing terminal hairs in a sea of male pattern baldness. The results of the study published in 1959 also refuted the then popular theory that AGA resulted from ischemia, the chronic activity of the scalp muscles, by branches of the facial nerves, causing shearing stresses in the dermis of the scalp.[10]

Since the development of punch graft hair transplantation for AGA and other alopecias, many improvements have been made in both instrumentation and technique. Physicians with diverse surgical training have entered the field of hair replacement surgery and expanded the surgical options to modalities other than punch grafting. Some innovations have endured, others have been abandoned, and others remain controversial. A review of some of the more significant advances follows.

TECHNIQUE ADVANCES

Saline infiltration of the donor area[11] improved graft harvesting, as did the introduction of sharper and motorized punches.[12] Closing donor sites with sutures rather than allowing them to heal by secondary intention reduced both healing time and patient discomfort in addition to improving the cosmetic appearance of the donor site scar.[13,14] Although the strip graft method introduced by Vallis[15] never became fully established, it may have been the first use of a double-bladed knife to obtain a strip of donor graft tissue, which is now a popular technique of donor harvesting.

The past five years have been a period of tremendous innovation and expansion in the field of hair replacement surgery. New techniques and improvements in surgical instrumentation have greatly increased the quality of the end aesthetic result and the skill and speed with which the transplant surgeon can operate. Surgical techniques and instrumentation have been so improved and refined that the transplantation of hundreds, and indeed thousands, of minigrafts and micrografts in a single session is not an unrealistic goal for the transplant surgeon.[16]

Strip donor harvesting, minigrafting and micrografting techniques, and laser surgery are some of the developments that have revolutionized office-based hair restoration surgery. The technique of harvesting conventional grafts containing 10 to 15 hairs with a motorized punch and placing them in neat rows in the bald recipient area has been largely replaced by the method of strip harvesting, followed by the random planting of hundreds of minigrafts and micrografts in the bald recipient area to mimic the natural, scattered pattern of hair growth.

PATIENT SELECTION

Most men and women with an area of significant balding and an adequate source of donor hair in the occipitotemporal region of the scalp are good candidates for hair transplants. The procedure can be performed in people of all races.[17] However, not all hair loss is androgenetic or of a type suitable for autograft correction. It is essential that an accurate diagnosis be made by patient history and by clinical and laboratory evaluation.[6,18] Laboratory studies of differential, contributory, and pathogenic factors operative in an AGA diagnosis include complete blood count (CBC) with differential, Venereal Disease Research Laboratory (VDRL) testing, bilirubin, alkaline phosphatase, cholesterol, triglycerides, serum glutamic-oxaloacetic transaminase (SGOT), uric acid, and creatinine levels; adrenal function tests, including cortisol and dehydroepiandrosterone sulfate; androgen function tests, including testosterone, sex hormone–binding globulin, and free testosterone index; and thyroid function tests, including free thyroid index (T_4 and T_3 uptake) and possibly T_3 and thyrotropic hormone (TSH). If menstrual irregularities or

signs of virilization are also present in the prospective female hair transplant patient, then determination of follicle-stimulating hormone (FSH), luteinizing hormone (LH), and prolactin levels may be indicated. Human immunodeficiency virus (HIV) and hepatitis B screening are recommended for all hair transplant candidates.

On the basis of the aforementioned principle of autograft dominance, hair transplantation is not suitable for patients with active hair loss caused by alopecia areata, lupus erythematosus, pseudopelade of Brocq, lichenplano pilaris, folliculitis or scleroderma and its variants, morphea and coup de sabre. On the other hand, "burnt-out" lupus morphea, and other cicatricial alopecias[19] can often be successfully treated with hair transplants. In these latter cases we recommend performing a test procedure involving a small number of grafts. Permanent baldness as a result of burns, trauma, or radiation can be corrected with transplants if adequate donor hair remains.

Patient evaluation requires that the general medical status of the patient is good, with particular emphasis given to identifying any bleeding diathesis or tendency to keloid formation. The recipient and donor site sizes, and the density, color, texture, and curl of the hair available for correction are evaluated to determine what degree of improvement is feasible. These findings, a proposed hairline, and the amount of bald scalp to be treated are then discussed with the patient.

Hair transplantation must never be urged on an unenthusiastic patient. If one is already satisfied with his or her appearance, the coaxing of an accompanying spouse or friend should not be allowed to sway the patient's feelings. If the patient is young and actively loosing hair, a family history may provide some insight into his or her eventual degree of baldness. The decision to start hair transplants early, even when the hair loss is progressing, is made with an awareness of the emotional makeup and needs of the patient. To prevent disappointment, both the patient and physician should have a realistic expectation of what is surgically possible. Sufficient time should be spent with a patient to allay any fears and to correct misunderstandings. The patient should be fully informed about the procedure, including its immediate and long-term postoperative consequences. The physician should avoid accepting a psychiatrically disturbed patient for surgery. If one is in doubt, postponing the procedure is a sensible decision. Alternatively, single test transplants to an inconspicuous area can be performed. This test is recommended for patients with keloid tendencies and is very useful for an apprehensive patient; a few minutes of surgery may provide more peace of mind than prolonged verbal reassurances.

PREOPERATIVE PREPARATION

After determining that a patient can be helped with transplants, other options for correction are also discussed, including flap and scalp reduction techniques. If a hair-piece is worn, the patient is advised that it can be used postoperatively as long as the attachment sites do not rest on any transplanted grafts. The social, recreational, cosmetic, and occupational limitations imposed by hair transplantation surgery and the postoperative healing period are reviewed. The approximate number of transplants for optimal correction, the cost, the number of grafts per procedure, the sites and the frequency of procedures, and the time required for appearance of first growth and then final regrowth are estimated and discussed with the patient in detail. The reasons for performing the transplants for each area in several or

multiple procedures are explained: Because diminished hair yield might result if all the grafts required were performed in one session, intergraft spacing must be planned so that an adequate blood supply reaches all the grafts.

In planning the procedure, a brief description of the sequence of events that the actual surgery will follow are reviewed with the patient. Local anesthesia, hair trimming of the donor sites, punch and/or strip harvesting techniques, and the placement of grafts are explained to the patient. Of greatest importance is the establishment of the hairline. The patient should be given a mirror to hold at eye level while a hairline is drawn in, reviewed with the patient, and agreed on. This decision is second in importance only to the determination that hair restoration surgery is indicated. Artfully reestablishing the frontal hairline is essential to avoid an unnatural appearance. In addition to exhibiting a natural frontal peak, the hairline must be suitable for both present and future decades. The direction, color, texture, and density of the hair to be transplanted may need to be reviewed at this time. To avoid hairs going awry, all grafts in the recipient area are oriented so that the hair follicles follow a natural pattern. This is usually centripetal on the dome of the

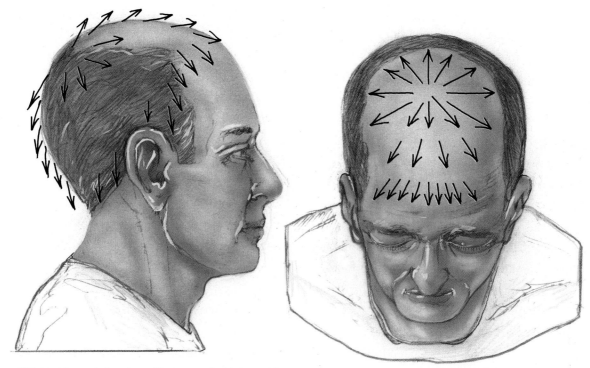

Figure 27-1. Natural direction of hair growth. (Adapted from *J Dermatol Surg Oncol.* 1985; 11(3):323.)

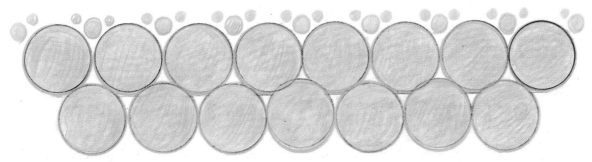

Figure 27–2. Smaller diameter plugs—minigrafts or micrografts at frontal hairline. (Adapted from *J Dermatol Surg Oncol.* 1985; 11(3):323.)

scalp and frontal on the anterior scalp (Fig. 27–1). In the past, when re-establishing the frontal hairline with conventional grafts, which measured 3.0 to 4.0 mm in diameter, the overlapping of grafts reduced the appearance of a scalloped edge. At present, smaller diameter minigrafts or micrografts may be used exclusively along the frontal hairline or interspersed between older conventional grafts to produce a more natural appearance (Fig. 27–2).

Minigrafting is an established concept with a new name. In 1970 Orentreich[20,21] described the use of small circular punch grafts to refine the frontal hairline. These minigrafts and micrografts were reincarnated in the early 1980s when Marritt[22] used them in eyelash transplantation, and Nordstrom[23] subdivided 4-mm punch grafts into micrografts, each containing two to four follicles, and inserted them into stab incisions. This work was further discussed by Marritt,[24] Bradshaw,[25] and Stough,[26] who bisected or quadrasected larger punch grafts and placed them into small punch holes or stab incisions.

Minigrafts consist of three to four hairs obtained by meticulously cutting a circular 4.0- to 4.5-mm punch graft into quadrants or by cutting a long strip of donor skin into multiple grafts each bearing three to four hairs. The minigrafts are then placed into 2.0-mm holes cut with a punch or into stab incisions made with a No. 15 scalpel blade.[27] Micrografts containing one to two hairs may be placed into 1.25-mm punch recipient sites or into stab incisions. Micrografts are essential to optimize the natural appearance of the frontal hairline.

After a decision to proceed is made, photographs of the recipient sites are taken, and the patient is advised to wear appropriate clothing for the day of surgery, the removal of which will not disturb the graft sites and postoperative dressings (i.e., no turtlenecks or clothing that must be pulled over the head). The patient is advised to shampoo the morning of the transplant procedure because shampooing is contraindicated for four to five days postoperatively. The use of styling products is contraindicated immediately before surgery. The patient is advised not to take anticoagulants or aspirin in any form for 14 days before and 10 days after surgery. Acetaminophen can be substituted. In addition, garlic supplements are thought to have anticoagulant properties, and this popular dietary supplement should be discontinued 14 days before and two days after surgery. No alcohol is advised for one to two days before and after surgery, and strenuous exercise 48 hours before surgery is best avoided. Patients are advised to let their hair grow long in advance of their surgery date to allow for adequate combing over the operative sites. The patient should be instructed not to fast before surgery and to eat a normal breakfast or lunch.

SURGICAL TECHNIQUE

Hair transplants may be performed with the patient in a recumbent or in a sitting position. If vasovagal syncope occurs, a motorized chair that can reposition the patient from the sitting position into the supine position is required. The upper clothing is removed, and the patient is draped for comfort and to avoid soiling. The operative sites and proposed hairline are reviewed with the patient.

PREOPERATIVE MEDICATION AND ANESTHESIA

Each surgeon will choose his or her own preferred method of sedation. Because we normally perform the procedure with the patient in a sitting position, we use oral diazepam or intramuscular midazolam, with or without nitrous oxide analgesia before injection of local anesthetic, which is usually 2% lidocaine with 1:100,000 epinephrine. Epinephrine is excluded in patients with certain cardiac conditions. Although allergy to lidocaine is extremely rare, a skin test is appropriate if the patient may be allergic. Administering the lidocaine slowly through a 30-gauge needle, with or without topical refrigeration of the injection site, minimizes patient discomfort. To avoid overdosing with lidocaine, especially when large areas are to be operated on, the donor site is anesthetized and harvested first. This removes some of the injected anesthetic and allows time for some metabolism of the lidocaine before the recipient site is injected. Vasovagal bradycardia can induce syncope and should be anticipated, especially on the first visit. Any time that syncope is imminent, the patient should be placed in the supine position and, if necessary, the legs should be elevated. Injecting epinephrine with the lidocaine helps counteract bradycardia and reduces bleeding. Carbonated colas or orange juice should be offered to the patient because they quickly correct the hypoglycemic effect of epinephrine.

Although large volumes of anesthetic sometimes make the procedure more tolerable for the patient, unnecessarily large volumes of fluid should be avoided in the frontal area. Large volumes may contribute to the formation of postsurgical edema and subcutaneous bleeding and generally cause postoperative care problems involving forehead and eyelid swelling. Elasticized bandaging of the forehead overnight and a short course of corticosteroids may ameliorate this problem. Keep in mind that providing music and conversing with the patient during the procedure always relieves anxiety.

HARVESTING THE GRAFTS

When selecting the donor site, the density, color, thickness, texture, and curl of the hair are considered to facilitate blending with the hair at the recipient sites. The hair covering that portion of the donor site to be excised is clipped to 3 mm but not shaved, to allow visualization of the implied angle and direction of the hair follicles in relation to the skin surface. This allows proper angling of the punch or multiblade scalpel when harvesting the grafts. Cutting across the hair follicles injures them and reduces the number of hairs that will grow from each graft (Fig. 27–3).

The Strip Harvesting Technique

For tumescence, sterile physiologic saline, administered with a 30- to 50-ml syringe, is injected into the subcutaneous tissue. Filling the area beneath the dermis increases the distance between the skin and the skull and reduces risk of injury to underlying neurovascular structures. The infiltration of saline into the donor sites makes the donor skin more rigid, thereby reducing distortion when cutting strips of donor tissue, hence reducing the chance of transecting hair follicles. The surgeon then matches the multibladed scalpel to the angle of the trimmed visible hair. The most important aspect of strip harvesting is controlling the scalpel blades so that they remain parallel to the changing angle of the hair shafts throughout the cutting process (Fig. 27–4A). The hair of a healthy donor strip should be intact from the follicle root to the skin surface. Mastering the intricate technique of cutting parallel to the donor scalp yields an optimal strip of viable hairs and is the surgeon's greatest challenge. The instructional video by James Arnold, M.D., is a useful primer for the transplant surgeon who hopes to master the technique of strip harvesting.[16]

On removal, the donor strips are cleansed of debris by gently rubbing between two pieces of saline-soaked gauze and then placing them in physiologic saline (Fig. 27–4B). Bleeding vessels are then cauterized, and the donor site is closed with sutures or staples. Staples and sutures are usually removed 7 days postoperatively.

The Punch Technique

Conventional grafts harvested with motorized punches are removed gently, because pulling with force can damage the

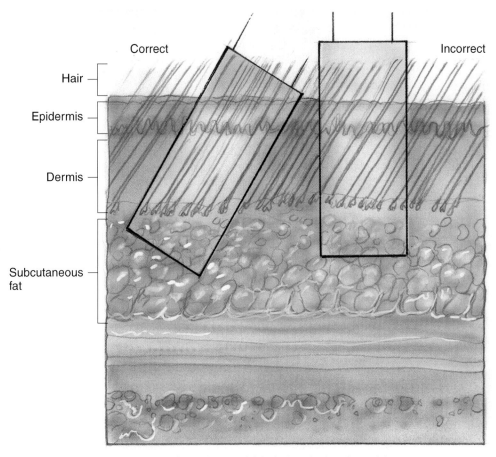

Figure 27-3. Proper angling of punch or multibladed scalpel. Adapted from *J Dermatol Surg Oncol.* 1985; 11(3):321.)

follicles and their papillae. If necessary, the donor graft tissue is freed of its fibrous band attachment by cutting with scissors well below the dermal papillae. After their removal, the grafts are immediately placed in physiologic saline solution. Because the donor site skin is 0.5 mm to 1.0 mm thicker than the alopecic recipient skin, donor grafts need to be trimmed of excess fat. Trimming reduces cobblestoning as does the cross stitching of conventionally sized harvested grafts. Spicules of hair must be removed to prevent foreign body reaction.[28] To camouflage the donor site, careful planning of graft spacing is necessary. Infiltration of anesthetic and large volumes of sterile, physiologic saline[27] into the donor sites makes the skin turgid and facilitates the accurate punching of grafts, in much the same way as it facilitates the cutting of strip grafts, reducing distortion and yielding an optimal number of grafts. To further optimize the quality of punched donor grafts, the motor-driven punches are resharpened for each procedure.

PREPARATION OF MINIGRAFTS AND MICROGRAFTS FROM HARVESTED STRIPS AND PUNCHES

A magnifier, a tongue blade soaked in saline as a cutting surface, Foerster™ forceps, and Personna™ surgical prep blades are the instruments required for graft preparation.[16] The visible excess fat is trimmed from a harvested strip or punch because it interferes with the eventual insertion of the prepared graft into the recipient site.

Minigrafts and micrografts prepared from punched donor tissue consist of meticulously cutting a circular 4.0- to 4.5-mm punch graft into quadrants (minigraft), and from there sectioning off a single hair graft (micrograft).

The preparation of minigrafts and micrografts from strip-harvested tissue necessitates alignment of the Personna surgical prep blade perpendicular to the graft (Fig. 27–4C). The blade is placed between two hairs and

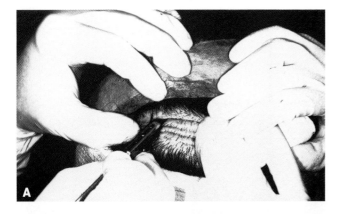

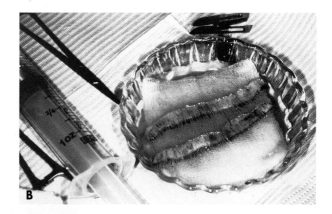

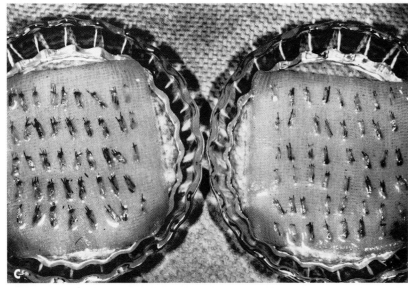

Figure 27–4. (A) Strip harvesting with multibladed scalpel. **(B)** Harvested strips of donor tissue. **(C)** Minigrafts and micrografts prepared from harvested strips.

just pressing downwards easily separates off a minigraft or micrograft. Lateral sawing motions are contraindicated when preparing the grafts because this action dulls the blade and interferes with graft alignment.[16]

PLANTING THE GRAFTS

Punched Recipient Sites

Recipient sites for minigrafts containing three to four hairs are made with a 2.0-mm surgical punch or by stab incision with a no. 15 scalpel blade. Care is taken to remove any fibrous tissue at the base of the recipient site to accommodate the thicker donor graft. Micrografts containing one to two hairs may be placed into 1.25-mm punch recipient sites or stab incisions. The recipient area can be grafted in three to four procedures without any grafts touching during any single procedure.

Slit Grafting

Tiny slit incisions (less than 2 mm), made with a No. 61 spear point-shaped blade, are used to create single hair micrograft recipient sites.[16] Slits heal easily and are undetectable when placed just along the hair line. Concentrating on their scattered and seemingly randomized placement, mimicking the natural growth of hair along the hair line is the goal. Micrografts can be placed between minigrafts and conventional grafts to create a more natural appearance. Rarely is any suturing of minigraft and micrograft recipient areas required.

Placement of Hair Graft

After the preparation of the recipient sites for their donor grafts, there follows the most labor-intensive part of the hair transplant procedure, which is the actual placement of the grafts. Two nurse-assistants can spend several hours inserting the minigrafts, micrografts, and conventional grafts. Foerster forceps are used for inserting conventional and minigrafts into their individual openings, and Foerster microforceps are used for micrograft insertion.[16] The use of cotton-tipped applicators to apply gentle pressure and to hold the graft in place facilitates insertion. Single hair micrografts can drop below the skin surface after insertion, and the 3-mm whisker of hair left in anticipation of this eventuality (when the donor hair was trimmed in preparation for harvesting), now proves useful. The whisker of hair acts as a marker for each graft and provides leverage for the nurse-assistant to pull the graft level with the surface.[16]

After hemostasis and cleansing are complete, an antibiotic ointment is applied. Proper draping, manual pressure, cotton applicators inserted into heavily bleeding holes, and bandaging minimizes bleeding and helps keep blood from the patient's view. When the recipient area is completely bald, the grafts can be taped down with Micropore to facilitate bandaging and postoperative care. As much cleaning as is feasible is done after the grafts are set to make the postoperative care period easier for the patient. A light spray of hydrogen peroxide facilitates this clean-up procedure.

If only a limited number of transplants are performed, it is possible for the patient to leave without a bandage. The donor site is prepared in such a way that the hair above camouflages the operative area. The recipient site can be left alone with just a thin layer of antibiotic ointment, and the surrounding hair may be styled over the site for cosmetic camouflage.

POSTOPERATIVE COURSE

Oral antibiotics, usually erythromycin or tetracycline, 250 mg, are usually prescribed for seven days postoperatively. The patient is instructed to apply a thin layer of antibiotic ointment to donor and recipient sites twice a day for 10 to 14 days to minimize dry crust formation and speed re-epithelialization. Patients with minigrafts and micrografts are instructed to apply the antibiotic ointment the day after surgery and twice daily thereafter until the surgical sites are healed. A 1-week course of anti-inflammatory corticosteroids is also prescribed to reduce swelling. Analgesics to reduce discomfort (usually acetaminophen with codeine or hydrocodone with acetaminophen) are prescribed. No alcoholic beverages should be taken for 48 hours and no aspirin for 10 days after surgery; the aforementioned aspirin substitutes are permitted.

If bleeding occurs, patients are instructed to apply firm moderate pressure directly to the area with gauze or a clean handkerchief for 15 minutes and then to gradually release pressure. This usually stops bleeding. Strenuous physical activity is contraindicated on the first 48 hours, and then only limited physical activity is allowed for the next 10 postoperative days. Edema and/or ecchymosis may develop in the recipient area in the first 24 to 48 hours after surgery and may last from 7 to 10 days. It may also spread to the forehead and eyelids. Patients are instructed to sit up as much as possible and to sleep with the head elevated to reduce swelling.

Donor site suture removal takes place seven days after surgery. Cross-stitch sutures placed over conventional grafts can be removed three to five days after surgery.[29]

Great care should be taken when combing or brushing the hair near the site of the grafts. Shampooing may begin on the third postoperative day and should be very gentle until healing is complete. Patients may soak their entire scalp in the shower with just a gentle spray, shampooing very delicately and carefully. Dried and crusting blood can be removed by soaking with a 3% hydrogen peroxide solution.

Postoperative pain is rare; in fact, temporary hypesthesia and paresthesia are not uncommon because sensory nerves are often severed. Patients should be reassured that these altered sensations are usually temporary and will normalize within 6 months. A patient should also be advised that any excessive swelling or pain, or any pulsation at the operative sites, should be brought promptly to the surgeon's attention. It may be desirable, although certainly not essential, for a patient to return the day after surgery for a checkup. At this time, with the aid of a hydrogen peroxide spray, the operative sites can be cleansed and checked. The donor site rarely needs redressing on this visit, and the recipient site, if not concealable by hair styling, can have a small nonadherent (with or without antibiotic ointment) dressing applied. A hair prosthesis can be worn if the attachment sites are placed so as not to cover any donor grafts. Whenever possible, the length and styling of the hair is planned in advance to conceal the operative sites.

If for any reason a graft falls out, patients are instructed to handle it carefully and to cleanse it in saline or an 8-ounce glass of tepid water plus a teaspoon of salt. They are further instructed to wrap the graft in a clean cloth saturated with the mildly salted water and to store it in the refrigerator for no more than four days within which period it can be reinserted. If a graft cannot be saved or reinserted in a timely fashion, the site can be regrafted at the next transplant visit.

The first procedure should be given a minimum of one month to heal before further grafting is undertaken. This allows for the return of vascularity and optimal hair growth and prevents avascular necrosis. If performing follow-up transplants after one month and before three months (which is the interval when the hairs from previous grafts have been shed and before the new hairs begin to grow), care must be taken not to inadvertently remove the sometimes difficult to detect previous grafts that are temporarily free of hair.[30] For best results, new hair growth should be evident (about three months postoperatively) before additional transplants are undertaken.

It is impossible to predict, with any degree of accuracy, the number of hairs in any given graft. The number is usually eight to fifteen for conventional grafts, two to four for minigrafts, and one to two for micrografts. It is important to convey to the patient that the visible portion of the transplanted hairs will be shed within one month. Occasionally, one or two of the hairs are not shed and continue to grow. Permanent hair growth starts about three to four months after surgery, the length of a typical telogen period. Because scalp hair normally grows

about half an inch per month, it will take three to six additional months (i.e., six to nine months postoperatively) for the full effect to be appreciated (Fig. 27–5).

COMPLICATION AND SEQUELAE

Cobblestoning or elevation of grafts can be treated by electrodesiccating the elevations, by cutting them flat with a blade, or rarely by dermabrasion. Hyperpigmentation can be treated by bleaching, cryotherapy, or dermabrasion. Hypopigmentation is common because the skin of the donor grafts has been relatively sun-protected and the recipient areas can be quite tan with actinic alterations. Tanning is slow but will eventually blend these sites.

The occasional bacterial infection requires appropriate antibiotic treatment. Inflammation should prompt a search for trapped hair spicules. In addition to bleeding, other rarely seen problems are aneurysms, arteriovenous fistulas,[31] and pyogenic granulomas. Avascular necrosis may occur if the grafts are too numerous and placed too close together or if donor site suturing is too tight. The unavoidable transection of nerves may produce temporary hypesthesia and, as they regenerate, paresthesia. Rarely a painful neuroma will develop; it can be treated with intralesional corticosteroid injections or excision.

Keloids, which occur very rarely, can be treated with intralesional corticosteroids. If a keloid occurs in a recipient site, it usually interferes with hair growth and may be a contraindication to further transplants.

ANCILLARY TECHNIQUES

Free scalp flaps were reported by Harri in 1974,[32] Juri introduced flaps at the 1975 International Congress of Plastic Surgeons in Paris,[33] and the technique has since been refined by others.[34–36] Bald scalp reduction, first reported by Blanchard and Blanchard,[37,38] and refined by others,[39–43] has become one of the most enduring and valuable adjuncts to grafting. Kabaker and others[35,44] have

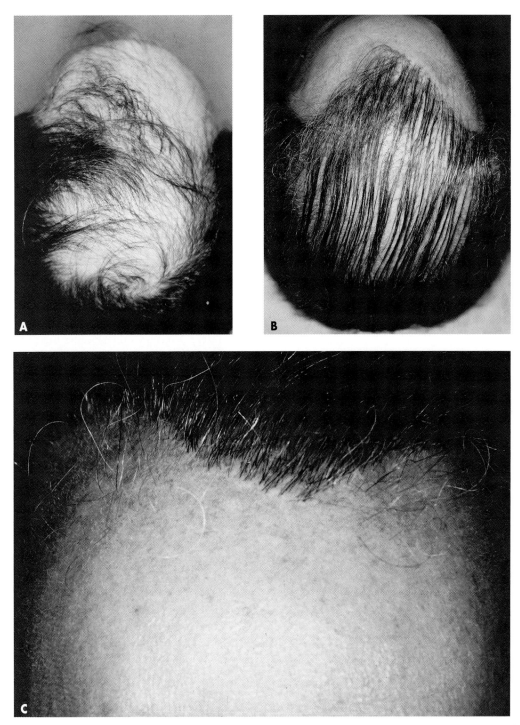

Figure 27–5. Cosmetically successful result without superextensive grafting. **(A)** Before. (B) After. **(C)** Close-up of the re-created natural peak and its subtle hairline.

demonstrated the usefulness of tissue expanders for bald scalp reduction. Frecht's method of scalp extension may duplicate the advantages of tissue expanders without the disadvantages.[45]

CONCLUSION

Hair transplantation is a safe and efficacious method of redistributing scalp hair into a cosmetically acceptable pattern.

With application of the aforementioned complementary techniques, cosmetically optimal results are even more accessible to today's patient with AGA. In the future the limiting factors of donor hair quantity and quality in hair restoration surgery may be overcome by hair follicle cloning, whereby the bald scalp may be populated by virtually unlimited numbers of test tube follicles.[46] Until a safe and effective method of regrowing the miniaturized follicles of AGA[47] is perfected, hair transplantation will continue to be used. For the AGA patient and for the patient needing hair growth in areas of alopecic scars, surgical measures that are both finite and permanent are clearly the treatment of choice.

The benefits of hair transplantation far outweigh the problems, making it a highly successful and gratifying procedure.

ACKNOWLEDGEMENT

This text appeared as part of Chapter 27 (Hair Transplantation). In: Krespi YP, ed. *Office-Based Surgery of the Head.* Philadelphia: Lippincott-Raven Publishers, 1998.

PEARLS

- Smaller grafts are better.
- Single hairs are best.
- Harvesting with minimal trauma to follicles is optimal.
- Angle of insertion should conform to natural hair whirls (calyces).
- Optimize recipient bed preparation.

REFERENCES

1. Okuda S. Klinische und experimentelle Untersuchungen uber die Transplantation von lebenden Haaren. *Jpn J Dermatol* 1939; 40:537 (Japanese).
2. Okuda S. Clinical and experimental studies of transplantation of living hairs. *Jpn J Dermatol Urol,* 1939; 46:135–138 (Japanese).
3. Orentreich N. Autografts in alopecias and other selected dermatological conditions. *Ann NY Acad Sci,* 1959; 83:463–479.
4. Kobori T, Montagna W, eds. *Biology and Disease of the Hair.* Baltimore: University Park Press; 1976.
5. Friederich HC. Indikation and Tecnik der Operativ-plastischen Behandlung des Haarverlustes. *Hautarzt.* 1970; 21:197–202.
6. Orentreich N. Pathogenesis of alopecia. *J Soc Cosmet Chem.* 1960; XI:479–499.
7. Orentreich N, Rizer RL. Medical treatment of androgenetic alopecia. In: Brown AC, Crounse RA, eds. *Hair, Trace Elements, and Human Illness.* Part 4. *Hirsutism and Alopecia.* New York: Praeger; 1980:294–304.
8. Norwood OT, Shiell RC. *Hair Transplant Surgery,* 2nd ed. Springfield, Illinois: Charles C. Thomas; 1984.
9. Hamilton JB. Patterned loss of hair in man: Types and incidence. *Ann NY Acad Sci.* 1951; 53:708–728.
10. Szasz TS, Robertson AM. The theory of the pathogenesis of ordinary human baldness. *Arch Dermatol Syphilol.* 1950; 61:34–48.
11. Frankel EB. Hair transplantation: Additional observations. *Cutis.* 1975; 15:545.
12. Tezel J. Miniature drill expedites hair transplantation. *Cutis.* 1969; 5:461.
13. Carreirao S, Lessa S. New technique for closing punch graft donor sites. *Plast Reconst Surg.* 1978; 61:455–456.
14. Pierce HE. An improved method for closure of donor sites in hair transplantation. *J Dermatol Surg Oncol.* 1979; 5:475–476.
15. Vallis CP. Surgical treatment of receding hairline. *Plast Reconstr Surg.* 1964; 33:247.
16. Arnold J. *500 micro and mini grafts before or after lunch. A primer for modern hair transplantation* (instructional video), 1995.
17. Selmanowitz VJ, Orentreich N. Hair transplantation in blacks. *J Natl Med Assoc.* 1973; 65:471–482.
18. Orentreich N. Hair Problems. *J Am Med Womens Assoc.* 1966; 21:481–486.
19. Stough DB, Berger RA, Orentreich N. Surgical improvement of cicatricial alopecia of diverse etiology. *Arch Dermatol.* 1968; 97:331–334.
20. Orentreich N. Hair transplants. In: Maddin S, ed. *Current Dermatologic Management.* St. Louis: C.V. Mosby; 1970:13–20.
21. Ayres S. Hair transplantation. In: Epstein E, ed. *Skin Surgery,* 3rd ed., Springfield, Ill: Charles C. Thomas; 1970.
22. Marritt E. Transplantation of single hairs from the scalp as eyelashes. *J Dermatol Surg Oncol.* 1980; 6:271–273.
23. Nordstrom REA. "Micrografts" for improvement of the frontal hairline after hair transplantation. *Aesth Plast Surg.* 1981; 5:97–101.
24. Marritt E. Single hair transplantation for hairline refinement: A practical solution. *J Dermatol Surg Oncol.* 1984; 10:962–6.
25. Bradshaw W. Quarter-grafts: A technique for mini-grafts. In: Unger WP, Nordstrom REA. eds. *Hair Transplantation,* 2nd ed. New York: Marcel Dekker; 1988:333–351.
26. Stough DB, Nelson BR, Stough DB. Incisional slit grafting. *J Dermatol Surg Oncol.* 1991; 17:53–60.

27. Norwood OT, Shiell RC. *Hair Transplant Surgery*, 2nd ed. Springfield, Ill: Charles C Thomas; 1984.

28. Altchek DD, Pearlstein HH. Granulomatous reaction to autologous hairs incarcerated during hair transplantation. *J Dermatol Surg Oncol.* 1978; 4:928.

29. Orentreich N, Orentreich D. Cross stitch suture technique for hair transplantation. *J Dermatol Surg Oncol.* 1984; 10:970–971.

30. Orentreich N, Orentreich D. Androgenetic alopecia and its treatment. In: Unger WP, ed. *Hair Transplantation*, 3rd ed rev Expanded. New York: Marcel Dekker; 1995.

31. Souder DE, Bercaw BL. Arteriovenous fistula secondary to hair transplantation. *N Engl J Med.* 1970; 283:473.

32. Harri K, Obmori K, Obmori S. Hair transplantation with free scalp flaps. *Plast Reconstr Surg.* 1974; 53:410.

33. Juri J. Use of parieto-occipital flaps in the surgical treatment of baldness. *Plast Reconstr Surg.* 1975; 55:456.

34. Elliott RA. Lateral scalp flaps for instant results in male pattern baldness. *Plast Reconstr Surg.* 1977; 60:669.

35. Kabaker S. Experiences with parieto-occipital flaps in hair transplantation. *Laryngoscope* 1978; 88:73.

36. Fleming RW, Mayer TG. Short vs. long flaps in the treatment of male pattern baldness. *Arch Otolaryngol.* 1981; 107:403.

37. Blanchard G, Blanchard B. La reduction tonsurale (detonsuration): Concept nouveau dans le traitement chirurgical de la calvite. *Rev Chir Esthet.* 1976; 4:5.

38. Blanchard G, Blanchard B. Obliteration of alopecia by hair-lifting: A new concept and technique. *J Natl Med Assoc.* 1977; 69:639.

39. Stough DB, Webster RC. Esthetics and Refinements in Hair Transplantation, *International Hair Transplantation Symposium*, Lucerne, Switzerland, Feb. 4, 1978.

40. Sparkuhl K. Scalp Reduction: Serial Excision of the Scalp with Flap Advancement, *The International Hair Transplant Symposium*, Lucerne, Switzerland, Feb. 4, 1978.

41. Unger MG, Unger WP. Management of alopecia of the scalp by a combination of excisions and transplantation. *J Dermatol Surg Oncol.* 1978; 4:670.

42. Bosley L, Hope CR, Montroy RE. Male Pattern Reduction (MPR) for surgical reduction of male pattern baldness. *Curr Ther Res.* 1979; 25:281.

43. Alt TH. Scalp reduction as an adjunct to hair transplantation: Review of relevant literature and presentation of an improved technique. *J Dermatol Surg Oncol.* 1980; 6:1011.

44. Kabaker S, Kridel R, Krugman N, Swenson R. Tissue expansion in the treatment of alopecia. *Arch Otolaryngol.* 1986; 112:720.

45. Frecht P. Scalp extension. *J Dermatol Surg Oncol.* 1993; 19:616–622.

46. Yang JS, Lavker RM, Sun T. Upper human hair follicle contains a sub population of keratinocytes with superior in vitro proliferative potential. *J Invest Dermatol.* 1993; 101:652–659.

47. Orentreich N, Durr NP. Biology of scalp hair growth. *Clin Plast Surg.* 1982; 197–205.

Clinical Cosmetology: an Adjunct to Aesthetic Facial Surgery

The chapter on cosmetology, appropriately begins the conclusion of this volume but is no less an integral component of a successful aesthetic patient surgical outcome than any previous chapter. The association and support of cosmetologists and colleagues in the beauty profession and industry sometimes makes the difference between success and failure in the final surgical result.

The article by Ms. Pazienza, an extraordinarily talented and licensed cosmetologist, demonstrates how a range of techniques from makeup to the use of hair prostheses and facial prostheses can be used to solve problems that in many cases simply cannot be addressed or solved by surgical solutions.

The article by Mr. Tricomi brings the fashion and beauty industry into the fold. The subtleties of aesthetics certainly go beyond scientific evaluation. In this vein, the beautician and companion industries have brought many products, techniques, and viewpoints that the successful facial surgeon needs to be well acquainted with and use at the outset.

Clinical Cosmetology: an Adjunct to Aesthetic Facial Surgery

Aesthetic Facial Plastic Surgery, edited by Thomas Romo, III, and Arthur L. Millman, Thieme Medical Publishers, Inc., New York, New York, Copyright © 2000.

CHAPTER 28

A Reconstructive Aesthetician's Perspective

LOUISA E. PAZIENZA

The most challenging and important part of any aesthetic surgery procedure is making an easy transition for the patient, preoperatively, intraoperatively, and postoperatively. This affords an exciting opportunity for the physician to work with a medical esthetician or cosmetologist as a team to optimize results with the proper preoperative and postoperative care,[1] easing patients into a normal work activity level as early as possible after surgery.

This chapter will address the relationship between the medical esthetician or cosmetologist and the surgeon. It will also cover the training and experience of a medical esthetician and insight into the field of aesthetic rehabilitation or clinical cosmetology as it is also known. In addition, this chapter will include techniques of skin camouflage followed by an appendix listing camouflage products and related information.

The concept of the esthetician or cosmetologist/medical team is unique, and like any successful team it requires a coordination of efforts; effective communication and compatible availability are essential. To understand the abilities and roles of the key players is critical to properly plan the best possible program for the patient. The patient, in return, is provided with an accurate picture of what these combined efforts can offer. Through time, patience, knowledge, and experience one can develop the requisite interpersonal skills for such professional relationships.[2]

Because it is not uncommon for the patient to be seen by one or more surgeons in preoperative consultation today, the medical esthetician is commonly present when discussing the options of camouflage, postoperative skin care, and cosmetology during wound healing. This provides a level of assurance and comfort with regard to the patients' concerns during the convalescent period. The result is a continuity of care, beginning with the primary surgeon and ending with the medical esthetician or cosmetologist. What is achieved is a maximizing of efforts on behalf of the patient, thereby ensuring the patient's long-term care and satisfaction.[2]

The role of the medical esthetician or cosmetologist is to evaluate the postoperative condition of the patient, explain the options to the patient, and provide a specialized service within the scope of their training and experience. In addition, the medical esthetician or cosmetologist should keep a professional appearance and demeanor as an extended care adjuvant. This also includes familiarizing oneself with the patient's medical history before providing services and to keep an open dialogue with the patient's physician and staff. It is the responsibility of the surgeon and the medical esthetician to discuss realistic expectations with the patient during the consultation. Computer imaging can be useful to establish client expectations.

CRITERIA FOR THE ESTHETICIAN OR COSMETOLOGIST

Skin camouflage techniques are used primarily by licensed estheticians or cosmetologists who have received

further training in this specialized area. There is not yet a supplementary licensing program for medical esthetics; however, postgraduate teaching facilities may offer training of this nature. It is not uncommon for a registered nurse or other health care provider to offer such services. When assembling your multidisciplinary team of specialists, and the medical esthetician, in particular, one should look for state board licensing, certificate of advanced training, work experience, and references. This criteria may vary according to the regulations of each state or country. The terms "camouflage therapist," "aesthetic rehabilitation specialist," "medical esthetician," and "clinical cosmetologist" are all used interchangeably to describe essentially the same services. Customs vary between regions and disciplines.

Advanced training is especially useful if it includes color theory, plastic surgery and dermatologic procedures and terminology, preoperative and postoperative skin care, interaction of topical and oral prescriptive medications, and advanced techniques of application. Further training may include scar chemistry, wound healing classification, burn scar formation, optical properties of light, and studies in human behavior or psychology.

The skin camouflage specialist should have an artist's skill in creating illusions in addition to a familiarity with different types of makeup application. Knowledge in theatrical and special effects makeup can enhance one's skill even further. Camouflage may also refer to scalp or facial hair replacement. Custom or prefabricated hair prostheses and accessories are available to address problematic hair loss, including eyebrows, mustaches, and beards. To apply camouflage techniques to the hair and scalp one needs a cosmetology license. One must be clear as to the extent of services a camouflage specialist offers. Hair replacement options will be discussed later in the chapter.

SKIN CAMOUFLAGE

Skin camouflage techniques use the mixing and customizing of opaque pigmented preparations and the application of these mixtures to the skin to normalize the appearance of a pigmentation or surface discrepancy. The skin camouflage specialist instructs the patients to apply the preparation either until the condition has healed or every day as for vitiligo (Fig. 28–1).

The first known use of camouflage techniques was in the United Kingdom after World War II for camou-

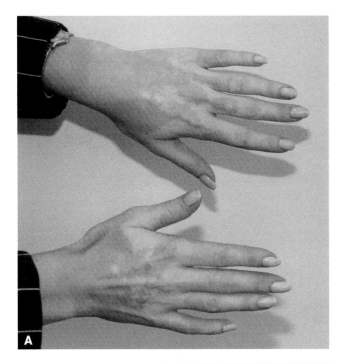

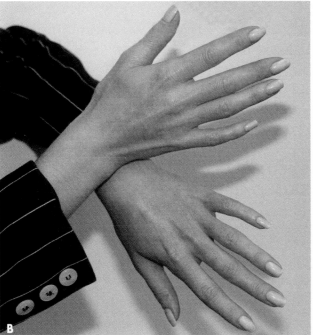

Figure 28-1. (A) Before and **(B)** after application of skin camouflage for vitiligo.

flaging serious burns on pilots.[3] As with many other disfiguring conditions, camouflage is the last option when patients are no longer candidates for surgery. Camouflage allows the patient to feel more comfortable in society, thus it slowly enables the patient to resume control of their lives after a trauma or after an elective surgical procedure. Camouflage technique addresses both the physical appearance of the condition and the psychological need of the patient.[4]

It is necessary to bring attention to the camouflage products themselves and the criteria demanded of them: (1) the product must be opaque to visible light and waterproof, (2) the hues must accurately represent those found in all ethnic variations, and (3) it must be natural in appearance, not obvious when applied. Although skill and experience are critical in obtaining successful results, the selection of products one chooses is equally important and greatly affects the client's satisfaction.

Conventional beauty cosmetics should not be confused with camouflage because their purpose is different in nature. They can, however, be combined as would be the case for everyday use as a concealer underneath or on top of conventional makeup. The term "cosmetics," when referring to camouflage, should be used selectively. Camouflage is manufactured for medical/rehabilitative purposes. The term "pigments" or "preparation" is a more comfortable term when discussing this option with some patients, particularly men. One's choice of terminology can remove the stigma associated with wearing "makeup" and allows men a therapeutic perspective when using it. The purpose of camouflage is to normalize one's appearance rather than to enhance it. Conventional cosmetics are manufactured for the purpose of enhancing facial features. These conventional products do not meet the above criteria and therefore are not adequate for camouflage purposes. Conventional cosmetics do, however, have a very special role that should be discussed with the patient preoperatively and postoperatively, to best accentuate their newly enhanced features. Many patients may not realize how helpful properly applied cosmetics can be

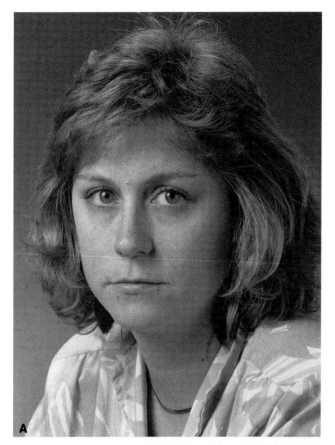
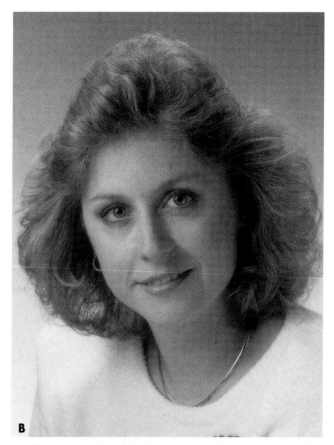

Figure 28–2. (A) Before and **(B)** after professional makeup application.

at any age. A professional makeup artist can turn one from frumpy to fabulous (Fig. 28–2) with the appropriate application of colors and hair style. Hair color and style are also important considerations.

Corrective techniques are also used to minimize poor features. They can highlight and contour to create illusions of symmetry. This effect is particularly useful to correct close-set or wide-set eyes, drop lip, or large or asymmetric nose. Regardless of the technique, makeup creates illusions, and these illusions affect how one is perceived by oneself and society. By improving one's appearance, one's self-esteem increases. Similarly, aesthetic surgery serves the same purpose to a different degree. The aesthetic surgeon, working in conjunction with the cosmetologist, provides a full range of complementary and therapeutic services to address appearance concerns of their patients.

INDICATIONS

Skin camouflage is indicated for a variety of conditions, including ecchymosis (Fig. 28–3A), erythema, erythematous lines of closure (Fig. 28–4A), postinflammatory hyperpigmentation (Fig. 28–4A), hypopigmentation, atrophic and hypertrophic scars (Fig. 28–5A), congenital markings, and tattoos (Fig. 28–6A).

PREOPERATIVE/POSTOPERATIVE SKIN CARE

Preoperatively, the surgeon will determine whether the procedure will leave residual or undesirable skin discoloration, noticeable suture lines, or hair loss, which may be of concern to the patient. It is at this time that the surgeon will call for the consultation of a medical esthetician, cosmetologist, or both to address these concerns. The medical esthetician will evaluate the patient's skin and determine the appropriate products and services

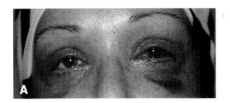
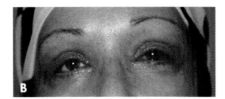

Figure 28-3. (A) Before and **(B)** after application of skin camouflage for ecchymosis.

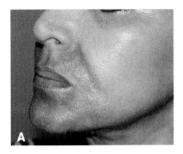
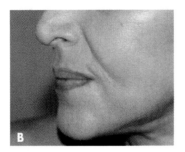

Figure 28-4. (A) Before and **(B)** after application of skin camouflage for erythematous lines of closure.

that will be beneficial to the patient during the healing stages of surgery and thereafter. She or he will also recommend preoperative services such as lymphatic drainage. The reason for this is to stimulate the purification of the blood before surgery, thus eliminating toxins and waste from the blood in preparation for the procedure. Because manual lymphatic drainage (MLD) brings improved function of the lymphatic system when performed regularly, it becomes a vital service in maintaining health enhancement, and therefore it is highly recommended preoperatively and postoperatively and thereafter. MLD reduces ecchymosis in nearly half the time of the naturally slow moving lymph. It also greatly accelerates the process of building new cells by carrying

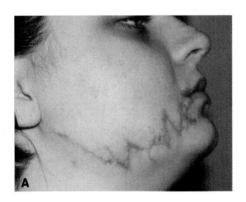
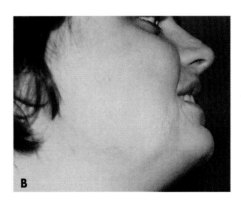

Figure 28-5. (A) Before and **(B)** after application of skin camouflage for scarring.

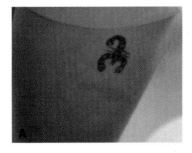
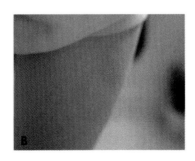

Figure 28-6. (A) Before and **(B)** after application of skin camouflage for a tattoo.

building substances to the cells and has a stimulating effect on the imune system.[5]

Because the lymph vessel system is located in the dermis, it is necessary to use a precise rhythmical and gentle manipulation to stimulate the function of the lymph. This method was first developed by Dr. Emil Vodder in France, whose success with MLD has been acclaimed throughout the world. Physicians, massage therapists, RNs, estheticians, and cosmetologists are eligible for training in MLD. Two methods of lymphatic drainage exist. The first and original is Vodder's method of manually manipulating the lymph. This method is highly effective yet physically taxing on the practitioner. In an attempt to encourage the use of this treatment, an easier method has been developed that uses a mechanical apparatus to consistently simulate the gentle pulsating technique in a pattern similar to that at Vodder. This method is combined with the application of biological products, thus creating a new science known as lymphobiology™.

Because MLD has a stimulating effect on the parasympathetic nervous system when applied properly, it has a calming and soothing effect on the patient. It is best applied during a facial treatment after a massage. Estheticians use lymphatic drainage for health enhancement. Certified MLD therapists use MLD to treat a variety of conditions such as acne, inflammation, edema, and other related conditions. Although this text merely introduces this therapeutic modality, other texts are available that describe the therapy practices, pathology, and physiology of MLD in detail.

Contraindications of MLD

Contraindications for MLD include acute inflammatory conditions resulting from poisons, viruses, bacteria, all malignant diseases, acute inflammation, embolism, and pulmonary edema. Relative contraindications, such as asthma, pregnancy, hyperthyroidism, low blood pressure, treated cancer, and tuberculosis, suggest that one should proceed only in certain areas.

TECHNIQUES

Skin camouflage techniques are based on color theory principles; techniques of application of pigmented, opaque preparations; and knowledge of wound healing phases. Aspects of color theory used are both complementary colors and color neutralization; thus to camouflage erythema, a shade of the complementary color green would be applied to counteract, then set with powder before applying the camouflage product. With a color wheel, one can learn to neutralize any color or mixture of colors with practice. A color wheel is shown in Figure 28–7. Another color theory principal is derived from pointillism. The practitioner will scan the colors in the palate to create a visual mixture of a skin color. Skin pigmentation and texture are a result of layers of intrinsic structures and extrinsic components such as hair, pores, furrows corresponding to folds in the dermis, and other markings. It is critical to the success of the application to

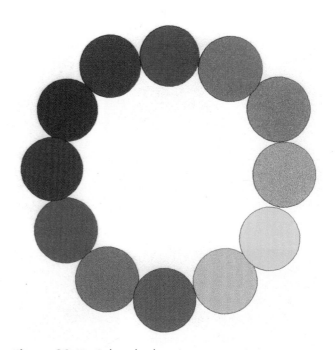

Figure 28–7. Color wheel.

recreate these natural elements of the skin after the application of the camouflage to achieve an aesthetically pleasing result. This is particularly important for men so they do not appear to be "masked." This precision demands the utmost skill. Having achieved this skill, the practitioner can enable the patient to wear the camouflage only where desired, and it should be virtually undetectable.

For surface changes such as an atrophic or hypertrophic scar, color theory principles of light and dark are used. These principals create optical illusions. When a sudden change in the plane of a surface, occurs, a hard edge and an apparent intensity of the shadow and the highlight also occurs. One should decrease the value of the highlight or create a lowlight so that the area appears less prominent. To complete this optical illusion, it is necessary to adjust the value (lightness and darkness) of the shadow. When mixed, applied, and blended by a skilled specialist, it will create the illusion of a more even surface (Fig. 28–8). The aerial perspective, recognized by the fourteenth century painter Ucello, demonstrates that centralization of value and intensity is inversely proportional to the nearness of the color to the eye. In other words the farther away the eye is, the less strongly differentiated the colors

become.[6] Up close, within 12 inches, an atrophic scar, now with appropriate dark and light principles applied, appears slightly noticeable, whereas at 36 inches, a comfortable social distance, it now appears flush with the surrounding skin and may disappear from sight completely.

One approaches hypopigmentation and hyperpigmentation with these principles in mind. Depending on the type of pigmentation, several additional principles of color theory may be considered and incorporated into the final method of camouflage. In most cases, color theory principles yield predictable results. In the cases that do not, one needs an experienced and highly skilled camouflage specialist to develop the method that best suits the condition and individual (Fig. 28–1A).

Once the camouflage method is completed, it is necessary to then "set" the application with a waterproof setting powder. This stabilizes the product and keeps it waterproof throughout the day. Typically, a camouflage session lasts between 1 and 2 hours, depending on the condition and how much instruction is needed for the patient. It is very possible that two sessions are needed for a standard camouflage, the second almost entirely to teach the patient application.

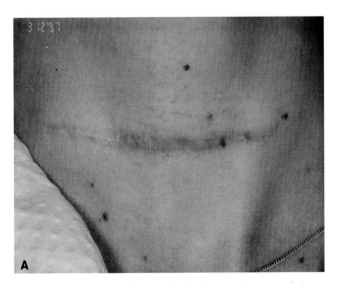 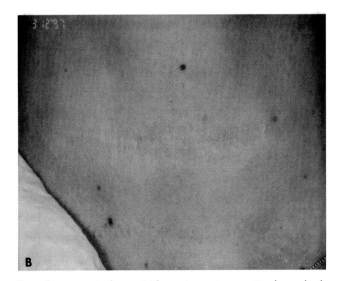

Figure 28–8. (A) Before and **(B)** after application of skin camouflage for a surgical scar. When pigments are mixed, applied, and blended correctly, it can create the illusion of a more even surface.

Physics and Light

The environment in which one renders pigmentation services must be abundantly illuminated with full spectrum or white light. The reason for this is that light alters our perception of color. If the light source does not contain full spectrum, it is unlikely one will achieve a match to the skin. To demonstrate this fact, visualize a port-wine stain in fluorescent light. Because fluorescent light does not contain red, the port-wine stain will appear much darker and deeper than it actually is. Now imagine applying color theories in fluorescent light. The result is a mess of thick cakey grayish camouflage when the patient leaves the office. This is not desirable. Similarly, incandescent light does not contain greens or blues, hence arterial and venous undertones and various melanin tones are not visible. The camouflage specialist can assist the patient in working around these problems when in different environments.

Active Ingredients

Many professional skin care products are manufactured more effectively today as a result of new active ingredients and more effective methods for combining them together. A partial list of these ingredients and their functions are described in Table 28–1.

Table 28–1 Active Ingredients of Skin Care Products

Active Ingredient	Function
Salicylic acid	Desquamates the skin by reducing oil and removing cellular debris
Hyaluronic acid	Superhydrator, helps to restore elasticity
Glycolic acid	Penetrates the "mortar" of the stratum corneum, thus allowing faster cellular renewal
Integral DNA	Antioxidant and moisturizer
Vitamins C and E	Antioxidants
Titanium dioxide	Ultraviolet A, B, and C radiation block

Retinoids and skin bleaching agents are sometimes combined into these active ingredients to create a more potent product. Potency is derived from quality. The grade quality of your ingredient affects the potency of the product. Just as extra virgin olive oil is the purest grade olive oil, so are pharmaceutical grade ingredients.

SKIN CARE MAINTENANCE

For medical estheticians or camouflage specialists, the skin is their canvas. The better condition the "canvas" is in the better the result of cosmetic or camouflage application. The importance of maintaining the skin preoperatively and postoperatively should not be underestimated. In fact, a regimen consisting of MLD not only expedites healing of postoperative ecchymosis, erythema, and edema but also helps to improve the overall function of the lymphatic system.[5]

A proper skin care regimen is critical in maintaining aesthetic facial surgery results by keeping the pores clean of follicular debris, keeping the surface smooth, and improving the overall health and vitality of the skin with the aid of pH balancing treatments, hydrating treatments, firming treatments, exfoliating treatments, and massage techniques. Although these are just a few of the treatments available, we will take a closer look at the principal procedures of a "facial" and its benefits.

Proper cleansing techniques help the patient learn how to use cleansers and which cleansers are appropriate for the property they are removing. Not all cleansers are made to remove the same properties. If a patient has to use friction to remove a product from their skin, is probably the wrong cleanser. Products referred to as removers are typically used for removing cosmetic products rather than cleansing the skin. The remover should be followed by a cleanser to cleanse any residue of the remover, excess oil, and dirt on the face. Deep cleansing refers to extracting debris and comedones from the pores and should only be performed by a licensed professional trained in comedone extraction, such as a licensed esthetician or physician. Massage is used to stimulate the blood circulation, reduce edema and pain, induce relaxation, reduce fat cells, and tone muscles. *Steaming* helps to prepare the skin for extraction and soothes and refreshes. *Extraction* also removes milia and allows the skin to heal faster. *Exfoliation* desquamates the dead cells on the surface of the skin promoting renewal of cells and creating an immediate and noticeable smoothness and glow. *Masks* are used for soothing, calming, refining, hydrating, and deep cleansing. Masks also stimulate, tighten, and firm the skin. Other treatments may include the use of high frequency for sterilization, galvanic current, and electric mask. *Specialty treatments* may include glycolic peels, specialty masks, firming treatments, and lymphatic drainage. Other benefits of facials include activating glandular activity, relaxing the nerves, maintaining muscle tone, strengthening weak muscle tissue, correcting minor skin disorders, preventing fine lines and wrinkles, and giving a youthful feeling and appearance.

POST LASER RESURFACING

Other treatments that are beneficial postoperatively include hydrating treatments and soothing masks. Postoperative skin care for laser resurfacing is very particular. No products should be used on freshly resurfaced skin unless they have been tested on freshly resurfaced or burned skin because it has not developed a tolerance to cosmetic ingredients and fragrances. One should wait at lease 8 weeks before giving exfoliating treatments to post-lasered skin. Post-laser skin care maintenance should consist of the mildest types of cleansers and moisturizers and a hydrating mist before applying moisturizer. These products, preferably, should be made for postsurgical and post-laser conditions. For the first 6 to 8 months, an Ultraviolet A, B, and C block (SPF30) is mandatory daily.

COMPLICATIONS

Very few complications are associated with camouflage application or products. Failure to observe necessary re-epithelielization time may result in irritation and tiny milia. This will cause physical and possibly emotional dis-

comfort for the patient. On freshly resurfaced skin, it is important to use only those products tested on freshly resurfaced skin, which has not built a tolerance to cosmetic ingredients. Milia and other infection can occur in suture holes if not allowed to close before applying camouflage. The greatest risk is referring a patient to an unqualified person. It is crucial to avoid applying camouflage on open lesions, herpes blisters, acute inflammation, poison ivy or oak, and infected conditions. Caution should be taken with severe actinic conditions. One should take care with ingredients known to cause allergic reactions or irritation.

CAMOUFLAGE FOR HAIR LOSS
INDICATIONS

Camouflage for hair loss is indicated for patients with alopecia (all types), including loss of facial and scalp hair; visible intraoperative and postoperative hardware (screws); lines of closure on scalp; thin or thinning hair; and male pattern baldness.

TECHNIQUES

Eyebrows are a very important facial feature and are unique to each individual. They give character, color, and symmetry to the face and serve as an architectural frame. The lack or position of eyebrows can affect how a person is perceived. Low, droopy eyebrows makes one appear unhappy, depressed, even angry, whereas raised eyebrows gives the appearance of health and well-being, even youth.

Fortunately, today's endoscopic forehead lift raises the brow without leaving obvious lines of closure and gives a natural appearance. Although natural, the effect of how one's disposition is perceived is dramatic and therefore greatly improves the patients' self-esteem.

The past popularity of tweezing eyebrows has left some with alopecia or remnants of what use to be beautiful brows. Cosmetology has long provided cosmetic remedies for thin or sparse brows as has hair graft surgery. The cosmetics used are pencils, usually waterproof, and powders that are drawn onto the skin or blended in with sparse hairs to create a desired shape.

In recent years, new technology in the area of cosmetology has provided another alternative. *Micropigmentation* (tattooing) is a method in which a desired color is implanted into the dermis. This technique is popular among women who choose to have permanent eyeliner, lipliner, lipstick, and eyebrows and throw away their conventional cosmetics. Other uses include areola reconstruction for postmastectomy patients and for camouflaging scars on the scalp. Prudence must be observed during patient selection for this technique. However, there may be complications associated with micropigmentation such as allergies to the dyes used and inability to achieve desired color. Natural cellular renewal causes a fading, which may then require additional treatments. Hypopigmentation, such as vitiligo, would not be appropriate for this treatment because it is difficult to match the surrounding skin and it has the tendency to spread. Conditions that do not have to be matched to a surrounding area are more appropriate. If the color does not match the surrounding skin, the patient must then under go a painful laser procedure to remove the dye. A licensed cosmetologist or medical esthetician must have an additional license or certification in micropigmentation to perform this technique.

Even though micropigmentation can permanently create eyebrows, it cannot replace the actual hair. Short of surgery, one final option exists. *Custom* or *prefabricated eyebrows* made from natural or synthetic hair (Fig. 28–9). Mustaches and beards can also be fabricated. This option is natural in appearance and easy to use and care for. In addition, the patient can choose the exact shape and color desired. With custom or prefabricated eyebrows patients can resume a normal, active lifestyle, including such activities as swimming.

Almost every race hair type can be created for replacement of eyebrows and scalp hair, also called cranial prostheses. For centuries wigs have been worn to

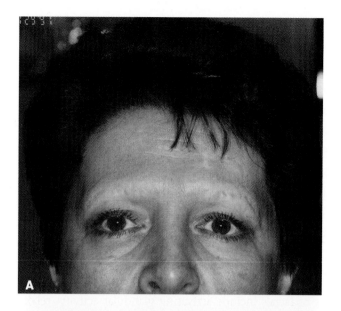
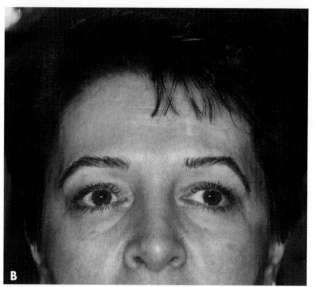

Figure 28–9. (A) Before and **(B)** after application of custom hand made eyebrows using natural hair.

cover the hair for various customs and fashions. Wigs are still worn for those reasons and are commonly worn for medical reasons. These medical reasons range from hair loss resulting from medical treatments such as chemotherapy to hair loss resulting from alopecia or to camouflage coronal and hairline incisions. Incisions and hardware such as that for endoscopic forehead lifting can be camouflaged either with the patients' own hair or with the use of an invention called HAIR-B-TWEENZ™.

HAIR-B-TWEENZ™ is a hair integration system that mixes with the clients' own hair. By snapping in the combs then sliding natural hair through the spaces between the wefts with the tail of a comb, it blends easily into the natural hair (Fig. 28–10). A hair color swatch makes it easy to find the right shade. Different base widths and hairlengths easily accommodate most hair styles. This is a practical option for men to fill in thinness

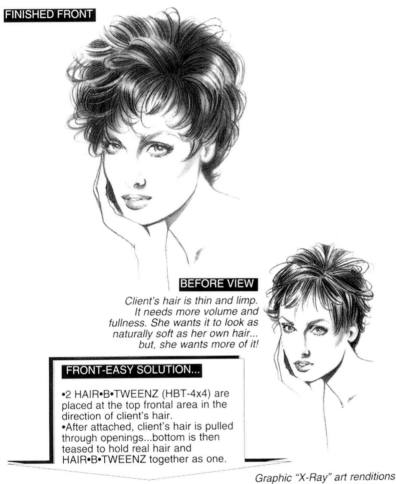

FINISHED FRONT

BEFORE VIEW

Client's hair is thin and limp. It needs more volume and fullness. She wants it to look as naturally soft as her own hair... but, she wants more of it!

FRONT-EASY SOLUTION...

•2 HAIR•B•TWEENZ (HBT-4x4) are placed at the top frontal area in the direction of client's hair.
•After attached, client's hair is pulled through openings...bottom is then teased to hold real hair and HAIR•B•TWEENZ together as one.

Graphic "X-Ray" art renditions show exactly where HBT's are placed to achieve above finished styles.

Figure 28-10. HAIR-B-TWEENZ™. By snapping in combs and sliding natural hair through the spaces between the wefts with the tail of a comb, the hairpiece blends easily into the natural hair. (From Look of Love Int. Catalog® 1995, with permission.)

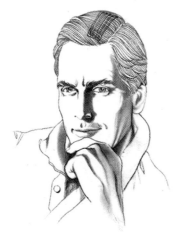

For side-parted styles, pull own hair through spaces, blend and cut to suit.

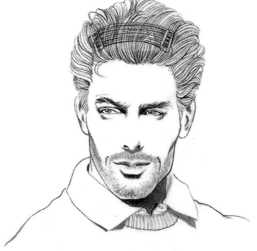

Even men could use them to fill-in thinness!

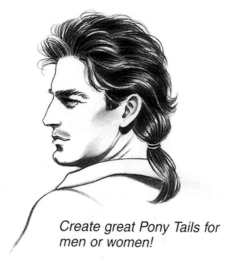

Create great Pony Tails for men or women!

Figure 28–11. Hairpieces for male clients. (From Look of Love Int. Catalog© 1995, with permission.)

and is also useful during postoperative healing (Fig. 28–11). HAIR-B-TWEENZ™ can be used to camouflage postoperative hardware, coronal incisions, grafts (interim delay), and staples. To blend larger areas, HONEYCOMB™ is used and creates fuller coverage (Fig. 28–12). Three base sizes accommodate most coverage needs. The manufacturer of these products is included in the appendix at the end of this chapter.

Be sure to work with a cosmetologist who is skilled at creating facial symmetry using hairstyling. Hairstyles directed toward the face can camouflage rhytidectomy and other hairline incision lines (Fig. 28–13). Prefabricated wigs are also helpful for temporary camouflage. For a sporty look, cloth headbands create a clever camouflage for hairline incision lines and come in an assortment of widths and fabrics. Terry cloth is most commonly used in sport bands for men and women.

Hypertrichosis or superfluous hair growth has more treatment options today than in the past. Electrolysis is still the leading method for permanent hair removal; although it is making room for the laser hair removal technology. Waxing is a good temporary method of hair removal, which usually lasts up to 6 weeks and is used in preparation for the Therma Laze laser, for permanent hair removal. Therma Laze laser is a form of YAG laser, the latter is used for removing tattoos and brown spots.

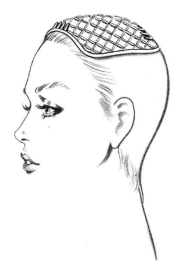

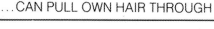
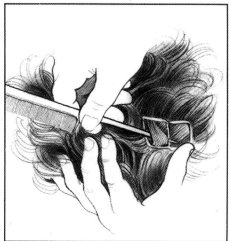
...CAN PULL OWN HAIR THROUGH

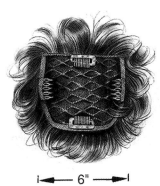
|← 6" →|

Figure 28-12. HONEYCOMB™ is used to create fuller coverage in clients with hair loss. (From Look of Love Int. Catalog© 1995, with permission.)

CONCLUSION

Helping a patient make an easy transition back into the workplace and social scene after aesthetic surgery presents a challenge to the surgeon. Becoming involved with a medical esthetician or cosmetologist will make this transition easier for the patient and more rewarding for the surgeon. It is the role of the medical esthetician or cosmetologist to evaluate the patient and determine which services will be necessary after surgery, explain the options to the patient, and provide any specialized service required by the patient. These services may include skin and hair camouflage techniques, skin care maintenance, and makeup application. Thus the medical esthetician or cosmetologist plays a key role in the postoperative course of the patient's self-image, which is key in a successful result.

PEARLS

- The role of the medical esthetician or clinical cosmetologist is to evaluate the postoperative condition of the patient, explain the options for camouflage, and provide specialized service within the scope of his or her training and experience.

- One's choice of terminology can remove the stigma associated with wearing cosmetics and allows men a therapeutic perspective when using them.

- Because MLD brings improved function of the lymphatic system when performed regularly, it becomes a vital service in maintaining healthy skin and so is recommended preoperatively and postoperatively.

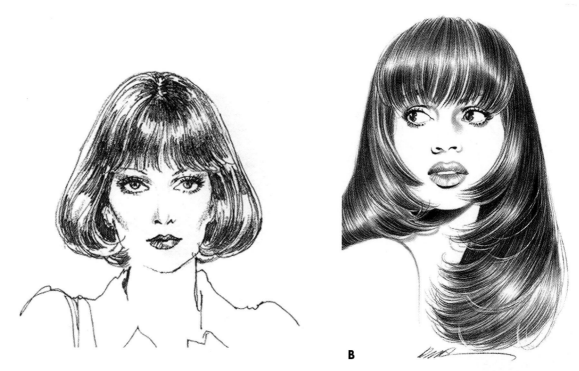

A   **B**

Figure 28–13. Prefabricated wigs can camouflage hair loss and surgery scars. (From Look of Love Int. Catalog© 1995, with permission.)

REFERENCES

1. Romo T, Millman A, Pazienza L. Camouflage following aesthetic laser resurfacing. *Dermascope.* Jul/Aug 1996.
2. Sherwyn J, Pazienza L. The patient/client experience. *Dermascope.* May/June 1996.
3. Allsworth J. *Skin Camouflage, a Guide to Remedial Techniques.* Cheltenham, United Kingdom: Stanley Thornes Ltd.; 1985.
4. Pazienza L. Making legislation work for you. *Dermascope.* 1993.
5. Wittlinger H, Wittlinger G. *Textbook of Dr. Vodder's Manual Lymph Drainage,* Vol. 1, 5th ed. Brussels: Haug; 1992.
6. Corson R. *Stage Makeup,* 8th ed. Englewood Cliffs, NJ: Prentice-Hall; 1989.
7. Pazienza L. Truest color with natural light. *Dermascope.* Jul/Aug 1995.
8. LoVerme P, Pazienza L. Dermabrasion, chemical peel and camouflage. *Dermascope.* Sept/Oct 1996.
9. Mayer R, Fleming R. *Aesthetic and Reconstructive Surgery of the Scalp.* St. Louis: Mosby; 1992.
10. Thomas J, Holt G. *Facial Scars, Incision, Revision and Camouflage.* St. Louis: Mosby; 1989.
11. Jewell D. *Making Up By Rex.* New York: Clarkson N. Potter; 1986.
12. Kibbe C. *Standard Textbook of Cosmetology.* Bronx, NY: Milady; 1982.

APPENDIX

This represents a partial list.

CAMOUFLAGE PRODUCTS

United States

Alcone Company Inc.
5-49 49th Avenue
Long Island City, NY 11101
Postoperative Make-up Department
1-800-466-7446

McMillan CosMedics
125 Marving Road
Middletown, NY 07748
732-706-0690
www.mcmillancosmedics.com
www.mcmillanpalette.com

Cinema Secrets
4400 Riverside Drive
Burbank, CA 91505

Natural Cover
7 West Aylesbury Road
Suite S
Timonium, MD 21093
1-410-308-0937

Canada

Kirsch Camouflage
Kirsch Cosmetic Clinic
257 Eglinton Avenue West
Toronto, Ontario
Canada, M4R 1B1
1-416-487-4887

Europe

Keromask
Innoxa LTD.
202 Terminus Road
Eastboume, Sussex BN21 3DF
England

HAIR REPLACEMENT AND ACCESSORIES

International

Look of Love Int.
1913 Route 27
Edison, NJ 08817
1-800-526-7627

United States

Center for Aesthetic Rehabilitation
150 Broadway
Suite 616
NY, NY 10038
732-706-0690

SKIN CARE PRODUCTS

Catherine Atzen Laboratories, Inc.
1129 Dell Avenue
Campbell, CA 95008
1-408-364-0295

ELTA SWISS SKIN CARE

Swiss American Products
4641 Nall Road
Dallas, Tx 75244
1-800-633-8872

AESTHETIC ORGANIZATIONS

American Aestheticians Education Association
1-214-394-1740
1-800-985-AAEA CST

Aesthetics International Association
1-800-961-3777

AESTHETIC PUBLICATIONS

Dermascope Magazine
Les Nouvelles Esthetique
Skin Inc.

Cosmetology: an Adjunct to Aesthetic Facial Surgery

Aesthetic Facial Plastic Surgery, edited by Thomas Romo, III, and Arthur L. Millman, Thieme Medical Publishers, Inc., New York, New York, Copyright © 2000.

Cosmetology

A Hairdresser's Perspective

EDWARD TRICOMI, JOEL WARREN, AND RENÉE GARNES

Like a gilded frame to an oil painting, haircut and color complement the face. The wrong hairstyle can counteract otherwise successful cosmetic surgery by insufficiently covering any possible scars or by creating an illusion that does not complement a newly shaped nose or jawline. The wrong hair color can draw attention to uneven skin tone or redness. In addition, hair, like skin, can reflect a patient's age, so it must look as young as your patient's new face. Therefore to achieve a successful final result to cosmetic surgery, it is in both the patient's and the surgeon's best interest that haircut and color receive almost as much attention as the surgery itself. A cosmetic surgeon who is eager for his patients to have a positive and successful experience should recognize the importance of working together with professionals in the beauty industry. A patient's satisfaction with her surgery will improve if her hair works with her new look.

Just as surgical technique has improved in the past decade, so has the technology of haircare products. Gentler shampoo and coloring formulas are readily available, and hair professionals have become better educated on how to cut and color hair in a manner that is sensitive to a client's special needs. Today's stylists and colorists understand the importance of postoperative care and the significance of the right haircut to set off a newly shaped face, and they recognize the caution that is required when working with chemicals, such as haircolor. In addition to gentler formulas, new techniques have been developed for haircolor application that reduce its contact with skin and scalp. With these improvements, cosmetic surgeons can trust in the expertise of hair professionals and can rely on them as an extension of their own service to the patient. A patient who desires cosmetic surgery to enhance aesthetic beauty needs to consider the skills of the hair professional as well. Because cosmetic surgery has so much to do with a patient's self-esteem, the role of the hairdresser cannot be ignored. During the postsurgery phase a hair professional can help a patient feel better about himself or herself with a change of hair color or an updated hair style. The cosmetic surgeon's guidance and recommendations will ensure that a patient meets with a skilled hair professional to put the finishing touches on the final look.

PATIENT SELECTION

Every patient can benefit from the services of a hair professional who understands the consequences of cosmetic surgery. Preoperative and postoperative beauty care in the form of a new haircut or color have a critical effect on a patient's psychologic and emotional response to the cosmetic surgery procedure. A client who chooses a facelift with the expectation of looking younger must consider making changes to his hair for this same purpose. To disregard these elements may result in disappointment with the surgery's results.

A patient's hairstyle should be taken into consideration when deciding on the placement of incision marks on and around the face. A patient who wears her hair very short and off the face probably will not want to change this style to disguise scars around the perimeter of the face. The surgeon should ask each patient how they wear their hair and if they have any plans to make drastic style changes in the future. A patient whose hair is thin and fine will not be able to disguise scars on the scalp as easily as one who has thick, textured hair. In these instances the hair cannot be relied on to hide any indications of surgery, such as the incisions made in an endoscopic forehead lift. In addition, a patient who regularly perms her hair must understand that she is prohibited from that chemical service for some time after surgery. This is also true for patients who regularly wear a hairpiece or hair extensions.

TIMING

The timing of the hair consultation and services, in relation to the date of the surgery, is critical. During a preoperative consultation with the surgeon (in conjunction with the hairstylist, if possible), the patient should explain how she wears her hair, and the surgeon should explain any scarring that might limit future hairstyles such as a new short (pixie) cut that may reveal scarring that was formerly hidden under a shoulder-length bob. A patient should have photographs taken immediately after a preoperative hair appointment to document for the surgeon how she wears her hair. This will assist the surgeon in producing flawless results. A patient will not want to be forced to change her hairstyle entirely to compensate for a new hair-growth pattern or visible scars that do not work with her regular hairstyle.

If a patient cannot coordinate a meeting with her surgeon and hairstylist simultaneously, the surgeon must explain to the patient in precise terms where incisions will be placed and the manner of facial changes that will occur. Armed with these exact details of the surgery, a patient can then consult with the hairstylist to discuss how to proceed with her hairstyle.

This consultation also ensures that the stylist knows what not to do to the patient's hair. A slight change in haircut may prepare the patient for her postoperative appearance. Before surgery, a patient should be advised to have her hair cut in the style that will work best for her after surgery. This has two benefits: It ensures that the patient's hair is at its best as her face heals, so that she sees the results in the optimal light; and for those patients who wish to keep their cosmetic surgery a secret, they can attribute their new, better look to their new haircut.

Hair color also needs to be refreshed or changed before surgery. Patients who will have incisions in the scalp area should be advised to have any hair-color treatment done no less than a week before surgery because this reduces the risk of infection. Patients whose hair color is dramatically different from that of their natural color (such as those with gray hair) should have their roots touched up no more than 1 week before surgery to ensure that no sizable amount of regrowth appears before they can next have a color treatment. If a patient is advised to refrain from coloring her hair for a significant amount of time, colorists can use hair mascara or hair-color sticks (crayons for the hair) to apply temporary color to the hair without applying chemicals to the scalp.

As haircolor formulas have improved and become gentler (many using natural ingredients rather than strong chemicals), haircolor treatments pose less threat to sensitive skin. A patient can visit her hair colorist a minimum of 4 weeks after surgery to receive a color service without fearing that the coloring product will harm her still-healing skin. In addition, haircoloring techniques such as off-scalp foiling and hair painting can produce the same natural-looking results without any skin product contact. Hair color treatment products such as shampoos and conditioners also have gentler formulas than ever before. Because hair color is damaged and stripped by aggressive cleansers, these new formulas are designed to

maintain the color for as long as possible. This same gentleness benefits the postsurgery patient because it is sure not to irritate the scalp as it heals.

PRECAUTIONS

A skilled hair professional can be relied on to help a patient get back to normal after surgery by showing him or her new hair styles and colors that may further enhance his or her new face. However, the hairstylist cannot be relied on to work around any unforeseen changes made to the hair-growth pattern as a result of incisions made during surgery. Problems that can arise include alopecia from hair follicles damaged by an incision. A patient who experiences some hair loss from damaged hair follicles will not be satisfied with the results of his or her surgery because they will have only traded one problem for another.

Another potential problem is redirected hair growth, resulting from inaccurately sewn skin. To avoid this, surgeons need to ensure that follicles are not bent in a manner that is not conducive to the patient's natural hair flow. As in the case of cowlicks, hair that goes against the overall growth pattern can be problematic for both the hairstylist and the patient and disrupt the usual hairstyle. This is especially problematic for a patient with thin, fine hair because the hair's weight cannot fight the new growth direction.

MAKEUP

Patients must understand that it takes some time before makeup can be used on skin that is still healing. Nevertheless, makeup is also a tool that helps a patient's overall self-esteem concerning his or her looks because it works effectively to cover the signs of surgery as soon as skin is able to withstand it. Surgeons must seek out professional makeup artists who have been educated in the special concerns of cosmetic surgery patients. Makeup artists who are sensitive to these clients can help them through the healing process and can reinforce such commonsense advice as avoiding the sun and drinking plenty of water to keep skin hydrated.

Maketip artists who are attune to the needs of the plastic surgery patient use gentle, natural solutions with soothing and anti-inflammatory properties, such as witch hazel. Makeup artists can supply a patient with camouflage makeup, which is heavier than a regular makeup formulation, and teach her how it is applied. Camouflage makeup tends to be oil-based to provide complete coverage; however, patients who have dry skin tend to prefer water-based makeup. The camouflage process requires a layering of makeup and specially formulated powder.

RELATIONSHIPS

Developing relationships with a roster of beauty professionals who understand the process and special concerns involved in cosmetic surgery can lead to increased success with every patient's surgery. Surgeons are well advised to seek out the most reputable salons in the area and invite stylists, colorists, and makeup artists to an informational seminar on the cosmetic surgery field. By educating beauty professionals, physicians can be certain that they will be attune to the needs of their patients and will not jeopardize the surgery's results by coloring too soon or applying products to unhealed skin. These same professionals can then explain to the physicians the extent of what they can do to enhance the surgery results and disguise any visible signs of surgery. Also, people in this field can provide excellent patient referrals because they too work in a field where their customer wants to improve her looks.

CONCLUSIONS

By developing an interdisciplinary partnership with hair and makeup professionals, plastic surgeons are taking an additional, yet sometimes forgotten, measure in ensuring the success of each patient's surgery results. Hairstylists, colorists, and makeup artists bring to the table a set of specialized skills that can enhance not only the aesthetic results but also the psychologic results of plastic surgery.

PEARLS

- Find reputable salons with which to establish working relationships.
- Offer classes for the hair and makeup professionals on the special needs and conditions of the plastic surgery patient; elicit discussion from class attendees on their concerns and knowledge.
- Ensure that your patient has met with her hair professional (or refer her to one with whom you have developed a relationship and whom you trust) before her surgery. Discuss how your patient wishes to wear his hair after surgery.
- Analyze your patient's hair growth patterns before surgery.
- Be cautious with respect to the hair growth patterns during surgery and not to cut any follicles.
- After surgery, advise your patient on when she can see her hairstylist and colorist and advise that she meets with a professional makeup artist who is skilled at working with plastic surgery patients.

The Pursuit of Excellence in Facial Plastic Surgery

This chapter is the grand finale of our book on aesthetic facial plastic surgery. In the final analysis every surgeon must review his or her results and techniques in the constant process of modification and advancement toward the goal of a perfect surgical result. The pursuit of excellence is a deeply personal matter and approached differently by every surgeon.

The article by Dr. Beraka, a plastic surgeon, is excellently written and demonstrates a deep commitment toward excellence in surgery. Dr. Beraka describes, in both philosophical and technical terms, what the pursuit of excellence embodies in facial plastic surgery.

Dr. Fagien, an oculoplastic surgeon, presents his experience and philosophy specifically with regard to midfacial surgery and blepharoplasty. His analysis of the subjective and philosophical components that go into aesthetics provide an indispensable component to successful cosmetic surgery.

Although no surgical techniques are specifically presented, we believe the reader will gain more from the understanding and incorporation of the pursuit of excellence into surgical technique, than in any specific chapter in this book.

The Pursuit of Excellence in Facial Plastic Surgery

Aesthetic Facial Plastic Surgery, edited by Thomas Romo, III, and Arthur L. Millman, Thieme Medical Publishers, Inc., New York, New York, Copyright © 2000.

CHAPTER 30

A Plastic Surgeon's Perspective

GEORGE J. BERAKA

If a man has good corn, or wood, or boards, or pigs, to sell, or can make better chairs or knives, crucibles or church organs, than anybody else, you will find a broad hard-beaten road to his house, though it be in the woods.

Emerson[1]

Although much emphasis is placed on new techniques and new technology in cosmetic surgery, the available fund of knowledge is adequate for most patients and can yield wonderful results. Often, the limiting factor in the outcome is the behavior of the individual surgeon. Perhaps we need to shift our focus a little: we need more excellent surgeons and better operations. More of our educational efforts should be directed at teaching the pursuit of excellence, which becomes crucial long before the operation begins. I like to tell residents that three things are necessary in a cosmetic surgeon: integrity, stamina, and a good eye.

INTEGRITY

Excellence in cosmetic surgery is more intangible and difficult to monitor than in other fields of medicine and there are two important reasons for this. The first is that people contemplating cosmetic surgery are perfectly healthy. No pathologic problem needs to be corrected. Therefore the procedures recommended by the surgeon and, in fact, the very decision to operate at all depend more on the surgeon's judgment and ethical standards.

The second reason is that the outcome of cosmetic surgery is so subjective. No functional criteria (i.e., a pain-free knee joint, improved vision) exist to define the success of an operation. Sometimes a cosmetic surgery patient is satisfied with mediocre results. If he or she is not satisfied but the surgeon retains the patient's trust, the patient will accept a mediocre result as "the best that could be done." Tissue committees and morbidity and mortality conferences are less useful in identifying problems and with so much aesthetic surgery performed in the surgeon's office, less peer review occurs. Therefore in cosmetic surgery the pursuit of excellence must be generated from within the surgeon. This is a tall order.

Excellence not only means striving for a good surgical result, it also means really doing what is best for the patient. Cosmetic surgery patients are not sick, but they are still patients who entrust their bodies to us. Our professional standards must not be those of the marketplace. We do have to "sell" ourselves to our prospective patients; we have to convince them of our competence. However, we should never try to sell motivation for surgery.[2]

The wonderful thing about our work is that virtue truly is its own reward, in both senses. A plastic surgeon who does his or her best for everyone and who truly treats patients the way he or she would like to be treated, assuming reasonable competence, will see his or her practice grow and good name spread. We do well by doing good.

STAMINA

Stamina is crucial in cosmetic surgery for similar reasons. Any surgeon who is not demented will perform a vascular anastomosis as well as he possibly can, regardless of how tired he is. The fruits of failure are swift and terrible; they enforce rectitude. How is the patient to know if his or her facelift is the best that the surgeon can do? A little extra effort or a few more minutes can make a real difference. The patient will live with the result for a long time. Most of our patients are healthy and anesthesia is now safe; so little reason exists to rush in the name of safety.

The surgeon should do every case as if the before and after pictures will be printed on the front page of *The New York Times* (or hometown newspaper).

AESTHETIC JUDGMENT OR "HAVING A GOOD EYE"

> *The painter draws with his eyes, not with his hands. Whatever he sees, if he sees it **clear**, he can put down. The putting of it down requires perhaps, much care and labor, but no more muscular agility than it takes for him to write his name. Seeing **clear** is the important thing.*
>
> Grosser, *The Painter's Eye*[3]

The third critical quality in a cosmetic surgeon is a good eye. The craft of cosmetic surgery is in the hands of the surgeon but the art of cosmetic surgery is in the eyes. The eye must be powerful and discriminating. Detecting subtle details and asymmetries, visualizing the changes that will make a face more attractive, assessing accurately the endpoint of the operation—these are the capacities of a good eye. Without this attribute, the surgeon does not know what the goal is and what has been achieved.

I once attended a rhinoplasty lecture given by a well-known surgeon. The before and after pictures started to flash on the screen, and it became apparent that many of his patients looked worse after surgery. However, this was not a lecture on complications. The speaker was clearly pleased with his results and he showed them proudly. Several members of the audience were obviously embarrassed.

How to explain this story? This is an extreme example of poor visual discrimination. This surgeon is intelligent and caring. He just could not tell the difference between a good rhinoplasty and bad one.

The capacity for aesthetic judgment varies widely in the population. It is the job of program directors to select residents with a good eye. However, it is also possible for the practicing surgeon to improve his aesthetic sense through conscious effort and practice. One invaluable exercise is to learn to draw the face. Some wonderful books provide guidance[4-6] (Fig. 30–1). If we cannot see something, we cannot draw it. Trying to draw forces us not just to look, but to see intensely and minutely, and this eventually becomes a habit.

Edwards' book is worth reading even if you do not want to learn to draw. She teaches a cognitive shift model of thinking from verbal, analytical (left hemisphere) processing toward a more global, intuitive (right hemisphere) mode. "The key to learning to draw therefore is to set up conditions that cause you to make a mental shift to a different mode of information processing—the slightly altered state of consciousness—that enables you to see well" (p. 5). Developing the capacity to consciously make this mental shift is particularly useful for surgeons, who tend to be rigid and linear.

Cosmetic surgeons devote surprisingly little attention to the work of "real" artists—sculptors and painters. These are the people who see what most of us cannot see. Detailed study of a few paintings can teach us to see better. For example, the work of Giovanni Bellini, Bronzino, and Ingres (Fig. 30–2) is valuable to students of the human face. Studying the faces of models and systematically analyzing high-quality black and white photographs of one's patients will gradually improve our aesthetic eye. This is an area tailor made for interactive computer programs.

Because harmony and symmetry are intuitive elements of beauty, since antiquity people have searched for geometric laws that describe a beautiful face.[7] The cosmetic surgeon should understand cephalometric analysis. A facial angle of about 100 degrees is associated with an attractive face.[8] However, ratios and angles are more useful in defining *normal* than beautiful. Beauty cannot be measured because it lies in endless combinations within the narrow limits of the normal.

SELECTION AND TRAINING OF RESIDENTS IN AESTHETIC SURGERY

Until recently, medical school grades and written test scores were the principal tools for surgical resident selection. Even today, pre-eminent training programs make no attempt to evaluate manual dexterity or spatial cognition in their applicants. However, awareness is growing that failures in plastic surgery are seldom intellectual failures. Therefore we are developing better screening for the complex functions that a plastic surgeon must perform.

Specific training in aesthetic surgery has improved dramatically. Some of today's leaders in plastic surgery learned little aesthetic surgery during their residency. They learned it at the wonderful Baker-Gordon Symposia in Miami (which are still invaluable). Now aesthetic surgery is an integral part of plastic surgery residency training, and programs with low aesthetic surgery case loads send their residents on aesthetic surgery rotations.

For example, at Lenox Hill Hospital in New York City, we provide aesthetic surgery training to residents from two other programs. The residents have their own cosmetic surgery clinic and perform many cosmetic operations with close attending supervision.

ANATOMY

Knowledge is power. The freedom given by these understandings [of anatomy] allows aesthetic considerations to define the procedure, not dated dicta of what is "safe."

Lambros[9]

Anatomy is the most critical discipline for a surgeon. Ignorance of anatomy leads to complications on the one

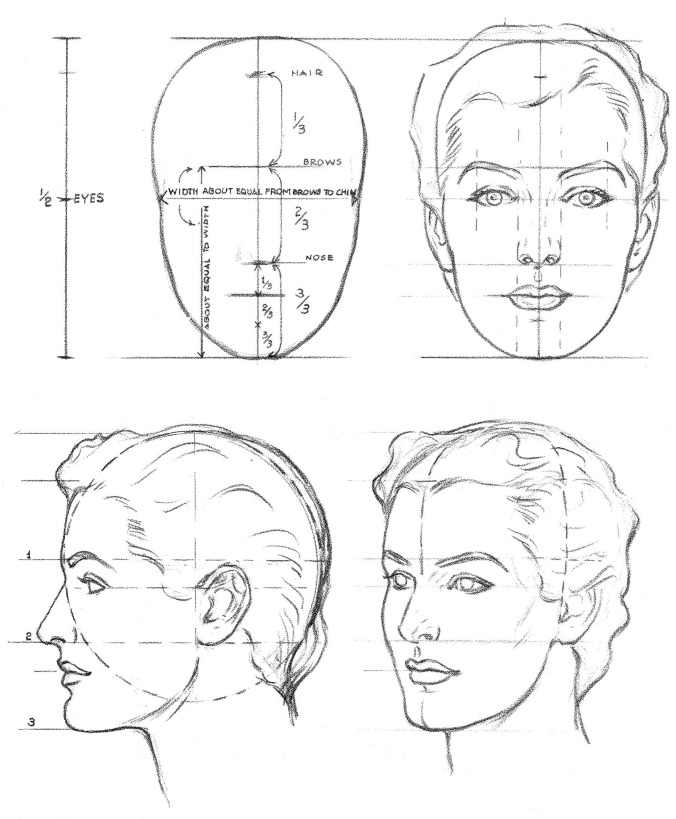

Figure 30–1. Drawing the Face. (From *Drawing the Head and Hands* by Andrew and Ethel Loomis. Copyright ©1956 by Andrew Loomis. Used by permission of Viking Penguin, a division of Penguin Books USA Inc.)

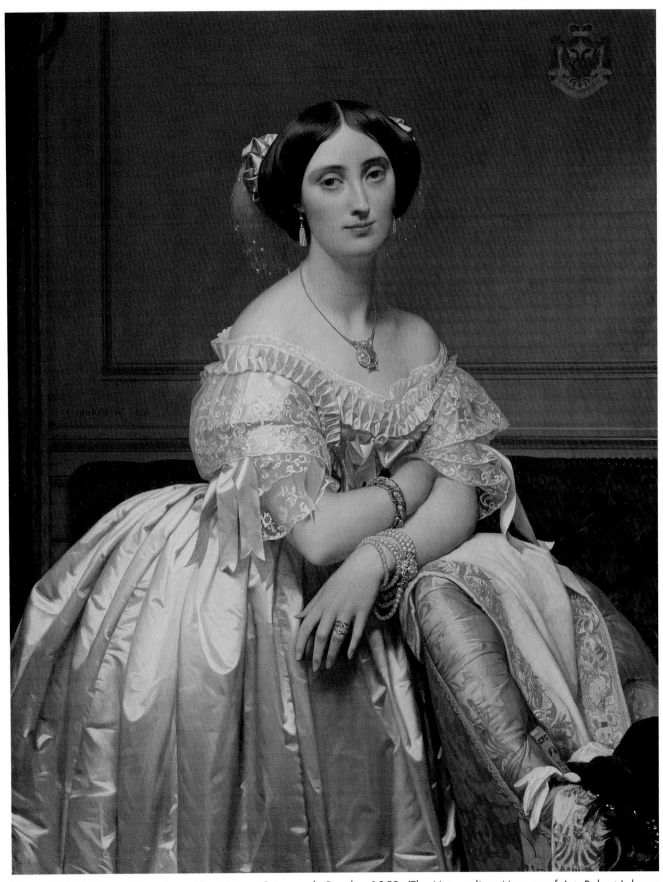

Figure 30–2. Ingres, Jean August Dominique. Princess de Broglie, 1853. (The Metropolitan Museum of Art, Robert Lehman Collection, 1975. [1975.1.186])

hand and to inadequate results because of fear of complications on the other. I went through my residency without doing a single cadaver dissection and that is a common experience. Detailed surgical anatomy must be studied regularly and systematically in training programs until the structures and their relationships are as unconsciously familiar as the streets of one's hometown.

The most serious obstacles to practical anatomic training are the logistics and expense of obtaining cadavers. Within the next few years, virtual reality programs may provide an accessible alternative to cadaver dissection.[10]

Spending 1 hour every week studying anatomy is one of the most educational pastimes for a surgeon. In addition to the standard anatomy texts, several excellent more specialized atlases are available.[11–15] Saban and Polselli's work "brings one close to actually going to the anatomy laboratory and sequentially dissecting a fresh cadaver head layer by layer with cosmetic procedures in mind"[16] (Fig. 30–3). Owsley's facelift book has several valuable anatomic descriptions and pictures.[17]

In the last several years a number of important contributions to our knowledge of facial anatomy have occurred. Knize described the course of the two branches of the supraorbital nerve.[18] The medial branch extends to the hairline; the lateral, more critical branch provides sensation to the frontal scalp and it lies deep and courses just superficial to the periosteum about 1 cm medial to the line of fusion (Fig. 30–4). Knize also has explained the various layers of the superficial temporal fascia and the relationship between galea and fat at the level of the eyebrows.[19] These anatomical details obviously have major implications for how we perform browlifts.

Isse[20] believes that the corrugator muscle is not a primary depressor of the medial brow and that isolated corrugator contraction does not produce the typical vertical glabellar furrows. The corrugator does tether the medial brow toward the midline and corrugator overresection leads to unattractive lateral displacement of the eyebrows often seen after browlifts. Isse advocates modification of the depressor supercilii. He also performs vertical inci-

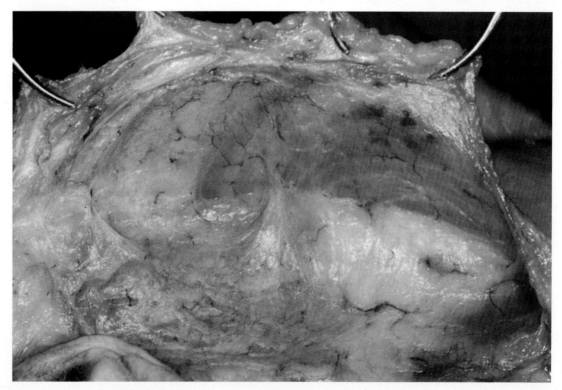

Figure 30–3. Elevation of SMAS-platysma layer in the parotid-masseteric area. Neck is on the right side of illustration. (From "Chapter 4: Parotid Area and Cheek" by Jose Saintini of the *Atlas of Surgical Anatomy of the Face and Neck*, edited by Yves Saban and Roberto Polselli. Copyright 1994, by Masson, Paris. Used by permission of Masson S.A. Paris, France.)

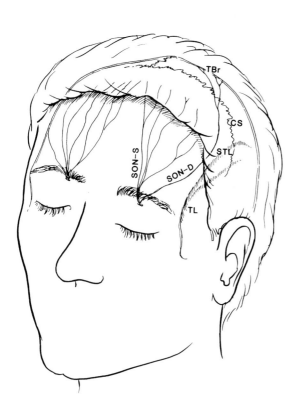

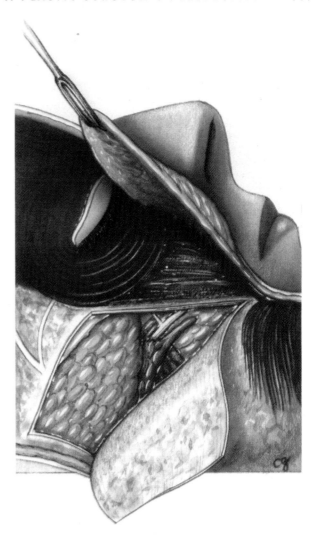

Figure 30–4. Diagram illustrating the courses of the deep (*SON-D*) and the superficial (*SON-S*) divisions of the supraorbital nerve trunk that form just after the trunk exits the supraorbital rim. The SON-D ran superiorly and obliquely across the forehead between the galea aponeurotica and the periosteum and, by the midforehead level, was always found running parallel to and between 0.5 and 1.5 cm medial to the superior temporal line (*STL*) of the skull. This relationship with the STL over the forehead continued onto the scalp area. Just before reaching the level of the coronal suture (*CS*), the SON-D typically bifurcated before forming the fine terminal branches (*TBr*) that pierced the galea aponeurotica and entered the frontoparietal scalp. The SON-S division formed branches that pass through the lower frontalis muscle at variable levels to run cephalad over this muscle and enter the anterior scalp. (From "A Study of the Supraorbital Nerve" by David M. Knize, on page 565 of *Plastic and Reconstructive Surgery*, 96:3, 1995.)

Figure 30–5. The malar fat pad has been separated from the underlying SMAS, which invests the orbicularis, zygomaticus, and levator muscles. Laterally, the SMAS has been incised and reflected caudally, exposing the underlying zygomatic branch of the facial nerve accompanied by the transverse facial artery and the parotid duct as they traverse the buccal space deep to the superficial facial muscles. The superficial location of the frontal branch cephalad to the zygomatic arch is indicated. (From "Lifting the Malar Fat Pad for Correction of Prominent Nasolabial Folds" by John Q. Owsley, on page 465 of *Plastic and Reconstructive Surgery*, 91:3, 1993.)

sions in the orbicularis oculi muscle at the level of the lateral eyebrow; these incisions are simultaneously *myotomies*, which weaken the depressor function of the orbicularis, and *neurotomies* of the small fibers of the frontal nerve supplying the glabellar musculature.

The recent rediscovery of the malar fat pad[21] has been a breakthrough in the treatment of central face sagging. It

is important to understand the independence of the malar fat pad from the superficial fascia (Fig. 30–5).

Loeb,[22] de la Plaza,[23] and Hamra[24] have made us realize that in many people lower lid bags are not caused by true fat excess, which should be resected. Depending on the circumstances, the fat can be redraped out of the orbit or it can be repositioned within the orbit (Fig. 30–6).

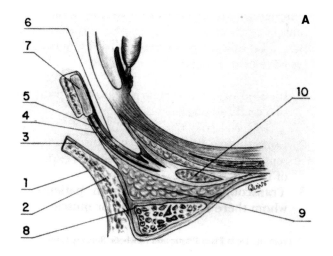

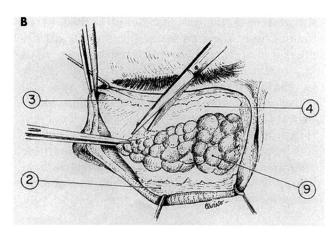

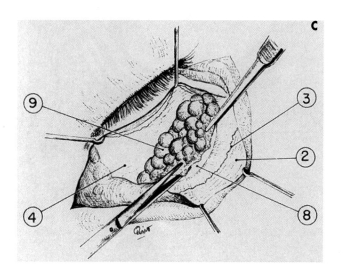

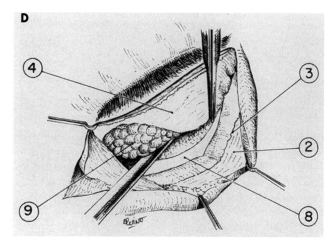

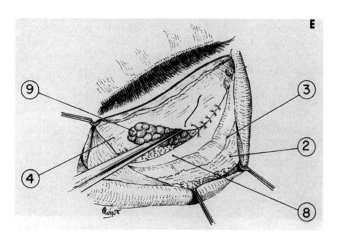

Figure 30–6. (A) Sagittal section of the lower eyelid showing the different anatomic layers: (1) skin, (2) orbicularis oculi muscle, (3) orbital septum, (4) capsulopalpebral fascia, (5) inferior tarsal muscle (Müller's muscle), (6) conjunctiva, (7) tarsus, (8) orbital rim, (9) orbital fat, and (10) inferior oblique muscle. (*Redrawn after Lester T. Jones.*) **(B)** Dissection of the fat from the septum and the capsulopalpebral fascia after exposure of the fat pad by opening the skin, orbicularis muscle, and septum. **(C)** Dissection of the fat from the lower part of the septum down to the orbital rim; the septum remains adherent to the posterior aspect of the orbicularis muscle. **(D)** Replacement of the fat in the orbital cavity. (E) Retention of the fat by continuous suture of the periosteum of the orbital rim to the lower portion of the capsulopalpebral fascia. (From "A New Technique for the treatment of Palpebral Bags" by Rafael de la Plaza, and Jose M. Arroyo, on pages 678-681 of *Plastic and Reconstructive Surgery*, 81:5, 1988.)

De la Plaza has also shown that the lower lid capsu-lopalpebral fascia is sufficiently lax and redundant that it can be anchored to the arcus marginalis with no restriction of globe mobility. Both extraorbital redraping and internal repositioning of the orbital fat can be performed through the transconjunctival approach.[25] Camirand[26] also points out that orbital fat herniation produces some enophthalmos, which may be corrected by repositioning the fat within the orbit (Fig. 30–7).

Hamra[27] redrapes the lower eyelid fat outside the orbit. The arcus marginalis is released along the inferior orbital rim. The orbital fat with the overlying septum orbitale is then sutured below the orbital rim (Fig. 30–8). This approach helps create a smooth eyelid-cheek transition.

The malar septum is an interesting structure that has been recently described and that may explain the malar bag.[28] Barton,[29] Stuzin,[30] and Yousif[31,32] have all conducted important anatomic studies of the deeper layers of the face, and their work is worth close study.

By far the single worst cause of anatomic insecurity in cosmetic facial surgery is the facial nerve, and only two relationships are possible with the facial nerve: complete avoidance or total familiarity. Unfortunately, avoidance is not compatible with the pursuit of excellence. A superficial subcutaneous facelift does not require knowledge of facial nerve anatomy and can in fact yield a good result in a woman with good bone structure and no facial fat. These were the women who had good facelift results in the 1960s.[33] However, a surgeon who limits himself or herself to this approach will produce many mediocre results.

So there is no choice: Anatomic dissection must be performed. Descriptions must be read and reread.[34,35] The peripheral course of the frontal branch and the marginal mandibular branch are fairly well understood. The buccal and zygomatic branches are more variable (Fig. 30–9). With the increasing popularity of deep plane facelifts, more facial nerve injuries are being seen, and these often involve the zygomatic or buccal branches. More aggressive dissection around the zygomaticus major muscle is most likely responsible for these injuries.

However, it is not just the pathways of the nerves that create uncertainty. Many surgeons are uncertain about how far a nerve is from the skin, how much deeper it is than the subcutaneous musculoaponeurotic system (SMAS), and how close it is to the zygomatic arch. It is this three-dimensional sense that must be mastered.[36]

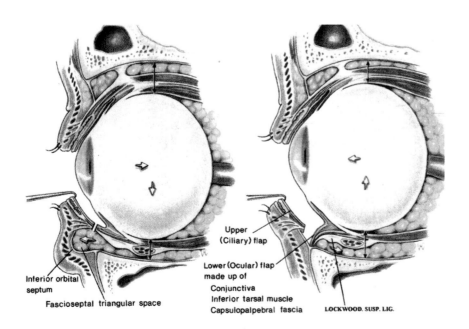

Inferior orbital septum

Fascioseptal triangular space

Upper (Ciliary) flap

Lower (Ocular) flap made up of
Conjunctiva
Inferior tarsal muscle
Capsulopalpebral fascia

LOCKWOOD. SUSP. LIG.

Figure 30–7. Herniation of the lower eyelid fat causes the globe to settle and creates an enophthalmia. The fat pad, when restored to its normal position, preserves the globe forward and up. (From the Panel Discussion: Management of the Lower Eyelid, on page 48 of *Aesthetic Surgery Journal*, Jan/Feb, 1997.)

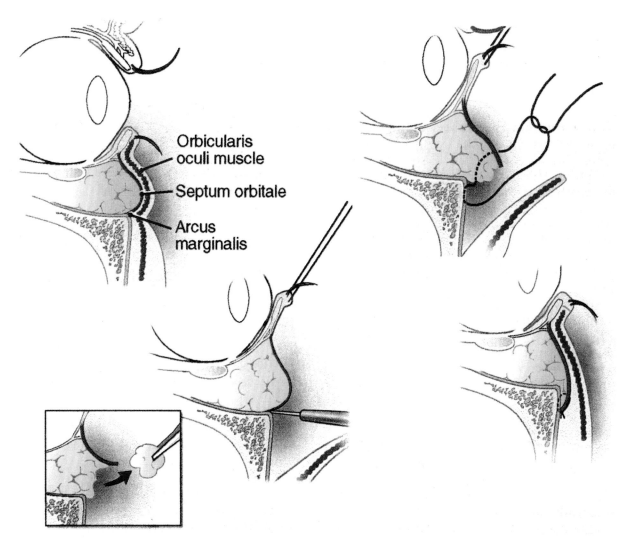

Figure 30–8. (*Above, left*) Side view of normal orbital anatomy. (*Below, left*) The arcus marginalis is released. Some fat may be removed if necessary. (*Above, right*) Sutures are placed between the inferior margin of the septum orbitale and soft tissue overlying the orbital rim. (*Below, right*) The septum including orbital fat is reset over the orbital rim. (From "The Zygorbicular Dissection in Composite Rhytidectomy: An Ideal Midface Plane" by Sam T. Hamra, on page 1651 of *Plastic and Reconstructive Surgery*, 102:5, 1998.)

PREOPERATIVE DIAGNOSIS

Every surgeon can become proficient in diagnosis. It is simply a matter of taking the time and paying attention to detail. Analysis of each part of the aging face leads to a successful surgical plan.

Beginning with the forehead, the height of the hairline should be noted. If the height is greater than 6 cm, the patient should probably undergo an open hairline browlift as opposed to an endoscopic browlift. (The following discussion is centered around the appearance of the female face.) If the central hairline is excessively high, the appearance of aging is accentuated and an illusion of baldness is present even if the patient has thick hair. The position and arch of the eyebrows should be noted; the medial eyebrow should be at the level of the orbital rim and the lateral eyebrow should be 1 cm above the orbital rim.

The distance between the medial eyebrows should be measured. If this distance is greater than 2.5 cm, corrugator resection should be very conservative, if done at all. Excessive corrugator resection can lead to separation of the eyebrows with an unattractive result. Horizontal forehead wrinkles are evidence of frontalis muscle hyperactivity,

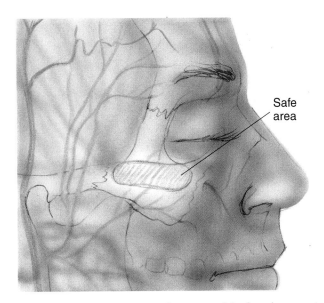

Figure 30–9. Representative dissection of the facial nerve. A small rectangular "safe area" is lateral to the orbit and above the origin of the zygomaticus muscles. Deep sutures can be placed in this "safe area," which lies between the frontal and the zygomatic branches of the nerve.

which is usually a result of brow ptosis. The frontalis muscle contracts to elevate the brows. After the brows are elevated surgically, the frontalis muscle will relax. The appearance of the brows and upper lids will reveal which muscles are contributing to brow ptosis. The actions of the orbicularis, the depressor supercilii, the corrugator, and the procerus should each be individually studied.[20]

In the temples, excessive distance between the lateral canthus and the temporal hairline gives an aged appearance.[37] A conventional temporal facelift incision will cause a lateral shift in temporal skin and increase this distance. The amount of lateral shift can be estimated by pinching the skin. If a traditional temporal incision will result in a lateral canthus to temporal hairline distance greater than 4 cm, then a hairline temporal incision may be indicated (Fig. 30–10).

A high sideburn because of a previous facelift may also dictate a hairline incision. The presence of visible

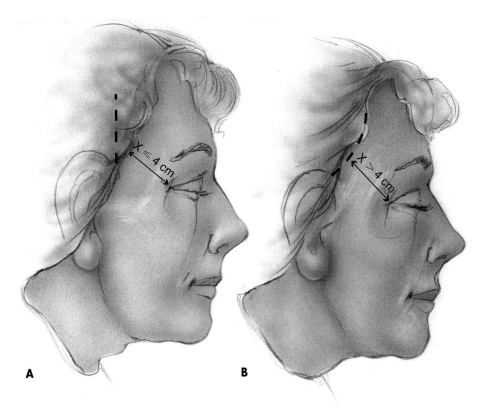

Figure 30–10. (A) If distance X will remain equal to or less than 4 cm after a facelift, a conventional temporal incision is used. **(B)** If distance X will exceed 4 cm after a facelift or if it exceeds 4 cm preoperatively, a hairline temporal incision should be considered.

subcutaneous veins in the temple should be noted in a patient who will undergo laser resurfacing. If these veins are present, only superficial resurfacing with a single laser pass should be performed. Otherwise these veins can become excessively visible and unsightly (Roberts, T. Personal communication, 1997). Thickness and density of the hair should be noted. In patients with thin, sparse hair, even carefully placed frontal scars may be noticeable.

In some patients, the brow glides upward freely on manual elevation, and in others the brow is quite adherent to the supraorbital rim. When the brow is adherent, a subgaleal browlift is more effective than a subperiosteal approach. Bear in mind, however, that the subgaleal browlift will further elevate the hairline.

Excess skin in the upper lids can be more apparent than real. The upper lids should be assessed after the brow is manually placed in an aesthetically ideal position. Hooding of the upper lid extending beyond the orbital rim is indicative of excess extraorbital fat (suborbicularis oculis fat). Upper lid ptosis and retraction should be noted.

Schirmer's test may be performed although other more sensitive tests can predict the risk of postoperative exposure keratitis. Pre-existing scleral show, a weak lower lid as determined by the snap back test, and malar hypoplasia are all danger signs.[38] The amount of herniated fat in each lower lid compartment should be assessed, and this is best done by gently compressing the globe with the patients' eyelids shut in forward gaze. Lower lid skin excess and wrinkling should be noted, and these suggest the need for laser resurfacing. A staring quality of the gaze and any tendency to exopthalmos can easily be made worse by excessive eyelid resection. Most important in the lower lid: *Does the patient need a canthopexy?*

All faces are asymmetric and in looking at the overall face, specific asymmetries should be noted. The bony prominences should be studied. Occasionally modification of the supraorbital rims with burring of bone is indicated. Quite frequently micrognathia is present and

should be treated. The appearance of moderate malar flatness in an aging face does not necessarily mean that malar implants are indicated. Very often repositioning the malar fat pad and sagging cheek superiorly will satisfactorily augment this area (Fig. 30–11). The skin of the face should be studied for sun damage and wrinkling. Dynamic and static wrinkles should be differentiated. Important features in the central face include sagging of the malar fat pad, depth of the nasolabial folds, marionette lines, and sagging of the oral commissures. The size and fat content of the jowls should be noted.

A "sideburn traction" test is useful in deciding how much deep dissection a given patient needs. If pulling up on the sideburn corrects the jowl, skin redraping may be enough. In other patients, upward sideburn traction has minimal effect on the jowl, and these are the patients in which platysma and SMAS repositioning is necessary.

In the neck alone dozens of features must be examined. The amount and elasticity of the skin, fat excess superficial to and deep to the platysma, degree of platysma looseness and banding, position and size of the submandibular glands, position of the hyoid bone, and hypertrophy of the anterior belly of the digastric muscles are some of the important anatomic variables.

This survey mentions only some features that need to be assessed before surgery. Literally hundreds of them exist. Yet the preoperative examination is often brief and cursory. If the surgeon does not individualize each patient's anatomy, the same operation is used for different problems. Predictably, the results will be widely variable.

PREOPERATIVE PREPARATION

Some surgeons go into the operating room with an improvisational attitude. They are willing to "wing it" to some extent. By so doing they introduce an unnecessary element of chance into the result. The importance of formulating a sound surgical plan in advance cannot be overstated.

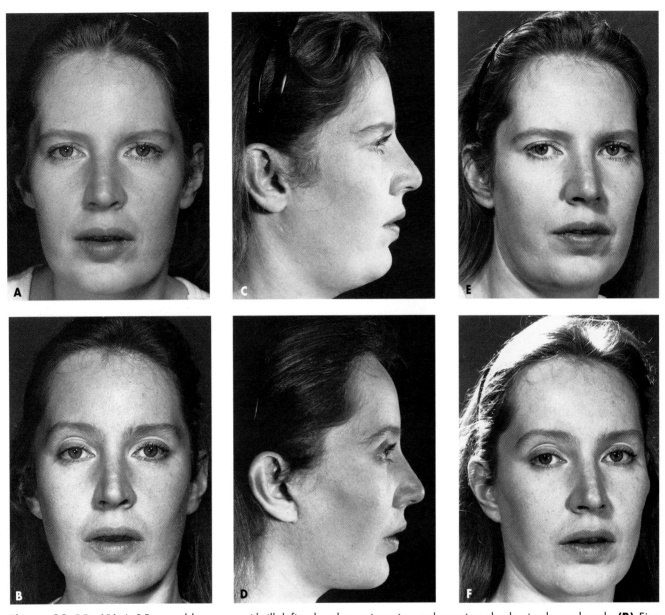

Figure 30–11. (A) A 35-year-old woman with ill-defined malar eminencies and sagging cheeks, jowls, and neck. **(B)** Five months postoperative view after malar fat pad elevation with deep-plane facelift and browlift. Note chiseled, enhanced midface. **(C)** Preoperative lateral view. **(D)** Postoperative lateral view. Note malar prominence. **(E)** Preoperative oblique "portrait" view. **(F)** Postoperative oblique view. Note more delicate cheek contour. Buccal fat pad not excised.

To make a good plan the surgeon needs an accurate diagnosis and a fine understanding of what the patient wants. The only need in cosmetic surgery is in the patient's mind and so it is worthwhile to spend time and effort to understand what the patient wants. Write down verbatim what the patient says about her appearance and the desired changes. A sensitive nurse is an invaluable asset in this regard because the patient may not be completely open with the surgeon. Meet with the patient more than once. A preoperative visit about 2 weeks before surgery is a good time to review the patient's goals, conduct another brief examination, review the preoperative photographs, and write down a detailed plan. This process ensures that no important step will be omitted and that surgery is tailored to the individual patient. Whether the surgeon is performing a facelift or a rhinoplasty, dozens of steps need to be decided on for a given patient, and a cookie-cutter approach is a straight road to mediocrity.

The step-by-step written plan should be placed next to the preoperative photographs in the operating room where it can be reviewed at a glance.

Just before surgery, with the patient alert and sitting upright, skin markings should be made with a surgical pen. Items to be marked include anatomic landmarks, nerve pathways, incision lines, redraping vectors, bulges, and creases. A few minutes spent on the markings will make for an easier and more successful procedure, and the surgeon must not allow himself or herself to be rushed. If the anesthesiologist and operating room staff understand the importance of marking the patient preoperatively, this important step will be integrated into the daily routine.

SOME TECHNICAL DETAILS

Excellent results can be achieved by virtually any technique provided the surgeon has a sound understanding of the anatomy, good aesthetic judgment and a sense of balance and proportion.

Turpin[39]

Individual progress also depends on the surgeon's ability to take advantage of innovations and to recognize quickly the false pathways.

Ristow[33]

Cosmetic surgery is as much an art as a science and for almost every statement made, there is a good surgeon who will disagree. In fact, this entire book is dedicated to diverse approaches. The point is not to endorse a particular technique but to encourage a scholarly attitude that is neither rigid nor flighty.

A young surgeon should become proficient in one technique, identify its limitations in his or her hands by studying his or her results, and then carefully and selectively try variations and innovations.

Progress is a double-edged sword and recent developments in facelifting are a good example of this. Excellent surgeons advocate widely different techniques.[17,40–42] There are at least five possible planes of dissection and many possible maneuvers. Controlled studies are essentially impossible. Techniques are adopted and discarded too quickly. Confusion is prevalent.

In addition, as if the scientific pace was not fast enough, we have to deal with market pressures. New procedures are oversold on television and in magazines and patients request them. If the surgeon is not "at the forefront," he risks losing credibility as an expert and he definitely risks losing the patient.

The following are some selective personal observations and suggestions regarding a wide variety of procedures.

THE BROW

All incisions within the scalp or at the hairline should be sharply beveled[43] so hair follicles are present in the wound surface (Fig. 30–12). Hair will grow through the subsequent scar and make it essentially invisible.

Browlifts should be performed only occasionally in men. Low brows look fine in men (look at Paul Newman.) It is very easy to feminize a man's appearance with a browlift. Many "good" results shown at meetings on close analysis really show a pretty face. In addition, brows in men should be relatively straight.

The surgeon should perform many browlifts on women (Fig. 30–13). Although low, normal brows are compatible with a vigorous, attractive look in youth, many older women look fresher with higher brows. Therefore it is not just a matter of replacing the brows where they were in youth. Sometimes, they should be higher after a browlift than when the patient was younger.[44] Be aware that patients need to be reassured that they will not look startled.

Do not overelevate the medial eyebrow. Browlifts can create a brow arch far from the ideal.[45] Do not overresect the corrugators; the medial brows will spring apart.

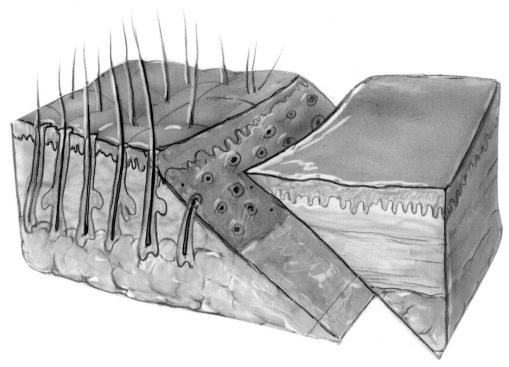

Figure 30–12. Incisions in the hairline or within the scalp should be sharply beveled. Hair will grow through and in front of the scar and camouflage it.

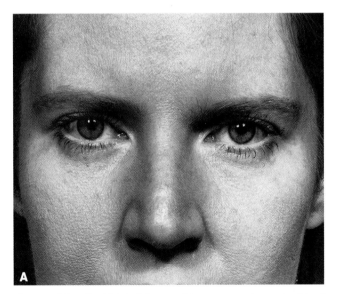 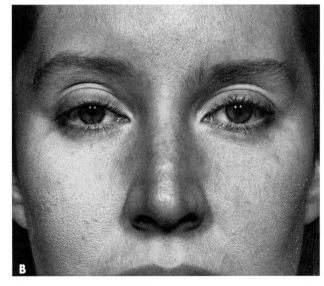

Figure 30–13. (A) A 35-year-old woman with ptosis of both medial and lateral brows. **(B)** Five months postoperative view after endoscopic browlift with complete periosteal release and with myotomies and neurotomies of brow depressors. No eyelid surgery was performed.

The endoscopic technique has made the browlift appealing to many more patients and has wide applicability.[46] It is reliable and easy. The endoscopic mid-facelift[20,47] is more difficult to learn and fewer patients are ideal candidates for it.

THE EYELIDS

When the brows are properly repositioned, fewer and less extensive upper eyelid procedures are necessary. Trimming the medial fat through a stab wound and tightening

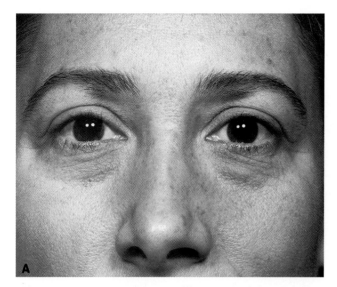 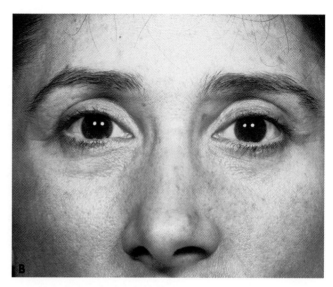

Figure 30–14. (A) A 39-year-old woman with herniated lower lid fat and some looseness and wrinkling of lower lid skin. **(B)** Ten months postoperative view after transconjunctival lower blepharoplasty with excision of subciliary skin strip. Note absence of scleral show. Patient also underwent upper blepharoplasty.

the skin with the carbon dioxide laser may be all that is needed. It is a mistake to resect excessive upper lid skin in a patient with ptotic brows. The result is unattractive and a subsequent browlift will produce lagophthalmos.

The transconjunctival blepharoplasty has produced improved results in lower lid surgery: fewer patients with round eyes and scleral show. In conjunction with transconjunctival fat trimming, a subciliary skin strip can be excised without undermining, leaving the orbicularis muscle and the septum intact (Fig. 30–14). Alternatively, the skin can be tightened with the carbon dioxide laser.

The surgeon should perform many lateral canthopexies. This is another area of anatomic insecurity. The upper lid approach to the lateral canthus described by Jelks[48] is easy and produces consistent results (Fig. 30–15). Although currently out of fashion, horizontal lower lid shortening (the modified Kuhnt-Szymanowski procedure) is simple and useful in patients with a lax lower lid and a stable lateral canthal ligament. The lower lid should *not* be shortened if the globe is prominent; the shortened lower lid will sink even lower below the globe's equator.

THE FACE

Before aiming for a 90-degree submental angle and obliteration of the nasolabial folds, the beginning surgeon should concentrate on *leaving the patient looking as if she did not have any surgery.* It is not the partial improvements that rankle. It is the patients who look strange and hard and surgical. These poor patients (and there are many) wear their failure on their face. They aspired to look better, to improve themselves. Instead, they acquired surgical stigmata. Many did not want to advertise their aspirations, but their new look tells the world of both their effort and their failure. The pathos of this circumstance must be difficult to bear.

The causes of the "surgical look" are fairly well understood. They include the levitating sideburn, the vanishing temporal hairline, pixie ears, widened mouth, submental hollow, and hanging submandibular glands. One of my favorite concepts is Connell's "angle of dangle": The earlobe should dangle freely at an angle 15 degrees posterior to the axis of the pinna.[37] Another useful principle is: If you cannot effectively lift the central face, do not overtighten the lateral face; it is this dispar-

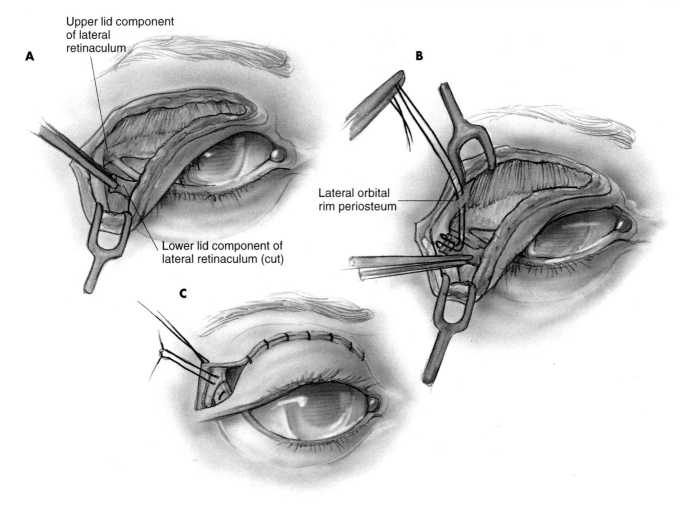

Figure 30–15. (A) Through the lateral aspect of an upper blepharoplasty incision the lateral retinaculum is identified. The inferior lower lid component of the retinaculum is incised and divided from the periosteum of the lateral orbital wall. **(B)** The isolated lower lid component of the lateral retinaculum is sutured to the inner aspect of the lateral orbital wall at a predetermined level. **(C)** Tightening the suture completes the canthoplasty and elevates the lower lid.

ity that can look grotesque. In nonhuman primates, it is only the central face (the face of expression) that is exposed. The lateral face (the face of mastication) is covered with hair. Furthermore do not think of the facelift as a pulling or tightening operation; think of it as a redraping and elevating of several layers of tissue (Fig. 30–16).

It is helpful to think of the skin part of a facelift as two large rotation flaps separated at the earlobe. The face flap rotates superiorly and the neck flap rotates posteriorly. Rotation produces asymmetric dog ears; do not be afraid to excise these.

All dissection should be performed under direct vision and transillumination of the flaps provides excellent visualization of the desired plane. The thickness of the flap can be gauged by the amount of light coming through the flap. In contrast, direct illumination with a headlight or fiberoptic retractor can create excessive glare, and it can be difficult to determine exactly where to cut along the uniform yellow fatty surface.

Another important technical point: As the dissection proceeds medially, only gentle retraction and elevation of the flap should be applied. Excessive "toeing-in" of

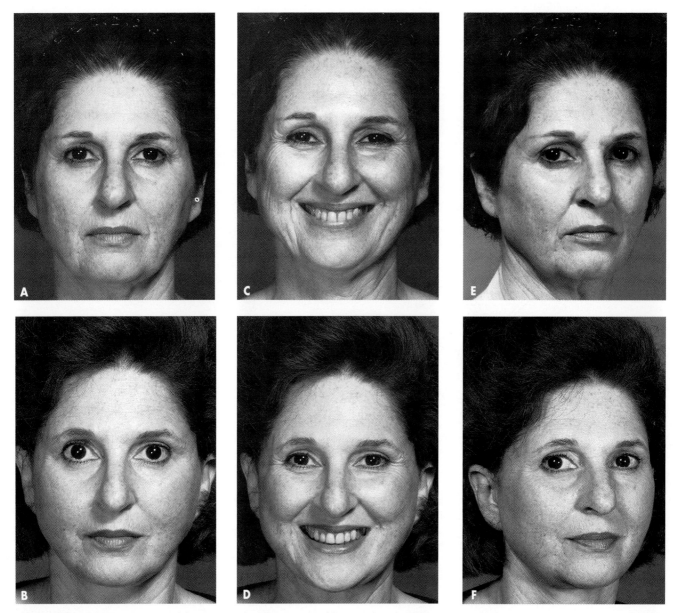

Figure 30–16. (A) A 54-year-old woman with diffuse aging of face and neck. **(B)** Fourteen months postoperative view after facelift. Note congruent appearance of central and lateral face. Patient had simultaneous blepharoplasty. **(C)** Preoperative smiling view. **(D)** Postoperative smiling view. Patient does not look "surgical." **(E)** Preoperative oblique view. **(F)** Postoperative oblique view.

the retractor will lift structures that must remain deep to the plane of dissection. This hazard can be vividly illustrated once the zygomaticus major muscle has been identified. Forceful retraction of the flap will lift this muscle up to 2 cm from the maxilla, and one does not want to dissect deep to the zygomaticus major.

Posterior rotation of the neck flap can leave a "step" or short interruption in the occipital hairline. Much has been written about the evils of this "step", but I do not

recall a single patient complaining about it.[49] (Patients will complain bitterly about a *low* mastoid scar or a hypertrophic scar in this area.) The occipital flap should be rotated posteriorly.[50]

In my own progress, the improvement of the neck with platysma surgery was a major breakthrough.[51]

Ristow's excellent review of milestones in facelift surgery is worth studying closely.[33] He emphasizes that in the single-layer facelift, the skin flap should be quite thick.

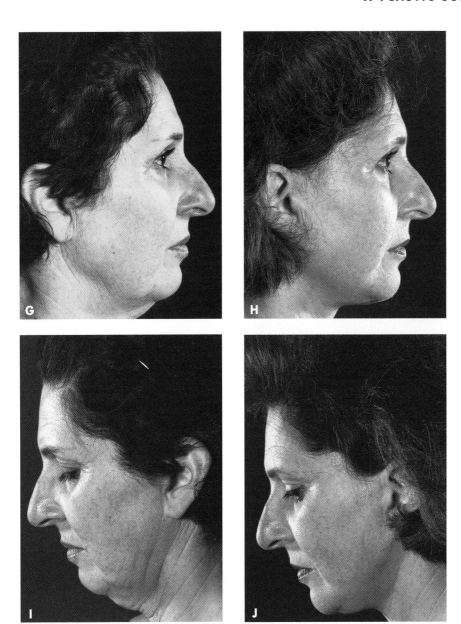

Figure 30-16. *(continued)*
(G) Preoperative right lateral view. Note marked jowling and oblique neck. **(H)** Postoperative right lateral view. Significant correction is possible without a pulled look. **(I)** Preoperative lateral "book in lap" view magnifies neck deformity. **(J)** Postoperative lateral "book in lap" view. Correction is maintained in this position because of superior redraping of fat and platysma.

When the SMAS is elevated as a separate layer, however, the skin flap must be thinner and is more fragile.

For the surgeon who is ready to plunge into the deeper planes, Owsley's systematic and lucid exposition of a step-by-step approach to the SMAS and the malar fat pad is very useful.[17] When studying another surgeon's work, the usual criteria of scientific proof are not available, and one runs into the specter of individualism: What if his good results are caused largely by his talent and not his specific technique? The work of some sur-

geons is more reproducible than that of others. In selecting a model, the student should rely on what he or she finds consistent and safe.

Hamra's concepts merit close study.[24,52] The August 1997 issue of *Plastic and Reconstructive Surgery* includes an editorial and three articles, which taken together comprise a strong and timely review of contemporary facelifting.[53–56]

The recent attention that has been given to the malar fat pad has been a real step forward; elevating this structure does wonders for the central face. A number of approaches to the malar fat pad have been described.[57] I find it simplest to leave the fat pad attached to the skin, dissecting between the pad and the zygomaticus major muscle.

In the deeper planes an occasional facial nerve injury can occur in the best of hands.[58] No amount of rejuvenation is worth long-term facial palsy. The individual surgeon must look at the individual patient and assess the expected improvement and the possible risk.

Facial skin resurfacing with the Ultrapulse carbon dioxide laser[59,60] represents progress and in my practice has largely replaced chemical peels (Fig. 30–17). In addition to producing improvements in wrinkling and pigmentation, impressive skin tightening is present. The most common applications are full-face laser resurfacing as an isolated procedure and laser resurfacing of the central face at the time of a facelift.

THE NECK

In selected younger patients with elastic skin, the neck can be improved through a submental incision without a facelift.[61,62] The platysma is tightened and excess fat both

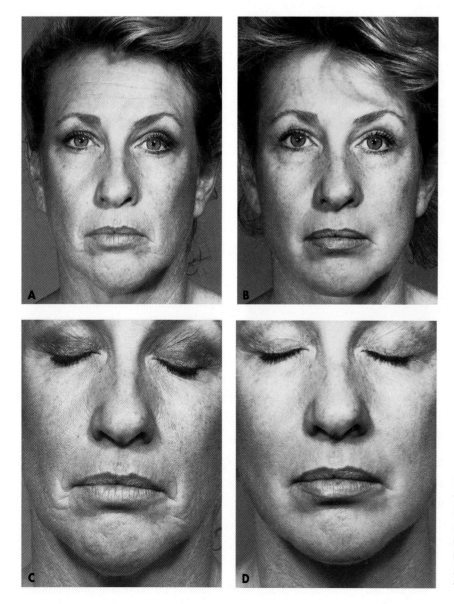

Figure 30–17. (A) A 41-year-old woman with significant perioral rhytids. **(B)** Ten months postoperative view after perioral carbon dioxide laser resurfacing. **(C)** Preoperative close-up view. **(D)** Postoperative close-up view. Note some skin tightening and improvement of wrinkles.

deep to and superficial to the platysma can be trimmed. Particularly in the neck, precise preoperative assessment is essential. The neck should be palpated with the platysma both contracted and relaxed. Having the patient push forward with her tongue against the posterior surface of the mandibular incisors helps to judge the thickness of the submental fat. If the patient had an obtuse neck when she

was young (evidence of a low-lying hyoid bone, subplatysma fat, ptotic submandibular glands), correction will predictably be more difficult.[62]

The occasional 40-year-old woman will get a remarkable improvement with liposuction of the neck alone (Fig. 30–18). However, liposuction tends to be overused. When performing a facelift, conservative

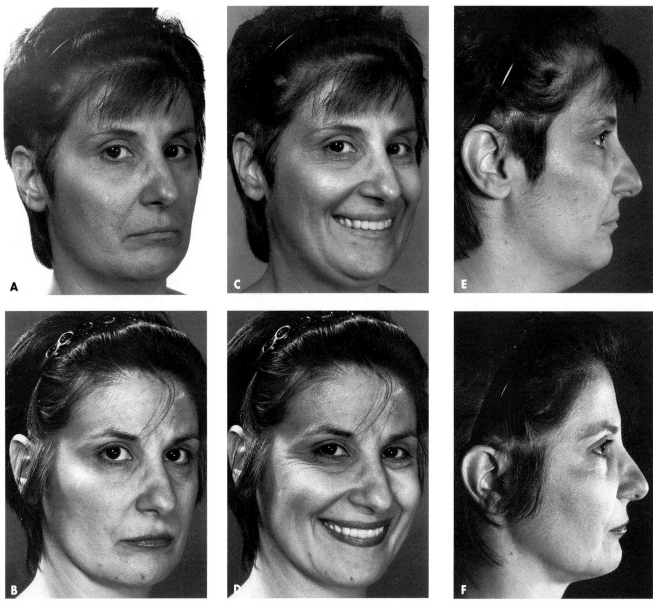

Figure 30–18. (A) A 43-year-old woman with subcutaneous fat deposits in lower face and neck. **(B)** Ten month postoperative view after superficial liposuction of the lower face and neck. Note good skin retraction. **(C)** Preoperative smiling view accentuates "double chin." **(D)** Postoperative smiling view. **(E)** Preoperative lateral view. **(F)** Postoperative lateral view. Note mandibular definition. Hyoid bone is in good position and no platysma bands are present.

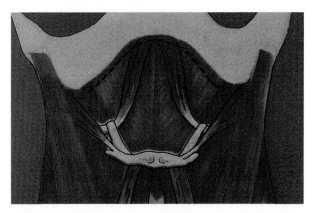

Figure 30–19. Illustration of the location of the myotomy, which goes through the anterior belly of the digastric, mylohyoid, and geniohyoid muscles at their attachment to the posterior surface of the mandibular symphysis. (From "Problem Neck, Hyoid Bone, and Submental Myotomy" by Bahman Guyuron, page 832 of *Plastic and Reconstructive Surgery,* 90:8;1992.)

superficial liposuction of the *jowls* with a 1.8-mm cannula is very useful. Lipectomy in the neck is best performed sharply under direct vision. This approach allows more control and prevents overresection. A layer of fat 4-mm thick should be left under the neck skin. Closed liposuction followed by flap elevation can lead to unsightly dermal adhesions. It is particularly important not to resect too much fat in the midline, because this leads to a submental hollow; lipectomy must be systematically extended laterally where it is more difficult to perform.

Another useful maneuver exists for the low anterior hyoid bone. The submental muscles are detached from the posterior aspect of the mandibular symphysis. This allows retraction of the posterior belly of the digastric muscles with consequent elevation of the hyoid[63] (Fig. 30–19).

BEHAVIOR IN THE OPERATING ROOM

A well-planned operation can founder on the shoals of operating room disorder. Regardless of legal theory, the surgeon had better behave as the captain of the ship if he wants a good result. He must strive to have a stable crew of anesthetist, assistant, scrub nurse, and circulating nurse. A good scrub nurse can double as the assistant. The team then knows the necessary equipment and instruments and the sequence of steps, so they can anticipate the surgeon's needs. When the surgeon operates in an unfamiliar environment, such as a hospital where he does not work regularly, a great deal of planning is required. Because surgery has become more technical, one cannot assume that the staff always understands how to assemble the endoscopic system or how to calibrate the laser. It is best to go over all the instruments with the nurse before scrubbing. The instruments can then be arranged on the stand in the order in which they will be used.

Hospital scissors, chisels, and rasps are often dull, and it is wise to carry one's own. Talk to the anesthesiologist before starting. Let him or her know at which points in the operation the patient needs to be deeply sedated. Tell him exactly how the endotracheal tube should be positioned and emphasize the importance of a smooth extubation.

To change metaphors, a good operation should run like a well-choreographed ballet, with each step seamlessly leading to the next. The procedure acquires a momentum of its own. When things are running smoothly, the surgeon can achieve a trancelike state beyond concentration where stress-free energy and intuitive knowledge guide the eyes and the hands.[64] This flow and momentum and ideal state of mind all crash to a standstill when the surgeon opens his palm to receive the next instrument and the nurse frantically runs out of the room to look for it.

However, despite the best planning, small crises will occur. To overcome these, the surgeon must cultivate equanimity and self-control. *Music* of the surgeon's choice playing in the operating room can help relieve stress and improve concentration.[65]

HOW I WOULD DO IT DIFFERENTLY NEXT TIME

Nothing differentiates the excellent surgeon from the mediocre one as much as the response to feedback—from colleagues, patients, and staff but, most importantly, from one's own observation and experience. Some surgeons thoughtfully and incrementally modify their techniques by retaining successful elements, identifying those that do not work, and solving frustrating steps with various solutions, whereas others blithely continue with the same procedures day after day, repeating their mistakes. This is why the term *an experienced surgeon* can be misleading, because some learn much more from experience than others.

The first step in improvement is a brutally honest and self-critical evaluation of one's results, even if this process occasionally interferes with peace of mind. Let your standards be higher than those of your patients. Postoperative follow-up must be long and systematic, with a recall program. High-quality postoperative photographs are taken 3 months after surgery or later and studied next to the preoperative set. An effort must be made to do this for *every* patient. We learn the most from our least successful results. The unhappy patient may drift elsewhere for further care and an "out of sight, out of mind" attitude prevails. She perhaps may be dismissed with a "that's-the-way-you-healed" attitude. It is the dissatisfied patient who should be followed most closely, and of course this is also the best approach to damage control.

Finally, keep written records of your progress. Memory is very selective. We tend to remember only our good results and the very rare catastrophe. A powerful tool can improve one's results and it can be made a daily habit (Spencer, F. Personal Communication, 1980). Keep a confidential notebook titled "How I Will Do It Differently Next Time." Immediately after each major operation, write or dictate a note to yourself about what you learned. In almost every case a small detail and occasionally a breakthrough exists.

PEARLS

- Excellence in the pursuit of facial plastic surgery is more difficult to monitor than in other fields of medicine because (1) the surgeon is operating on a healthy patient and (2) the outcome of a facial plastic procedure is very subjective.

- One very valuable exercise that a surgeon may use to improve his or her aesthetic sense is to learn to draw the face. Drawing will force the surgeon not just to look but to *see*.

- The fear of complications and inadequate results can be reduced by studying the anatomy of the face. Studying facial anatomy for 1 hour every week is an excellent educational pastime for the surgeon.

- Preoperative planning requires an accurate diagnosis and complete understanding of the patient's wishes.

- A stable group of operating room staff, including anesthetist, assistant, scrub nurse, and circulating nurse, will help a procedure run more smoothly by anticipating the surgeon's needs and being familiar with the technique.

REFERENCES

1. Emerson RW. *Journal*. February 1855.
2. Fredricks S. Commentary: Ultrasound-Assisted Lipoplasty Panel, ASAPS Meeting, New York City, May 1997.
3. Grosser M. *The Painter's Eye*. New York: Holt, Rhinehart & Winston; 1951:17.
4. Loomis A. *Drawing The Head And Hands*. New York: Viking Press; 1956:75–87.
5. Samuels M, Samuels N. *Seeing With The Mind's Eye*. New York: Random House; 1975:24–25.
6. Edwards B. *Drawing On The Right Side Of The Brain*. Los Angeles: J.P. Tarcher, Inc; 1979:4–5.
7. Fischer R. Aesthetics and the biology of the fleeting moment. *Perspect Biol Med*. 1965; 8:210–212.
8. Peck H, Peck S. A concept of facial aesthetics. *Angle Orthod*. 1970; 40:284–318.
9. Lambros V. Fat contouring in the face and neck. *Clin Plast Surg*. 1992; 19:401–414.

10. Saul A. Virtual reality training: Will computers replace cadavers? *Plast Surg News.* 1997; 3:1.

11. Saban Y, Polselli R. *Atlas Of Surgical Anatomy Of The Face And Neck.* Paris: Masson Publishers; 1994:41–65.

12. Larrabee, Jr WF, Makielski KH. *Surgical Anatomy Of The Face.* New York: Raven Press; 1993:3–206.

13. McMinn RMH, Hutchings RT, Logan BM. *Color Atlas Of Head And Neck Anatomy.* Chicago: Yearbook Medical Publishers; 1981:72–89.

14. Zide BM, Jelks GW. *Surgical Anatomy Of The Orbit.* New York: Raven Press; 1985:1–12.

15. Tardy ME, Brown RJ. *Surgical Anatomy Of The Nose.* New York: Raven Press; 1990:33–37.

16. Whetzel TP. Review of Saban Y and Polselli R: Atlas of surgical anatomy of the face and neck. *Plast Reconstr Surg.* 1996; 97:241–244.

17. Owsley JQ. *Aesthetic Facial Surgery.* Philadelphia: W.B. Saunders Co; 1994:1–195.

18. Knize DM. A study of the supraorbital nerve. *Plast Reconstr Surg.* 1995; 96:564–569.

19. Knize DM. An anatomically based study of the mechanism of eyebrow ptosis. *Plast Reconstr Surg.* 1996; 97:1321–1333.

20. Isse NG. Endoscopic facial rejuvenation. *Clin Plast Surg.* 1997; 24:213–231.

21. Owsley JQ. Lifting the malar fat pad for the correction of prominent nasolabial folds. *Plast Reconstr Surg.* 1993; 91: 463–476.

22. Loeb R. Fat pad sliding and fat grafting for leveling lid depressions. *Clin Plast Surg.* 1981; 8:757–776.

23. de la Plaza R, Arroyo JM. A new technique for the treatment of palpebral bags. *Plast Reconstr Surg.* 1988; 81:677–685.

24. Hamra ST. Arcus marginalis release and orbital fat preservation in the midface rejuvenation. *Plast Reconstr Surg.* 1995; 96:354–362.

25. de la Plaza R, de la Cruz L. Extension of the indications for the transconjunctival approach in blepharoplasty. *Int Video-J Plast Aesthe Surg.* 1996; 3:2.

26. Camirand A. Panel discussion on management of the lower eyelid. *Aesthetic Surg J.* 1997; 17:45–52.

27. Hamra ST. The zygorbicular dissection in composite rhytidectomy: An ideal midface plane. *Plast Reconstr Surg.* 1998; 102:1646–1657.

28. Pessa JE, Garza JR. The malar septum: The anatomic basis of malar mounds and malar edema. *Aesthetic Surg J.* 1997; 17:45–52.

29. Barton FE. Rhytidectomy and the nasolabial fold. *Plast Reconstr Surg.* 1992; 90:601–607.

30. Stuzin JM, Baker TJ, Gordon HL. The relationship of the superficial and deep facial fascias: Relevance to rhytidectomy and aging. *Plast Reconstr Surg.* 1992; 89:441–449.

31. Yousif NJ, Gosain A, Matloub HS, et al. The nasolabial fold: An anatomic and histologic reappraisal. *Plast Reconstr Surg.* 1994; 93:60–69.

32. Yousif NJ, Mendelson BC. Anatomy of the midface. *Clin Plast Surg.* 1995; 22:227–240.

33. Ristow B. Milestones in the evolution of facelift techniques. In: Grotting JC, ed. *Reoperative Aesthetic and Reconstructive Plastic Surgery.* St. Louis: Quality Medical Publishing; 1995:181–204.

34. Bernstein L, Nelson RH. Surgical anatomy of the extraparotid distribution of the facial nerve. *Arch Otolaryngol.* 1984; 110:177–183.

35. Gosain AK. Surgical anatomy of the facial nerve. *Clin Plast Surg.* 1995; 22:241–251.

36. Rudolph R. Depth of the facial nerve in the facelift dissection. *Plast Reconstr Surg.* 1990; 85:537–544.

37. Connell BF, Marten TJ. Deep-layer techniques in cervicofacial rejuvenation. In: Psillakis, JM, ed. *Deep Face-lifting Techniques.* New York: Thieme; 1994:161–190.

38. Rees TD, La Trenta GS. The role of the Schirmer's test and orbital morphology in predicting dry-eye syndrome after blepharoplasty. *Plast Reconstr Surg.* 1988; 82:619–625.

39. Turpin IM. The modern rhytidectomy. *Clin Plast Surg.* 1992; 19:383–400.

40. Duffy MJ, Friedland JA. The superficial plane rhytidectomy revisited. *Plast Reconstr Surg.* 1994; 93:1392–1403.

41. Hamra ST. Composite rhytidectomy. *Plast Reconstr Surg.* 1992; 90:1–13.

42. Ramirez OM. Endoscopic full face lift. *Aesth Plast Surg.* 1994; 18:363–371.

43. Camirand A, Doucet J. A comparison between parallel hairline incisions and perpendicular incisions when performing a face lift. *Plast Reconstr Surg.* 1997; 99:10–15.

44. Isse NG. Endoscopic facial rejuvenation: endo-forehead, the functional lift. *Aesth Plast Surg.* 1994; 18:21–29.

45. Freund RM, Nolan WB III. Correlation between brow lift outcomes and aesthetic ideals for eyebrow height and shape in females. *Plast Reconstr Surg.* 1996; 97:1343–1348.

46. Daniel RK, Tirkanits B. Endoscopic forehead lift: An operative technique. *Plast Reconstr Surg.* 1996; 98:1148–1157.

47. Byrd HS, Andochick SE. The deep temporal lift: A multiplanar, lateral brow, temporal, and upper facelift. *Plast Reconstr Surg.* 1996; 97:928–937.

48. Jelks GW, Glat PM, Jelks EB, Longaker MT. The inferior retinacular lateral canthopexy: A new technique. *Plast Reconstr Surg.* 1997; 100:1262–1270.

49. Kaye BL. The extended neck lift: The "bottom line." *Plast Reconstr Surg.* 1980; 65:429–435.

50. Marten TJ. Facelift-planning and technique. *Clin Plast Surg.* 1997; 24:269–308.

51. Aston SJ. Platysma-SMAS cervicofacial rhytidoplasty. *Clin Plast Surg.* 1983; 10:507–520.

52. Hamra ST. Repositioning the orbicularis oculi muscle in the composite rhytidectomy. *Plast Reconstr Surg.* 1992; 90:14–22.

53. Miller TA. Facelift: Which technique? *Plast Reconstr Surg.* 1997; 100:501.

54. Baker TJ, Stuzin JM. Personal technique of face lifting. *Plast Reconstr Surg.* 1997; 100:502–508.

55. Baker DC. Lateral SMASectomy. *Plast Reconstr Surg.* 1997; 100:509–513.

56. Owsley JQ. Face lift. *Plast Reconstr Surg.* 1997; 100:514–519.

57. Barton FE Jr, Kenkel JM. Direct fixation of the malar pad. *Clin Plast Surg.* 1997; 24:329–335.

58. Baker DC. Deep dissection rhytidectomy: A plea for caution. *Plast Reconstr Surg.* 1994; 93:1498–1499.

59. Weinstein C, Alster TS. Skin resurfacing with high-energy, pulsed carbon dioxide lasers. In: Alster TS, Apfelberg DB, eds. *Cosmetic Laser Surgery.* New York: Wiley-Liss; 1995: 9–27.

60. Weinstein C, Roberts TL III. Aesthetic skin resurfacing with the high-energy ultrapulsed carbon dioxide laser. *Clin Plast Surg.* 1997; 24:379–405.

61. Feldman J. Corset platysmaplasty. *Clin Plast Surg.* 1992; 19:369–382.

62. Ramirez OM. Cervicoplasty: Non-excisional anterior approach. *Plast Reconstr Surg.* 1997; 99:1576–1585.

63. Guyuron B. Problem neck, hyoid bone, and submental myotomy. *Plast Reconstr Surg.* 1992; 90:830–837.

64. Csikszentmihalyi M. *Finding Flow: The Psychology of Engagement with Everyday Life.* New York: HarperCollins; 1997:28–34.

65. Thompson JF, Kam PCA. Music in the operating theatre. *B J Surg.* 1995; 82:1586–1587.

The Pursuit of Excellence in Facial Plastic Surgery

Aesthetic Facial Plastic Surgery, edited by Thomas Romo, III, and Arthur L. Millman, Thieme Medical Publishers, Inc., New York, New York, Copyright © 2000.

CHAPTER 31

An Oculoplastic Surgeon's Perspective

STEVEN FAGIEN

When I was asked to write on my perspectives regarding aesthetic facial plastic surgery, I had to look within, regarding my own personal practice, and evaluate the evolution of aesthetic surgery as it relates to where I am today.

The authors who have contributed to this text come from a wide variety of specialties, backgrounds, and training. How then, could we all come together in a collaborative effort to create a multidisciplinary product on the topic of aesthetic surgery that had any cohesiveness? I believe that this is because many of us have similar philosophies and practice ethics that have kept us true to our training and most importantly to ourselves and our patients.

Achieving excellence comes from a combination of attributes discussed in this chapter but ultimately is derived from searching for the truth in our abilities as a scientist, a surgeon, an artist, and, above all, a caring and, compassionate fellow human.

DEFINING EXCELLENCE

Is achieving excellence in aesthetic facial plastic surgery a formidable task? To answer one must first define *excellence* in this regard. On the surface we would simply answer that excellence is achieved by producing *great results*. As we probe deeply into this question, however, we find that the answer is not quite so simple and actually cannot be considered in such a broad generic sense. We can evaluate parameters that are indicators of excellence such as superb aesthetic results, but even this aspect of excellence must be further subdivided into parameters that measure consistency, which would include not only continuous reproducible results but would also have to be categorized by particular facial areas (i.e., Does an excellent cosmetic surgeon who performs consistently great results in facial rhytidectomy deliver results of equal magnitude in rhinoplasty or blepharoplasty?). To this end how do we define or measure one's ability to achieve excellent aesthetic results? This, too, in itself is quite complicated because it can be measured by peer review, patient satisfaction, regional or national reputation, personal wealth, and so forth. We can also factor in, to some extent, financial success or possibly frequency of publication or invitation as guest speaker/faculty and even length of waiting time for patients to be seen in consultation or surgery (how "busy" the surgeon is). However, these factors may actually play little or no role in the determination of true excellence. Patients often flaunt results that many of us may silently criticize; at other times the most bitter complaints are by those whose results appear to approach perfection. What then makes one surgeon better than his or her colleagues or competitors? And ultimately, who becomes the official judge of aesthetics?

Many forces drive the pursuit of excellence in all of us. Ego is rarely associated with positive attributes of an individual but, if appropriately directed, can be a valuable factor in this pursuit. This quality, at times, can raise the standards of excellence with regard to peer and public (community) scrutiny because individuals desire to maintain excellent reputations whatever their true motivations are. Ego can also build and maintain confidence in facing surgical challenges and daring to improve on established methods and procedures. However, internal conflict and counterproduction may exist, precipitated by misplaced ego in situations where the drive is to do as much surgery as possible, possibly, in part, for the financial rewards. This approach can, at times, force a lesser ability to individualize and attend to detail with the result a somewhat formulized method ("one size fits all"). In these situations excellent aesthetic results can be achieved only when the patient "fits" the procedure, and lesser results are obtained in those who do not. In addition, at times the dogma can be blinding, where despite repeated difficulties with any particular procedure the surgeon cannot see this or fails to acknowledge the pitfalls.

Most excellence in surgical results begins with a thoughtful evaluation and treatment plan (much like in other areas of surgery), taking into serious consideration the patient's desires and concerns, a thorough evaluation of the patient, most often followed by an indepth explanation of the proposed surgical procedure(s), and a review of realistic expectations. At times, in attempting to enhance the thought process and to improve the patient experience, the treating physician or staff may schedule follow-up visits or telephone calls to answer any questions and concerns that may arise. Pretreatment and posttreatment routines (if applicable) are discussed at length not only to inform the patient of what to expect and to optimize results but also to allow the patient to plan appropriately with regard to activities that may be integral components of their life, including employment. The patient scrutinizes and values the entire experience with the relationship with their surgeon and his or her office. Each step in the process must be carefully analyzed and continuously amended to meet patients' needs and expectations.

SKILL

The basic *skills* of an individual procedure are assumed to be, if not mastered, well within the scope of the surgeon's capabilities. This not only allows for adequate execution of the procedure but can facilitate intraoperative changes in original surgical planning that might avoid complications or improve results. How the postoperative period is handled, especially in the presence of complications or perhaps poorly prepared patients, can be as crucial as the execution of surgical skills. This may require excess hand holding and frequent office visits to alleviate anxiety that is often associated with surgical procedures. We are all aware of those individuals who repeatedly have more than their fair share of complications that are, however, handled with impeccable grace and care in the postoperative period, which not only avoids litigation but also succeeds in maintaining an uninjured reputation in the community.

VISION

Technically speaking, we must dissect each patient during our evaluation. We need the *vision* to see where the patient wants to be and where you the surgeon wants the patient to be and to synthesize in your mind as you examine the patient how you will get there. This exercise must be executed for each particular area of the face that is to be addressed and finally a harmonious balance must be achieved to maximize overall aesthetic outcome. You *must* construct a pretty good "picture" of not only what the patient will look like (not necessarily by computer imaging) after surgery but also what you will likely encounter during surgery, including the integrity of the soft tissue to be mobilized. If not, the potential exists that the lack of vision will culminate in a suboptimal result.

Vision begins with an understanding of the effects and causation of facial aging followed by a broad knowledge of how to reverse or improve them. A sophisticated knowledge of the pertinent functional anatomy is crucial to understanding the various methods of facial rejuvenation. This not only allows for a better method and treatment plan but can aid in avoiding complications. Vision also encompasses individualization and the ability to understand which aesthetic displeasures are most suited to a wide selection of procedures. This must be understood on both a microscopic and macroscopic viewpoint.

KNOWLEDGE

We can simply divide age-related aesthetic changes into three categories: qualitative, qualitative, and malpositional changes. Traditionally, surgery for rejuvenation of the aged face was approached primarily from a macroscopic *malpositional* standpoint: the lift. Facelifts, browlifts, and necklifts are classic evidence for this and are still among the most common facial aesthetic procedures performed today. Lifts are typically associated with removal of "excessive" tissue (*quantitative*) such as skin, subcutaneous tissue, and muscle as evidenced in blepharoplasty, rhytidectomy, and traditional browlifts. The art of rhytidectomy has evolved significantly with better understanding of the anatomy of aging that has yielded more sophisticated procedures such as composite lifting and attention to the deeper facial components of aging, such as in the extended subcutaneous musculoapneurotic system (SMAS) surgery[1] and positional changes in facial fat, the mid-face or "cheek lift"[2] for midfacial rejuvenation, and endoscopic approaches to the forehead and brows.[3]

Pursuant to my expertise in ophthalmic plastic surgery, many nuances in this field have fueled the evolution of cosmetic eyelid plastic surgery into a field of its own. Lower blepharoplasty has also evolved in sophistication with our ability to achieve greater effects with better control of the lower eyelid position, tension, and canthal integrity with a host of canthoplasty procedures. An elaboration of each of these procedures is beyond the scope of this chapter. Suffice it to say that improved approaches to canthoplasty have derived themselves from the fact that more than 90% of the complications of blepharoplasty have been said to occur in the lower eyelid.[4] Our understanding of the role of each of the canthoplasty procedures has segregated our surgical procedures to adopt each technique for the appropriate patient. Horizontal shortening procedures such as the lateral tarsal strip[5] are now mostly reserved for the horizontally elongated lower eyelid in cases where significant lower eyelid laxity is present (Fig. 31–1). Failures of this procedure relate to long-term and short-term complications, including prolonged inflammation, canthal dystopia, and long-term diminshment of the horizontal palpebral aperture. Newer techniques in canthoplasty such as the inferior retinacular canthoplasty,[6] the lateral retinacular suspension[7,8] (Fig. 31–2), and the dermal

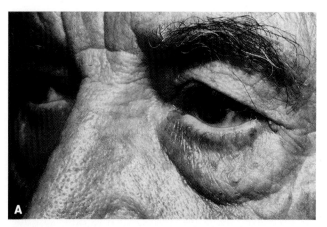
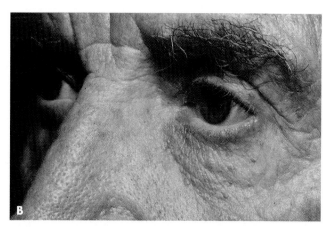

Figure 31–1. (A) This patient presented for cosmetic blepharoplasty. The examination revealed significant lower eyelid laxity and horizontal lid length in the presence of dermatochalasis and herniated orbital fat. **(B)** Less than 1 year after four-quadrant blepharoplasty using a horizontal shortening lateral tarsal strip procedure. Note the loss of horizontal palpebral width often seen with cantholytic canthoplasty.

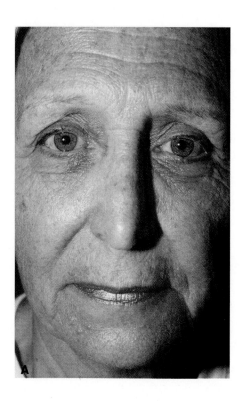
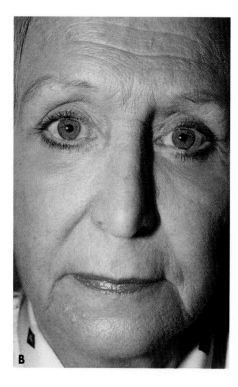

Figure 31–2. (A) This patient presented for periorbital rejuvenation. Examination revealed brow ptosis, upper and lower eyelid dermatochalasis with significant lower eyelid rhytides, and a moderate degree of lower eyelid laxity. **(B)** Four months after browlift, upper and lower (transconjunctival) blepharoplasty, lower eyelid skin CO_2 laser resurfacing, and transpalpebral lateral retinacular suspension.

orbicular pennant[9] herald advantages of preserving the lateral commissure and are used in particular situations as detected on physical examination. Transconjunctival blepharoplasty has also experienced the transition of being a procedure solely for the individual with lower eyelid herniated orbital fat (Fig. 31–3) to a procedure that can be used in a host of situations of varied anterior eyelid lamellae pathologic conditions caused in part by the technology of laser abrasion and chemoexfoliation combined with the various techniques in canthoplasty (Fig. 31–4).

Recently, a recrudescence of awareness of the *qualitative* aspects of the aging skin have been brought forth with laser technology[10] (with simplifications that have been, in part, market driven, which has allowed the permeation of essentially all medical and surgical specialty fields to enter the world of cosmetic surgery). Skin peeling by other methods (chemoexfoliation) has been widely accepted as a method of rejuvenation (Fig. 31–5) for more than 30 years.[11] We have benefited from this history and from those with advanced and immense experience in skin care and skin peeling by a variety of methods.[12]

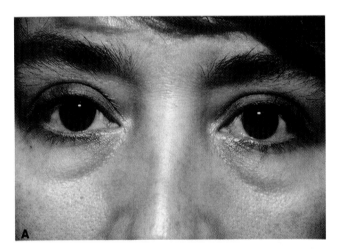
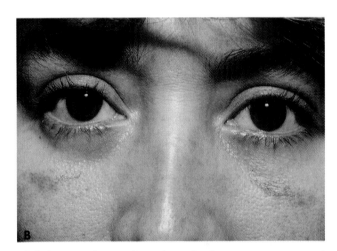

Figure 31–3. (A) This patient presents with complaints of lower eyelid "bags" only. **(B)** Three days after lower transconjunctival blepharoplasty. Note that subtle changes in lower eyelid position (albeit mostly transient) can be seen with this approach.

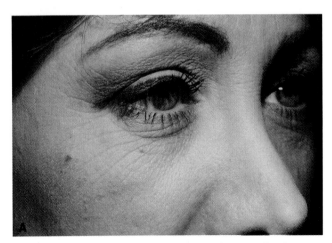
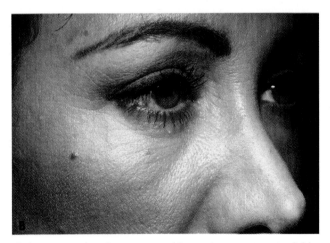

Figure 31–4. (A) This patient presents for periorbital rejuvenation. **(B)** Four months after upper and lower (transconjunctival) blepharoplasty, lateral retinacular suspension, and lower eyelid skin CO_2 laser resurfacing.

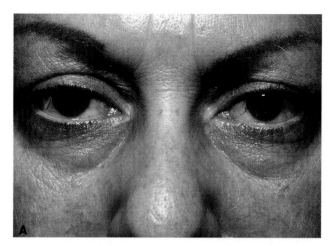
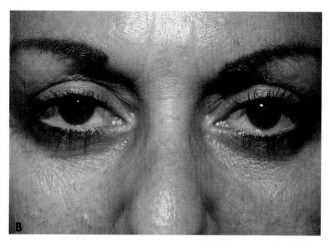

Figure 31–5. (A) Preoperative photo. **(B)** One year after upper and lower (transconjunctival) blepharoplasty with TCA application to the lower eyelid skin. Note the improvement but noneradication (recurrence) of lower eyelid rhytids at 1 year postoperatively.

We have also begun to understand another dimension of *qualitative* soft tissue changes with age, such as the depletion of dermal collagen (and other microscopic dermal components) and subcutaneous fat. Over the past two decades a search has been undertaken for an ideal substance for dermal and subcutaneous soft tissue augmentation, beginning with the use of atelopeptide bovine and porcine collagen in an attempt to replace depleted human dermal collagen.[13] Although obvious benefits occurred with this exercise regarding the appre-ciation of the value of soft tissue augmentation and the evolution of other useful products, it became increasingly clear that although a small risk of immunogenicity (including allergy) existed with injectable foreign animal protein, the stability and longevity of the heterologous dermal implant had never been established. Longer lasting and safe injectable dermal implants, such as Autologen® (Fig. 31–6) and Dermalogen®,[14–17] and better techniques in subcutaneous augmentation with the use of microlipoinjection techniques with fat[18] have

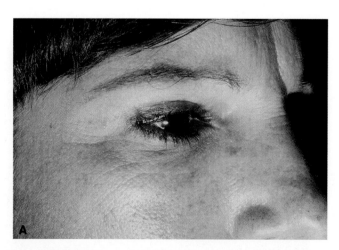
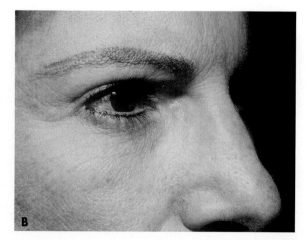

Figure 31–6. (A) Preoperative photo revealing a deep glabellar forehead furrow. **(B)** Four years after four injections of autologous collagen (Autologen®) injections to this region. The collagen (in part) was derived from skin obtained during upper blepharoplasty.

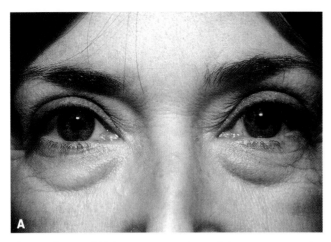 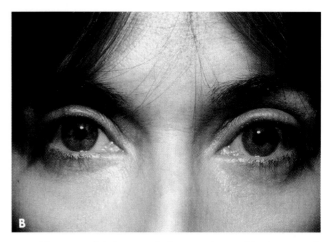

Figure 31–7. (A) Preoperative photo of this patient revealing upper and lower eyelid dermatochalasis and steatoblepharon with marked hyperfunction lateral canthal rhytids. **(B)** Four months after upper and lower (transconjunctival) blepharoplasty, lateral retinacular suspension, and lower eyelid skin CO_2 laser resurfacing. Botox was administered to the lateral canthus 1 week before surgery.

evolved to a highly acceptable level. Attempts at developing an alloplastic (off the shelf) surgically implantable[19] or injectable agent[20] continue to meet with frustration for risk of infection, migration, extrusion, and possibly equally as important lack of aesthetics.

Chemodenervation with botulinum toxin type A (Botox) has also proven useful as an adjunctive and possibly synergistic component to surgery, skin exfoliation (Fig. 31–7), and soft tissue augmentation.[21–23] The use

of chemodenervation for the treatment of dynamic facial lines and facial soft tissue malposition has evolved into an art of its own (Fig. 31–8).

PURSUIT

We have also benefited from the multidisciplinary approach to facial aesthetic surgery as each subspecialty has brought with it a point of view that could be shared

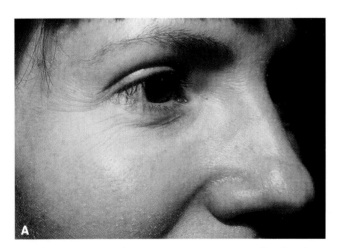 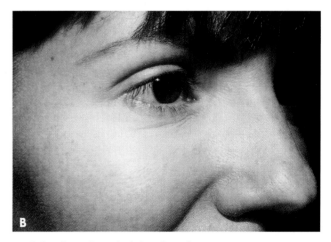

Figure 31–8. (A) This young patient presented with unhappiness with her lateral canthal rhytids with any animation. **(B)** One week after application of Botox to the lateral canthus. This effect lasted approximately 6 months.

or at least acknowledged by those in other specialties. The learned surgeon not only balances the many aspects of facial aging and their remedies in combination with individualization but continues to seek better ways to improve outcomes that are derived from an enhanced appreciation of causation and adaptation of the most effective methods in *the pursuit of excellence in aesthetic surgery*.

PEARLS

- Defining excellence in facial plastic surgery is nearly impossible because the factors involved in defining it are numerous, perhaps extending beyond the surgeon to the patient and the surgeon's colleagues.
- A surgeon's skill must extend beyond the operating room to his or her handling of patients. Handling complications with grace and care avoids lawsuits and upholds the surgeon's reputation.
- A surgeon's ability to understand facial anatomy and the causes and effects of aging not only enable the surgeon to more accurately predict the postoperative result but also help to avoid complications.
- One of the best ways for the surgeon to excell is to learn from his or her colleagues in the various disciplines.

REFERENCES

1. Stuzin JM, Baker TJ, Gordon HL. The relationship of the superficial and deep facial fascias: Relevance to rhytidectomy and aging. *Plast Reconstr Surg.* 1992; 89:441.
2. Hester TR, Codner MA, McCord CD. The "centrofacial" approach for correction of facial aging using the transblepharoplasty subperiosteal cheek lift. *Aesthet Surg Q.* 1996; Spring; 51–58.
3. Rohrich RJ, Beran SJ. Evolving fixation methods in endoscopically assisted forehead rejuvenation: Controversies and rationale. *Plast Reconstr Surg.* 1997; 100:1575.
4. Glat PM, Jelks GW, Jelks EB, et al. Evolution of the lateral canthoplasty: Techniques and indications [Discussion by James H. Carraway]. *Plast Reconstr Surg.* 1997; 100:1406.
5. Anderson RL, Gordy DD. The tarsal strip procedure. *Arch Ophthalmol.* 1979; 97:2192.
6. Jelks GW, Glat PM, Jelks EB, Longaker MT. The inferior retinacular lateral canthoplasty: A new technique. *Plast Reconstr Surg.* 1997; 100:1262.
7. Fagien S. Lower eyelid rejuvenation via transconjunctival blepharoplasty and a simplified transpalpebral lateral retinacular suspension (suture canthopexy): An algorithm for treatment of the anterior lower eyelid lamella. *Operative Techniques Plast Reconstr Surg.* 1998; 121–128.
8. Fagien S. Algorithm for canthoplasty: The lateral retinacular suspension. A simplified suture canthopexy. *Plast Reconst Surg.* 1999; 103:2042.
9. Jelks GW, Jelks EB. Repair of lower lid deformities. *Clin Plast Surg.* 1993; 20:417.
10. Fitzpatrick RE, Goldman MP, Satur NM, Tope WD. Pulsed carbon dioxide laser resurfacing of photoaged facial skin. *Arch Dermatol.* 1996; 132:395.
11. Baker TJ. Chemical face peeling and rhytidectomy. A combined approach for facial rejuvenation. *Plast Reconstr Surg.* 1962; 29:199.
12. Rubin M. *Manual of Chemical Peels.* Philadephia: J.B. Lippincott; 1995.
13. Knapp TR, Kaplan EN, Daniels JR. Injectable collagen for soft tissue augmentation. *Plast Reconstr Surg.* 1977; 60:398.
14. Fagien S. Autologous collagen injections to treat deep glabellar furrows. *Plast Reconstr Surg.* 1994; 93:642.
15. Fagien S. Autologen™ and Dermalogen™. In: Klein AW, ed. *Tissue Augmentation in Clinical Practice: Procedures and Techniques.* New York: Marcel Dekker; 1998:87–124.
16. Fagien S. Facial soft tissue augmentation with autologous injectable collagen. In: Putterman AM, ed. *Cosmetic Oculoplastic Surgery: Eyelid, Forehead, and Facial Techniques.* 3rd ed. Philiadelphia: W.B. Saunders; 1998.
17. Fagien S. Facial soft tissue augmentation with autologous and allogeneic human tissue collagen matrix (autologen and dermalogen). *Plast Reconstr Surg.* (in press).
18. Coleman SR. Long-term survival of fat transplants: Controlled demonstrations. *Aesthet Plast Surg.* 1995: 19:421.
19. Maas CS, Gnepp DR, Bumpous J. Expanded polytetrafluoroethylene (Gore-tex soft tissue patch) in facial augmentation. *Arch Otolaryngol Head Neck Surg.* 1993; 119:1008.
20. Lemperle G, Hazan-Gauthier N, Lemperle N. PMMA microspheres (Artecoll) for skin soft-tissue augmentation. Part II: Clinical investigations. Twelfth International Congress of International Society of Aesthetic Plastic Surgery, Paris, France, September 1993.
21. Fagien S. Extended use of botulinum toxin type a in facial aesthetic surgery. *Aesthet Surg J.* 1998; 18:215.
22. Fagien S. Treatment of hyperkinetic facial lines with botulinum toxin. In: Putterman AM, ed. *Cosmetic Oculoplastic Surgery: Eyelid, Forehead, and Facial techniques,* 3rd ed. Philadelphia: W.B. Saunders; 1998.
23. Fagien S. Botox for the treatment of dynamic and hyperkinetic facial lines and furrows: Adjunctive use in facial aesthetic surgery. *Plast Reconstr Surg.* 1999; 103:701.

Afterword

The surgical practice of aesthetic facial plastic surgery is a work in progress. This textbook demonstrates the dramatic evolution of the philosophy, method, technology, and surgical techniques in this area in the last three decades. And by the time the reader has completed this textbook, there will no doubt be additional changes in the method and approach to aesthetic facial plastic surgery. We look forward to participating in this evolution in the new millenium.

Thomas Romo, III   Arthur L. Millman

INDEX